PATHOLOGY OF LABORATORY RODENTS AND RABBITS

FOURTH EDITION

PATHOLOGY OF LABORATORY RODENTS AND RABBITS

Stephen W. Barthold, DVM, MS, PhD, Dipl. ACVP
Distinguished Professor Emeritus
Veterinary and Medical Pathology
University of California
Davis, CA

Stephen M. Griffey, DVM, PhD
Clinical Professor of Laboratory Animal Pathology
Director of the Comparative Pathology Laboratory
School of Veterinary Medicine
University of California
Davis, CA

Dean H. Percy, DVM, MSc, PhD, Dipl. ACVP
Professor Emeritus
Pathobiology Department
Ontario Veterinary College
Guelph, Ontario

WILEY Blackwell

Contents

Preface

The Fourth Edition of *Pathology of Laboratory Rodents and Rabbits* has been extensively revised in response to reviewers' and colleagues' comments, as well as addition of new material that has arisen since the Third edition was published in 2007. In particular, the chapter on rabbits has been significantly revised and expanded. A resounding message from reviewers and colleagues was to publish this edition in color. Technology has advanced such that color images are not only possible but also cost-effective. The images in this text are non-pareil, and have been generously contributed by colleagues, gleaned from the recent literature, and derived from personal collections of the authors.

Also notable in this edition is the change in authorship. Dean Percy has fully retired as an active author of this text, but his significant input remains throughout the text from previous editions. This book was his dream, and its long-term success since publication of the First Edition in 1993 can be largely attributed to his vision, energy, and perseverance. Stephen Barthold stepped up to the leadership for this edition, with the considerable assistance of his friend and colleague, Stephen Griffey. Reviewers suggested a third, younger author (Dr. Griffey) to carry on the tradition of this text in future editions. Dr. Griffey, like Drs. Percy and Barthold, is a veterinary pathologist with extensive experience and expertise in laboratory animal pathology.

Delving into the literature has been a thought-provoking journey down memory lane. Many of the contributors to the laboratory animal pathology field are deceased. Unfortunately, younger members of our profession must forego the privilege of personally knowing these giants upon whose shoulders our field has been built. Discovery of new diseases continues, but not at the pace that took place in the 1970s and 1980s.

This book is dedicated to our families, our mentors, our colleagues, and our students . . . past, present, and future. It is especially dedicated to the subjects of this text: laboratory rodents and rabbits. They contribute enormously to biomedical and veterinary science, and deserve our respect and full support.

About the Companion Website

This book is accompanied by a companion website:

www.wiley.com/go/Barthold/Pathology

The website includes downloadable photographs and illustrations from the book.

1 Mouse

INTRODUCTION

Apart from the many inbred strains, substrains, spontaneous mutants, and outbred stocks of laboratory mice, the mouse has been, and continues to be, central to molecular genomics, with worldwide efforts continuing to "knock out" every functional gene in the mouse genome and define the relationship between genotype and phenotype. In addition to understanding the genome, various mouse strains and stocks, as well as the genetically engineered mouse (GEM), play critical roles in hypothesis-driven biomedical research. These trends have created rich opportunities and critical demand for comparative pathologists who are knowledgeable in mouse pathobiology. Unfortunately, the scientific literature is replete with erroneous interpretation of phenotype by scientists (as well as pathologists) lacking expertise in mouse pathology. Effective mouse pathology requires a global understanding of mouse biology, euphemistically termed "Muromics" (see Barthold 2002).

It is impossible for the pathologist to command in-depth knowledge of all strains, stocks, and mutant types of mice, and in many cases there is little baseline data to draw upon. Nevertheless, the mouse pathologist must be cognizant of general patterns of mouse pathology, as well as strain- and GEM-specific nuances. Recommended references (Frith & Ward, 1988; Maronpot et al. 1999; McInnes 2012; Mohr 2001; Mohr et al. 1996; Ward et al. 2000) provide thorough pictorial coverage of spontaneous mouse pathology in several common inbred strains of mice. The incidence and prevalence of strain-specific pathology are highly dependent upon genetic and environmental influences, including diet, bedding, infectious disease, age, sex, and other factors. Compared to the above-cited references, our coverage of the esoterica of spontaneous mouse pathology is relatively superficial.

We herein emphasize general patterns of disease, while attempting to address important strain-, mutant-, and GEM-specific diseases when appropriate. There are a growing number of internet-accessible resources for mouse phenotyping and pathology of strains, stocks, and GEMs. A listing of these web resources is available through various sources (Bolon 2006; Brayton 2013; Fox et al. 2007, 2015). Although not specifically listed in this text, it is worth "surfing" through these cited websites that provide a plethora of information at multiple levels.

The unique qualities of the laboratory mouse and the precision of mouse-related research make infectious agents, even those with minimal (or no) pathogenicity, major concerns due to their potential and sometimes significant impact upon research reproducibility, including phenotype. A challenge that is unique to the mouse is the difficulty in drawing the line between commensalistic, opportunistic, or overtly pathogenic microorganisms. Since the last edition, a wide variety of immune-deficient GEMs have been created, thereby raising the status of several relatively innocuous infectious agents to the level of pathogens. Immune-deficient mice and new molecular methods of detection continue to reveal previously unrecognized mouse "pathogens," such as a number of *Helicobacter* spp., norovirus, and most recently, astrovirus. Furthermore, the unrestricted traffic of GEMs among institutions and the pressure to reduce costs of maintenance at the expense of quality control have resulted in the re-emergence of several infectious agents that have not been seen in several decades. We, therefore, unabashedly emphasize mouse infectious diseases in this chapter. Despite advances in husbandry and diagnostic surveillance, we are reluctant to discard entities that may seem to have disappeared from laboratory mouse populations because of their likelihood of return.

Pathology of Laboratory Rodents and Rabbits, Fourth Edition. Stephen W. Barthold, Stephen M. Griffey, and Dean H. Percy.
© 2016 John Wiley & Sons, Inc. Published 2016 by John Wiley & Sons, Inc.

MOUSE GENETICS AND GENOMICS

The laboratory mouse is an artificial creation, and there is no true "wild-type" laboratory mouse. Furthermore, there is no such thing as "normal" microflora, since laboratory mice are often maintained in microbially pristine environments devoid of pathogens and opportunistic pathogens, as well as other commensal flora/fauna. Laboratory mice are largely derived from domesticated "fancy mice" that arose from many years of trading mouse variants among fanciers in Europe, Asia, North America, and Australia. The laboratory mouse genome is, therefore, a mosaic derived from different subspecies of the *Mus musculus* (house mouse) complex, including *M.m. domesticus*, *M.m. musculus*, *M.m. castaneus*, *M.m. molossinus* (a natural hybrid of *M.m. musculus* and *M.m. castaneus*), and others. The genome of *M.m. domesticus* is the predominant contributor to most strains of mice, but many inbred strains share a common "Eve" with a mitochondrial genome of *M.m. musculus* origin and a common "Adam" that contributed their Y chromosome from *M.m. castaneus*. In addition, there is evidence that other *Mus* species, outside of the *M. musculus* complex, have contributed to the genome of some, but not all, laboratory mouse strains. For example, the C57BL mouse genome contains a contribution from *M. spretus*. Perhaps the only laboratory mouse that is derived from a single *M.m. domesticus* species (subspecies) is the "Swiss" mouse. Several *Mus* species that are outside of the *M. musculus* complex, such as *M. spretus*, have been inbred. Thus, the laboratory mouse genome is not uniform among strains and mouse strains are not entirely within the *M. musculus* clade.

There are over 450 inbred strains of laboratory mice that have arisen during the last century, and these strains, which were selectively inbred to pan-genomic homozygosity for purposes entirely unrelated to modern research, are the foundation upon which literally thousands of spontaneous mutants and GEMs have been built. Additional inbred strains have been developed from wild mice (*M.m. castaneus*, *M. spretus*, etc.). Furthermore, "outbred" mice (mostly Swiss mice) are highly homozygous and nearly inbred. In addition to historical inbreeding that may be intentional or the inadvertent result of maintaining small populations of mice, rederivation of a mouse population results in genetic bottlenecks as well. There is no such thing as a truly "outbred" laboratory mouse with a fully heterozygous genome representative of wild-type *M. musculus*, and there is no wild mouse genetic counterpart of the laboratory mouse. Recently, an octaparental Diversity Outbred (DO) mouse stock was developed from eight disparately related inbred strains of mice, but this stock is not extensively utilized. When working with mice, the pathologist must also become facile with strains, substrains, sub-sub-strains, hybrids, congenics, insipient congenics, coisogenics, consomics, conplastics, recombinant inbreds, recombinant congenics, spontaneous mutants, random induced (radiation, chemical, retroviral, gene trap) mutants, transgenics (random insertions), and targeted mutant mice, each with relatively unique, predictable, and sometimes unpredictable phenotypes and patterns of disease whose expression is modified by environmental and microbial variables.

The inherent value of the laboratory mouse is its inbred genome, but maintaining the genetic stability of inbred strains of mice is a challenge. Since the advent of GEMs, there has been widespread genetic mismanagement of mouse strains by investigators with considerable skill in mouse genomics but limited expertise in mouse genetics. Even with the best of intentions, continuous inbreeding leads to substrain divergence among different populations of the same parental origin due to spontaneous mutations, retrotransposon integrations, or residual heterozygosity. Genetic contamination is also a surprisingly frequent event in both commercial and academic breeding colonies of mice. Within a few generations, substrain divergence can result in significant differences in phenotype, including response to research variables. The variable genetic contributions of different origins of mice and selective inbreeding for strain characteristics, such as coat color or neoplasia, are especially important when considering retroelements, which make up 37% of the mouse genome. Retroelements are highly dynamic within the context of the inbred mouse genome. They are present in the genomes of all mammals but have become artificially important in the homozygous genome of the laboratory mouse, and in fact had much to do with development of original inbred strains of mice with unique phenotypes, especially coat color and neoplasia. It is difficult to ignore their impact on mouse pathology, and thus retroelements are discussed later in this chapter (see Section "Retroelements and Retroviral Infections").

NOMENCLATURE

The details of mouse nomenclature are beyond the scope of this book, but it is critically important that the full and correct strain, substrain, and mutant allelic or transgene nomenclature be utilized when evaluating pathology and in publications for maximal reproducibility of results. Being able to "read" the nomenclature of a mouse that is submitted for evaluation is critical for interpreting pathology. Guidelines for mouse nomenclature are available at the *International Mouse Nomenclature* home page (http://www.informatics.jax.org/mgihome/nomen/). *The Mouse in Biomedical Research: History, Genetics, and Wild Mice* (Fox et al. 2007), the mouse chapter in *Laboratory Animal Medicine* (Fox et al. 2015), and *Mouse Genetics* (L.M. Silver 1995) are also useful sources of information on mouse genetics, genomics, and nomenclature.

COMMON INBRED STRAINS

Among the many inbred strains, the great majority of biomedical research, including genomic research, is based on a relatively few mouse strains, including C57BL/6, BALB/c, C3H/He, 129, FVB, and outbred Swiss stocks. This is fortuitous for the pathologist, as familiarity with this relatively small list of strains provides a good basis for approaching the general pathology of mice. Despite emphasis on mouse strains, there are significant genotypic and phenotypic differences among substrains of any given strain, such as C57BL/6J versus C57BL/6N and among the various strains of 129 mice. An overview of characteristics among inbred strains has been developed by Festing (http://www.informatics.jax.org/external/festing/mouse/STRAINS.shtml) and The Mouse Phenome Database provides comprehensive information on many strains of mice (http://www.phenome.jax.org).

The reader is referred to other sources for more comprehensive information regarding the myriad possibilities of background pathology among laboratory mice (see Section "General References on Diseases of Mice"). This text is not intended to provide such depth of coverage, but herein provides a brief synopsis of important disease characteristics of the major strains/stocks of mice. The specific lesions are described further in later sections of this chapter.

C57BL/6 (B6) mice are the gold standard "background strain" for GEMs created by homologous recombination. Many mutant alleles and transgenes are backcrossed onto this strain. There are a number of other related "black" strains, including C57BL/10 (B10). B6 mice were initially bred for their longevity. Their melanism is manifested by their coat color, as well as melanin pigment in heart valves, splenic capsule and trabeculae, meninges, cerebral vessels, Harderian glands, and parathyroid glands. Common strain-related spontaneous diseases include hydrocephalus, hippocampal neurodegeneration, microphthalmia and anophthalmia, age-related cochlear degeneration and hearing loss, and malocclusion. B6 mice are predisposed to barbering or trichotillomania, which renders them susceptible to alopecia and staphylococcal ulcerative dermatitis. Aged B6 mice develop acidophilic macrophage pneumonia and epithelial hyalinosis, which are rapidly accelerated in B6 mice with the moth-eaten and various other mutations. B6 mice may develop late-onset amyloidosis, but this is highly dependent upon environmental and infectious factors (e.g., dermatitis). The most common B6 neoplasms are lymphoma, hemangiosarcoma, and pituitary adenoma.

BALB/c mice (BALB/c, BALB/cBy, et al.) are albinos. Mature males are rather pugilistic, requiring separate housing for particularly fractious individuals. Dystrophic epicardial mineralization of the right ventricular free wall is common, and they are prone to development of myocardial degeneration and auricular thrombosis. Corneal opacities are commonly found, and they often develop conjunctivitis, blepharitis, and periorbital abscesses. Hypocallosity (corpus callosal aplasia) is frequent, and they develop age-related hearing loss. BALB mice are remarkably resistant to spontaneous amyloidosis, in contrast to other mouse strains. The livers of normal BALB mice feature a moderate amount of hepatocellular fatty change. The most common tumors of BALB mice are pulmonary adenomas, lymphomas, Harderian gland tumors, and adrenal adenomas. Myoepitheliomas of salivary, preputial, and other exocrine glands are also relatively common in this strain.

C3H/He mice are agouti mice that are blind due to *rd1* mutation (*Pde6b^{rd1}*) and are also prone to corneal opacities and hearing loss later in life. They frequently develop focal myocardial and skeletal mineralization and myocardial degeneration. C3H/HeJ mice develop alopecia areata as they age. They are susceptible to exogenous murine mammary tumor virus (MMTV)-induced mammary tumors and develop a relatively high incidence of mammary neoplasia later in life due to endogenous MMTV. Other relatively common tumors include hepatocellular tumors.

129 mice rank high in the panoply of mousedom as the most frequent source of embryonic stem (ES) cells, from which most targeted mutant mice are derived. The 129 mouse is not a single strain, and in fact "129" is represented by 16 recognized strains and substrains. This is due to accidental and intentional genetic contamination of the original 129 strain by various laboratories. Thus, the designation 129 is followed by P, S, T, or X, and other designations, in addition to substrain determinants. Genetic differences between the targeting construct and the ES cells can significantly influence efficiency of homologous recombination. The differences among 129 mice are not subtle, with variation in coat color, behavior, and other characteristics, including patterns of pathology. Hypocallosity is relatively common in many 129 mice. 129 mice, like B6 mice, are prone to pulmonary proteinosis and epithelial hyalinosis. Megaesophagus occurs in some types of 129 mice. Blepharitis and conjunctivitis are common in 129P3 mice. 129/Sv mice are renown for development of testicular teratomas (aka embryonal carcinomas). Other common neoplasms in 129 mice are lung tumors, Harderian gland tumors, ovarian tumors, and hemangiosarcomas.

FVB/N mice are inbred Swiss mice that gained popularity for creation of transgenic mice in an inbred genetic background. They are blind due to homozygosity of *rd1* allele (*Pde6b^{rd1}*) and prone to seizures. Many lines of FVB mice develop persistent mammary hyperplasia and hyperplasia or adenomas of prolactin-secreting cells in the anterior pituitary, but mammary tumors are rare (unless through transgenesis). Common neoplasms include tumors of lung, pituitary, Harderian gland, liver, lymphomas, and pheochromocytomas.

NOD mice are inbred Swiss mice that were selectively bred for cataracts, and during that process were found to develop type 1 diabetes (nonobese diabetes (NOD)). This strain develops a number of other autoimmune disorders that are genetically determined at multiple loci. Notably, they have functional defects in macrophage and dendritic cell function, NK cells, NKT cells, regulatory CD4+CD25+ cells, and are C5a deficient. Their susceptibility to diabetes is highest when they are maintained in relatively germ-free environments, and is much lower in conventional environments. The NOD strain was genetically modified through backcrossing to create a xenotransplant host that is globally defective in NK cells, macrophage and dendritic cells (NOD characteristics), T and B cells (*Prkdc^scid*), and IL-2-receptor γ (*IL-2rγ^{tm1Wjl}*). The resultant strain, NOD.Cg*Prkdc^scid IL2rγ^{tm1Wjl}*/SvJ (*NSG*) has become the optimal host for xenogeneic transplants, particularly human stem cell and T-cell engraftment. As a result, graft versus host disease (GVHD) arises in engrafted mice, characterized by human T-cell infiltration of skin, liver, intestine, lungs, and kidneys (see discussion of GVHD in Section "Aging, Degenerative, and Miscellaneous Disorders"). Because of their global immunodeficiency, mice of this strain are uniquely susceptible to opportunistic infections.

Outbred Swiss mice are all closely related derivatives of a small gene pool of founder animals that were inbred for many generations in various laboratories before outbreeding, primarily by commercial vendors. Outbred Swiss mice are often erroneously considered "wild-type" for comparison with inbred mice. As noted previously, they are far from outbred and differ genetically from inbred mice. Many, but not all, Swiss mouse stocks have retinal *rd1* degeneration (homozygous recessive), reflecting their high degree of homozygosity. Swiss mice are particularly prone to amyloidosis, which is a major life-limiting disease. They develop a variety of incidental lesions, and the most common tumors are lymphomas, pulmonary adenomas, liver tumors, pituitary adenomas, and hemangiomas/sarcomas, among others.

GENOMIC CONSIDERATIONS FOR THE PATHOLOGIST

Having stressed the importance of strain and substrain, it is notable that the mouse genomic community does not utilize a single strain of mouse, and when they do use a similar strain, it is often a different substrain. GEMs are created in a variety of ways, including random mutagenesis (chemical mutagenesis, radiation, random transgenesis, gene trapping, retroviral transgenesis) and targeted mutagenesis (homologous recombination). Issues relevant to the pathologist with the most common means of creating GEMs, random transgenesis and targeted mutations, are discussed below.

Random insertion of transgenes is accomplished through pronuclear microinjection of zygotes with ectopic DNA (transgenes). This has generally been achieved using hybrid zygotes of 2 inbred parental strains, outbred Swiss mice, or from inbred Swiss FVB/N mice to take advantage of hybrid vigor to compensate for the trauma of microinjection and facilitate the process of microinjection by providing large pronuclei. Transgenes become randomly integrated throughout the genome, often in tandem repeats, so that each pup within a litter arising from microinjected zygotes is hemizygous for the transgene, but is genetically distinct from its littermates. The degree of transgene expression (phenotype) varies with the location of the transgene within the genome. Each founder line of the same transgene represents a unique and nonreproducible genotype and, therefore, phenotype. Transgenes tend to be genetically unstable, and copies may be lost in subsequent generations, resulting in ephemeral phenotypes. Transgene insertions can also lead to unanticipated altered function of genes through insertional mutagenesis, or regulation by flanking genes within the area of insertion. Unanticipated phenotypes, such as immunodeficiency or other effects, can therefore occur. The use of hybrids or outbred mice as founders requires selective inbreeding to attain a useful model. This can be circumvented by using inbred founders, such as FVB/N mice. Maintaining the transgene on an outbred genetic background or incompletely backcrossed background poses problems with uncontrolled modifier and compensatory genes that may unpredictably influence phenotype.

The discipline of mouse genomics has lent itself to incredible precision through homologous recombination, with the ability to alter not only specific genes but also gene function at specific time points during development or life stage, create tissue-specific gene alterations, gain of function, loss of function, and targeted integration of transgenes that allow customized development of mouse models of human disease that would not ordinarily arise within the context of the indigenous mouse genome. Targeted mutant mice are often created in one of several types of 129 ES cells, and once germline transmission has been effected, the 129-type mutant mouse is usually backcrossed to a more utilitarian mouse strain, such as B6. Full backcrossing to congenic status requires 3–4 years, which is seldom fulfilled. In constructs that require cre-lox technology, mutant mice are further crossed with cre transgenic mice, which may be of another strain, substrain, or stock background. Thus, despite superb precision in altering a gene of interest, the rest of the mouse's genome can remain highly heterogeneous, which defeats the inherent value of the GEM for research, or at least limits its full potential.

ES cells, and the mutations that they carry, are most often derived from one of the 129-type mouse strains, and ES cells become mice through the generation of chimeric progeny. Insufficient backcrossing, with retention of 129 characteristics, may result in erroneous assumptions about the phenotype of the targeted gene. There is considerable genetic variation among different 129 ES cell lines, which can be a potential problem for comparing phenotypes of the same gene alteration among different 129 ES cell-derived mice. The process of creating chimeric mice, which is an essential step involving microinjection of 129 ES cells into a recipient blastocyst, has consequences. Most ES cell lines are "male" (XY), but blastocysts are either male or female. Hermaphroditism is quite common in chimeric mice arising from XY and XX cells. XX/XY chimeras are usually phenotypically male, but may have testicular hypoplasia and lower fertility. XX/XY chimeras may also have cystic Muellerian duct remnants, an ovary and a testis, and/or ovotestes. In addition to gonadal teratomas that are inherent in many 129 mouse strains, extragonadal teratomas arising from 129 cells in chimeric mice can develop in perigenital regions and the midline.

Because of the highly inbred nature of laboratory mice, experimental mutation of many genes often leads to embryonic or fetal death that precludes evaluation of phenotype in adult mice. Thus, pathologists are being increasingly called upon to familiarize themselves with fetal development and evaluate developmental defects. Fetal pathology is beyond the scope of this text, but the reader can access several excellent sources of information (see Kaufman 1995; Kaufman and Bard 1999; Rossant and Tam 2002; Ward et al. 2000). Embryonic/fetal viability is most often influenced by abnormalities in placentation, liver function, or cardiovascular function (including hematopoiesis). Particular attention should be paid to these factors. Depending upon genetic background, lethality can vary. Gene expression, and therefore circumvention of events such as embryonic lethality, can be controlled temporally and quantitatively by tissue-specific promoters with drug-regulated transcription systems and with cre/lox deletion, in which cre recombinase can be controlled with transcription techniques. Temporal and quantitative control of transgenes poses unique challenges to pathologists when evaluating phenotype.

In addition to predicted phenotypes, GEMs often manifest unique pathology that is not present in parental strains. Genetic constructs are usually inserted into the genome with a promoter to enhance expression, to target expression within a specific tissue, or to conditionally express the transgene, but promoters can affect phenotype as much as the gene of interest. Promoters are seldom totally tissue-specific and can impact upon other types of tissue. Conversely, overexpression of transgenes, regardless of their nature, can result in abnormalities in normal cell function. Tumors, particularly malignant tumors of mesenchyme, including hemangiosarcomas, lymphangiosarcomas, fibrosarcomas, rhabdomyosarcomas, osteosarcomas, histiocytic sarcomas, and anaplastic sarcomas, are frequent spontaneous lesions in transgenic

mice that are relatively rare in parental strains of mice. Lymphoreticular tumors, which are quite common in parental strains of mice, reach epic proportions in GEMs. In some cases, relatively rare forms of lymphoma, such as marginal zone lymphomas, arise frequently in GEMs. Tumor phenotypes found in transgenic mice bearing *myc*, *ras*, and *neu* are distinctive and found only in mice with these transgenes. Many gene alterations have specifically targeted immune response genes, but others have unintentional effects upon immune response. When the immune responsiveness of the mouse is altered, opportunistic pathogens become an important factor in phenotype. Phenotypes have been known to disappear when mutant mice are rederived and rid of their adventitious pathogens.

Consequently, the pathologist must be cognizant of general mouse pathology, strain-related patterns of spontaneous pathology, infectious disease pathology, developmental pathology, comparative pathology (to validate the model), methodology used to create the mice, predicted outcomes of the gene alteration (including effects of the promoter), potential but unexpected outcomes of the gene alteration, and Mendelian genetics. The pathologist must also resist temptation to overemphasize a desired phenotype, underemphasize an undesired phenotype, or proselytize a phenotype as a model for human disease when it isn't. There is no better person to be the gatekeeper of reality in the world of functional genomics than the comparative pathologist.

ANATOMIC FEATURES

The laboratory mouse has several unique characteristics, and there are vast differences in normal anatomy, physiology, and behavior among different strains of mice, many of which represent abnormalities arising from homozygosity of recessive or mutant traits in inbred mice.

Integumentary System
The history of the laboratory mouse is steeped in selective breeding for variation in coat color and consistency, with many defined mutants. Hair growth occurs in cyclic waves, beginning cranially and progressing caudally. Examination of mouse skin mandates awareness of the growth cycle and location examined. Melanin pigment is restricted to the hair follicular epithelium and hair shaft, with minimal pigmentation of the interfollicular epidermis. Thus, newborn mice, regardless of their ultimate coat color, are uniformly pink until hair growth begins.

Hematology and Hematopoeitic System
Mouse hematology has been recently reviewed (Everds 2007). Strain-specific data and comparisons among inbred mouse strains are available through the Mouse Phenome Database. Recommended approaches to

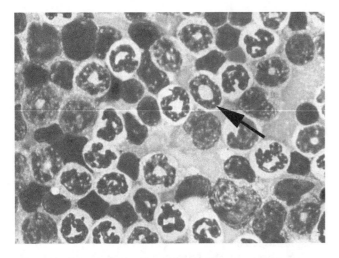

FIG. 1.1. *Ring-shaped nuclei (arrow) of myeloid progenitor cells in the bone marrow of a normal mouse.*

evaluation of GEMs with hematological phenotypes are also available (Car and Eng 2001). Mouse erythrocytes are small, with a high reticulocyte count, moderate polychromasia, and anisocytosis. Lymphocytes are the predominant circulating leukocyte and constitute approximately three-fourths of the total differential count. Mature male mice have significantly higher granulocyte counts than do female mice. Peripheral blood granulocytes tend to be hypersegmented, and band cells are rare, except when mice have chronic suppurative infections. Granulocytes in tissues and bone marrow often have ring-shaped nuclei (Fig. 1.1). Ring-shaped nuclei can be visualized as early as the progranulocyte stage in bone marrow, spleen, and liver, and only rarely can be found in peripheral blood. They also occur in cells of the monocytic lineage. Mice have circulating basophils, but they are extremely rare. Mice possess a very large platelet mass, due to high platelet numbers and relatively low mean volume, although some platelets can be as large as erythrocytes. The spleen is a major hematopoietic organ throughout life in the mouse, and hematopoiesis is found in the liver up to weaning age but may return in adults during disease states. Hepatic hematopoiesis can be misconstrued as inflammation. Hematopoiesis remains active in long bones throughout life.

Respiratory System

Cross sections of the nose reveal prominent vomeronasal organs, which are important in pheromone sensing and are frequent targets of viral attack. Virus-associated vomeronasal and olfactory rhinitis in neonatal mice can result in failure to suckle. Respiratory epithelium may contain eosinophilic secretory inclusions (hyalinosis), which are especially obvious in B6 and 129 mice. The lungs have a single left lobe and 4 right lobes. Cartilage surrounds only the extrapulmonary airways in mice, rats, and hamsters. Thus, primary bronchi are extrapulmonary. Respiratory bronchioles are

short or nonexistent. Cardiac muscle surrounds major branches of pulmonary veins and should not be misconstrued as medial hypertrophy. Bronchus-associated lymphoid tissue is normally present only at the hilus of the lung, except in hamsters. Lymphoid accumulations are present on the visceral pleura of mice, within interlobar clefts. These are organized lymphoid structures that are contiguous with the underlying lung tissue and are similar to "milkspots" in the peritoneum. Although not a normal finding, focal intra-alveolar hemorrhage is a consistent agonal finding in lungs of mice, regardless of the means of euthanasia. As in other species, focal subpleural accumulation of alveolar macrophages (alveolar histiocytosis) is common (see Rat chapter 2, "alveolar histiocytosis").

Gastrointestinal System

Mice are coprophagic, with approximately one-third of their dietary intake being feces. Stomach contents will reflect this behavior. Incisive foramina, located posterior to the upper incisors, communicate between the roof of the mouth and the anterior nasal cavity. Incisors grow continuously, but cheek teeth are rooted. Mice have no deciduous teeth, and their incisors are pigmented due to deposition of iron beneath the enamel layer. One of several sexual dimorphisms in the mouse is found in the salivary glands. The submandibular salivary glands in sexually mature males are nearly twice the size as females and parotid salivary glands are also larger. Male submandibular glands have increased secretory granules in the cytoplasm of serous cells (Fig. 1.2). These glands undergo similar masculinization in pregnant and lactating females. The intestine is simple. Gut-associated lymphoid tissue (Peyer's patches) is present in both the

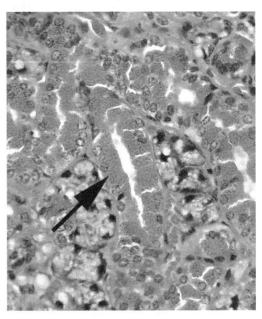

FIG. 1.2. *Submandibular (submaxillary) salivary gland from an adult male mouse. Note the prominent secretory granules (arrow) in the cytoplasm of epithelial cells.*

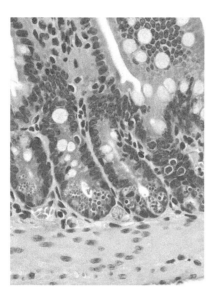

FIG. 1.3. *Ileal mucosa of a mouse illustrating the distinct cytoplasmic granules within Paneth cells at the base of the crypts.*

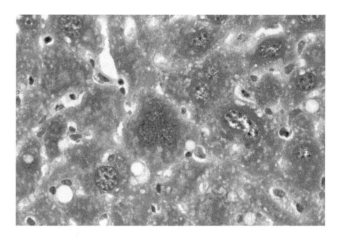

FIG. 1.5. *Polykarya and megalokarya, indicative of polyploidy, are commonly found in the liver and increase with age and disease states.*

small and large intestine. Paneth cells occupy crypt bases in the small intestine. These specialized enterocytes have prominent eosinophilic cytoplasmic granules (Fig. 1.3), which are larger in mice than in other laboratory rodents. Pregnant and lactating mice have noticeably thickened bowel walls due to physiological mucosal hyperplasia. Mice have a very short (1–2 mm) rectum, which is the terminal portion of the large bowel that is not enveloped in serosa. Because of this feature, mice are prone to rectal prolapse, especially if they have colitis.

The intestine of neonatal mice has several unique features. Neonatal small intestinal enterocytes are vacuolated and may contain eosinophilic inclusions due to the presence of the apical–tubular system, which is involved in uptake of macromolecules (Fig. 1.4). It

disappears as the intestine undergoes maturation. The neonatal mouse bowel has very shallow crypts of Leiberkuhn populated with mitotically inactive stem cells and very long villi that are populated with terminally differentiated, absorptive epithelium. Intestinal cell turnover kinetics are slow in the neonate, making neonates highly vulnerable to acute cytolytic viruses. Turnover kinetics accelerate with acquisition of microflora and dietary stimuli.

The liver of mice has variable lobation. Polyploidy is common in mouse liver cells. Hepatocytes frequently display cytomegaly, anisokaryosis, polykarya, and karyomegaly (Fig. 1.5). Cytoplasmic invagination into the nucleus is frequent, giving the appearance of nuclear inclusion bodies (Fig. 1.6). Hematopoiesis normally occurs in the infant liver (Fig. 1.7) but wanes by weaning age, although islands of myelopoiesis or erythropoiesis can be found in hepatic sinusoids of older mice,

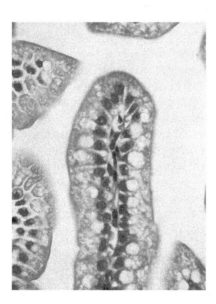

FIG. 1.4. *Enteric mucosa of a neonatal mouse, illustrating the vacuolated appearance of villus enterocytes.*

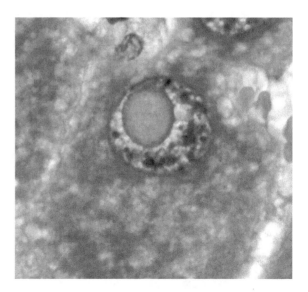

FIG. 1.6. *Cytoplasmic invagination into the nucleus of a hepatocyte, a common finding in rodents that has been misinterpreted as viral inclusions.*

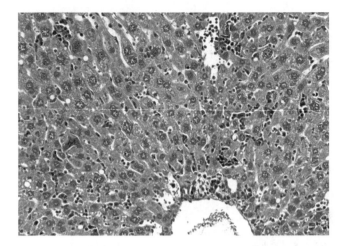

FIG. 1.7.   *Liver from a newborn mouse. There are numerous hematopoietic cells in the sinusoidal regions.*

particularly in disease states (Fig. 1.8). Hepatocytes frequently contain cytoplasmic fat vacuoles. Some strains, such as BALB mice, normally have diffuse hepatocellular fatty change, resulting in grossly pallid livers, compared with the mahogany-colored livers of other mouse strains.

Genitourinary System

Female mice have a large clitoris, or genital papillus, with the urethral opening near its tip, which is located anterior to the vaginal orifice. Females that develop in utero between male fetuses are somewhat masculinized, reflected by an increased anogenital distance and behavior. Tissues of the adult uterine wall are normally infiltrated with eosinophils, which wax and wane cyclically and disappear during pregnancy. Eosinophils increase in number in response to semen. Mice have hemochorial placentation. Males have large redundant testes that readily retract into the abdominal cavity through open inguinal canals, particularly when the mice are picked up by the tail. Both sexes have well-developed preputial (or clitoral) glands, and males have

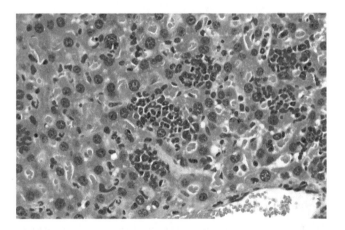

FIG. 1.8.   *Liver from an adult mouse with suppurative pyelonephritis, illustrating marked hepatic myelopoiesis.*

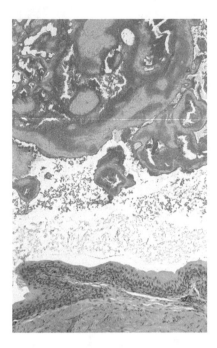

FIG. 1.9.   *Copulatory plug in the urinary bladder of a male mouse. The presence of ejaculate coagulum is common in the urethra and bladder as an agonal finding, although antemortem ejaculation may result in urinary obstruction.*

conspicuous accessory sex glands, including large seminal vesicles, coagulating glands, and prostate. Ejaculation results in formation of a coagulum, or copulatory plug. This frequently occurs agonally. Coagulum can be found in urinary bladder or urethra as a normal incidental finding at necropsy (Fig. 1.9) and must not be misconstrued as a calculus or obstruction. However, copulatory plugs can and do cause obstructive uropathy. Sexual maturity in males results in several sexual dimorphic features, including larger kidneys, larger renal cortices, larger cells in proximal convoluted tubules, larger renal corpuscles, and cuboidal epithelium lining the parietal layer of Bowman's capsule, resembling tubular epithelium (Fig. 1.10). This is not absolute, since some glomeruli of male mice are surrounded by flat epithelium and some glomeruli of female mice are surrounded by cuboidal epithelium. Mice are endowed with relatively large numbers of glomeruli per unit area, compared with other species, such as the rat. Mice have a single, long renal papilla that extends into the upper ureter. Proteinuria is also normal in mice, with highest levels in sexually mature male mice. Major contributors to proteinuria in male mice are "mouse urinary proteins," which function as pheromones. In particular, MUP-1 is highly antigenic and a major cause of occupational allergies among animal handlers.

Endocrine System

The mouse adrenal gland has several notable features. The adrenals of male mice tend to be smaller and have less lipid than those of females. Accessory adrenals, either partial or complete, are very common in the

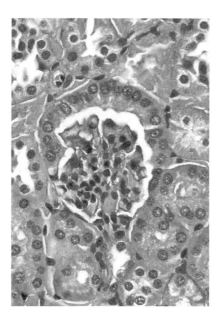

FIG. 1.10. *Renal cortex from an adult male mouse, illustrating the cuboidal epithelium lining the parietal surface of Bowman's capsule.*

adrenal capsule or surrounding connective tissue. The zona reticularis of the adrenal cortex is not discernible from the zona fasciculata. Proliferation of subcortical spindle cells, with displacement of the cortex, is common in mice of all ages (Fig. 1.11). The function of these cells is not known. A unique feature of the mouse adrenal is the X zone of the cortex, which surrounds the medulla. The X zone is composed of basophilic cells and appears in mice around 10 days of age. When males reach sexual maturity and females undergo their first pregnancy, the X zone disappears. The X zone disappears gradually in virgin females. During involution, the X zone undergoes marked vacuolation in females

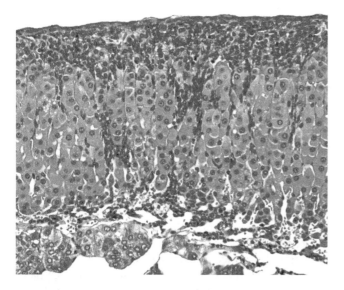

FIG. 1.11. *Subcapsular spindle cell proliferation in the adrenal gland of a normal adult mouse. This change is common, but its significance is not known.*

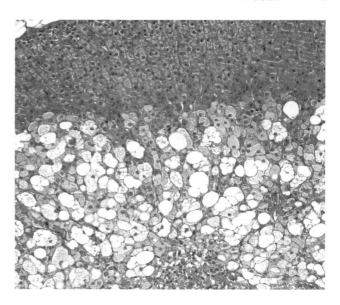

FIG. 1.12. *Vacuolating degeneration of the involuting X zone at the corticomedullary junction of the adrenal gland of an adult female mouse.*

(Fig. 1.12) but not in males. Residual cells accumulate ceroid. Pancreatic islets are highly variable in size, including giant islets that can be confused with hyperplasia or adenomas.

Skeletal System

Bones of mice, like those of rats and hamsters, do not have Haversian systems, and ossification of physeal plates with age is variable and incomplete, depending upon mouse genotype.

Lymphoid System

Rodents do not have tonsils, but have nasal-associated lymphoid tissue (NALT). Germinal centers are not well defined in lymph nodes. The thymus does not involute in adults. Hassall's corpuscles are indistinct. Islands of ectopic parathyroid tissue may be encountered in the septal or surface connective tissue of the thymus, and, conversely, thymic tissue may occur in thyroid and parathyroid glands. Epithelial-lined cysts are also common. The splenic red pulp is an active hematopoietic site throughout life (Fig. 1.13). During disease states and pregnancy, increased hematopoiesis can result in splenomegaly. Lymphocytes tend to accumulate around renal interlobular arteries, salivary gland ducts, urinary bladder submucosa, and other sites, increasing with age. These sites are often involved in generalized lymphoproliferative disorders. Melanosis of the splenic capsule and trabeculae is common in melanotic strains of mice (Fig. 1.14). This must be differentiated from iron (hemosiderin) pigment (Fig. 1.15), which tends to accumulate in the red pulp as mice age, particularly in multiparous females. Mast cells can be frequent in the spleen of some mouse strains, such as A strain mice.

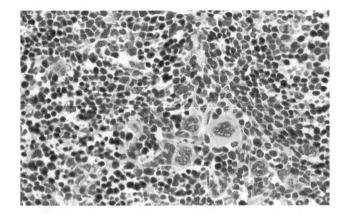

FIG. 1.13. *Spleen from an adult mouse, illustrating the large numbers of hematopoietic cells, including megakaryocytes, in the sinusoids, a common finding throughout life.*

Other Anatomic Features

The brain and spinal cord are larger in mature male mice compared to females. Melanosis occurs in the antero-ventral meninges of the olfactory bulbs, optic nerves, parathyroid glands, heart valves, and spleens of mela-notic mouse strains, such as B6 mice. Foci of cartilage or bone can be found within the base of the aorta. These foci are not an os cordis but rather occur within the wall of the aorta. Mice have 3 pectoral and 2 inguinal pairs of mammary glands, with mammary tissue enveloping much of the subcutis, including the neck. Mammary tissue can be found immediately adjacent to salivary glands, which is especially apparent during lactation. Nipple development is hormonally regulated in mice, and nipples are quite small in males. Mammary tissue of males totally involutes during development. Remark-ably, virgin female mice can be induced to lactate by the presence of other females nursing litters. Mammary glands normally involute between pregnancies, but they do not involute in multiparous FVB mice, due to a tendency to develop hyperplasia of prolactin-produc-ing cells and pituitary adenomas. Brown fat is prominent as a subcutaneous fat pad over the shoulders and is also present in the neck, axillae, and peritoneal tissue.

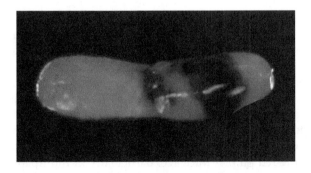

FIG. 1.14. *Splenic melanosis in a melantotic (C57BL) mouse. Note the patches of pigmented capsule.*

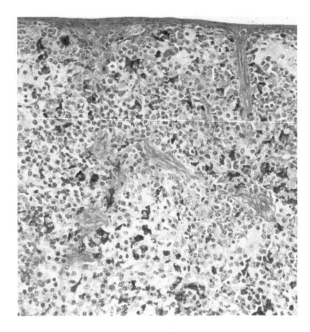

FIG. 1.15. *Iron pigment (hemosiderin) in the spleen of an adult female mouse (Perl's stain).*

Immunologic Idiosyncracies

Neonatal mice are globally immunodeficient. Different components of the innate and acquired immune response subsequently evolve at differing rates, depend-ing upon genetic background. Although mice are gener-ally immunocompetent at weaning, they are not fully so until 6–12 weeks of age. Neonates depend upon acquisi-tion of maternal antibody to protect them during early life. Maternal IgG is transferred in utero through Fc yolk sac receptors, and postnatally through IgG receptors in the small intestine, which actively acquire immuno-globulin up to 2 weeks of age. Milk-borne IgA is also important in protecting suckling mice, but neither IgA nor IgM are absorbed. Passive immunity is a critical component in understanding the outcome of viral infec-tions in mouse populations. Epizootic infections can be devastating in naïve populations of neonates, but once the infection becomes enzootic within a population, maternal antibody protects suckling mice during their period of age-related vulnerability. Maternal antibody generally persists in the serum of pups for about 6 weeks.

The immune response can vary considerably among different strains of mice. An often-cited feature is the Th1-Th2 polarized T-cell response, in which BALB/c mice tend to respond to antigenic stimuli with a Th2 skewed response and B6 mice with Th1 skewed responses. This is far from absolute, but there seems to be truth in the concept that B6 mice deal more efficiently with viral infections. B6, B10, SJL, and NOD mice have their own unique immunoglobulin isotype, IgG2c, in lieu of, but distinct from, IgG2a. IgG2c is not an allelic variant of IgG2a, since in these strains the IgG2a gene is completely absent, and in IgG2a-positive strains, the IgG2c gene is absent. This may impact accurate measurements of humoral responses. The mouse genome possesses approximately 40 histocompatibility loci, and the major histocompatibility (MHC) loci are located on chromosome 17 within the MHC complex, known as the *H-2* complex. Each inbred strain of mouse has a defined *H-2* haplotype, or combinations of alleles, which are well-recognized determinants of strain-specific immune responses, including responses to infectious disease. Because of the inbred nature of laboratory mouse strains, *H-2* haplotype is a singularly important strain characteristic.

Various stressors, including dehydration, hypothermia, and acute infections, may result in massive corticosteroid-induced lymphocytic apoptosis. This is accompanied by generalized lymphoid depletion and transient nonspecific alterations of immune responsiveness. This is especially apparent in the thymus and is a frequent and rapid onset lesion in "water bottle accidents," when mice become hypothermic or dehydrated. Recently rederived and xenobiotic mice have lymphoid hypoplasia, accompanied by functional hyporesponsiveness.

Genetic engineering has given rise to many immunologic mutants of mice, and other naturally arising immune mutants have also been popularized, such as nude (T-cell-deficient), SCID (B- and T-cell-deficient), and beige (NK cell-deficient) mice. The preeminent immunodeficient mouse is the NSG mouse, discussed above. Immunodeficient mice must never be considered to be simply missing a single functional component of the immune system, since they typically have compensatorily activated innate and acquired immune responses compared to wild-type. Homozygous immunodeficient inbred mouse mutants that are progeny of the heterozygous (immunocompetent) parental matings or through embryo transfer into immunocompetent recipients can acquire functional immunoglobulin-secreting B cells from their immunocompetent dams. They can also acquire functional B cells postnatally through foster nursing. The chimeric cells may remain functional for at least several months.

Less obvious and often overlooked immunologic idiosyncrasies also exist among common inbred strains. All strains of adult male mice manifest a sexual dimorphism in which serum levels of both C4 and C5 are higher than in females, and male SJL mice have a significantly higher level of C5 compared to males of other strains. In addition, inadvertent consequences have arisen from inbreeding and selection for other characteristics. One such common defect is a 2 base pair gene deletion in the 5th component of complement (C5). This mutation results in C5 deficiency in many inbred strains of mice, including AKR, SWR, DBA/2J, A/J, A/HeJ, NOD, and RF, among others. SJL mice are NK cell-deficient. NOD mice have multiple immune defects (see above). Substrain divergence due to spontaneous

acquisition of mutations can give rise to novel new substrain phenotypes, such as the LPS unresponsiveness of C3H/HeJ and C57BL/10ScN mice, which is attributed to a mutation of toll-like receptor 4 (TLR4). All strains of mice lack functional TLR10 due to genetic disruption by a retroviral insertion. CBA/CaN (CBA/N), but not other CBA mice, have an X-linked defect in humoral immunity, with impaired maturation of B cells, diminished immunoglobulin production, and impaired T-independent immune responses. Thus, knowledge of specific strain and substrain characteristics greatly improves the understanding of responses to experimental variables.

BIBLIOGRAPHY FOR INTRODUCTION THROUGH ANATOMIC FEATURES

Adamson, S.L., Lu, Y., Whiteley, K.J., Holmyard, D., Hemberger, M., Pfarrer, C., & Cross, J.C. (2002) Interactions between trophoblast cells and the maternal and fetal circulation in the mouse placenta. *Developmental Biology* 250:35–73.

Arvola, M., Gustafsson, E., Svensson, L., Jansson, L., Holmdahl, R., Heyman, B., Okabe, M., & Mattsson, R. (2000) Immunoglobulin-secreting cells of maternal origin can be detected in B cell-deficient mice. *Biology of Reproduction* 63:1817–1824.

Baba, A., Fujita, T., & Tamura, N. (1984) Sexual dimorphism of the fifth component of mouse complement. *Journal of Experimental Medicine* 160:411–419.

Barthold, S.W. (2002) "Muromics": genomics from the perspective of the laboratory mouse. *Comparative Medicine* 52:206–223.

Beck, J.A., Lloyd, S., Hafezparast, M., Lennon-Pierce, M., Eppig, J.T., Festing, M.F., & Fisher, E.M. (2000) Geneologies of mouse inbred strains. *Nature Genetics* 24:23–25.

Biermann, H., Pietz, B., Dreier, R., Schmid, K.W., Sorg, C., & Sunderkotter, C. (1999) Murine leukocytes with ring-shaped nuclei include granulocytes, monocytes, and their precursors. *Journal of Leukocyte Biology* 65:217–231.

Bolon, B. (2006) Internet resources for phenotyping engineered rodents. *ILAR Journal* 47:163–171.

Car, B.D. & Eng, V.M. (2001) Special considerations in the evaluation of the hematology and hemostasis of mutant mice. *Veterinary Pathology* 38:20–30.

Cinader, B., Dubiski, S., & Wardlaw, A.C. (1964) Distribution, inheritance, and properties of an antigen, MUB1, and its relation to hemolytic complement. *Journal of Experimental Medicine* 120:897–924.

De, M.K., Choudhuri, R., & Wood, G.W. (1991) Determination of the number and distribution of macrophages, lymphocytes, and granulocytes in the mouse uterus from mating through implantation. *Journal of Leukocyte Biology* 50:252–262.

Everds, N.E. (2007) Hematology of the laboratory mouse. In: *The Mouse in Biomedical Research*, Vol. 3 (eds. J.G. Fox, S.W. Barthold, M.T. Davisson, C.E. Newcomer, F. W. Quimby, & A. L. Smith), pp. 133–170. Academic Press, New York.

Hasan, U., Chaffois, C., Gaillard, C., Saulnier, V., Merck, E., Tancredi, S., Guiet, C., Briere, F., Vlach, J., Legecque, S., Trinchieri, G., & Bates, E.E. (2005) Human TLR10 is a functional receptor, expressed by B cells and plasmacytoid dendritic cells, which activates gene transcription through MyD88. *Journal of Immunology* 174:2942–2950.

Kaufman, M.H. (1995) *The Atlas of Mouse Development*. Academic Press, San Diego.

Kaufman, M.H. & Bard, J.B.L. (1999) *The Anatomical Basis of Mouse Development*. Academic Press, San Diego.

Kramer, A.W. & Marks, L.S. (1965) The occurrence of cardiac muscle in the pulmonary veins of Rodentia. *Journal of Morphology* 117:135–150.

Linder, C.C. (2006) Genetic variables that influence phenotype. *ILAR Journal* 47:132–140.

Lynch, D.M. & Kay, P.H. (1995) Studies on the polymorphism of the fifth component of complement in laboratory mice. *Experimental and Clinical Immunogenetics* 12:253–260.

Martin, R.M., Brady, J.L., & Lew, A.M. (1998) The need for IgG2c specific antiserum when isotyping antibodies from C57BL/6 and NOD mice. *Journal of Immunological Methods* 212:187–192.

Qureshi, S.T., Lariviere, L., Leveque, G., Clermont, S., Moore, K.J., Gros, P., & Malo, D. (1999) Endotoxin-tolerant mice have mutations in toll-like receptor 4 (Tlr4). *Journal of Experimental Medicine* 189:615–625.

Robertson, S.A., Mau, V.J., Tremellen, K.P., & Seamark, R.F. (1996) Role of high molecular weight seminal vesicle proteins in eliciting the uterine inflammatory response to semen in mice. *Journal of Reproduction and Fertility* 107:265–277.

Rossant J. & Tam, P.P.L. (2002) *Mouse Development: Patterning, Morphogenesis, and Organogenesis*. Academic Press, New York.

Scher, I. (1982) CBA/N immune defective mice; evidence for the failure of a B cell subpopulation to be expressed. *Immunological Reviews* 64:117–136.

Silver, L.M. (1995) *Mouse Genetics*. Oxford University Press. Out of print, available at http://www.informatics.jax.org/silver/index.shtml

Simpson, E.M., Linder, C.C., Sargent, E.E., Davisson, M.T., Mobraaten, L.E., & Sharp, J.J. (1997) Genetic variation among 129 substrains: importance for targeted mutagenesis in mice. *Nature Genetics* 16:19–27.

Staley, M.W. & Trier, J.S. (1965) Morphologic heterogeneity of mouse Paneth cell granules before and after secretory stimulation. *American Journal of Anatomy* 117:365–383.

Ward, J.M., Elmore, S.A., & Foley, J.F. (2012) Pathology methods for the evaluation of embryonic and perinatal developmental defects and lethality in genetically engineered mice. *Veterinary Pathology* 49:71–84.

Wetsel, R.A., Fleischer, D.T., & Haviland, D.L. (1980) Deficiency of the murine fifth complement component (C5): a 2-base pair gene deletion in a 59-exon. *Journal of Biological Chemistry* 265:2435–2440.

Wicks, L.F. (1941) Sex and proteinuria in mice. *Proceedings of the Society for Experimental Biology and Medicine* 48:395–400.

GENERAL REFERENCES ON DISEASES OF MICE

This text has used the following references extensively as sources of information. Many of these citations have multiple authors embedded within, but for the sake of space, individual authors within review books are not cited. Various sections of this chapter refer back to these basic general references, rather than repeat them for each section.

Brayton, C. (2007) Spontaneous diseases in commonly used mouse strains. In: *The Mouse in Biomedical Research. Diseases*, 2nd edn (eds. J.G. Fox, S.W. Barthold, M.T. Davisson, C.E. Newcomer, F.W. Quimby, & A.L. Smith), pp. 623–717. Academic Press, New York.

Chandra, M. & Frith, C.H. (1994) Spontaneous lesions in CD-1 and B6C3F1 mice. *Experimental Toxicologic Pathology* 46:189–198.

Fox, J.G., Barthold, S.W., Davisson, M.T., Newcomer, C.E., Quimby, F.W., & Smith, A.L. (2007) *The Mouse in Biomedical Research*, Vols. 1–4. Academic Press, New York.

Frith, C.H. & Ward, J.M. (1988) *Color Atlas of Neoplastic and Non-Neoplastic Lesions in Aging Mice*. Elsevier, Amsterdam. Out of print, available at http://www.informatics.jax.org/frithbook/

Frith, C.H., Highman, B., Burger, G., & Sheldon, W.D. (1983) Spontaneous lesions in virgin and retired breeder BALB/c and C57BL/6 mice. *Laboratory Animal Science* 33:273–286.

Haines, D.C., Chattopadhyay, S., & Ward, J.M. (2001) Pathology of aging B6;129 mice. *Toxicologic Pathology* 29:653–661.

Jones, T.C., Capen, C.C., & Mohr, U. (1996) *Respiratory System*, Monographs on Pathology of Laboratory Animals, 2nd edn. Springer, New York.

Jones, T.C., Capen, C.C., & Mohr, U. (1996) *Endocrine System*, Monographs on Pathology of Laboratory Animals, 2nd edn. Springer, New York.

Jones, T.C., Hard, G.C., & Mohr, U. (1998) *Urinary System*, Monographs on Pathology of Laboratory Animals, 2nd edn. Springer, New York.

Jones, T.C., Mohr, U., & Hunt, R.E. (1988) *Nervous System*, Monographs on Pathology of Laboratory Animals, 2nd edn. Springer, New York.

Jones, T.C., Mohr, U., & Popp, J.A. (1997) *Hemopoietic System*, Monographs on Pathology of Laboratory Animals, 2nd edn. Springer, New York.

Jones, T.C., Popp, J.A., & Mohr, U. (1997) *Digestive System*, Monographs on Pathology of Laboratory Animals, 2nd edn. Springer, New York.

Mahler, J.F., Stokes, W., Mann, P.C., Takaoka, M., & Maronpot, R.R. (1996) Spontaneous lesions in aging FVB/N mice. *Toxicologic Pathology* 24:710–716.

Maronpot, R.R., Boorman, G.A., & Gaul, B.W. (1999) *Pathology of the Mouse: Reference and Atlas*. Cache River Press, Vienna, IL.

McInnes, E.F. (2012) *Background Lesions in Laboratory Animals: A Color Atlas*. Elsevier.

Mohr, U. (2001) *International Classification of Rodent Tumors: The Mouse*. Springer, Berlin.

Mohr, U., Dungworth, D.L., Capen, C.C., Carlton, W.W., Sundberg, J.P., & Ward, J.M. (1996) *Pathobiology of the Aging Mouse*, Vols. 1 and 2. ILSI Press, Washington, DC.

Renne, R., Brix, A., Harkema, J., Herbert, R., Kittel, B., Lewis, D., March, T., Nagano, K., Pino, M., Rittinghausen, S., Rosenbruch, M., Tellier, P., & Wohrmann, T. (2009) Proliferative and non-proliferative lesions of the rat and mouse respiratory tract. *Toxicologic Pathology* 37:5S–73S.

Smith, R.S. (2002) *Systematic Evaluation of the Mouse Eye: Anatomy, Pathology and Biomethods*. CRC Press, Boca Raton, FL.

Thoolen, B., Maronpot, R.R., Harada, T., Nyska, A., Rousseaux, C., Nolte, T., Malarkey, D.E., Kaufman, W., Kuttler, K., Deschl, U., Nakae, D., Gregson, R., Vinlove, M.P., Brix, A.E., Singh, B., Belpoggi, F., & Ward, J.W. (2010) Proliferative and nonproliferative lesions of the rat and mouse hepatobiliary system. *Toxicologic Pathology* 38:5S–81S.

Ward, J.M., Mahler, J.F., Maronpot, R.R., Sundberg, J.P., & Frederickson, R.M. (2000) *Pathology of Genetically Engineered Mice*. Iowa State University Press, Ames, IA.

Whary, M.T., Baumgarth, N., Fox, J.G., & Barthold, S.W. (2015) Biology and diseases of mice. In: *Laboratory Animal Medicine* (eds. J.G. Fox, L.C. Anderson, G.M. Otto, K.R. Pritchett-Corning, & M.T. Whary). Academic Press, New York.

INFECTIONS OF LABORATORY MICE: EFFECTS ON RESEARCH

Laboratory mice are host to a large spectrum of over 60 different infectious agents that may, under some circumstances, be pathogens. Many of these agents have been eliminated from contemporary mouse colonies but may re-emerge periodically. Declaring an infectious agent a pathogen in the laboratory mouse can be a challenge. Some agents produce no discernible pathology, even in immunodeficient mice (e.g., astrovirus); some are opportunistic pathogens (e.g., *Pseudomonas*); and others (e.g., mouse hepatitis virus) can be overtly pathogenic in naïve neonatal mice or immunodeficient mice, and yet produce minimal or no signs when enzootic within a population or when infecting genetically resistant mice. These features create a challenge for educating the investigator about the significance of infectious agents in the mouse and convincing institutional officials of the need to provide core support for surveillance and diagnostic programs that ensure the health and welfare of research animals, as well as protecting the research investment. There are 3 major reasons for being concerned about infectious agents in the mouse: jeopardy of unique colonies, zoonotic risk, and effects on research. Effects on research are significant and varied, and there is growing documentation of infectious agents obscuring phenotypes in GEMs.

This text emphasizes all known naturally occurring infections of laboratory mice that have the potential for producing either lesions in mice or effects upon research, even those that have largely disappeared from contemporary mouse populations. This is because of the expanding use of immunologically deficient mice, burgeoning (and overcrowded) mouse populations, variable or inadequate microbial control practices, infestation of animal facilities by feral mice, and the re-emergence of rare infectious agents due to unrestricted traffic of GEMs among institutions. Microbial quality control is often a casualty in the face of financial austerity, imposed by declining National Institutes of Health budgets, rising husbandry costs, and increasingly onerous government and institutional regulations. All of these factors are contributing to the re-emergence of infectious disease among laboratory mice.

Disease expression is significantly influenced by age, genotype, immune status, and environment of the mouse. Genetic manipulation has introduced additional and often unexpected variables that may influence disease expression. Under most circumstances, even the most pathogenic murine viral agents cause minimal clinical disease. However, under select circumstances, the same agents can have devastating consequences. Genetically immunodeficient mice and infant mice less than 2 weeks of age that have not benefited from maternal immunity are highly susceptible to viral disease. Mouse strain genetic background, including *H-2* haplotype, is an important factor in host susceptibility, with growing nuances contributed by experimentally induced gene alterations. Different viruses, and different strains of virus, vary considerably in their contagiousness and virulence, which impacts sampling size for surveillance and recognition of disease. Housing methods, including ventilated cages and microisolator cages, complicate detection and significantly influence the contagion dynamics within a population. Infectious agents can be introduced to mouse colonies through feral mice, unrestricted traffic of personnel, biologic material, including transplantable tumors, ES cells, and iatrogenic introductions of mouse pathogens when used as models for human disease.

Investigation of host–agent epizootiology by the astute diagnostician must encompass all of these factors. Animals submitted for necropsy should be accompanied by thorough clinical history, including microbial surveillance data of the colony, accurate nomenclature, genetic background, and genetic manipulation. Mice must be carefully selected to provide maximal opportunity for diagnosis. Clinically ill animals or live cagemates of deceased or ill mice are optimal, since they would be most likely to have active infections or lesions. Diagnosis of infections in a rodent colony should not be solely dependent upon gross and microscopic pathology. A useful adjunct is serology, but this should never be used alone for diagnosis. Mice may be seronegative if actively infected with acutely cytolytic viruses, such as mouse hepatitis virus (MHV), and will be seropositive during or following recovery. Conversely, mice may be seropositive yet actively infected with a second strain of the same agent, as is the case with MHV. Young mice can be seropositive due to passively derived maternal antibody but not actively infected with the agent in question. Some virus infections, such as Sendai virus, induce immune-mediated disease. Thus, mice may not become clinically ill until a week or more into infection. Therefore, positive seroreactivity would be confirmatory in clinically ill mice infected with Sendai virus. These examples underscore that seroconversion to an agent does not imply a cause and effect relationship with disease, unless epizootiology, pathology, and serology are considered collectively. Finally, molecular methods of detection are increasing in use but must be accompanied by appropriate positive and negative controls, and positive results must always be confirmed by sequencing or other methods.

BIBLIOGRAPHY FOR INFECTIONS OF LABORATORY MICE: EFFECTS ON RESEARCH

Baker, D.G. (2003) *Natural Pathogens of Laboratory Animals: Their Effects on Research.* ASM Press, Washington, DC.

Barthold, S.W. (2002) "Muromics": Mouse genomics from the perspective of the laboratory mouse. *Comparative Medicine* 52:206–223.

Barthold, S.W. (2004) Genetically altered mice: phenotypes, no phenotypes, and faux phenotypes. *Genetica* 122:75–88.

Barthold, S.W. (2004) Intercurrent infections in genetically engineered mice. In: *Mouse Models of Human Cancer* (ed. E.C. Holland), pp. 31–41. Wiley-Liss, Hoboken, NJ.

Bhatt, P.N., Jacoby, R.O., Morse, H.C., III, & New, A.E. (1986) *Viral and Mycoplasmal Infections of Laboratory Rodents: Effects on Biomedical Research.* Academic Press, New York.

Franklin, C.L. (2006) Microbial considerations in genetically engineered mouse research. *ILAR Journal* 47:141–155.

Lindsey, J.R., Boorman, G.A., Collins, M.J., Jr., Hsu, C.-K., Van Hoosier, G.L., Jr., & Wagner, J.E. (1991) *Infectious Diseases of Mice and Rats*. National Academy Press, Washington, DC.

Newcomer, C.E. & Fox, J.G. (2007) Zoonoses and other human health hazards. In: *The Mouse in Biomedical Research: Diseases* (eds. J.G. Fox, S.W Barthold, M.T. Davisson, C.E. Newcomer, F. W. Quimby, & A. L. Smith), Vol. 2, pp. 721–747. Academic Press, New York.

DNA VIRAL INFECTIONS

Adenovirus Infections

Mice are host to 2 distinct adenoviruses, murine adenovirus-1 (MAdV-1) and murine adenovirus-2 (MAdV-2), which should be more accurately termed mouse adenovirus 1 and 2. MAdV-1 and MAV-2 can be differentiated from each other genetically, serologically, and by pathology. MAdV-1 and MAdV-2 differ significantly at the DNA level, with MAdV-2 having a distinctly larger genome. Adenoviruses are nonenveloped DNA viruses that replicate in the nucleus. Infection results in pathognomonic intranuclear inclusions.

Epizootiology and Pathogenesis

MAdV-1 (previously FL) was initially discovered as a contaminating cytopathic agent during attempts to establish Friend leukemia (FL) virus in tissue culture. Infection is transmitted by direct contact through urine, feces, and nasal secretions. Serologic surveys have indicated that MAdV-1 was at one time common in laboratory mouse colonies, but it is now rare or nonexistent in laboratory mice from North America and Europe. Naturally occurring clinical disease or lesions due to MAdV-1 have not been described, but experimental intraperitoneal inoculation of neonatal, suckling, and immunodeficient mice with MAdV-1 results in viremia and a fatal, multisystemic infection within 10 days. MAdV-1 infects cells of the monocyte–macrophage lineage, microvascular endothelial cells, respiratory epithelium, adrenal cortical cells, and renal distal tubular cells. Experimental inoculation of weanling or adult mice results in multisystemic infection with leukocyte-associated viremia and prolonged viruria. There are marked mouse strain differences in susceptibility to experimental infection. Mice less than 3 weeks of age are universally susceptible to experimental disease, and adult C57BL/6, DBA/2, SJL, SWR, and outbred CD-1 mice tend to be susceptible to lethal experimental disease, whereas BALB/c, C3H/HeJ, and most other inbred strains tested are disease resistant. Susceptible strains develop hemorrhagic encephalitis, which does not occur in resistant strains. The nature of infection of immunodeficient strains of mice depends upon strain genetic background. BALB-*scid* and BALB-*scid/beige* mice develop fatal disseminated infection with focal hemorrhagic enteritis and microvesicular fatty change in the liver, consistent with Reye's-like syndrome, but no neurologic involvement. B6-*Rag1* mice develop disseminated disease with hemorrhagic encephalomyelitis.

Athymic C3H/HeN-*nude* mice develop a progressive wasting disease with disseminated infection and duodenal hemorrhage, but no central nervous system involvement. Thus, genetic background is a major determinant of susceptibility to lesions in the central nervous system. Lymphoid B cells are critical for controlling disseminated infection, and T cells are required for recovery from infection but also contribute to pathology.

MAdV-2 (K87) was initially isolated from feces of an otherwise healthy mouse. In contrast to MAdV-1, MAdV-2 is principally enterotropic, regardless of route of inoculation, mouse strain, or immunosufficiency. Following oral inoculation of mice less than 4 weeks of age, MAdV-2 is excreted in feces for 3 or more weeks with peak infection between 7 and 14 days. Immunocompetent mice apparently recover. Seroconversion of rats to MAdV-2 has been noted, but they are not susceptible to experimental inoculation with the mouse virus, suggesting that they are host to a related, but different, adenovirus (see Rat Chapter 2, Rat Adenovirus Infection).

Pathology

Natural infection of immmunocompetent adult mice with MAdV-1 is typically subclinical, but the growing number and use of immunodeficient strains of mice warrant awareness of experimental findings. Mice experimentally inoculated with MAdV-1 develop runting, dehydration, thymic involution, and grossly evident foci of necrosis in liver, spleen, and other organs. Intranuclear inclusions can be found within foci of necrosis and hemorrhage in multiple organs, including brown fat, myocardium, cardiac valves, adrenal gland (Fig. 1.16), spleen, brain, pancreas, liver, intestine,

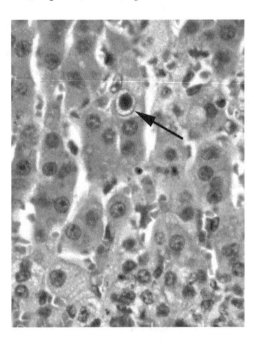

FIG. 1.16.   *Adrenal cortex from a mouse experimentally infected with mouse adenovirus MAdV-1. A single intranuclear inclusion (arrow) is present in the cortical epithelium.*

salivary glands, and renal distal tubular epithelium. Peribronchiolar and pulmonary interstitial infiltration with mononuclear leukocytes have been found in adult B6 mice following intranasal inoculation. Focal hemorrhagic enteritis has also been noted in some genotypes of mice following experimental inoculation. Gastrointestinal tracts can be empty, with segmental inflammation and hemorrhage in the distal duodenum and jejunum. Inclusions in intestinal lesions tend to be difficult to visualize. Hemorrhagic foci may occur throughout the central nervous system but especially in the white matter of susceptible mouse strains. Endothelial cell necrosis is prominent in these foci, but inclusions are rare except in Purkinje cells. Central nervous system lesions can be clinically manifest as rigid tails, hypermetria, paraphimosis, ataxia, and urinary bladder distention.

Clinical signs are usually absent in MAdV-2 infected mice, but runting of suckling mice has been observed in natural infections. Naturally infected athymic nude mice are clinically normal. Gross lesions of MAdV-2 infection are not evident, except that juvenile mice may be bloated and runted. Mice naturally or experimentally infected with MAdV-2 develop intranuclear inclusions in mucosal epithelial cells of the small intestine, especially in the distal segments, and the cecum. Inclusions are most plentiful in infant mice but can also be found in smaller numbers in the mucosa of adult mice, especially dams that are suckling infected infants. Similar inclusions have been noted in adult nude mice without other detectable lesions. Typically, inclusion-bearing nuclei are located in the apical portions of cells, rather than in their normal basal location (Fig. 1.17).

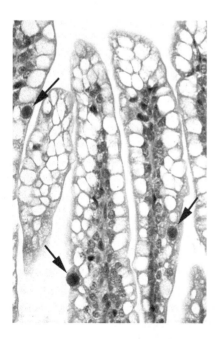

FIG. 1.17. *Small intestine from a juvenile mouse infected with mouse adenovirus MAdV-2. Note the distinct intranuclear inclusion bodies (arrows) in a few enterocytes lining the villi.*

Diagnosis

Serology is the most effective means of screening mouse populations for MAdV infection. These agents partially cross-react serologically, depending on method, in a one-way relationship with antiserum to MAdV-2 cross-reacting with MAdV-1, but not conversely. Since MAdV-1 is quite rare in laboratory mice, MAdV-2 antigen should be used. Differential diagnoses for MAdV-1 include multisystemic infections that produce intranuclear inclusions, such as polyoma virus and cytomegalovirus. Intestinal epithelial MAdV-2 inclusions are pathognomonic, but not always apparent. They are not induced by any other known agent, although K virus can form inclusions in intestinal endothelial cells. Inclusions in the apical region of enterocytes must be differentiated from mitotic cells and intraepithelial lymphocytes. Success at finding MAdV-2 inclusions is maximized in infant mice. MAdV strain-specific PCR can also be used.

Herpesvirus Infections

Mice are host to two members of the family Herpesviridae, subfamily Betaherpesvirinae and genus *Muromegalovirus*, including mouse cytomegalovirus (MCMV) and mouse thymic virus (MTV). Neither is common among contemporary laboratory mouse populations, but may contaminate archival biological products.

Mouse Cytomegalovirus Infection

MCMV is a mouse-specific virus that was originally isolated by M.G. Smith from salivary glands of naturally infected laboratory mice. Cytomegaloviruses replicate in the nucleus and cause cytomegalic inclusion disease, characterized by enlarged cells bearing both intranuclear and intracytoplasmic inclusions, particularly in salivary glands. MCMV has been studied extensively as an animal model of human CMV (HCMV) infection, but significant biological differences exist between MCMV and HCMV. Most laboratory studies have utilized the original Smith strain of MCMV, or derivatives thereof, and may not accurately reflect the natural biology of other MCMV strains. Nevertheless, the intense scrutiny of MCMV as a prototype model system has shed considerable light on its pathogenesis.

Epizootiology and Pathogenesis

Wild mice are commonly infected with MCMV. There are multiple genetically diverse MCMV strains within wild mouse populations, and mixed infections of single mice are common. Laboratory studies have found that infection-induced immunity to one strain does not preclude infection with a second strain. MCMV is transmitted oronasally by direct contact and is excreted in saliva, tears, urine, and semen. Experimental infection is significantly influenced by virus strain, dose, route of inoculation, and host factors (age, genotype). Neonates of all mouse strains are universally susceptible to severe disease, and resistance to lethal disease evolves after weaning and increases until about 8 weeks of age. Genetically resistant mouse strains include B6, B10, CBA, and C3H mice, and susceptible strains include BALB/c and A strain mice. Resistance is associated with *H-2k* haplotype, but non-*H-2* associated factors also exist, including a resistance factor that is linked to loci on chromosome 6 within the natural killer (NK) cell complex. This region encodes a receptor expressed on NK cells that binds to a glycoprotein of MCMV, but MCMV isolates from wild mice have naturally occurring mutations that fail to activate NK cells through this receptor. NK cells interact with MCMV in other ways that are linked to the *H-2k* haplotype.

Following experimental inoculation of infant mice, viremia and multisystemic dissemination occur within 1 week, with infection of lung, heart, liver, spleen, salivary glands, and gonads. Macrophages are major targets of the virus, and blood monocytes are important for the viremic phase of infection. Following dissemination, virus is rapidly cleared from tissues, except from salivary gland. Infection of NK-deficient beige mice, or mice depleted of NK cells, significantly prevents virus clearance. Adaptive immune responses, including CD4 and CD8 cells, are also important in clearing infection from most sites. Athymic or SCID mice fail to control active infection, but B-cell-deficient mice can recover from acute infection. Curiously, despite functional innate and acquired immune responses in fully immunocompetent mice, including NK, CD4, CD8, and B cells, MCMV continues to persist and replicate in salivary gland tissues. A number of MCMV genes function to control the innate and acquired immune responses, in addition to determining cell tropism and inhibiting apoptosis. Most of these genes are not essential for virus replication in vitro, and therefore provide selective advantages for virus persistence in vivo. An important feature of MCMV (and other herpesviruses) is latent infection, in which virus persists in a nonreplicative state, but can be reactivated by immunosuppression or stress. Based upon tissue explanting and PCR, latency of MCMV has been documented in various organs, including salivary glands, lung, spleen, liver, heart, kidney, adrenal glands, and myeloid cells. This state of latency can persist for the life of the mouse.

Unlike HCMV, MCMV does not readily cross the placenta, and in utero transmission does not usually take place in naturally and experimentally infected mice. Infection of pregnant mice may cause fetal death and resorption, delayed birth, and runted pups, but these are nonspecific events. Nevertheless, latently infected dams have been documented to transmit low-level or latent infection to fetuses in utero. MCMV infects cells in the epididymis, seminal vesicles, testes, including Leydig cells and spermatozoa, as well as ovarian stromal cells. Experimental transmission by artificial insemination has been reported. Thus, sexual transmission is likely.

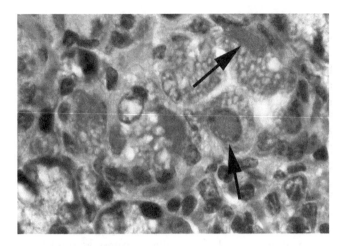

FIG. 1.18. *Submaxillary salivary gland from a wild mouse infected with mouse cytomegalovirus. Intranuclear inclusions (arrows) are present in acinar epithelial cells.*

Pathology

Overt disease and disseminated lesions do not usually occur in naturally infected mice. The most frequently encountered lesions occur in the submandibular salivary glands and, rarely, in the parotid glands. Eosinophilic intranuclear and intracytoplasmic inclusions are present in acinar epithelial cells with cytomegaly (Fig. 1.18) and lymphoplasmacytic infiltration of interstitium. During the acute disseminated phase in experimentally inoculated infant mice or T-cell-deficient mice, focal necrosis, cytomegaly, inclusions, and inflammation occur in many tissues, including salivary glands, lacrimal glands, brain, liver, spleen, thymus, lymph nodes, peritoneum, lung, skin, kidney, bowel, pancreas, adrenal, skeletal and cardiac muscle, cartilage, and brown fat. Diffuse interstitial pneumonitis has been described in BALB/c mice that were immunosuppressed by a variety of methods, and athymic mice develop progressive multifocal nodular pulmonary inflammation. Athymic mice also develop progressive destruction of adrenals. Arteritis of the pulmonary artery and aorta (at the base of the heart) has been documented during experimental MCMV infection in B6 and BALB/c mice, but no virus was confirmed within the lesions. A single case of naturally occurring MCMV disseminated infection has been reported in an aged laboratory mouse. MCMV has been shown to have a synergistic effect with *Pseudomonas aeruginosa*.

Diagnosis

Lesions in salivary glands are typical of cytomegalovirus, but are not always present in infected animals. Serology is the method of choice for colony surveillance, but detection of infection in immunodeficient mice that do not seroconvert must be accomplished through nucleic acid detection, including in situ hybridization and PCR. These methods can also be used to detect latent infection. Differential diagnosis for sialoadenitis with inclusion bodies must include polyoma virus. Other viruses that infect salivary glands include reovirus 3, mouse thymic virus, and mammary tumor virus, but these viruses do not induce inclusions.

Mouse Thymic Virus Infection

Detailed information about mouse thymic virus (MTV) is generally lacking, since in vitro methods of propagation have not been identified and little experimental work has been performed. Virtually nothing is known about its genome. Synonyms include thymic necrosis virus, thymic agent, and mouse T-lymphotropic virus. The prevalence of MTV in laboratory mouse populations is extremely rare, but it is very common among wild mice. MTV can be a contaminant of MCMV stocks prepared from salivary glands. Because of its lymphocytotropism, MTV infection may result in significantly altered immune responses.

Epizootiology and Pathogenesis

MTV was first discovered when inoculated newborn Swiss mice developed thymic necrosis following serial passage of mammary tumor homogenates. This feature of MTV has been emphasized in subsequent studies, but MTV infects salivary glands as its primary target. Outcome of experimental infection is strikingly age dependent and also influenced by mouse genotype. Intraperitoneal as well as oronasal inoculation of newborn mice results in acute thymic necrosis, which is visible grossly as diminished thymic mass, within 1–2 weeks. Subsequently, the thymus returns to normal, but mice remain persistently infected. Age-related susceptibility to thymic necrosis decreases progressively until 6 days of age, at which point mice are no longer susceptible to thymic necrosis. Although largely an experimental phenomenon, thymic necrosis has been encountered in infant mice from naturally infected mouse colonies. CD4+8+ and CD4+8– T cells are selectively targeted by MTV, although virus replication also occurs in thymic epithelial cells and macrophages. Newborn mice develop viremia, with MTV detectable in multiple organs. Mice of all ages develop infection of salivary glands, with persistent virus shedding in saliva for several months or more. Athymic mice, which lack the T-cell substrate for virus replication, tend to shed virus less consistently. The mode of MTV transmission is presumed to be primarily through the saliva, and MTV is readily transmitted by direct contact. MTV has also been isolated from mammary tissue of an infected mother and from mammary tumor extracts, suggesting another possible route of transmission. Vertical (in utero) transmission has not been documented.

Pathology

MTV infection of infant mice results in the formation of intranuclear inclusion bodies and necrosis of thymocytes and, to a lesser extent, cells in lymph nodes and spleens. During recovery, there is granuloma formation. Lesions in salivary glands have not been noted. BALB/c and A strain mice, but not B6, C3H, or DBA/2 mice, when inoculated as neonates develop gastritis. Mice of other strains develop oophoritis and antibodies to thyroglobulin. These phenomena are believed to be autoimmune in origin, via nonspecific activation and expansion of self-reactive T cells, and not related to MTV in these tissues.

Diagnosis

Seroconversion can be detected using infected salivary tissue as antigen. Mice infected as neonates may not seroconvert, probably due to immune tolerance. The mouse antibody production (MAP) test can be useful, but PCR is now available for testing mouse tissue and biologic products. Differential diagnoses include coronavirus or stress, which may cause thymic necrosis, but not inclusions. A bioassay has been used to detect MTV, in which inoculated infant mice develop thymic necrosis.

Parvovirus Infections

Laboratory mice are subject to infection with two different autonomously replicating types of viruses in the family Parvoviridae: minute virus of mice (MVM) and mouse parvovirus (MPV). The official and generally unaccepted name for MVM is mice minute virus (MMV), which will not be used in this text. MVM and MPV, including dual infections, are among the most prevalent viruses in contemporary laboratory mouse populations. MPV strains represent the predominant type (75%) in parvovirus-positive populations. Clinical disease is seldom present in immunocompetent mice, but these viruses have significant immunomodulatory effects, and they are remarkably refractory to effective eradication from contaminated mouse colonies.

MVM and MPV share considerable homology among genes that encode 2 antigenically cross-reactive (among all mouse parvoviruses) nonstructural proteins, NS1 and NS2, but display variation among genes that encode structural capsid proteins, VP1, VP2, and VP3. VP2, in particular, contributes to significant antigenic and biologic differences among mouse parvoviruses. Sequence analysis, differential PCR, and restriction fragment length polymorphism analysis have lent clarity to the rodent parvovirus interrelationships. The MVM group contains MVMp, MVMi, MVMm, and MVMc, and the MPV group contains a cluster of closely related MPV-1a, MPV-1b, MPV-1c, a somewhat disparate cluster containing MPV-2, and another cluster containing MPV-3 and a closely related hamster parvovirus that is closely related to MPV-3 and likely to be of mouse origin. The mouse parvoviruses are distinctly different from the parvoviruses of rats. More isolates and strains are likely to be discovered, and therefore it is most expedient to discuss the two major phylogenetic groups.

Epizootiology and Pathogenesis

Mouse parvoviruses are transmitted through feces and urine by oronasal exposure with a slow rate of cage-to-cage spread. In general, parvoviruses of all host species are dependent upon the S phase of the cell cycle for virus replication, and therefore induce cytolytic disease only in dividing tissues (including lymphoid tissues undergoing antigenic stimulation). However, virus replication, and therefore patterns of disease, is limited to certain cell types that bear the appropriate viral receptors. For example, many parvoviruses replicate in intestinal crypt epithelium, but rodent parvoviruses do not target that cell population, and therefore do not induce intestinal disease.

Following oral inoculation, mouse parvoviruses initially replicate in intraepithelial lymphocytes, lamina propria, and endothelium of the small intestine, and then disseminate to multiple organs, including kidney, intestine, lymphoid tissues, liver, and, to a much lesser extent, lung, with tropism for endothelial cells, hematopoietic cells, and lymphoreticular cells. Viremic dissemination is likely related to the high degree of lymphocytotropism of these viruses, but MVM viremia is also erythrocyte associated. Both types of virus target small intestine and lymphoid tissue, and MVM also replicates in kidney. MVM infection of both infant and adult immunocompetent mice is limited in duration, with recovery. In contrast, MPV infection is typically persistent following infection of mice of all ages, but juvenile mice may transmit virus more efficiently. Neonatal mice are protected from infection by maternal antibody in enzootically infected colonies. Mice resist reinfection with the homotypic virus, but are fully susceptible to infection with the heterotypic serotype, thus explaining the naturally high frequency of dual MVM and MPV infections.

Pathology

Natural infection of immunocompetent mice is clinically silent, regardless of age or strain of mice. Experimental infection of neonatal BALB/c, SWR, SJL, CBA, and C3H mice with MVMi has been shown to cause mortality due to hemorrhage, hematopoietic involution, and renal papillary infarction. DBA/2 neonates also developed intestinal hemorrhage and more rapid hepatic hematopoietic involution, whereas B6 neonates are resistant to vascular and hematopoietic diseases. MVM is more pathogenic for hematopoietic tissues than MPV. Infection of neonatal BALB/c mice with MVMi revealed replication and a significant decrease in bone marrow and splenic cellularity, with depressed myelopoiesis. MVM infection of SCID and neonatal mice has been found to induce lethal leukopenia, due to virus replication in primordial hematopoietic cells, with severe depletion of granulomacrophagic cells and compensatory erythropoiesis in bone marrow. Natural MVM-related disease has been observed in

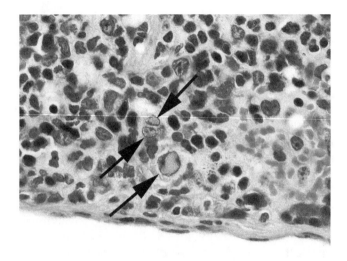

FIG. 1.19. *Intranuclear inclusions (arrows) in mononuclear cells of the spleen in an immunodeficient mouse naturally infected with minute virus of mice (MVM). (Source: Franklin 2006. Reproduced with permission from Oxford University Press.)*

NOD.Cg-*H2^{H4}*-*Igh-6* null mice with leukopenia and anemia. Intranuclear inclusions were present in mononuclear cells of spleens (Fig. 1.19) and bone marrow. Experimental exposure of infant mice with MVM, including intranasal inoculation and contact exposure, results in virus replication in the cells of the subventricular zone, subependymal zone of the olfactory bulb, and the dentate gyrus of the hippocampus. These are the 3 main germinal centers in postpartum neurogenesis of the mouse. MVM also targets the outer granular layer of the cerebellum, with cytolysis of cells that have migrated to the internal granular layer, resulting in granuloprival cerebellar hypoplasia. In experimentally infected pregnant mice, MVM replication may occur in various tissues, including placenta and fetus, without histological evidence of lesions.

Diagnosis

MVM and MPV infection is usually diagnosed by seroconversion, but colony surveillance can be challenging due to the inefficient cage-to-cage transmission of these viruses, thereby requiring large sample sizes for surveillance. Indeed, the inefficient cage-to-cage transmission has made it possible to test and cull as a means of eliminating infection from a population. Furthermore, experimental inoculation of adult ICR, BALB/c, C3H/HeN, C57BL/6, and DBA/2 mice with different doses of MPV has revealed marked differences in serologic response, with antibody detection in all C3H mice, some but not all ICR, BALB, and DBA mice, and none of the B6 mice, except when inoculated with very high doses of virus. ELISAs utilize the extensive cross-reactive recombinant NS1 antigen to detect antibody to both MVM and MPV, and recombinant VP2 antigen or empty capsids can be used to differentiate antibodies between

MVM and MPV. Caution is advised, since antibodies to new isolates or strains that are more distantly related to MVM or MPV may not be detected. PCR primers for detection of conserved and group-specific regions of the genome are available for detection of virus in tissues and feces. The mesenteric lymph node is an optimal tissue for PCR-based detection of mouse parvoviruses. A comparison of sensitivity of testing procedures resulted in the following percentage of positives: mesenteric lymph node PCR (93%), serologic immunofluorescence assay (68%), direct fecal PCR (10%), and cage fecal PCR (5%). The MAP test and virus isolation, including tissue explant cultures, are more labor-intensive methods that can also be utilized.

Papillomavirus Infections

A papillomavirus (MusPV) was discovered in an inbred NMRI-*nude* mouse colony, in which the mice developed florid papillomas at the mucocutaneous junctions of their nose and mouth. The agent induced papillomas in T-cell-deficient (athymic nude and SCID) strains of mice. MusPV is infectious, but not oncogenic, in a variety of immunocompetent strains of mice, which display varying degrees of susceptibility. MusPV is genetically closely related to the rat papillomavirus virus. Another *M. musculus* papillomavirus has since been reported from normal ear skin tissue of wild mice in Europe. Although these viruses are rare in laboratory mouse populations, they are likely to attain popularity as research models, with subsequent iatrogenic introduction to laboratory mouse populations.

Polyomavirus Infections

Mice are hosts to two genetically distinct polyomaviruses: polyoma virus (PyV) and K virus. They belong to the family Polyomaviridae, which contains a number of related viruses (macaque SV-40 virus, human BK and JC viruses, hamster polyomavirus, rat polyomavirus, and rabbit kidney vaculolating virus). These viruses once belonged to the family Papovaviridae, but that family has been disbanded and split into Polyomaviridae and Papillomaviridae. PyV encodes a middle T antigen that is important in oncogenesis. The K virus genome is similar to that of PyV, but lacks the middle T antigen of PyV. Both viruses are rare or nonexistent in contemporary laboratory mouse populations, but PyV continues to be used as an experimental oncogenic virus that on occasion results in iatrogenic introductions to susceptible mouse colonies.

Polyoma Virus Infection

PyV was originally termed the "Stewart-Eddy (SE) polyoma virus" and the "parotid tumor virus." The virus has been extensively studied as an oncogenic virus that induces many (poly) types of tumor (-oma). The name is well deserved, as tumors arise from more than a dozen different cell types. Under experimental conditions, it is

oncogenic in several different species. The oncogenic activity for which this virus is so well known is largely an experimental phenomenon, requiring parenteral inoculation of genetically susceptible strains of mice within the first 24 hours of life with high titers of selected isolates virus with high oncogenic activity. The relevance of PyV to the laboratory mouse has risen with the use of PyV middle T (PyV-MT) gene as a component of transgenic constructs. PyV is known to contaminate transplantable tumors and cell lines, which in turn have served as inadvertent sources of contamination of mouse stocks.

Epizootiology and Pathogenesis

PyV was initially discovered by Ludwig Gross, when newborn mice unexpectedly developed salivary gland tumors following inoculation with filtered extracts of mouse leukemia tissue. PyV is an environmentally stable virus that is shed primarily in saliva, urine, and feces. Infection is most efficiently acquired intranasally. Infection of a mouse population requires a continuous source of exposure, which is provided by repeatedly utilized nesting sites of wild mice. The virus fails to survive under laboratory mouse husbandry conditions and is, therefore, quite rare in contemporary mouse colonies. Oronasal inoculation of neonatal mice results in virus replication in the nasal mucosa, submaxillary salivary glands, and lungs, followed by viremic dissemination to multiple organs, including kidneys. Mortality can be high at this stage. By day 12, the virus is cleared by the host immune response from most sites but persists in the lung and especially kidney for months, where virus replicates in renal tubular epithelial cells. Infection of older mice is more rapidly cleared, with inefficient virus excretion for shorter periods. Transplacental transmission does not seem to occur naturally, but virus can be reactivated in the kidneys of adult mice during pregnancy if they were infected as neonates. Since PyV is a widely used experimental virus, iatrogenic contamination of laboratory mice can take place, but consequences are limited for the reasons just cited. Thus, under natural conditions, maternal antibody from immune dams, coupled with the low level of environmental contamination in a laboratory mouse facility, precludes successful infection of neonatal mice and attenuates survival of the virus in the population.

The oncogenic characteristics of PyV have been extensively studied and are herein reviewed because pathologists may encounter mice that are either experimentally infected with the virus, inadvertently exposed to the virus as immunodeficient strains, or derived from PyV transgenic constructs. Not all strains or isolates of the virus are oncogenic, including many "wild-type" isolates. Virus strains that produce "large plaques" in cell culture can induce tumors in 100% of susceptible mice, whereas other strains, which produce "small plaques," induce few or no tumors. If genetically susceptible mice are experimentally inoculated parenterally with oncogenic virus at less than 24 hours of age, microscopic foci of cellular transformation arise in multiple tissues. Most of these foci remain microscopic, but others grow rapidly into large tumors within 3 months. Tumors arising in mice inoculated with less oncogenic strains may not arise until 6–12 months, and the tumors that arise are usually mesenchymal, rather than epithelial in origin.

The genetic basis of susceptibility to PyV oncogenesis has been extensively studied in more than 40 inbred strains and F1 hybrids, with susceptibility ranging from 100% to complete resistance, with many intermediate phenotypes. Resistance can be determined by both immunological and nonimmunological factors. For example, C57BL mice are highly resistant due to effective antiviral and antitumor immunity, which can be abrogated by neonatal thymectomy, irradiation, or immunosuppression. C57BR mice are susceptible to infection as neonates but do not develop tumors. Other strains of mice are resistant to tumor induction, even when immunosuppressed. Susceptibility to tumor induction has been linked to *H-2k* haplotypes. C3H/BiDa (*H-2k*) are fully susceptible, whereas DBA/2 and BALB/c mice (*H-2d*) are resistant. In addition, susceptibility is conferred in many mouse strains by an endogenous mouse mammary tumor provirus, *Mtv-7*. *Mtv-7* encodes a superantigen (Sag) that, when expressed, results in deletion of Vß6+ T cells. This abrogates the ability of these mice to mount an effective antitumor cytotoxic T-cell response. Another, non-Sag mechanism for susceptibility has recently been discovered in wild-derived inbred mice.

The biological characteristics of PyV are uniquely suited for disseminated, polytropic infection and neoplasia. The virus protein VP1 nonselectively binds universally to sialic acid of cell surfaces, contributing to polytropism. The virus also possesses multivalent enhancer regions that enable it to be transcribed and replicate in many cell types. The virus encodes three T (tumor) antigens that interact with various cell factors and growth signaling pathways. PyV-MT antigen is the major transforming protein that binds and activates protein kinase pp60 (*c-Src*) and other members of the *c-Src* family. PyV-MT antigen can transform cells by itself and is therefore a popular component of transgenic constructs for neoplasia research. Many transgenic lines of mice possess PyV-MT contributions to their genome.

Pathology

Under natural conditions, lesions are not likely to be encountered, except in immunodeficient mice. Nude mice have been shown to develop multifocal necrosis and inflammation, followed by tumor formation in multiple tissues reminiscent of experimentally inoculated neonatal mice. Microscopic examination of tissues from neonatally inoculated mice has revealed foci of

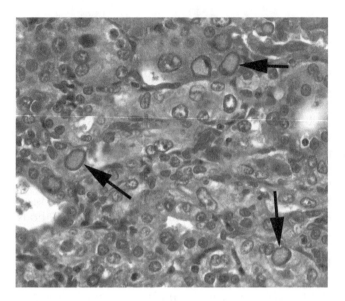

FIG. 1.20.   *Intranuclear inclusions in the renal tubular epithelium (arrows) of a mouse experimentally infected with polyoma virus.*

virus replication in over 40 different cell types, underscoring the virus polytropism. Intranuclear inclusions can be observed with difficulty in cytolytic lesions and are most apparent in renal tubular epithelium (Fig. 1.20). Many of these foci give rise to transformed cells without virus replication. Cytopathic and proliferative changes are especially apparent in bronchiolar, renal pelvic, and ureteral epithelium. When genetically susceptible neonatal mice are experimentally infected with oncogenic strains of the virus, tumors arise most commonly from mammary gland, salivary gland, and thymus. Multiple skin tumors of hair follicle origin (with notable similarity to the skin tumors that occur in hamsters under natural conditions when exposed to hamster polyomavirus) are frequently observed. Tumors of mesenchymal origin are also common, including renal sarcomas, osteosarcomas, hemangiomas, and fibrosarcomas. Experimentally infected mice develop runting syndrome, polyarteritis, and enhanced autoimmune disease.

Accidental infection of nude mice has been shown to result in multisystemic wasting disease, with paralysis and development of multiple tumors, particularly of uterus and bone. Experimental infections of nude mice yielded a very high prevalence of mammary adenocarcinomas among females and osteosarcomas among males. Nude mice can also develop infection of oligodendroglia with demyelination, similar to progressive multifocal leukoencephalopathy (PML) in immmunocompromised humans infected with BK and JC viruses, and macaques infected with SV-40 virus. Paralysis in nude mice is due to vertebral tumors as well as demyelination. A single report examined the effects of intraperitoneal inoculation of C.B-17-*scid* and B6-*scid* mice. Mice of both types became acutely ill and died within 2 weeks, with cutaneous hemorrhages and splenomegaly. The mice were thrombocytopenic, with depletion of megakaryocytes in spleen and bone marrow, and developed marked extramedullary myelopoiesis in the spleen, which was misinterpreted as "myeloproliferative disease." If PyV gains access to other types of immunodeficient mice, it is likely to behave in a manner that is dictated by the properties of the virus, genetic background of the mouse strain, and nature of the immunodeficiency, but the rarity and inefficient transmission of PyV have limited the chances of natural exposure.

Diagnosis

The presence of PyV in immunocompetent mouse populations is best detected serologically, but PCR has been developed for detecting virus in tissues and other biological products. Differential diagnoses of nude mice with wasting disease include primarily mouse hepatitis virus, *Pneumocystis murina*, Sendai virus, and pneumonia virus of mice (PVM). Microscopic lesions containing intranuclear inclusion bodies must be differentiated from lesions caused by K virus, MAdV, and MCMV.

K Virus Infection

For all practical purposes, K virus is of historical interest and occurs rarely, if at all, in contemporary laboratory mouse colonies. Unlike PyV, K virus has no oncogenic action, either naturally or experimentally, in keeping with the absence of middle T antigen.

Epizootiology and Pathogenesis

K virus was initially discovered by Lawrence Kilham (thus the K) following intracerebral inoculation of infant mice with tissue extracts from an adult mouse during experiments on the mammary tumor virus. K virus is spread by the oronasal route. When orally inoculated into neonatal mice, the virus initially replicates in intestinal capillary endothelium and then disseminates hematogenously to other organs, including lung, liver, spleen, kidney, and brain, where it replicates in vascular endothelium. There appears to be strong tropism for pulmonary endothelium. At 6–15 days after inoculation of neonatal mice, there is a sudden onset of dyspnea due to pulmonary vascular edema and hemorrhage, resulting in rapid death. Pulmonary disease does not occur when older mice are inoculated, with complete resistance evolving between 12 and 18 days of age. Older mice mount an early and effective immune response that prevents the viremic phase of infection. Infection of nude mice results in disease similar to that seen in suckling mice. Regardless of age, mice remain persistently infected, and the site for virus persistence is renal tubular epithelium, which is typical of other members of the polyomavirus group. In naturally infected colonies, clinical signs are absent, with dams conferring passive immunity to litters during the disease-susceptible neonatal period.

Pathology

Gross lesions are restricted to lungs of neonatal or immunodeficient mice. Microscopically, intranuclear inclusions are present in vascular endothelium of jejunum, ileum, lung, liver, and occasionally brain. Inclusions are poorly discernible and require optimal fixation, especially in the intestine. Pulmonary lesions consist of congestion, edema, hemorrhage, atelectasis, and septal thickening. Livers of neonatal mice can have sinusoidal leukocytic infiltration and nuclear ballooning of cells lining sinusoids. Lymphocytic infiltrates (including interstitial pneumonia) arise in recovering mice. Inclusions may be found in renal tubular epithelial cells, frequently in groups of 2 or more, associated with foci of interstitial inflammation.

Diagnosis

Recognition of diagnostic lesions is difficult at best and is most likely in neonatally infected mice. Serological surveillance can be carried out by a variety of methods. PCR has been utilized to detect virus in infected mouse tissues. Differential diagnosis of multisystemic infection with intranuclear inclusions should include PyV, MAdV-1, and MCMV.

Poxvirus Infection: Ectromelia Virus Infection; Mousepox

No virus of laboratory mice conjures up an image of ruin like ectromelia virus (ECTV). Some of this reputation is justified, but most is human in origin. ECTV is a large DNA virus of the family Poxviridae and genus *Orthopox*, to which vaccinia, variola, monkeypox, cowpox, and others also belong. Orthopoxviruses share extensive antigenic cross-reactivity. Each is a distinct species, but the host range can be broad. Marchal reported an epizootic disease with high mortality in adult mice and termed it "infectious ectromelia," because of the frequency of limb amputation (ectromelia) in surviving mice. Frank Fenner performed seminal work on pathogenesis of the agent "ectromelia virus," which causes the disease "mousepox," although the terms are often erroneously interchanged. Outbreaks in the United States have stimulated renewed interest in the pathogenesis of mousepox. Mousepox was originally studied as a model for human smallpox, and that interest re-emerged with bioterrorism research.

Epizootiology and Pathogenesis

The origin of ectromelia virus remains an enigma, since it has never been found in wild populations of *M. musculus*. Unsubstantiated evidence has suggested infection of wild non-*Mus* rodents in Europe, but it has not been confirmed by appropriate sequence analysis and may actually reflect infection with cowpox virus. Ectromelia virus was at one time common among mouse colonies in Europe and may be enzootic in laboratory mice in China. In the past, outbreaks in the United States have been due to introduction of infected mice or mouse products from Europe. In more recent outbreaks of mousepox, the source of the virus was traced to commercial mouse sera either collected from mice in the United States or imported from China. Strains of ECTV, including Hampstead, Moscow, NIH-79, Washington University, St. Louis 69, Beijing 70, Ishibashi I–III, and NAV, vary in virulence, but are serologically and genetically homogeneous. The NAV strain, which was isolated from mice infected with commercial mouse serum from China, is essentially the same virus as the original Hampstead virus. These findings strongly suggest that ECTV has not had a long or widespread enzootic history among commensal or domestic mice. ECTV is not highly contagious. It can be experimentally transmitted via a number of routes, but the primary means of natural transmission is believed to be through cutaneous trauma, which requires direct contact, and transmission has been shown to be facilitated by handling. Young mice suckling immune dams are protected by maternal antibody from disease but not from infection. ECTV readily infects the placenta and fetuses, but infected fetuses die and are not a source for vertical transmission within a population.

The hypothetical model of infection involves invasion through skin or mucous membranes, local replication, spread to regional lymph nodes, primary viremia, and then replication in spleen and liver. Between 3 and 4 days after exposure, a secondary viremia ensues, inducing replication of virus in skin, kidney, lung, intestine, and other organs. There is increasing evolution of lesions (disease) on days 7–11, including cutaneous rash. This scenario differs markedly between mouse genotypes. Susceptible mouse strains, such as C3H, A, DBA, SWR, CBA, and BALB/c, die acutely with minimal opportunity for virus excretion. Several other mouse strains develop illness but survive long enough to develop cutaneous lesions with maximal opportunity for virus shedding. Others, such as B6 and AKR mice, are remarkably resistant to disease and, therefore, allow inefficient virus replication and excretion. Thus, a textbook mousepox epizootic requires a select combination of introduction, suitable mouse strains for transmission, and the presence of susceptible strains for disease expression. Immunosuppression will exacerbate disease in mildly or subclinically infected mice. For these reasons, classic outbreaks of high mortality are often not seen in genetically homogeneous colonies of mice. Immunologically competent mice recover completely from infection and do not generally serve as carriers. Therefore, rederivation of virus-free mouse populations can be achieved from immmunocompetent mice. Immunodeficient mice cannot clear virus and are likely to be highly susceptible to fatal disease. Susceptibility to ECTV is dependent upon age, sex, strain, and immune status of the host and the virus strain. Interferons, NK cells, T cells, and B cells are all important. The genetics of resistance are complex and polygenic and not linked to *H-2* haplotype. Resistance

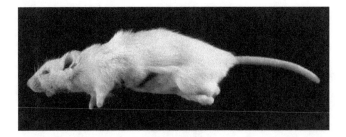

FIG. 1.21.   *Healed amputating lesions of the distal extremities (ectromelia) from a mouse that survived natural infection with ectromelia virus. (Source: R. Feinstein, The National Veterinary Institute, Sweden. Reproduced with permission from R. Feinstein.)*

factors have been mapped to loci on chromosome 6 that includes the NK cell complex, chromosome 2 that includes the gene for C5, chromosome 17, and chromosome 1.

Pathology

Expression of lesions is dependent upon factors discussed above. Clinical signs range from subclinical infection to sudden death. External lesions during the acute phase of infection in susceptible surviving mice include conjunctivitis, alopecia, cutaneous erythema and erosions (rash), and swelling and dry gangrene of extremities, which result in "ectromelia" in surviving mice (Fig. 1.21). Internally, livers may be swollen, friable, and mottled with multiple pinpoint white to coalescing hemorrhagic foci (Fig. 1.22). Spleens, lymph nodes, and Peyer's patches may be enlarged, with patchy pale or

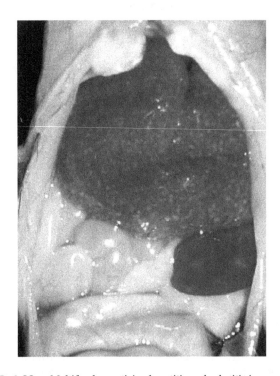

FIG. 1.22.   *Multifocal necrotizing hepatitis and splenitis in a mouse during the acute phase of mousepox. (Source: Labelle et al. 2009. Reproduced with permission from American Association for Laboratory Animal Science.)*

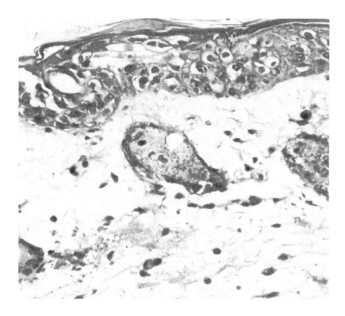

FIG. 1.23. *Skin from a mouse infected with ectromelia virus. Note ballooning degeneration and intracytoplasmic inclusions in the epidermis, with underlying dermal edema.*

hemorrhagic areas. Intestinal hemorrhage, particularly in the upper small intestine, is common. Microscopic lesions consist of focal coagulative necrosis in the liver, spleen, lymph nodes, Peyer's patches, and thymus, as well as other organs. Multiple basophilic to eosinophilic intracytoplasmic inclusion bodies (1.5–6 µm) are evident in infected cells, especially hepatocytes at the periphery of necrotic foci. These inclusions are poorly discernible with routine staining, but can be enhanced by doubling hematoxylin-staining time. Lymphoid tissue can be hyperplastic and/or focally necrotic, with occasional eosinophilic cytoplasmic inclusion bodies (type A pox inclusions or Marchal bodies). Erosive enteritis, often in association with Peyer's patches, is common, with type A inclusions in enterocytes. Skin lesions consist of focal epidermal hyperplasia, with hypertrophy and ballooning of epithelial cells and formation of numerous prominent large type A inclusions (Fig. 1.23). Later, skin lesions become erosive and inflammatory in character. Inclusions, inflammation, and erosion are also found in conjunctiva, vagina, and nasal mucosa. The conjunctival mucosa is a preferred area to search for inclusion bodies. Recovered mice often have fibrosis of the spleen and can have amputated tails and digits.

Diagnosis
The variable clinical signs and lesions can be problematic, but careful selection of clinically ill mice will enhance an accurate diagnosis. The complex of liver, spleen, and epithelial lesions bearing typical inclusions is pathognomonic. Splenic fibrosis in recovered mice is also a unique feature of this disease. Confirmation can be achieved by electron microscopic identification of the strikingly large poxvirus particles, immunohistochemistry, PCR, or virus isolation. Serology is a useful diagnostic adjunct in recovered mice and is an important surveillance tool for monitoring mouse populations. Serologic testing is likely to be of little value during the early stages of the infection. Vaccination is variably practiced and can interfere with interpretation of serology results. It should also be noted that vaccination protects mice from severe disease, but still allows active infection. Differential diagnoses must include agents that cause hepatitis in adult mice, such as MHV, Tyzzer's disease, salmonellosis, and others. Skin lesions must be differentiated from bite wounds, trichotillomania, hypersensitivity, and other forms of dermatitis. Gangrene and amputation of digits or tail can also occur due to trauma or "ringtail." Draconian depopulation measures to eliminate ECTV from mouse populations are probably not necessary if a rational approach to quarantine, testing, and rederivation is taken based upon the biology of this virus.

RNA VIRAL INFECTIONS

Arenavirus Infection: Lymphocytic Choriomeningitis Virus Infection
Mus musculus is the natural reservoir host for lymphocytic choriomeningitis virus (LCMV), and mice have carried this virus throughout the world from their original Old World niche. LCMV is a significant pathogen of humans, and was initially discovered during investigation of St. Louis encephalitis in 1933, when human brain material was injected into the brains of monkeys and mice, which developed lymphocytic choriomeningitis. The lesion, lymphocytic choriomeningitis, is not a feature of natural infection in mice. LCMV belongs to the family Arenaviridae, which includes a single genus *Arenavirus*, named because of the granular-appearing (Latin arenosus, "sandy") ribosomes within virions. If for no other reason, LCMV is important because of its significant zoonotic potential. LCMV has been studied extensively as a model system of immune-mediated disease, virus persistence, and immune tolerance, resulting in emphasis on aspects of infection that are not necessarily relevant to natural infection. LCMV has also been used as a model of noncytolytic viral disruption of differentiated cell function, resulting in disease without lesions (a claim that has not involved pathologists). LCMV is an unacceptable agent in laboratory animal facilities, and its eradication should be aggressively effected. The polytropic nature of LCMV and its wide host range allow this virus to readily infect transplantable tumors and cell lines, which can serve as a source of contamination for mouse colonies.

Epizootiology and Pathogenesis
LCMV is not ubiquitous, in that isolated mouse populations may or may not be enzootically infected. It is fortunately rare among contemporary laboratory mouse

populations, but may be a contaminant of biological products derived from mice. LCMV has also been found in pet mice and colonies of mice raised for feeding other species, including non-human primates. LCMV can naturally infect a variety of other mammals, including hamsters, guinea pigs, cotton rats, chinchillas, canids, and primates, including humans. Newborn rats can be infected experimentally, but this species seems to be refractory to natural infection. Among mice, the highly labile virus can be transmitted by direct contact and aerosol through nasal secretions as well as urine and saliva.

Enzootic infection in a mouse population is maintained by vertical transmission from dam to fetus and neonates. Infection of the fetus occurs during early pregnancy, and ova can be infected prior to implantation. There is no evidence for transmission by coitus. Nearly every cell in the fetus may become infected noncytolytically, with no significant adverse effect, although reduced litter sizes and runted pups may occur. The widely disseminated fetal infection involves the immature thymus, resulting in selective immune tolerance, with negative selection and depletion of LCMV-responsive CD8 T cells. This state of tolerance is highly LCMV selective, with otherwise normal immune responsiveness to other antigens. A similar scenario can occur if pups are infected as neonates. The state of LCMV immune tolerance allows multisystemic, persistent, subclinical infection, with the mice growing to reproductive maturity and perpetuating the cycle to the next generation. Immune-tolerant adult females that were infected as neonates can not only infect their own young in utero but also do not confer passive immunity to neonates, which further facilitates spread of the virus due to communal nursing behavior. Tolerance is not absolute, as mice develop LCMV-specific antibody, but antibody is non-neutralizing and complexed with excess viral antigen, which tends to be deposited in tissues, including arterial walls, choroid plexus, and glomeruli. Eventually, tolerance breaks down further, resulting in chronic lymphocytic infiltrates in multiple tissues and immune complex glomerulonephritis (late disease). The onset of late disease varies with genetic strain of mice. This phenomenon is irrelevant in wild mice, since mice become ill at an age in which their reproductive contributions to the population are no longer essential. LCMV immune-tolerant mice with disseminated infection can also develop a number of endocrine disorders due to diminished secretion of growth hormone with hypoglycemia, diabetes with hyperglycemia and abnormal glucose tolerance, and decreased thyroxine and thyroglobulin. These phenomenas are due to noncytolytic infection of endocrine organs, resulting in disturbance of cell function.

In contrast, natural or experimental infection of adult, immunocompetent mice follows a distinctly different course. Experimental infection results in a wide variety of disease manifestations, depending upon host and virus factors. Following natural exposure, or natural routes of experimental inoculation (intranasal or oral), immunocompetent adult mice typically develop short-term, acute infections from which they recover and seroconvert. However, parenteral inoculation with "aggressive" strains of virus results in disseminated infection of multiple organs, followed by a host immune response with CD8 T-cell-mediated disease. When virus is inoculated intracerebrally, disease is characterized by immune-mediated lymphocytic choriomeningitis (especially with "neurotropic" strains), whereas intraperitoneal inoculation results in immune-mediated hepatitis. In contrast, inoculation of mice with high doses of virus that are "docile" and "viscerotropic" results in immune exhaustion (in contrast to immune tolerance) and therefore mice develop no clinical, T-cell-mediated disease (thus, the term "docile"). The mechanism for immune exhaustion is selective targeting and high affinity for alpha-dystroglycan receptors on dendritic cells. The virus thus initially targets dendritic cells in the marginal zones of the spleen and lymph nodes, and then spreads to T-cell regions, with subsequent T-cell-mediated immune destruction of infected lymphoid tissue. This cycle of infection and destruction results in massive depletion of lymphoid tissues, including thymus, spleen, and T-cell regions of lymph nodes. This immune exhaustion results in global immunodeficiency, in contrast to the selective immune tolerance that takes place in fetally or neonatally infected mice. In both scenarios, virus infection is persistent.

LCMV strains and isolates cannot be differentiated serologically, as LCMV is a monotypic quasispecies. Nevertheless, there are a number of clonal laboratory strains with differing experimental tissue tropism and biological behavior, including Armstrong, Traub, WE, Pasteur, and others. Experimental disease is dependent upon virus strain, dose, route of inoculation, and host factors, including age, strain, and immunocompetence. A significant determinant of susceptibility to the adult, immune-mediated form of experimental disease is linked to the *H-2* locus. Mice with *H-2q/q* (e.g., SWR) or *H-2q/k* (e.g., C3H.Q) haplotypes are disease susceptible, whereas mice of the *H-2k/k* haplotype (e.g., C3H/He) are disease resistant. *H-2* haplotype is associated with CD8 T-cell responsiveness, but CD4 T cells, B cells, NK cells, and interferons, among other factors, contribute to LCMV immunity. The adult form of infection following parenteral inoculation is largely an experimental phenomenon, but it provides insight into the outcome of inoculation of mice with contaminated biological material. LCMV is a frequent contaminant of transplantable tumors. Considering the wide variety of immune-deficient mice being utilized today, and the many immune factors that are determinants of controlling outcome of infection or disease, awareness of the full spectrum of LCMV biology is useful.

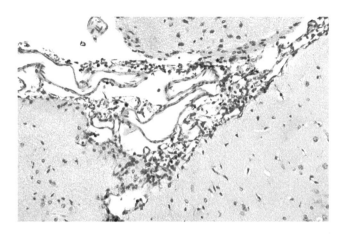

FIG. 1.24. *Lymphocytic infiltration of meninges of a mouse inoculated intracerebrally with lymphocytic choriomeningitis virus (LCMV).*

Pathology
Clinical signs of natural LCMV infection are minimal, but can include runting in infant mice, reduced litter size, and chronic wasting in older mice if infection is occurring in utero within the colony. Microscopic lesions are likewise nonspecific and most likely to be found in persistently infected aged mice, which may develop vasculitis, glomerulonephritis, and lymphocytic infiltration in multiple tissues, including brain, liver, adrenal, kidney, and lung. Acute disease is largely an experimental phenomenon arising from parenteral inoculation with high doses of virus. Infection with "aggressive" strains of virus results in generalized lymph-adenopathy with lymphoid hyperplasia, lymphocytic infiltrates in multiple tissues, necrotizing hepatitis, and lymphocytic choriomeningitis (especially if inoculated intracerebrally) (Fig. 1.24). Infection with "docile" strains of virus results in severe generalized lymphoid depletion in T-cell regions of the thymus, spleen, and lymph nodes. Although natural infection of nude mice has been documented, pathology was not described.

Diagnosis
Definitive diagnosis of LCMV infection cannot be based on pathology. Serology with recombinant nucleoprotein antigen has circumvented the hazards of growing the virus for antigen. However, serology may be problematic, since horizontal infection among adult mice is inefficient and likely to cause seroconversion among a very few mice within a population. Mice infected in utero or as neonates are immune-tolerant to LCMV and do not efficiently seroconvert, or circulating antibody is complexed with antigen. Adult mice infected with docile types of virus may have immune exhaustion, and not seroconvert. Thus, serological testing must be applied to a large sample size and can be enhanced by cohousing adult sentinel mice with mice suspected to be persistently infected. LCMV can be confirmed in suspect tissues with a variety of bioassay approaches, such as

MAP testing, but this has been supplanted by PCR. Differential diagnoses for runting in infant mice include a number of other viral infections. Chronic illness in older mice must be differentiated from generalized lymphoproliferative disorders, amyloidosis, glomerulonephritis, and chronic renal disease of aging mice.

Arterivirus Infection: Lactate Dehydrogenase-Elevating Virus Infection
Lactate dehydrogenase-elevating virus (LDV) belongs to the family Arteriviridae. LDV was initially discovered as a contaminant of a transplantable tumor that caused significant elevation of lactate dehydrogenase (LDH) in plasma of inoculated mice. LDV significantly alters macrophage function and immune responsiveness, including enhancement or suppression of tumorigenesis, and other effects. LDV is highly mouse specific, is inefficiently transmitted among mice, and can be easily eradicated, but it remains one of the most frequent contaminants of murine transplantable tumors, including hybridomas.

Epizootiology and Pathogenesis
The prevalence of LDV among contemporary mouse colonies is unknown, since serological surveillance seldom includes this agent. It is endemic, but not universal, in wild mouse populations throughout the world. LDV is highly specific to the mouse and also has a very restricted cell tropism for a specific subset of macrophages (F4/80-positive) and, under some circumstances, neural tissue. The primary means of natural transmission is through bite wounds among fighting mice, but studies also suggest that it can be sexually transmitted. In addition, LDV is inefficiently transmitted by direct contact, even though the virus is excreted in feces, urine, milk, saliva, and semen. Maternal transmission to the fetus can occur, but occurs only during the acute, high-viremic stage and is regulated by maternal immune status, developmental stage of the fetus, and a strong gradient of placental and umbilical cord trapping of virus immune complexes. Infection of the fetus is favored at 13–14 days or more of gestation. Fetal susceptibility is due to development of susceptible F4/80-positive macrophages. For these reasons, LDV seldom infects fetuses under natural conditions.

Different quasispecies of LDV exist, including LDV-P and LDV-vx, which prevail in laboratory mice. Closely related viruses, with similar genetic, phenotypic, and biological characteristics, have been isolated from wild mice. LDV-P and LDV-vx induce persistent, life-long infections in immunocompetent mice. Persistent infection is maintained by selective infection of a continually renewable subpopulation of mature macrophages that express F4/80 cell surface antigen that is present only on mature macrophages and not on progenitor stages. Virus attains extremely high titer within 12–14 hours after infection due to cytolysis and massive release of virions.

At this stage, antigen and RNA-positive cells are present in many tissues. There is rapid exhaustion of the target cell population, resulting in subsequent attenuation of the level of viremia, which persists at a lower level throughout life. At this stage, there are few or no infected cells in most tissues, with the exception of spleen, lymph node, and testes. The drop in levels of viremia occurs prior to acquired immunity and has similar kinetics in athymic nude mice and chemically immunosuppressed mice. There is also immunosuppression due to clonal exhaustion of cytotoxic T cells as well as virus-induced inhibition of IL-4 with suppression of helper T cells. Depletion of the target subpopulation of macrophages results in impaired clearance of plasma enzymes, including LDH, with 5- to 10-fold elevations. This phenomenon is not specific to LDH, as several other enzymes are also significantly elevated. Immune clearance of the virus is precluded due to the presence of 3 large N-linked polylactosaminoglycan chains on the short ectodomain of the envelope glycoprotein, VP-3P, which carries the neutralization epitope. These persistent viruses, therefore, are resistant to neutralizing antibody. LDV infection stimulates a strong polyclonal antibody response, with the formation of immune complexes, but immune complex disease does not seem to occur.

Some variants of LDV, such as LDV-C and LDV-v, infect not only macrophages but also anterior horn neurons of C58, AKR, C3H/Fg, and PL mice. The ectodomains of these LDV variants lack 2 N-terminal N-glycosylation sites, which confers upon them tropism for alternate receptors on neurons but also renders them susceptible to neutralizing antibody and immune clearance. Specific strains of mice (noted above) develop a paralytic syndrome, age-dependent poliomyelitis (ADPM), that has been touted as a model of amyotrophic lateral sclerosis (ALS). ADPM requires suppressed host immunity that can result from old age, immunodeficiency, or chemical immunosuppression. Immunosuppression favors persistent infection with these neutralizing antibody-susceptible variants of virus, which can then infect neurons. ADPM also requires interaction with ecotropic murine leukemia virus (MuLV) that is endogenous in ADPM-susceptible strains of mice. Susceptible mouse strains possess N-ecotropic MuLV and are homozygous at the $Fv-1^n$ locus. Ecotropic MuLV is expressed in glial cells and neurons of the central nervous system. Through as yet unknown mechanisms, MuLV infection of anterior horn neurons renders these cells susceptible to cytolytic infection when they are coinfected with LDV, thereby resulting in ADPM.

Pathology

Clinical signs or lesions are not seen in naturally infected mice, and lesions are minimal in experimentally infected immunodeficient mice. Experimentally inoculated mice develop transient necrosis of T-cell areas of lymphoid tissues, pyknosis of reticuloendothelial cells, and leukopenia within 72 hours after inoculation. As infection proceeds, these changes disappear, and there is generalized splenomegaly and lymphadenomegaly with expanded germinal center formation due to polyclonal B-cell activation. Central nervous system disease in experimentally infected, immunosuppressed C58, AKR, C3H/Fg, and PL mice consists of mononuclear leukocytic infiltrates in the ventral, and to a lesser extent dorsal, horns of the spinal cord, scattered neuronolysis with apoptosis, and perivasculitis. C57BL mice infected with LDV develop mild to moderate nonsuppurative leptomeningitis, myelitis, and occasionally radiculitis without clinical signs. A natural outbreak of poliomyelitis has been reported in $Fv-1^n$ homozygous ICR-scid mice following inoculation with contaminated biological material.

Diagnosis

Serological methods for LDV antibody have not been generally used because of difficulties with antigen–antibody complexes and polyclonal B-cell activation. Nevertheless, antibody can be effectively detected using purified LDV virions or infected cells as antigen. LDV replicates in primary macrophage cell cultures but causes no cytopathic effect. The gold standard for LDV diagnosis in the past has been measurement of plasma LDH enzymes in mice given serial dilutions of test material, but now PCR is used for confirmation, since LDH is not specific for LDV infection. Differential diagnoses include any agent or disease that causes enzyme elevations, but other enzyme elevations are not as high or persistent. Neurologic LDV lesions must be distinguished from spinal cord lesions induced by mouse encephalomyelitis virus (MEV), MHV, or retrovirus. LDV can be eliminated from transplantable tumors by growth in vitro, or by passage in athymic rats, both of which lack the necessary mouse macrophage subpopulations needed to sustain infection.

Astrovirus Infection

Astroviruses are small, nonenveloped, positive-sense, single-stranded RNA viruses that are associated with enteric disease in a wide variety of birds and mammals, including humans. Using a metagenomic approach, several strains of astrovirus have been identified in laboratory mice and wild murids. Further studies with PCR have shown that astrovirus infection is geographically widespread and common among laboratory mice in academic and commercial institutions in the United States and Japan. A wide variety of immunocompetent and immunodeficient strains of mice have been found to be infected. Experimental infection has been shown to be restricted to intestine in immunocompetent mice, but systemic involvement of liver and kidney has been documented in Rag-1-deficient mice. Infection is controlled by both innate and acquired immune responses, and Infection is persistent in immunodeficient mice. Infection is clinically silent, and no lesions, including histopathologic lesions, have been found, regardless of immune status. The significance, if any, of astroviruses in laboratory mice remains unknown.

Coronavirus Infection: Mouse Hepatitis Virus Infection

Mouse hepatitis virus (MHV) belongs to the family Coronaviridae. MHV is very common among wild and conventionally housed mouse populations, and is represented by numerous antigenically and genetically related strains that vary considerably in their virulence and organotropism. This is due to the high propensity of coronaviruses to mutate and recombine. Despite "hepatitis" in its name, MHV is not always hepatotropic. MHV shares antigenic cross-reactivity with other (Group 2) coronaviruses, which includes human coronavirus OC43, bovine coronavirus, rat coronavirus, and hemagglutinating encephalomyelitis virus of swine. Although the role of these related viruses is often questioned as sources of unexplained MHV outbreaks, there is no evidence that MHV comes from anywhere but mice and mouse products. The polytropism of some MHV strains contributes to their propensity to infect a variety of mouse-derived biological products, including transplantable tumors, cell lines, ES cells, and hybridomas. MHV has protean effects upon a wide variety of research variables, particularly immune response.

Epizootiology and Pathogenesis

MHV was initially recognized in mice with neurologic disease in 1949 and subsequently isolated from a variety of cell cultures, tumors, clinically ill mice with a variety of disease manifestations, and mice with abnormal responses to research variables. Despite its prevalence and potential pathogenicity, clinical MHV disease is not common. The outcome of infection depends upon the interaction of different MHV strains on host variables, which include age, genotype, and immune status, including maternally derived antibody.

MHV strains can be divided into two biologically distinct but overlapping groups. Respiratory strains possess primary tropism for upper respiratory mucosa and enterotropic strains have primary tropism for enterocytes. Those strains with respiratory tropism initially replicate in nasal mucosa and disseminate to a variety of other organs because of their polytropic nature. Representatives of this type of MHV include the prototype strains MHV-JHM, MHV-A59, MHV-S, and MHV-3, among others. Disseminated infection to multiple organs is favored by virulent strains of virus, mice less than 2 weeks of age, genetically susceptible strains of mice, or immunocompromised mice. Dissemination of MHV from the nose occurs via the blood and lymphatics to pulmonary vascular endothelium and draining lymph nodes, respectively. Secondary viremia disseminates

virus to multiple organs, with virus replication and cytolytic lesions in central nervous system, liver, lymphoid tissues, bone marrow, and other sites. Infection of central nervous system by viremic dissemination occurs primarily in neonatal or immunodeficient mice but not older, immunocompetent mice. Direct infection of adult mouse brain can also occur by extension of the virus along olfactory neural pathways, even in the absence of dissemination to other organs. After approximately 5–7 days, immune-mediated clearance of the virus begins, with no persistence or carrier state beyond 3–4 weeks. Infection of mice after weaning age is usually subclinical, particularly in natural infections caused by generally nonvirulent strains of virus. The obvious exception is immunodeficient mice, which cannot clear the virus and develop progressively severe disease. They can die acutely or develop chronic wasting disease if infected with relatively avirulent strains of MHV.

Mouse genetic susceptibility and resistance to polytropic MHV has been studied extensively. BALB/c mice are generally quite susceptible to MHV, whereas SJL mice are remarkably resistant. Susceptibility to MHV-A59 and MHV-JHM has been linked to allelic variation of carcinoembryonic antigen-related cell adhesion molecule 1 (CEACAM1). MHV does not necessarily respect such clear explanations, since these differences are quite virus strain-specific, and other MHV strains utilize alternative cellular receptors. MHV-3 is widely known to be highly virulent in genetically susceptible BALB/c and DBA/2 mice, but is less virulent in semisusceptible C3H and disease-resistant A/J mice. MHV-3 disease severity is determined by thrombosis and coagulation necrosis due to induction of procoagulant activity by macrophages in susceptible, but not resistant, mice. Most polytropic MHV strains display neurotropism following intranasal inoculation of various mouse genotypes, including A, BALB/c, CBA, C3H/He, and C3H/Rv but not SJL mice. These experimental examples emphasize the point that the biologic behavior of wild-type MHV is likely to be unpredictable.

Enterotropic MHV strains tend to selectively infect intestinal mucosal epithelium, with minimal or no dissemination to other organs, even in immunodeficient mice. Enterotropic strains that have been described include MHV-S/CDC, MHV-Y, MHV-RI, and MHV-D, among others. Early descriptions of lethal intestinal virus of infant mice (LIVIM) are consistent with enterotropic MHV, but the LIVIM agent was lost before it could be fully characterized. All ages and strains of mice are susceptible to enterotropic MHV infection, including SJL mice, which are resistant to polytropic MHV. Disease occurs only in infant mice due to their intestinal mucosal proliferative kinetics. Infection of neonatal mice results in severe necrotizing enterocolitis with high mortality within 48 hours after inoculation. Mortality and lesion severity diminish rapidly with advancing age at inoculation. Adult mice develop minimal lesions, but replication of equal or higher titers of virus occurs, compared with neonates. The severity of intestinal disease is associated with age-related intestinal mucosal proliferative kinetics, rather than immune-related susceptibility. To underscore this point, disease is minimal in nude or SCID mice infected as adults. Recovery from enterotropic MHV is immune-mediated and requires functional T cells. No persistent carrier state seems to occur in recovered, immunocompetent mice, but persistent infection and virus shedding in feces can occur in T- and B-cell-immunodeficient mice, as well as transgenic mice without known immune dysfunction. Thus, biologic behavior, in particular duration of infection, is unpredictable in GEMs. Enterotropic MHV infections are often complicated by other opportunistic pathogens, including *Escherichia coli* and *Spironucleus muris*.

Host immunity to MHV is strongly MHV strain specific. Recovery from one MHV strain provides strong resistance to re-exposure with the homotypic strain, but only partial or no resistance to infection with an antigenically heterotypic strain. Innate immunity and both cellular and humoral arms of the acquired immune response are important in controlling infection, but T cells are critical for virus clearance and recovery from infection. Maternally derived passive immunity is critically important in MHV epizootiology. The highly contagious nature of some MHV strains, particularly enterotropic MHV, within naïve mouse populations can result in high mortality among neonatal mice. Pups suckling immune dams, on the other hand, are completely protected from infection, and subsequently acquire infection at an age in which they are not apt to develop severe clinical disease. Maternal protection against polytropic MHV strains is mediated through serum IgG that is passed in utero to the fetus or postnatally through intestinal IgG receptors. In contrast, maternal protection against enterotropic MHV is mediated through luminal whey containing IgA and IgG. Maternally derived passive immunity, like active immunity, is also MHV strain specific, providing protection against homotypic, but only partial or no protection against heterotypic strains of MHV. In spite of the fact that most MHV infections at the level of a single mouse are acute with recovery, the high rate of MHV mutation within an infected population and the strain-specific nature of active and passive immunity contribute to and actually select for persistence of virus within a population.

Vertical transmission from infected dams to fetuses has been documented experimentally, but is highly unlikely to occur naturally. This would require infection of a virus-naïve genetically susceptible mouse with a relatively virulent, polytropic strain of MHV during pregnancy. Even if such events take place, fetal infection would be fatal, so live offspring would not be an issue. The zona pellucida is an effective barrier to MHV infection. However, introduction of MHV through ES cells or

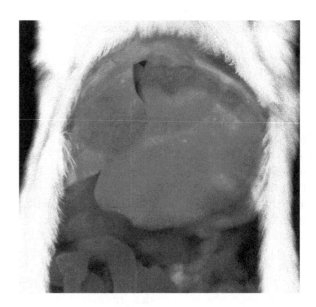

FIG. 1.25.   *Multifocal hepatitis in a BALB/c mouse infected with mouse hepatitis virus (MHV).*

germplasm into naïve mouse colonies represents a greater concern. MHV has a well-documented ability to persistently infect cell lines without cytopathic effect, including ES cell lines.

Pathology

The majority of natural polytropic MHV infections are subclinical, with mild or no gross lesions. Immunocompetent mice may have grossly discernable white foci on the surface of the liver (Fig. 1.25), which can be profoundly obvious and often hemorrhagic in immunodeficient mice (Fig. 1.26). In immunodeficient mice infected with relatively low virulence MHV strains, mice may survive long enough to develop hepatic nodular hyperplasia with parenchymal collapse and fibrosis. Foci

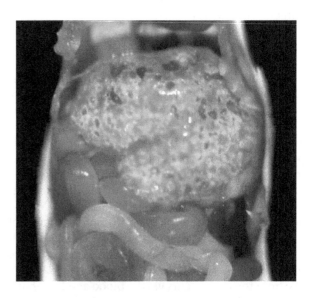

FIG. 1.26.   *Severe multifocal coalescing hepatic necrosis in a SCID mouse infected with MHV.*

of splenic necrosis, with splenomegaly due to extramedullary hematopoiesis, are often present in immunodeficient mice. Neurologic manifestations may be observed in immunodeficient mice, and rarely in immunocompetent mice, including vestibular signs and posterior paresis.

Microscopic findings in mice infected with polytropic MHV strains are characterized by focal acute necrosis and syncytia of parenchymal cells and vascular endothelium in multiple organs, including liver, splenic red and white pulp, lymph nodes, gut-associated lymphoid tissue, thymus, and bone marrow. Focal peritonitis may also be present. Hallmark syncytia are not as obvious in immunocompetent mice, but residua of syncytia may be found in liver, characterized by large degenerating cells at the periphery of necrotic foci with dense basophilic apoptotic nuclear bodies. Syncytia are common in lesions of immunodeficient mice, which allow lesions to reach their fullest potential (Figs. 1.27 A and B). Syncytia of pulmonary vascular endothelium are common in immunodeficient mice (Fig. 1.28). Pancytopenia has been documented in mice experimentally infected with polytropic MHV, and probably occurs in severe natural infections. Bone marrow necrosis, syncytia,

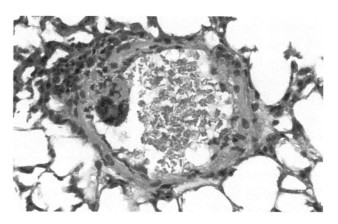

FIG. 1.28. *Endothelial syncytium in a pulmonary vessel of an immunodeficient mouse infected with MHV.*

and compensatory hematopoietic hyperplasia can be found in naturally infected mice, accounting for the splenomegaly that occurs in immunodeficient mice. Neonatally infected mice and immunodeficient mice can have vascular-oriented necrotizing encephalitis (Fig. 1.29). Mice may also develop nasoencephalitis due to localized infection of olfactory mucosa, olfactory nerves, olfactory bulbs, and olfactory tracts of the brain, with meningoencephalitis and demyelination. This pattern of infection occurs regularly after intranasal inoculation of many MHV strains, but is a relatively rare event by natural exposure.

Lesions due to enterotropic MHV depend primarily upon age of the host. Neonatal mice in naïve mouse colonies can experience massive outbreaks of high mortality, presenting as dehydrated, runted pups. These mice have segmentally distributed areas of villus attenuation, enterocytic syncytia (balloon cells), and mucosal necrosis (Fig. 1.30). Eosinophilic intracytoplasmic inclusions may be present, but are not as diagnostic as syncytia. Mesenteric lymph nodes usually contain lymphocytic syncytia, and mesenteric vessels may contain endothelial syncytia.

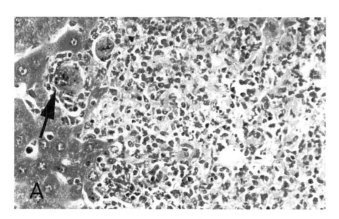
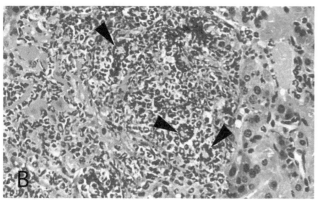

FIG. 1.27. *(A and B) Focal hepatitis in mice infected with MHV. Note the degenerated syncytium (arrow) at the periphery of a necrotic focus in an immunocompetent mouse (A), in contrast to the prominent syncytia (arrowheads) that are obvious in the liver of an immunodeficient mouse (B).*

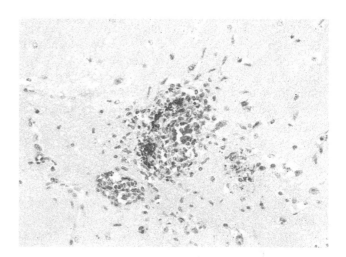

FIG. 1.29. *Vascular-oriented encephalitis from an immunodeficient mouse naturally infected with MHV.*

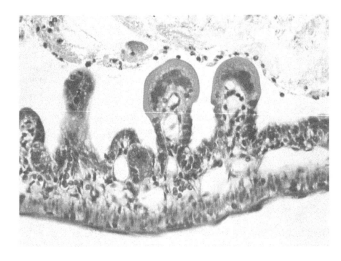

FIG. 1.30.   *Small intestine of a neonatal mouse infected with enterotropic MHV. Villi are markedly attenuated, with prominent syncytia of villus enterocytes.*

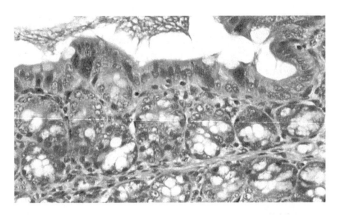

FIG. 1.31.   *Ascending colon from a mouse with MHV infection. Syncytia are present on the mucosal surface. The ascending colon is the most common site to find MHV syncytia in adult mice.*

Surviving mice develop compensatory intestinal mucosal hyperplasia. Lesions are most likely to be found in the terminal small intestine, cecum, and ascending colon. Lesions are progressively milder with increasing age at the time of exposure. Adult mice have minimal lesions, except for enterocytic syncytia in surface mucosa, particularly in cecum and ascending colon (Fig. 1.31). Immunodeficient mice develop similar but progressive lesions, depending upon age at inoculation. Natural enterotropic MHV infection has been described in adult nude mice with chronic hyperplastic typhlocolitis and mesenteric lymphadenopathy. More typically, intestinal lesions in immunodeficient mice, including naturally infected nude mice, are remarkably mild with minimal hyperplasia. Enterotropic MHV strains do not generally disseminate, but hepatitis and encephalitis can occur with some virus strains in certain mouse genotypes.

Residual lesions in mice that have recovered from infection may include reactive hyperplasia of lymph nodes and spleen, hematopoietic hyperplasia, perivascular lymphocytic infiltrates in the lung, and foci of inflammation in liver. Residual brain lesions are usually found in the brain stem and characterized by perivascular cuffing of lymphocytes and vacuolization. Demyelination is a much emphasized feature of experimental brain infections, but is rare under natural circumstances. Unusual presentations may occur in MHV-infected GEMs with specific gene defects. Granulomatous serositis (Fig. 1.32), with or without hepatitis or intestinal lesions, has been found in interferon-gamma and interferon-gamma receptor null mice, but this pattern of disease has also been observed in mice with other targeted mutations. The serosal exudates contain numerous syncytia (Fig. 1.33) and MHV antigen. It is unknown if this syndrome is related to polytropic or enterotropic MHV.

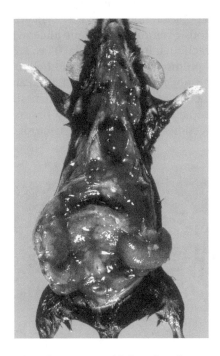

FIG. 1.32.   *Granulomatous serositis in an interferon-gamma null mouse naturally infected with MHV. (Source: France et al. 1999. Reproduced with permission from John Wiley & Sons Limited.)*

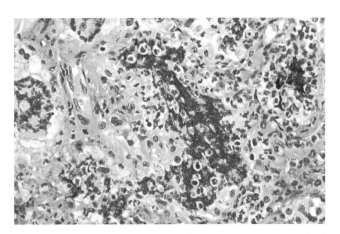

FIG. 1.33.   *Syncytia in the serosal exudate of an immunodeficient mouse with granulomatous serositis due to MHV infection.*

Diagnosis

Diagnosis during the acute stage of MHV infection can be made by visualization of characteristic lesions with syncytia in target tissues, but clinical signs and lesions can be highly variable for reasons discussed above. Active infection can be confirmed by immunohistochemistry, by virus isolation, or PCR. Recovered mice may have perivascular lymphocytic infiltrates in the lung and microgranulomas in the liver. In general, respiratory strains of MHV are polytropic and grow in a number of established cell lines in vitro, but enterotropic MHV strains are far more restrictive and fastidious in vitro. Virus in suspect tissue can be confirmed by a variety of bioassay methods, such as MAP testing or infant or nude mouse inoculation. Amplification by passage in immunodeficient mice will increase the likelihood of in vitro isolation from infected tissue. PCR can be utilized to detect MHV in feces or tissue of infected mice. Serology is the most useful means of surveillance for retrospective infection in a colony. Seropositive mice are poor candidates for pathology workup, since they are likely to have recovered, but on occasion they can be actively infected with a second strain of virus. Nude mice can develop antibody, although their antibody response is unpredictable. There is little merit in attempting to identify MHV strains serologically, since all strains are broadly cross-reactive and antigenic relatedness does not predict virulence or organotropism. Differential diagnoses include salmonellosis, Tyzzer's disease, and mousepox in adult mice, as well as reovirus, cytomegalovirus, and adenovirus in infant mice. Mice with enteritis must be differentiated from epizootic diarrhea of infant mice (EDIM), salmonellosis, Tyzzer's disease, and reovirus infection. Demyelinating lesions must be differentiated from those caused by mouse encephalomyelitis virus, LDV in immunosuppressed AKR or C58 mice, or polyoma virus in immunodeficient mice.

Norovirus Infection

Mouse norovirus (MNV) belongs to the family Caliciviridae, genus *Norovirus*. *Noroviruses* are of particular importance because approximately 90% of viral gastroenteritis in humans worldwide is attributed to norovirus infections. The first recognized norovirus was the Norwalk virus, from which the name "norovirus" was derived. A newly recognized murine norovirus (MNV-1) was identified and reported in 2003, and since then over 35 new isolates have been found among laboratory mouse colonies throughout the world. MNVs are highly prevalent in contemporary mouse populations, with the potential of disrupting research outcomes. MNVs belong to a single serogroup, but display different biological phenotypes. MNV is unique among noroviruses in that it is the only norovirus that can be replicated in cell culture.

Epizootiology and Pathogenesis

Human noroviruses are famous for the rapid spread of illness among cruise ship passengers and the difficulty in decontaminating ships following outbreaks. These features may be important in understanding the epizootiology and control of MNV in animal facilities. However, unlike human noroviruses, MNV is remarkably nonpathogenic, except under highly specific circumstances. MNV infection is lethal in GEMs with STAT1 deficiency, including STAT1 null mice with intact B and T cells, STAT1 null mice lacking B and T cells (RAG null), and STAT1 null mice lacking RNA-dependent protein kinase (PKR null). Infection of 129, B6, RAG1, RAG2, interferon alpha/beta receptor null, interferon gamma receptor null, iNOS null, or PKR null mice with functional STAT1 resulted in no clinical disease. Following oral or intranasal inoculation of susceptible STAT1 null mice, persistent levels of viral RNA were detected in a variety of tissues, including lung, liver, spleen, intestine, blood, and brain. Virus antigen is present in liver Kupffer cells. In the spleen, antigen is found in the red pulp and marginal zones, but also in nonlymphoid cells in the white pulp. This pattern is suggestive of tropism for macrophages and dendritic cells, which has been confirmed in vitro. In immunodeficient mice, MNV-1 RNA has been detected in the feces for several days postinoculation, and in the mesenteric lymph nodes, spleen, and small intestine for up to 5 weeks postexposure. Macrophages in tissues such as lung, liver, and lymphoid organs are primary sites for MNV-1 replication. In view of the biology of other noroviruses, it is likely that the orofecal route is an important means of natural transmission of MNV-1. Immune-competent mice recover from MNV-1 infection, with seroconversion by day 21, whereas RAG null mice remain persistently infected. These features may be biased by the tissue culture adaptation of MNV-1, as infection of immunocompetent mice with new field isolates, including MNV-2, MNV-3, and MNV-4, resulted in persistent fecal shedding of virus.

Pathology

Microscopic lesions in STAT1 null mice inoculated per os or intranasally include alveolitis, pulmonary edema, and multifocal areas of coagulation necrosis in the liver, with minimal or no inflammatory cell response. There is a striking necrotizing splenitis with disruption of the normal architecture. In STAT1 null mice inoculated intracerebrally with MNV-1, endothelial hypertrophy with focal mononuclear cell infiltration in the neuropil and leptomeninges are present. In another study, lesions encountered in several strains of immunodeficient mice naturally infected with MNV were variable to absent, depending on the strain under study. Changes described included multifocal hepatitis with mononuclear and scattered polymorphonuclear cell infiltration, multifocal interstitial pneumonia, pleuritis, and peritonitis. In mesenteric lymph nodes, degeneration of scattered lymphocytes with focal fibrosis was occasionally observed. In sections stained by immunohistochemistry, intracytoplasmic viral antigen was demonstrated in mononuclear cells scattered in the liver, spleen, intestinal lymphoid tissue, lamina propria of the intestine, and intravascular mononuclear cells.

Diagnosis

Serology for MNV is based upon recombinant baculovirus MNV-1 capsid protein virus-like particles, and the antigen is effective at detecting antibody to all MNV isolates. Immunohistochemistry to demonstrate viral antigen in target tissues and PCR to detect MNV RNA in tissues or feces are useful diagnostic procedures. Negative-staining electron microscopy has also been used to visualize virus in infected tissues. Mesenteric lymph nodes appear to be an optimal site for detection and isolation of MNV.

Paramyxovirus Infections

Mice are susceptible to respiratory tract infections with two members of the Paramyxovirus family, including pneumonia virus of mice, which belongs to the genus *Pneumovirus*, and Sendai virus, which belongs to the genus *Respirovirus*. Both viruses may be associated with clinical disease, depending upon immune competence of the host.

Pneumonia Virus of Mice Infection

Pneumonia virus of mice (PVM) was originally discovered following serial blind lung passages in mice, which ultimately produced an agent capable of causing pneumonia. Under natural conditions, PVM is relatively innocuous in immunocompetent mice, but it has increased in significance with the advent of immunodeficient mice, in which it causes significant disease.

Epizootiology and Pathogenesis

PVM is a highly labile virus with a low degree of contagion, requiring close contact between mice. PVM infection occurs in laboratory rodents throughout the world, but its prevalence is declining. Clinical disease caused by natural infections with PVM has never been reported, except in immunodeficient mice. Among BALB/cBy, DBA/2, 129Sv, SJL, C3H/HeN, and B6 mice that were experimentally inoculated with a pathogenic strain of PVM, SJL mice were highly resistant, BALB/c and B6 mice displayed intermediate susceptibility, and DBA/2, C3H/HeN, and 129Sv mice were the most susceptible, based upon virus titer and pulmonary disease. Intranasal inoculation of immunocompetent BALB/c mice with a pathogenic PVM strain results in clinical illness with nonsuppurative perivascular and interstitial inflammation as well as bronchiolar desquamation and inflammation, which peak within 2 weeks and undergo resolution within 3 weeks. Virus replication occurs in alveolar lining cells, possibly alveolar macrophages, and to a lesser extent in bronchiolar epithelium. Natural isolates of PVM are typically nonpathogenic. Replication is restricted largely to the nasal mucosal epithelium, with minimal pathology. The low pathogenicity of PVM allows immunodeficient mice to develop progressively severe interstitial pneumonia with wasting syndrome without succumbing acutely. In these mice, PVM antigen is confined to alveolar type 2 cells and occasionally bronchiolar epithelial cells. SCID mice that were naturally infected with *P. murina*, then inoculated with a normally nonpathogenic isolate of PVM, developed more severe *Pneumocystis* pneumonia and higher *Pneumocystis* cyst counts, whereas PVM-infected, but *Pneumocystis*-free, SCID mice survived for 2 months despite high PVM titers in lung. Thus, PVM-related pneumonia in immunodeficient mice is often complicated by *Pneumocystis*, and vice versa, since both may be common agents in some mouse colonies.

Pathology

Clinical signs of disease and gross lesions are absent in natural PVM infections of immunocompetent mice. Microscopic lesions in intranasally inoculated experimental mice consist of mild necrotizing rhinitis, necrotizing bronchiolitis, and nonsuppurative interstitial pneumonia. Infiltrating leukocytes include neutrophils, but lymphocytes and macrophages predominate. Residual perivascular infiltrates of lymphocytes and plasma cells can persist for several weeks after virus is cleared. Immunodeficient mice manifest chronic wasting with cyanosis and dyspnea. Lungs are pale, fleshy, and firm and do not collapse. Microscopically, alveolar septa are thickened with edema and infiltrating macrophages and leukocytes, and alveolar spaces are collapsed and filled with fibrin, blood, macrophages, and large polygonal mononuclear cells, representing detached alveolar type 2 cells (Fig. 1.34). In sections stained by immunohistochemistry, viral antigen can be demonstrated within infected pneumocytes.

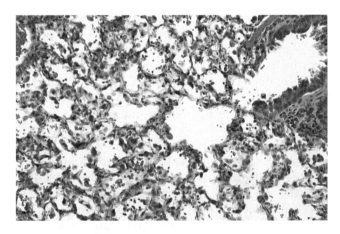

FIG. 1.34. *Progressive interstitial pneumonia in a SCID mouse infected with pneumonia virus of mice (PVM).*

Diagnosis

Most PVM infections are detected retrospectively by seroconversion. Because PVM is not highly contagious, the number of seropositive mice within a colony can be small. Seropositive mice often have mild pulmonary perivascular lymphoplasmacytic infiltrates. Differential diagnoses for pulmonary disease and wasting syndrome in immunodeficient mice include Sendai virus and *Pneumocystis murina* infections, which also cause progressive pulmonary disease. PVM lesions are similar to Sendai viral lesions microscopically, but PVM tends not to induce bronchiolar hypertrophy like Sendai virus. During active infection, PVM can be identified by immunohistochemistry, virus isolation, PCR, or MAP testing of suspect tissues. Nude mice do not seroconvert to PVM.

Sendai Virus Infection

Sendai virus was once common in laboratory rodent (mouse, rat, hamster, guinea pig) populations throughout the world, but is now rare. It is closely related antigenically to parainfluenza virus 1 of humans. It is named after Sendai, Japan, where it was first isolated from laboratory mice inoculated with human lung suspensions and later isolated from naturally infected mice. Because of Sendai virus' close relationship with human parainfluenza 1 virus, there has been a long-held debate as to the human or mouse origin of Sendai virus, or if humans are naturally susceptible to Sendai viral infection. Studies have indicated that Sendai virus and human parainfluenza virus 1 replicate equally well in the upper and lower respiratory tracts of both African green monkeys and chimpanzees, suggesting that Sendai virus lacks a significant host range restriction and could very well be an anthropozoonotic agent. Sendai virus stands out among other murine viruses as an agent that is capable of causing significant clinical illness in adult, immunocompetent mice. Sendai infections may alter the prevalence of pulmonary neoplasms in experimental carcinogenesis studies. The squamous metaplasia that is found in recovering lungs has been misconstrued as neoplasia. Sendai virus is also known to perturb a variety of immune responses.

Epizootiology and Pathogenesis

Sendai virus is a labile but highly contagious virus that is contact-transmitted by aerosol. Sendai virus prevalence appeared to increase during the 1960s and 1970s, when it was among the most common infectious disease agents of laboratory mouse populations, but has declined in the last few decades. Sendai viral epizootics had a peculiar seasonal pattern of unexplained origin. Although purely speculation, such a pattern could be explained if the virus were of human origin and circulating within the global human population.

Mice develop a descending infection of respiratory epithelium, which is abrogated by a cell-mediated immune response that clears the infection, but also generates disease. The level to which the infection extends within the respiratory tree is determined by mouse genotypic differences in mucociliary clearance, virus burden, and kinetics of immune response. Certain strains of mice, such as DBA/2, infant, and aged mice, are exquisitely susceptible to severe disease. These animals have an effective but delayed immune response to the virus, allowing infection to extend deep into the lung, but then mount a zealous response that results in severe disease. Other mouse strains, such as B6 mice, often have subclinical infections because of their rapid immune response, which precludes lower respiratory tract infection. In a comparative study among 19 inbred strains and 4 outbred Swiss stocks of mice, 129, DBA, and C3H mice were highly susceptible to lethal disease, whereas B6, AKR, SJL, and Swiss mice were resistant.

Sendai virus productively infects respiratory epithelium in the nose, trachea, bronchi, and bronchioles, as well as epithelium of the middle ears. It also spreads to type 2 alveolar cells. Cellular receptors for Sendai virus are widely distributed in many tissues, but respiratory tropism is dictated by the dependence of the virus to bud apically from respiratory epithelium and depend upon respiratory proteases to cleave its fusion glycoprotein into a biologically active form. Without the proteases, virus replication is restricted to a single cycle. Mutant strains of virus, with altered protease specificity and the ability to bud from basolateral cell membranes, can cause disseminated disease, but these (so far) are experimentally selected mutants. Following intranasal infection, virus titers appear in lung within a few days, then peak around days 6–8, at which time they rapidly decline due to the adaptive immune response. A transient viremia is present, reflecting the peak of virus activity in the lung. In the preimmune phase, Sendai virus is only mildly cytopathic. As the acquired immune response mounts, there is infiltration of CD4 and CD8 T cells, resulting in CD8-triggered apoptosis of infected nasal, tracheal, bronchial, and bronchiolar epithelial cells with nonuniform exfoliation of epithelium and erosion. If infection has extended to the lower respiratory tract, there is interstitial alveolar inflammation. Infection is acute, with no persistent carrier state, except in immune-deficient mice.

A number of innate and acquired components of the immune response are engaged during Sendai virus infection. Detectable seroconversion to Sendai virus appears around 10–12 days after infection and coincides with onset of immune-mediated clinical disease. Thus, in the preimmune phase of infection, mice may be mildly ill, but acute disease and mortality are associated with cytotoxic T-cell-mediated necrotizing bronchiolitis and alveolitis. Immunodeficient mice, particularly T-cell-deficient mice, develop progressive pneumonia. Maternal passive immunity is strongly protective for suckling pups when infection is enzootic within a population; it attenuates disease severity in postweaning mice that are exposed when passive antibody is waning.

Sendai virus infection is also associated with a number of infectious paraphenomena in mice and rats. It can predispose to the development of bacterial otitis media and interna, as well as precipitate *Mycoplasma*-associated lower respiratory disease in previously subclinically infected mice. Outbreaks of vestibular disease and pneumonia due to *Mycoplasma* or other bacteria can often be associated with recent activity of Sendai virus within the population. Although vertical transmission does not occur, Sendai viral infection of dams is associated with fetal resorption, prolonged gestation, and fetal death.

Pathology

Severely affected mice are dyspneic and have plum-colored consolidation of sharply demarcated foci, pulmonary hilus, anteroventral lung, or entire lung lobes (Fig. 1.35). These consolidated areas may turn gray in surviving mice. Microscopic changes during the immune phase of disease consist of segmental, necrotizing inflammation of nasal and airway epithelium (Fig. 1.36), as well as foci of interstitial pneumonia associated with terminal airways. Infiltrating cells vary with stage of infection, but include neutrophils, lymphocytes, and macrophages (Fig. 1.37). Alveolar spaces may be filled with fibrin, leukocytes, and necrotic cells, with atelectasis. Prior to immune-mediated necrosis, bronchiolar epithelium may be hypertrophic and hyperplastic, contain virus-induced syncytia, and may possess intracytoplasmic eosinophilic inclusions representing accumulation of viral nucleocapsid material. Intranuclear inclusions have been reported in nude mice. These virus-related changes are most apt to be seen in immature or immunologically deficient mice, since they are rapidly obscured by immune-mediated necrosis. During resolution, sloughed airway epithelium is replaced by proliferating hyperplastic epithelium, which

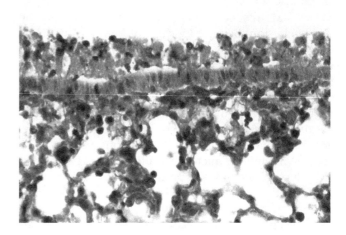

FIG. 1.36.   *Lung from a DBA mouse with Sendai viral infection. Note the acute necrotizing bronchiolitis.*

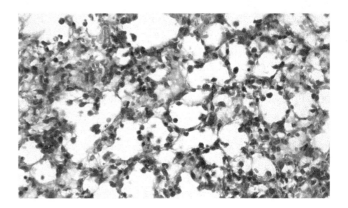

FIG. 1.37.   *Lung from a DBA mouse with Sendai virus infection, illustrating nonsuppurative interstitial pneumonitis.*

may undergo transient but marked nonkeratinizing squamous metaplasia. Alveoli become lined by cuboidal epithelium (Fig. 1.38) or filled with metaplastic squamous epithelium. Increased lymphoid cells populate the bronchial tree, adventitia of adjacent blood vessels, and

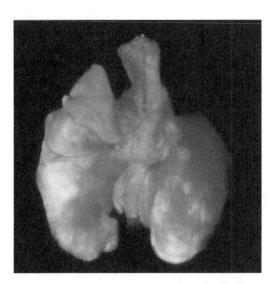

FIG. 1.35.   *Lung from a DBA mouse infected with Sendai virus. Note the dark areas around the hilus of both lungs consistent with congestion and early consolidation.*

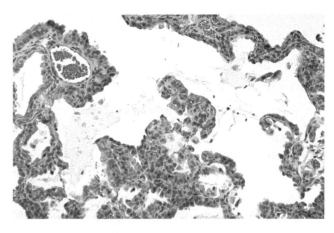

FIG. 1.38.   *Lung from a mouse in the reparative phase following recovery from Sendai virus infection. Note the cuboidal metaplasia of pneumocytes lining alveolar septa.*

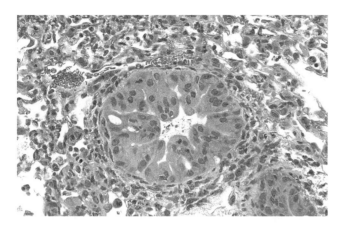

FIG. 1.39. *Lung from a SCID mouse infected with Sendai virus. There is marked hypertrophy and hyperplasia of bronchiolar epithelial cells that occur in the absence of immune-mediated necrosis.*

alveolar septa. All of these changes completely resolve by the 3rd or 4th week. Severely affected lungs, in which progenitor alveolar cells have been destroyed, may have foci of fibrosing alveolitis and bronchiolitis obliterans. T-cell-immunodeficient mice develop progressive pulmonary consolidation with wasting. Their lungs tend to be pale, firm, and do not collapse. Because immunodeficient mice cannot mount an effective immune response, necrotizing changes are minimal, and airway epithelium is typically hypertrophic and hyperplastic (Fig. 1.39). These mice develop progressively severe, diffuse alveolitis, similar to progressive PVM pneumonia in immunodeficient mice.

Diagnosis

The clinical and microscopic features of Sendai viral pneumonia in immunocompetent adult mice are diagnostic and can be confirmed by seroconversion, which generally occurs coincidentally with clinical disease. Differential diagnoses include other causes of respiratory disease, such as *Mycoplasma* and *Corynebacterium kutscheri*. Mild respiratory tract lesions can also occur with PVM or MHV. Immunodeficient mice can develop wasting disease with progressive pneumonia, which must be differentiated from pneumonia caused by PVM or *P. murina*. Sendai virus and PVM lesions in nude and SCID mice are similar, although in SCID mice, bronchial and bronchiolar lesions are more extensive with Sendai virus infection. Immunodeficient mice infected with PVM do not have the hypertrophic and hyperplastic changes in their respiratory epithelium that are characteristic of Sendai viral infections.

Picornavirus Infection: Mouse Encephalomyelitis Virus Infection

Mouse encephalomyelitis virus (MEV) belongs to the family Picornaviridae, genus *Cardiovirus*, which also includes the serologically related encephalomyocarditis virus (EMCV). EMCV has a less-selective host range and can infect wild mice, but is not known to infect laboratory mice. MEV is commonly referred to as mouse poliovirus or Theiler's virus, after its initial discoverer, Max Theiler. There are numerous strains of MEV that infect mice, including TO (Theiler's original), GDVII, FA, BeAn, and DA, among others. Some of these strains have been studied extensively as models for viral encephalitis and demyelination, resulting in emphasis on neurologic disease, which is only rarely a component of natural infection.

Epizootiology and Pathogenesis

MEV is a widespread infectious agent among wild and laboratory mice throughout the world. MEV is regarded as a mouse virus, but sera from rats and guinea pigs may react with MEV due to infection with related viruses. MEV was initially isolated from paralytic mice in the 1930s by Max Theiler. In spite of the emphasis on neurovirulence, MEVs are primarily enteric viruses. Virus excretion from the intestine is highly variable among mice, but it is often prolonged and intermittent. Transmission is inefficient, often with only a small percentage of seropositive mice within a population. In utero infection does not occur, and maternal antibody plays an important role in protecting pups. Infected mice develop a transient viremia that is limited by host immune response. Occasionally, virus gains access to the central nervous system. Vascular endothelial cells appear to serve as a conduit for entry into the brain, but there is also evidence for axonal transport of virus.

MEVs can be divided into two groups, based upon their experimental neurovirulence. Virulent strains of virus, such as GDVII or FA, induce severe fatal encephalitis, regardless of route of inoculation. Most other strains are less virulent and can cause biphasic disease, consisting initially of acute poliomyelitis, followed later by late-onset demyelinating disease. Virus can persist in the central nervous system for over a year, but virus titers decline markedly, and residual virus is restricted to white matter, where it replicates in macrophages, leukocytes, astrocytes, and oligodendrocytes. Immune attack on infected white matter results in demyelination and motor dysfunction, with gait disorders, tremors, ataxia, extensor spasm, urinary incontinence, and other signs. The neurological manifestations of MEV are grossly over-emphasized because of their experimental value. Under natural conditions, usually only 1 in 1,000–10,000 infected immunocompetent mice develops clinical signs of the nervous system, and this is invariably flaccid paralysis associated with the acute, poliomyelitis phase. However, in immunodeficient mice, exposure to MEV may result in high morbidity and mortality. Experimental susceptibility to MEV-induced demyelinating disease has been demonstrated in SJL, DBA/2, C3H/He, SWR, and PLJ strains, whereas BALB/c, B6, A, and 129 strains are resistant. Genetic susceptibility to demyelination is polygenic, but linked to *H-2d* haplotype in some strains.

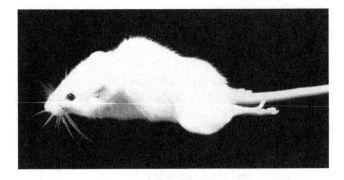

FIG. 1.40. *Mouse with posterior paresis due to natural infection with mouse encephalomyelitis virus (MEV).*

Pathology

MEV replicates in enterocytes, but intestinal lesions are not present. During the acute central nervous system (poliomyelitis) phase, mice may present with posterior paresis (Fig. 1.40). Virus attacks neurons and glia of the hippocampus, thalamus, brain stem, and spinal cord. Neuronolysis, neuronophagia, microgliosis, nonsuppurative meningitis, and perivasculitis are typical changes seen microscopically. These changes are most prevalent in the brain stem and ventral horns of the spinal cord (Fig. 1.41). During the demyelinating phase of experimental disease, foci of demyelination are present in the white matter of the spinal cord, brain stem, and cerebellum. Demyelinating lesions are not a likely component of natural infections. Acute myositis and focal myocarditis were observed in mice inoculated intraperitoneally with the DA strain of MEV, emphasizing the polytropism of the virus. The naturally occurring disease is much more devastating in immunodeficient mice, with high morbidity and mortality. In SCID mice, lesions are characterized by marked vacuolation and enlargement of affected neurons, particularly in the brain stem and ventral horn region of the spinal cord. Vacuolation of adjacent astrocytes and oligodendrocytes, with minimal to no inflammatory cell response, is another feature of

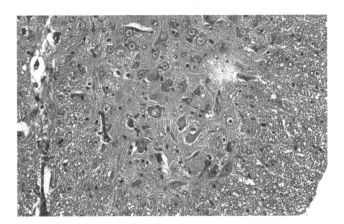

FIG. 1.41. *Spinal cord from the mouse depicted in the previous figure. There is acute neuronolysis in the ventral horn.*

the disease in SCID mice. Similar changes have been observed in the gray and white matter of nude mice.

Diagnosis

MEV infection is usually diagnosed serologically. There is extensive antigenic cross-reactivity between EMCV and MEV, but the former is not prevalent in laboratory mice. Antibodies to the two groups of virus can be differentially discriminated by serum neutralization. This method can also be used to discriminate between MEV strains, but that has no practical value. Seropositive mice should be considered to be actively infected with virus. Diagnosis can also be achieved by neurological signs and lesions in the small percentage of infected mice that develop central nervous system disease. MEV is not very contagious, requiring large sample sizes to accurately detect infection within a colony. Virus can be grown in cell culture, but isolation is difficult from adult mice. PCR amplification from tissue, particularly intestine and mesenteric lymph node, can also be used to diagnose active infection. Because of its low contagious potential, MEV can be eliminated from a colony of immunocompetent mice over time by test-and-slaughter at the cage level, if appropriate safeguards are taken against contamination of mice in adjacent cages. Differential diagnoses for neurological disease include trauma, neoplasia, otitis, MHV, LDV in immunodeficient C58 or AKR mice, and polyoma virus.

Reovirus Infection

Reoviruses that infect mice belong to the family Reoviridae and subgroup 1 of the genus *Orthoreovirus*. The name reovirus (respiratory enteric orphan virus) was proposed for a group of viruses associated with respiratory and enteric infections in humans. Reoviruses have since been isolated from a wide variety of mammals, birds, reptiles, insects, and other species. In fact, reovirus infection has been documented in every mammalian species tested. Mammalian orthoreoviruses are divided into 3 serotypes, based upon hemagglutination inhibition and neutralization tests. They are commonly referred to as reovirus 1, reovirus 2, and reovirus 3, although they actually represent a spectrum of viruses that are antigenically cross-reactive and genetically related. Although disease is rare, reovirus 3 has been incriminated as a pathogen in mice, and so it receives the most emphasis. Reoviruses frequently contaminate biological materials.

Epizootiology and Pathogenesis

Reovirus seroconversion is a frequent finding among wild mice and laboratory mice. Because reovirus 3 serotypes are the most common in laboratory mice, and only that serotype has been associated with natural disease in mice, reovirus 3 is emphasized and used as antigen. Seroconversion, however, reflects exposure to viruses from any of the serotypes. Reoviruses are transmitted by the orofecal route. Transmission among mice seems to occur primarily by direct contact among young mice. Contact transmission between adult mice is inefficient. Mice of all ages are susceptible to experimental infection by a variety of routes, but only mice infected as neonates develop disease. Strain-related differences in susceptibility have not been reported. Following oral inoculation of neonatal mice, virus enters through the M cells of Peyer's patches with dissemination to multiple organs via hematogenous, lymphatic, and/or neural spread. Reovirus 3 replication occurs in multiple organs of neonatal mice in the absence of significant lesions, until around day 10–12, when mice become clinically ill and develop lesions in multiple tissues, followed by recovery. This suggests an immune-mediated mechanism for development of lesions during the process of recovery, but this mechanism has not been defined. Pups born to immune dams do not develop disease. Oral inoculation of C.B-17-*scid* mice with reovirus 1 or 3 resulted in a lethal infection due to necrotizing hepatitis, with virus, but not lesions, detectable in multiple other organs.

Pathology

Disease and lesions occur only in infant mice from colonies previously unexposed to reovirus. At around 2 weeks of age, mice may be runted, jaundiced, and uncoordinated and have matted hair due to steatorrhea, which has been termed "oily hair effect." Surviving mice may remain runted and have transient dorsal alopecia. The most significant microscopic lesion is acute diffuse encephalitis that has a vascular distribution. Mice also develop focal necrotizing myocarditis, variable necrosis of lymphoid tissue, focal necrotizing hepatitis, portal hepatitis, acinar pancreatitis, and sialodacryoadenitis. C.B-17-*scid* mice infected with reovirus 1 or 3 developed progressive, necrotizing hepatitis, without lesions in other organs. Experimental inoculation of neonatal mice with prototype reovirus 1, 2, or 3 revealed different patterns of disease, but those differences do not necessarily reflect all members of each serotype.

Diagnosis

Reovirus infection is usually detected in a mouse population serologically, in the absence of disease, although outbreaks of disease have been reported among neonates. Some of the disease manifestations that have been reported in the early literature may be due to other infectious agents, such as MHV. Virus can be isolated from infected tissues, antigen can be visualized by immunohistochemistry, and tissues or biologic products can be tested by PCR. Lesions are nonspecific. Differential diagnoses of neonatal disease with steatorrhea include MHV, EDIM virus, and *Salmonella* infections.

Rotavirus Infection: Epizootic Diarrhea of Infant Mice

Epizootic diarrhea of infant mice (EDIM) virus belongs to the family Reoviridae, genus *Rotavirus*. The rotavirus A group encompasses viruses of humans, nonhuman primates, cattle, sheep, horses, pigs, dogs, cats, turkeys, chickens, and rabbits that are closely related genetically and antigenically. Each of these viruses has relative host specificity, but interspecies infection can be shown experimentally with high doses of inocula. They share a common propensity to cause enteritis and diarrhea in infants. EDIM has been studied as an animal model for rotaviral infections in other species. A number of group A rotaviruses have been isolated from mice, of which EDIM virus is a single strain. However, the term "EDIM" has been generally accepted as the inclusive name for intestinal rotavirus infection in mice and its agent.

Epizootiology and Pathogenesis

EDIM virus is highly contagious and prevalent in both laboratory and wild mice. Disease manifestations are relatively rare once infection is enzootic, due to protection of clinically susceptible infant mice by maternal IgA. Typically, clinical signs of EDIM occur in naïve breeding populations, but once infection is enzootic within the colony, EDIM disease is no longer apparent, although EDIM virus remains. Rotaviruses are shed copiously in feces, and transmission is by the orofecal route. Clinical disease ranges from inapparent to severe, depending primarily upon age. All ages of mice are susceptible to infection; however, disease is limited to mice less than 2 weeks of age. Virus selectively infects terminally differentiated enterocytes of villi and surface mucosa of the small and large intestine, respectively. These cells are most plentiful and widespread in the neonatal bowel and diminish in number, distribution, and degree of terminal differentiation as mucosal proliferative kinetics accelerate with acquisition of intestinal microflora. Viremia is detectable during peak virus replication, but virus replication is restricted to intestinal mucosa. All ages of mice are susceptible to productive infection, but the target cell population in adults is limited. Thus, functional disturbances tend not to be noted in older mice. Regardless of age at infection, recovery from diarrhea occurs at 14–17 days of age, with complete recovery from infection. Susceptibility to infection and disease may have a genetic basis, with BALB/c mice relatively susceptible, and B6 mice resistant. Infection of SCID mice follows the same age-related pattern of disease as immunocompetent mice. B cells, CD4 T cells, and CD8 T cells all contribute to resolution of infection, with persistent shedding of virus in B-cell-deficient and SCID mice.

During the first few days of infection, there is fluid accumulation and dilation of the small intestine. Diarrhea is induced by a combination of factors, including apoptosis and loss of absorptive epithelium, replacement of lost cells with immature nonabsorptive cells, altered carbohydrate absorption, osmotic effects related to luminal carbohydrate and bacterial fermentation, and active secretion of fluid and electrolytes. The secretory

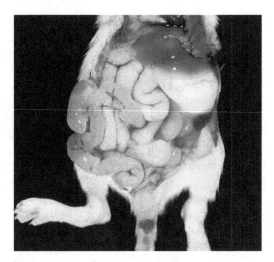

FIG. 1.42. *Infant mouse with epizootic diarrhea of infant mice (EDIM), caused by rotavirus. Note the full stomach, the flaccid and dilated small intestine, and pasting of the tail base with soft feces.*

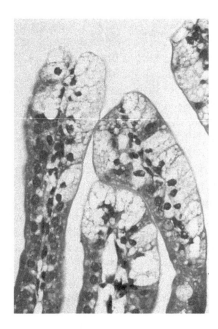

FIG. 1.43. *Small intestine of an infant mouse infected with rotavirus. Note the cytoplasmic swelling of enterocytes at the tips of the villi. Microscopic lesions are often subtle and may not be readily apparent.*

stimulus appears to be mediated by an enterotoxic effect of the viral nonstructural protein 4, which can be evoked with inactivated virus or recombinant protein, and activation of the enteric nervous system. Overgrowth of *E. coli*, and its atypical abundance in the upper small intestine, accompany the malabsorptive effects of the virus.

Pathology

Infection is often silent, but clinically affected mice can be runted and potbellied, with loose, mustard-colored feces staining the perineum. Steatorrhea with oily hair may also be apparent. The bowel is flaccid and distended with fluid and gas (Fig. 1.42), but mice continue to suckle. Some deaths may occur due to obstipation caused by fecal caking around the anus. In infant mice, EDIM virus causes hydropic change and vacuolation of terminally differentiated enterocytes at the tips of villi (Fig. 1.43) and large intestinal surface mucosa. Some nuclei may be pyknotic. Acidophilic intracytoplasmic inclusions have been described but are not diagnostic. In addition, the lamina propria may be edematous and lymphatics dilated, although inflammation is minimal. These changes are difficult to discern under the best of circumstances and are not apparent in mice older than 14 days of age. Remarkably, mice may manifest significant diarrhea with minimal microscopic lesions. Infected infant mice often have severe stress-related thymic necrosis.

Diagnosis

EDIM can be diagnosed presumptively on the basis of age, clinical signs, and lesions. Differential diagnoses include enterotropic MHV, MAdV-2, reovirus, salmonellosis, Tyzzer's disease, and Clostridial enteropathy. Vacuolation and intracytoplasmic inclusions must be differentiated from absorption vacuoles of the neonatal

apical tubular system that occur in the distal small intestine, which may contain solitary eosinophilic globules. Definitive diagnosis can be achieved by electron microscopy of intestinal mucosa or feces. Rotavirus antigen can be detected in feces by ELISA, and RNA can be detected by PCR. Antigen detection can be accomplished with commercially available rotavirus diagnostic kits, but false-positive reactions can occur with certain mouse diets. Careful controls are therefore advised. Serology for EDIM virus antibody is useful for surveillance and retrospective confirmation of infection.

RETROELEMENTS AND RETROVIRUS INFECTIONS

Retroviruses are the phylogenetic pinnacle of a diverse assemblage of related entities known collectively as retroelements, which occupy over 37% of the mouse genome. Most of these elements can be considered genetic parasites or fossil DNA, but they play a significant role in laboratory mouse strain characteristics and disease. Despite their significance, retroelements are often unfortunately ignored in texts on mouse biology. The reader is therefore herein subjected to an overview of retrovirus biology in order to better appreciate the role of retroelements in pathogenesis of disease and phenotypes in the laboratory mouse.

The mouse genome is replete with literally thousands of copies of endogenous integrated retroelements that require reverse transcription from RNA to DNA. Among the retroelements are replication-competent endogenous retroviruses whose genomes encode *gag, pro, pol,* and *env* genes that are flanked on their 5'- and 3'- ends by long terminal repeats (LTRs). Endogenous retroviruses include murine leukemia viruses (MuLVs) and murine mammary tumor viruses (MMTVs), which are genetically unrelated. MMTVs have a slightly longer genome than MuLVs, and their LTR regions encode a critically important gene: *Sag* (superantigen). Endogenous MuLVs and MMTVs are autonomous, in that they encode their own reverse transcriptase. Endogenous retroviruses are integrated as DNA within the genome, wherein they are termed "proviruses." The majority of endogenous retroviruses (proviruses) are defective, ranging from being one base pair substitution away from an active provirus to having multiple stop codons, frameshifts, and deletions that render them incapable of expression as a replication-competent virus. Furthermore, most proviruses are methylated and transcriptionally silent. Other autonomous retroelement families that are flanked by LTRs include intracisternal A particles (IAPs), MusD elements, VL30 elements, glutathione tRNA primer binding sites (GLNs), and murine endogenous retroelements (MuERVs), which include MuERVC, murine retrovirus-related sequences (MuRRS), and murine repeated viruses on Y chromosome (MuRVYs). These elements are missing significant parts of their genome (especially *env*) or encode no open reading frames at all. They are related to retroviruses because of similarities within their LTRs, and each family of retroelements has its own unique LTR sequences. There are also autonomous retroelements that lack LTRs, known as long interspersed nucleotide sequences (LINEs), which make up 20% of the mouse genome. Related retroelements that are nonautonomous, and therefore must borrow reverse transcriptase function from autonomous retroelements, are termed "retrotranscripts." These elements encode no proteins, but are usually flanked by LTRs. They include early transposons (ETns) and short interspersed nuclear elements (SINEs), which make up 8% of the genome. Finally, there are numerous solo LTRs, which are devoid of internal reading frames.

Replication-competent, endogenous MuLVs and MMTVs are closely related to exogenous MuLVs and MMTVs, which are not integrated within the mouse genome. Exogenous retroviruses are transmitted horizontally as conventional viruses. Exogenous viruses exist within wild mouse populations, but they have been eliminated (unless purposely reintroduced) from laboratory mice by cesarean rederivation and/or foster nursing. The well-studied Friend, Moloney, and Rauscher (FMR) group of MuLVs and the Bittner milk agent (MMTV-S) are exogenous retroviruses. The small number of replication-competent endogenous viruses can also be horizontally transmitted to other mice, if the mice possess the appropriate susceptibility factors.

Retroviruses and retroelements are highly promiscuous. Retroviruses possess a diploid genome, which incorporates two RNA genome strands. Virion assembly within host cells that are coinfected with either exogenous or endogenous retroviruses often results in acquisition of 2 different viral genomes within a virion. Reverse transcriptase readily jumps from homologous regions of one strand to the other, thereby creating recombinant forms of viral genomes. In this way, otherwise defective endogenous retroviruses, and even retroelements such as MuRRS and ETns, can contribute to generation of new replication-competent recombinant forms of virus with altered biological behavior. Some retroelements, such as VL30s, are frequently incorporated as passengers (parasitic RNA) during MuLV virion packaging and have a high recombination rate with retroviruses. Although most endogenous retroelements are defective, they represent mobile DNA species that can reintegrate in other regions of the genome during cell division without virion assembly and re-infection. These are known as retrotransposons.

Occasionally, retroviral integrations within the host genome result in usurping components of the host DNA, which becomes incorporated in the viral genome. These regions of host DNA tend to result in loss of critical viral sequences, and the virus becomes defective. Acute transforming MuLVs and murine sarcoma viruses (MuSVs) are viruses that have incorporated a host cellular proto-oncogene (*c-onc*) that directly alters cell division. Once in the viral genome, the *c-onc* is referred to as viral oncogene (*v-onc*). Often, *v-oncs* are mutated, which increases their pathogenicity. Acute transforming retroviruses are so named because they carry their own *v-onc* that induces rapid transformation and evolution of neoplasia (in contrast to chronic retroviruses that induce neoplasia by random insertional mutagenesis). Examples of acute transforming retroviruses are Abelson MuLV (the *v-onc* is *abl*) and Moloney MuSV (the *v-onc* is *mos*). Since acute transforming MuLVs and MuSVs are experimental tools, and do not appear to contribute to natural disease, they will not be discussed further. Defective proviruses, including acute transforming MuLVs and MuSVs, can be rendered infectious through assistance of helper viruses, which contribute the missing structural elements for virion assembly, particularly envelope proteins, and/or LTR elements that confer tissue specificity.

Each inbred strain of mouse has its own characteristic "signature" of endogenous retrovirus and retroelement sites of integration in its genome. Related mouse strains share similarity in these patterns of integrated proviruses. Furthermore, different families of retroviruses have contributed to the mosaicism of the laboratory mouse genome from different *Mus* species and at different times during the evolution of the mouse. Based upon genome sequence comparison among *Mus* species, retrovirus-like elements, such as Etns, probably entered the mouse genome 5–10 million years ago, whereas MuLVs and MMTVs entered the genome within the last 1.5 million years and are still in the process of entry in some cases. A progressive chronology of integration helps to explain retrovirus biology. Older elements represent "fossil" DNA with sequences that are quite divergent from more recent families of retrovirus. They tend to be highly methylated and have major sequence deletions, stop codons, frameshifts, and other characteristics that make them defective. The most recent acquisitions are the MuLVs and MMTVs, which also may exist in multiple copies throughout the genome, most of which are also transcriptionally silent or defective. Only a relative few are transcribed as replicating viruses capable of infecting other cells. These are the viruses that will be emphasized, but it must be recognized that even defective retrovirus-like elements can become reintegrated within the dividing cell genome as retrotransposons. This process takes place within the nuclear context of the dividing cell, in contrast to replicating viruses, which leave the cell and enter another. This explains the acquisition of multiple copies of these older elements throughout the genome. For example, there are 100–200 copies of VL30s, and 1,000–2,000 copies of ETns in the mouse genome that have arisen from retrotransposon activity.

Retroviruses of the mouse can best be described as "mother nature's transgenes," with a major component of their biology involving integration within the genome of dividing cells through viral reverse transcriptase. When integration involves somatic cells, the outcome can be variable, but integration in germ cells results in passage of the provirus within the genome to subsequent mouse generations. Integration is random and usually phenotypically silent, but integration in other sites can result in insertional mutagenesis. Retroelements and their mouse host have evolved a remarkable state of détente. Endogenous retroviruses have undergone adaptations that render them relatively innocuous to their hosts. They tend to be nonpathogenic and replicate poorly. Many show their phylogenetic age and are defective and transcriptionally silent. The host has also evolved to cope with their presence by mutation or loss of key viral receptors and other factors, thereby precluding reinfection (and reintegration in other sites of the genome that may result in deleterious effects).

Finally, an introduction to mouse retrovirus biology is not complete without understanding virus tissue and host species tropism. LTRs contain coding sequences, including enhancers and promoters, which dictate transcriptional activity and tissue specificity. The MMTV LTR, for example, confers tropism for mammary tissue, which is why MMTV LTR is often used in transgenic constructs for mammary cancer research. Endogenous MuLVs are generally classified biologically by their host species tropism. Ecotropic MuLVs have tropism for mouse cells, but not cells of other species. Furthermore, ecotropic viruses display differential tropism for cells of different mouse strains, through allelic variation of the $Fv-1$ gene. $Fv-1$ has 2 major allelic variants, $Fv-1^n$ and

$Fv-1^b$, that are codominant. Mice that are homozygous for $Fv-1^n$ are permissive for infection with N-tropic ecotropic viruses, whereas mice that are homozygous for $Fv-1^b$ are permissive for infection with B-tropic ecotropic viruses, and $Fv-1^{b/n}$ heterozygous mice are permissive to both types of ecotropic virus. $Fv-1^n$ mouse genotypes include AKR, CBA, C3H, C57L, C57BR, C58, and SWR strains, among others. $Fv-1^b$ mouse genotypes include A, BALB/c, C57BL/6, C57BL/10, FVB, and others. A third Fv-1 allele, $Fv-1^{nr}$, is found in AKR, NZB, NZW, and RF mice. Mice that carry ecotropic MuLV can effectively control ecotropic infection through the $Fv-1$ locus. For example, BALB mice carry an endogenous N-ecotropic virus, but it cannot replicate (and re-infect and re-integrate) within BALB mice. Xenotropic MuLVs have tropism for cells of other species but not mouse cells. This is an apparent example of the mouse evolving away from susceptibility to these endogenous viruses, as mice have lost or mutated the functional cellular receptor. Polytropic viruses have tropism for mouse, as well as other species. Based upon LTR sequences, the polytropic group has two subgroups: polytropic and modified polytropic viruses. Both have LTR insertions derived from MuRRS, but all endogenous polytropic viruses are defective.

Additional types of MuLV and retroelements exist in wild, but not laboratory, mice. A fourth group of viruses, known as amphotropic viruses, have tropism for cells of mice and other species, but they differ from polytropic viruses in their LTR sequences and receptor specificity and represent a family of viruses that are found in wild, but not laboratory, mice. It is generally believed that the Friend, Moloney, and Rausher MuLVs are related to the amphotropic group. Wild mice may also have exogenous ecotropic MuLV that is unrelated to the endogenous ecotropic viruses in laboratory mice. $Fv-4$ is another extensively studied resistance determinant for MuLV replication, but it has been found only in wild mice and is apparently not represented in the strains of laboratory mice that have been examined. It, like $Fv-1$, is derived from retrovirus sequences.

Ecotropic proviruses represent the most recent acquisitions into the mouse genome, and their presence varies among laboratory mouse strains. Several mouse strains, including 129, NZB, NFS, C57L, SWR, and CBA, are ecotropic virus-negative. Others, including BALB/c, A, C3H/He, and CBA, possess a single ecotropic virus, with low expression, and C57BL/6, C57BL/10, and C57BR possess a different, single ecotropic virus. A few exceptional mouse strains, most notably AKR, C58, and HRS, have multiple genome-length ecotropic proviruses, with high levels of expression. Ecotropic proviruses are given gene names ($Emv-1$, $Emv-2$, etc.). The multicopy Emv, formerly called Akv, that is present in AKR, C58, and HRS but not other strains of mice is a genetic contribution from $M. molossinus$. Xenotropic viruses are present in multiple copies in all mouse strains, but with generally low expression levels as replication-competent virus, with one exception being the NZB mouse, which expresses high levels of xenotropic virus in its tissues. Xenotropic proviruses are given the gene designation *Xmv* (*Xmv*-1, *Xmv*-2, etc.). Polytropic retroviruses, which probably represent the oldest of the endogenous retrovirus family in terms of germline acquisition, are present in all strains of mice, but all polytropic viruses are defective. Polytropic provirus genes are named *Pmv* and modified polytropic provirus genes are named *Mpmv*. There are over 50 MMTV proviral loci, designated *Mtv*-1 to *Mtv*-56, in various strains of mice. The majority of these proviruses do not produce infectious virus, with the notable exception of *Mtv*-1, which is present in DBA and C3H mice, and *Mtv*-2, which is present in GRS mice. Every chromosome of the mouse genome has multiple endogenous *Emv*, *Xmv*, *Pmv*, *Mpmv*, or *Mtv* proviruses. Some populations of wild mice have been found that lack both exogenous and endogenous MMTV.

Germline Insertional Mutagenesis

Reintegration of endogenous retroviruses or transposition of retroelements can and do result in spontaneous mutations among inbred mice. Examples of retrovirus integrations that have resulted in spontaneous mutations include the dilute (*d*) mutation of DBA mice due to insertion of an ecotropic virus into the *Myo5a* locus, the hairless (*hr*) mouse mutation due to a polytropic virus integration in the *hr* locus, and the rodless retina (*rd1*) mutation due to integration of a xenotropic virus into the *Pde6b* locus. Germline integrations of IAPs and ETns have also contributed to nearly 15% of all known spontaneous mutations, resulting in a wide variety of overt phenotypes, including athymia (*Foxn1*), stargazer (*Cacng2*), obese (*Lep*), and albino (*Tyr*), among many others. Like transgenes, spontaneous phenotypic revertants can occur when the offending retrovirus element is excised by DNA repair. Retrovirus integrations are usually random (although there are "hot spots" within the genome), and the resulting integrated DNA within the genome is "hemizygous," analogous to a transgene. Ecotropic viruses are responsible for the greatest number of novel proviral integrations in the germline. The artificial process of inbreeding laboratory mice has made these hemizygous integrations homozygous and thus they have been given gene names. Examination of the genomes of various substrains derived from parental strains has revealed both acquisition and loss of proviruses over the course of recent mouse history, contributing significantly to substrain genetic divergence and emphasizing the dynamic nature of retroviruses and retroelements.

Modulation of the Host Immune Response by MuLVs and MMTVs

Endogenous retroviruses and retroelements that encode proteins during the life of a mouse may elicit varying degrees of host immunity. Viruses that are expressed in high titer and in all tissues during early development are likely to induce immunological tolerance, particularly if expressed in the thymus. The superantigens (SAgs) of some MMTVs stimulate and deplete specific Vß T-cell subsets (see "MMTVs," later in this chapter). However, endogenous retroviruses or retroelements may not be expressed in tissues until later in life, and thus are likely to stimulate a host immune response, albeit weak. Proviruses may be transcriptionally silent until there is a stimulus for cell division, at which time they may be expressed and stimulate a host response. Thus, the host's immune response to its load of endogenous retroviruses is variable, but often results in the evolution of immune complexes as mice age that are suspected to contribute to the development of spontaneous vasculitis and glomerulonephritis. These disease syndromes, not surprisingly, vary in severity among different mouse strains. Expression of endogenous retroviruses in pancreatic islets of NOD mice is associated with the evolution of immune-mediated insulitis, and some have speculated that retroviruses may contribute to autoimmune disease in NZB x NZW hybrid mice.

Murine Leukemia Viruses

Exogenous MuLVs and replication-competent endogenous MuLVs are transmitted through milk and to a lesser extent semen, saliva, venereal transmission, perinatal infection, or transplacental transmission. Germline integration by MuLVs tends to be primarily through infection of dividing ova rather than male gametes. Reintegration of MuLVs into the genome of somatic cells results in random insertional mutagenesis, and neoplasia is favored when integration takes place near host proto-oncogenes.

The most extensively studied system for endogenous MuLV pathogenesis has been the AKR mouse (also C58 and HRS strains). AKR mice develop nearly 100% thymic lymphomas of T-cell origin within 6–12 months of age (Fig. 1.44). The AKR mouse genome contains over 40 provirus integrations, including 3 critical parental proviruses. All tissues express high levels of replication-competent ecotropic virus (*Emv*-11) early in life. This virus is B-tropic and incapable of infecting AKR cells, which are $Fv\text{-}1^{n/n}$ homozygous. However, high-level expression in cells that are coexpressing xenotropic virus results in genetic recombinant viruses with altered LTR sequences derived from the xenotropic parent. These recombinant viruses are expressed in cells that also coexpress a polytropic virus, which donates altered envelope (*env*) sequences and allows infection of thymic cells. These recombinant viruses undergo duplication of enhanced LTR sequences, with high levels of replication in the thymus, which favors insertional mutagenesis. The proximal viral pathogen, which represents a recombinant of 3 parental endogenous ecotropic, xenotropic, and polytropic parents, possesses the ability to induce foci in mink cells. It is thus called a mink cell focus (MCF)

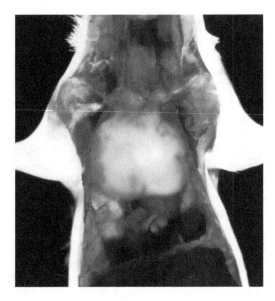

FIG. 1.44. *Thymic lymphoma in an AKR mouse due to naturally occurring recombination of endogenous retroviruses. Nearly all mice of this strain develop thymic lymphoma between 6 and 12 months of age.*

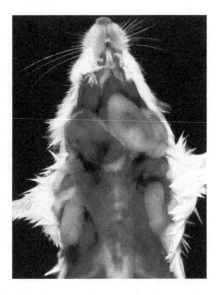

FIG. 1.45. *Multicentric lymphoma in a BALB/c mouse due to naturally occurring recombination of endogenous retroviruses. Note the markedly enlarged cervical and axillary lymph nodes.*

forming virus. MCF viruses are the product of in vivo recombination and do not exist as natural germline proviruses. These events are highly artificial laboratory mouse consequence from selective breeding for the thymic lymphoma phenotype and inbreeding. There is no evidence for MCFs among wild mice.

The majority of mouse lymphomas are of B or pre-B-cell origin and tend to arise in the spleen. They arise in 40% of NFS mice, which lack ectropic virus, but with a longer latency period and lower grade than mice carrying ectropic virus. Neonatal thymectomy of AKR mice results in B-cell lymphomas arising from the spleen, and congenic mice derived from ectropic virus-free NFS mouse background that have been backcrossed with the AKR *Emv* provirus locus develop splenic B-cell tumors. B-cell tumors with ectropic virus integrations result from random integration of the ectropic virus and are not necessarily associated with activation of host oncogenes. The virus is believed to be functioning to increase the rate of clones and speed the evolution of lymphomas that would otherwise arise but at a slower pace. BALB/c mice develop a late-onset lymphoma that is multicentric (Fig. 1.45). They carry nononcogenic, N-ectropic, and xenotropic viruses that form recombinants that are oncogenic and B-ectropic, resulting in infection of lymphoid cells, integration, and late-onset lymphoma. Each mouse strain possesses its own set of proviruses and host factors, with varying degrees of MuLV expression and disease that are mouse strain-, age-, tissue-, and cell type-specific.

Not all outcomes of MuLV infection are neoplastic, and in fact most are phenotypically silent. Other reported syndromes include altered coat color and consistency, hairlessness, central nervous system disease (see Arterivirus, LDV Infection in this chapter),

premature graying, and potentially any other phenotype resulting from random integration or infection with expression of viral gene products. The most widely studied MuLV-related neurologic syndrome has been observed in feral Lake Casitas mice, which naturally develop hind limb paralysis. The syndrome is caused by MuLV CasBr-E, an ectropic virus that is distinct from ectropic MuLVs of laboratory mice. Disease is readily reproduced by inoculation of $Fv-1^{n/n}$ laboratory mice. Diseased mice manifest neuronal loss with proliferation and hypertrophy of microglia, vacuolation, and spongiosis, particularly in the ventral horns of the lumbar spinal cord.

Murine Mammary Tumor Viruses

Although MMTVs are generally associated with mammary gland neoplasia, their lymphocytotropism and ability to transform lymphoid cells through insertional mutagenesis is an equally important aspect of their biology. Like MuLVs, MMTVs are either exogenous or endogenous. Exogenous and replication-competent endogenous MMTVs are transmitted primarily in the milk, and to a lesser extent saliva. Exogenous MMTV, which is known as MMTV-S (Standard), the "extrachromosomal milk factor," or the "Bittner agent," has been eliminated from modern mouse populations by cesarean rederivation or foster nursing, unless intentionally maintained for experimental purposes. In contrast, all strains of laboratory mice possess varying numbers of endogenous MMTV provirus (*Mtv*) in their genome. All exogenous and some endogenous MMTVs are expressed in mammary tissue and lymphoid tissue, but some endogenous MMTVs, including *Mtv*-7 and *Mtv*-9, are not expressed in mammary tissue. Like MuLVs, most MMTV endogenous proviruses are defective, but can recombine with replication-competent MMTVs.

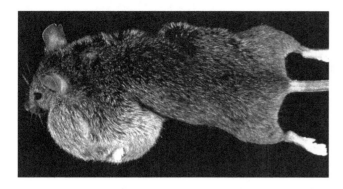

FIG. 1.46.   *Mammary neoplasia in a C3H mouse due to naturally occurring expression of endogenous mouse mammary tumor virus (MMTV).*

As their name implies, MMTVs are associated with mammary neoplasia through random integration. Genetically susceptible strains of mice, such as C3H, infected with exogenous MMTV-S, develop a high prevalence and early onset of mammary tumors. Mice that carry replication-competent endogenous *Mtv*-1 (C3H, DBA) or *Mtv*-2 (GRS) also develop mammary neoplasia (Fig. 1.46), but onset is delayed. MMTV dual lymphoid and mammary tropism, enhanced by LTR factors, favors this event. Exogenous MMTV (and replication-competent endogenous MMTV) is transmitted primarily from infected dams to nursing pups through the milk. Virus initially infects gut-associated M cells and dendritic cells and then replicates in B cells of Peyer's patches. Infected B cells express viral LTR-encoded superantigen (SAg) in the context of MHC class II on T cells, which results in stimulation and proliferation of T cells through recognition by specific Vß T-cell receptors. Activated T cells release lymphokines that further stimulate proliferation of bystander B cells. Dividing B cells are requisite for retrovirus infection, thereby amplifying virus-infected B lymphocytes, which subsequently transport MMTV to mammary tissue. The role of SAg is critical in MMTV biology, as the more the virus produced, the greater the efficiency of transmission in the milk. Once virus enters the mammary gland via infected lymphocytes, it further replicates extensively within mammary tissue. Mammary tropism is favored by promoters and enhancers in the LTR region, thereby amplifying virus and favoring transmission in the milk. High titers of the virus within mammary tissue increase the chance of proviral integration near a site of a cellular protooncogene, with subsequent oncogenesis. There is a high correlation between virus titer in milk and mammary tumor incidence within a mouse strain. MMTV also utilizes other mechanisms that favor its replication by circumventing the host innate immune response.

In contrast to mice exposed to exogenous MMTV, mice that express SAg from an endogenous MMTV develop selective deletion of the corresponding Vß T-cell subset. These mice resist infection with exogenous MMTV with the same SAg specificity, since the exogenous virus cannot effectively amplify itself in the Peyer's patches. In addition, Vß6 T-cell depletion in mice with endogenous *Mtv*-7 is a major factor for polyoma virus-induced neoplasia susceptibility in C3H/Bi, C58, CBA, AKR, and RF mice. Mice that are resistant to polyoma virus neoplasia, such as C57BR, C3H/He, and CBA, lack *Mtv*-7, but possess other *Mtvs* with different SAg specificity. Lack of appropriate Vß6 T-cell subset, induced by *Mtv*-7 SAg, precludes host T-cell immunity against polyoma virus-induced tumors.

Alternatively, MMTV proviruses may not be expressed until later in life, so there is no early Vß T-cell deletion. SJL mice, for example, carry endogenous *Mtv*-29 that is initially transcriptionally silent but expressed later in life when Peyer's patches are stimulated antigenically. Over 90% of SJL mice develop MMTV-associated lymphoma by 13 months of age. Expression of SAg results in massive T-cell-mediated B-cell proliferation, with B-cell lymphoma arising in Peyer's patches, mesenteric lymph nodes (Fig. 1.47), and subsequently other sites. The ensuing follicular center cell lymphoma is characteristic of this strain of mouse. A similar pattern of follicular center cell lymphoma arising from gut-associated lymphoid tissue is seen in other strains of mice, but later in life. For example, C57L mice also express *Mtv*-29, but suppress development of lymphomas by NK cells, whereas SJL mice develop a high prevalence and earlier onset of lymphomas because they are NK cell-deficient. MMTV can also be associated with T-cell lymphomas of the thymus in GR and other strains of mice. MMTVs derived from these

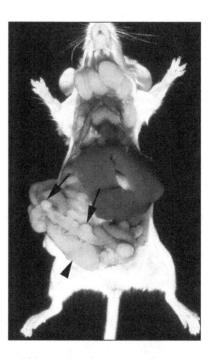

FIG. 1.47.   *Multicentric lymphoma arising from gut-associated lymphoid tissue in a SJL mouse due to naturally occurring expression of endogenous MMTV. Note the prominent Peyer's patches (arrows) and enlarged mesenteric lymph node (arrowhead).*

tumors have undergone a change in cell tropism from B cells to T cells, which is mediated through rearrangements in their LTR regions.

Diagnosis

Diagnosis of MuLV or MMTV is not necessary, since all mice are infected or have provirus sequences within their genome. Electron microscopic examination of normal and neoplastic mouse tissues frequently reveals C-type (MuLV), A-type (IAP), and B-type (MMTV) particles as an incidental findings.

Significance

MuLVs and MMTVs are an integral and important part of mouse biology and inseparable features of the laboratory mouse. They are valuable models for retrovirus pathogenesis. They become significant as natural pathogens when they induce life-limiting disease and cause spontaneous mutations and substrain divergence. For example, the emergence of an ecotropic MuLV in a colony of CFW Swiss mice has resulted in a high incidence of lymphoma in a stock that was previously characterized as having a low incidence of spontaneous lymphoma. The consequences of recombinant retroviruses arising from microinjection of ES cells into blastocysts of different mouse strain background have not been fully realized in chimeras and their progeny. MuLVs are known to recombine with HIV in SCID-*hu* mice, which limits the value of this model.

BIBLIOGRAPHY FOR VIRAL INFECTIONS

General References for Infectious Diseases

Fox, J.G., Barthold, S.W., Davisson, M.T., Newcomer, C.E., Quimby, F.W., & Smith, A.L. (2007) *The Mouse in Biomedical Research. Diseases*, Vol. 2, 2nd edn. Academic Press, New York.

Franklin, C.L. (2006) Microbial considerations in genetically engineered mouse research. *ILAR Journal* 47:141–155.

Lindsey, J.R., Boorman, G.A., Collins, M.J., Jr., Hsu, C.-K., Van Hoosier, G.L., Jr., & Wagner, J.E. (1991) *Infectious Diseases of Mice and Rats*. National Academy Press, Washington, DC.

Nicklas, W., Kraft, V., & Meyer, B. (1993) Contamination of transplantable tumors, cell lines, and monoclonal antibodies with rodent viruses. *Laboratory Animal Science* 43:296–300.

Whary, M.T., Baumgarth, N., Fox, J.G., & Barthold, S.W. (2015) Biology and diseases of mice. In: *Laboratory Animal Medicine*, 3rd edn (eds. J.G. Fox, L.C. Anderson, G.M. Otto, K. R. Pritchett-Corning, & M. T. Whary). Academic Press, New York.

DNA Viral Infections

Adenovirus Infection

Blaillock, Z.R., Rabin, E.R., & Melnick, J.L. (1967) Adenovirus endocarditis in mice. *Science* 157:69–70.

Charles, P.C., Guida, J.D., Brosnan, C.F., & Horwitz, M.S. (1998) Mouse adenovirus type-1 replication is restricted to vascular endothelium in the CNS of susceptible strains of mice. *Virology* 245:216–228.

Ginder, D.R. (1964) Increased susceptibility of mice infected with mouse adenovirus to *Escherichia coli*-induced pyelonephritis. *Journal of Experimental Medicine* 120:1117–1128.

Guida, J.D., Fejer, G., Pirofski, L.-A., Brosnan, C.F., & Horwitz, M.S. (1995) Mouse adenovirus type 1 causes a fatal hemorrhagic encephalomyelitis in adult C57BL/6 but not BALB/c mice. *Journal of Virology* 69:7674–7681.

Hashimoto, K., Sugiyama, T., & Saski, S. (1966) An adenovirus isolated from feces of mice. I. Isolation and identification. *Japanese Journal of Microbiology* 10:115–125.

Kajon, A.E., Brown, C.C., & Spindler, K.R. (1998) Distribution of mouse adenovirus type I in intraperitoneally and intranasally infected adult outbred mice. *Journal of Virology* 72:1219–1223.

Kring, S.C., King, C.S., & Spindler, K.R. (1995) Susceptibility and signs associated with mouse adenovirus type 1 infection of adult outbred Swiss mice. *Journal of Virology* 69:8084–8088.

Lenaerts, L., Verbeken, E., De Clercq, E., & Naesens, L. (2005) Mouse adenovirus type 1 infection in SCID mice: an experimental model for antiviral therapy of systemic adenovirus infections. *Antimicrobial Agents and Chemotherapy* 49:4689–4699.

Leuthans, T.N. & Wagner, J.E. (1983) A naturally occurring intestinal mouse adenovirus infection associated with negative serologic findings. *Laboratory Animal Science* 33:270–272.

Lussier, G., Smith, A.L., Guenette, D., & Descoteaux, J.-P. (1987) Serological relationship between mouse adenovirus strains FL and K87. *Laboratory Animal Science* 37:55–57.

Margolis, G., Kilham, L., & Hoenig, E.M. (1974) Experimental adenovirus infection of the mouse adrenal gland. I. Light microscopic observations. *American Journal of Pathology* 75:363–372.

Moore, M.L., McKissic, E.L., Brown, C.C., Wilkinson, J.E., & Spindler, J.R. (2004) Fatal disseminated mouse adenovirus type 1 infection in mice lacking B cells or Bruton's tyrosine kinase. *Journal of Virology* 78:5584–5590.

Pirofski, L., Horwitz, M.S., Scharff, M.D., & Factor, S.M. (1991) Murine adenovirus infection of SCID mice induces hepatic lesions that resemble human Reye's syndrome. *Proceedings of the National Academy of Science of the United States of America* 88:4358–4362.

Smith, A.L. & Barthold, S.W. (1987) Factors influencing susceptibility of laboratory rodents to infection with mouse adenovirus strains K87 and FL. *Archives of Virology* 95:143–148.

Smith, A.L., Winograd, D.F., & Burrage, T.G. (1986) Comparative biological characterization of mouse adenovirus strains FL and K87 and seroprevalence in laboratory rodents. *Archives of Virology* 91:233–246.

Weinberg, J.B., Stempfle, G.S., Wilkinson, J.E., Younger, J.G., & Spindler, K.R. (2005) Acute respiratory infection with mouse adenovirus type 1. *Virology* 340:245–254.

Winters, A.L. & Brown, H.K. (1980) Duodenal lesions associated with adenovirus infection in athymic "nude" mice. *Proceedings of the Society for Experimental Biology and Medicine* 164:280–286.

Mouse Cytomegalovirus Infection

Booth, T.W., Scalzo, A.A., Carrello, C., Lyons, P.A., Farrell, H.E., Singleton, G.R., & Shellam, G.R. (1993) Molecular and biological characterization of new strains of murine cytomegalovirus isolated from wild mice. *Archives of Virology* 132:209–220.

Brautigam, A.R., Dutko, F.J., Olding, L.B., & Oldstone, M.B.A. (1979) Pathogenesis of murine cytomegalovirus infection: the macrophage as a permissive cell for cytomegalovirus infection, replication and latency. *Journal of General Virology* 44:349–359.

Brody, A.R. & Craighead, J.E. (1974) Pathogenesis of pulmonary cytomegalovirus infection in immunosuppressed mice. *Journal of Infectious Diseases* 129:677–689.

Chen, H.C. & Cover, C.E. (1988) Spontaneous disseminated cytomegalic inclusion disease in an ageing laboratory mouse. *Journal of Comparative Pathology* 98:489–493.

Dangler, C.A., Baker, S.E., Karinki Njenga, M., & Chia, S.H. (1995) Murine cytomegalovirus-associated arteritis. *Veterinary Pathology* 32:127–133.

Gardner, M.B., Officer, J.E., Parker, J., Estes, J.D., & Rongey, R.W. (1974) Induction of disseminated virulent cytomegalovirus infection by immunosuppression of naturally chronically infected wild mice. *Infection and Immunity* 10:966–969.

Hamilton, J.R. & Overall, J.C., Jr., (1978) Synergistic infection with murine cytomegalovirus and *Pseudomonas aeruginosa* in mice. *Journal of Infectious Diseases* 137:775–782.

Jordan, M.C. (1978) Interstitial pneumonia and subclinical infection after intranasal inoculation of murine cytomegalovirus. *Infection and Immunity* 21:275–280.

Mims, C.A. & Gould, J. (1979) Infection of salivary glands, kidneys, adrenals, ovaries and epithelia by murine cytomegalovirus. *Journal of Medical Microbiology* 12:113–122.

Olding, L.B., Kingsbury, D.T., & Oldstone, M.B.A. (1976) Pathogenesis of cytomegalovirus infection: distribution of viral products, immune complexes and autoimmunity during latent murine infection. *Journal of General Virology* 33:267–280.

Reynolds, R.P., Rahija, R.J., Schenkman, D.I., & Richter, C.B. (1993) Experimental murine cytomegalovirus infection in severe combined immunodeficient mice. *Laboratory Animal Science* 43:291–295.

Shanley, J.D. & Pesanti, E.L. (1986) Murine cytomegalovirus adrenalitis in nude mice. *Archives of Virology* 88:27–35.

Shanley, J.D., Thrall, R.S., & Forman, S.J. (1997) Murine cytomegalovirus replication in the lungs of athymic BALB/c nude mice. *Journal of Infectious Diseases* 175:309–315.

Mouse Thymic Virus Infection

Athanassious, R., Brunet, & Lussier, G. (1993) Ultrastructural study of mouse thymus virus replication. *Acta Virologica* 37:175–180.

Cohen, P.L., Cross, S., & Mosier, D. (1975) Immunologic effects of neonatal infection with mouse thymic virus. *Journal of Immunology* 115:706–710.

Cross, S.S., Morse, H.C., & Asofsky, R. (1976) Neonatal infection with mouse thymic virus: differential effects on T cells mediating the graft-versus-host reaction. *Journal of Immunology* 117:635–638.

Cross, S.S., Parker, J., Rowe, W., & Robbins, M. (1979) Biology of mouse thymic virus, a herpesvirus of mice, and the antigenic relationship to mouse cytomegalovirus. *Infection and Immunity* 26:1186–1195.

Morse, S.S. (1988) Mouse thymic virus (MTLV; murid herpesvirus 3) infection in athymic nude mice: evidence for a T lymphocyte requirement. *Virology* 163:255–258.

Morse, S.S. (1989) Thymic necrosis following oral inoculation of mouse thymic virus. *Laboratory Animal Science* 39:571–574.

Morse, S.S. (1990) Comparative sensitivity of infectivity assay and mouse antibody production (MAP) test for detection of mouse thymic virus (MTLV). *Journal of Virological Methods* 28:15–23.

Morse, S.S. & Valinsky, J.E. (1989) Mouse thymic virus (MTLV): a mammalian herpesvirus cytolytic for CD4+ (L3T4+) T lymphocytes. *Journal of Experimental Medicine* 169:591–596.

Morse, S.S., Sakaguchi, N., & Sakaguchi, S. (1999) Virus and autoimmunity: induction of autoimmune disease in mice by mouse T lymphotropic virus (MTLV) destroying CD4+ T cells. *Journal of Immunology* 162:5309–5316.

Rowe, W.P. & Capps, W.I. (1961) A new mouse virus causing necrosis of the thymus in newborn mice. *Journal of Experimental Medicine* 113:831–844.

St-Pierre, Y., Potworowski, E.F., & Lussier, G. (1987) Transmission of mouse thymic virus. *Journal of General Virology* 68:1173–1176.

Wood, B.A., Dutz, W., & Cross, S.S. (1981) Neonatal infection with mouse thymic virus: spleen and lymph node necrosis. *Journal of General Virology* 57:139–147.

Parvovirus Infections

Besselsen, D.G. (1998) Detection of rodent parvoviruses by PCR. *Methods in Molecular Biology* 92:31–37.

Besselsen, D.G., Pintel, D.J., Purdy, G.A., Besch-Williford, C.L., Franklin, C.L., Hook, R.R., Jr., & Riley, L.K. (1996) Molecular characterization of newly recognized rodent parvoviruses. *Journal of General Virology* 77:899–911.

Besselsen, D.G., Romero, M.J., Wagner, A.M., Henderson, K.S., & Livingston, R.S. (2006) Identification of novel murine parvovirus strains by epidemiological analysis of naturally infected mice. *Journal of General Virology* 87:1543–1556.

Besselsen, D.G., Wagner, A.M., & Loganbill, J.K. (2000) Effect of mouse strain and age on detection of mouse parvovirus 1 by use of serologic testing and polymerase chain reaction analysis. *Comparative Medicine* 50:498–502.

Brownstein, D.G., Smith, A.L., Jacoby, R.O., Johnson, E.A., Hansen, G., & Tattersall, P. (1991) Pathogenesis of infection with a virulent allotropic variant of minute virus of mice and regulation by host genotype. *Laboratory Investigation* 65:357–364.

Christie, R.D. Marcus, E.C., Wagner, A.M., & Besselsen, D.G. (2010) Experimental infection of mice with hamster parvovirus: evidence for interspecies transmission of mouse parvovirus 3. *Comparative Medicine* 60:123–129.

Hanson, G.M., Paturzo, F.X., & Smith, A.L. (1999) Humoral immunity and protection of mice challenged with homotypic or heterotypic parvovirus. *Laboratory Animal Science* 49:380–384.

Harris, R.E., Coleman, P.H., & Morahan, P.S. (1974) Erythrocyte association and interferon production of minute virus of mice. *Proceedings of the Society for Experimental Biology and Medicine* 145:1288–1292.

Jacoby, R.O., Ball-Goodrich, L.J., Besselsen, D.G., McKisic, M.D., Riley, L.K., & Smith, A.L. (1996) Rodent parvovirus infections. *Laboratory Animal Science* 46:292–299.

Kilham, L. & Margolis, G. (1970) Pathogenicity of minute virus of mice (MVM) for rats, mice and hamsters. *Proceedings of the Society for Experimental Biology and Medicine* 133:1447–1452.

Kilham, L. & Margolis, G. (1971) Fetal infections of hamsters, rats, and mice induced with the minute virus of mice (MVM). *Teratology* 4:43–62.

Livingston, R.S., Besselsen, D.G., Steffen, E.K., Besch-Williford, C.L., Franklin, C.L., & Riley, L.K. (2002) Serodiagnosis of mice minute virus and mouse parvovirus infections in mice by enzyme-linked immunosorbent assay with baculovirus-expressed recombinant VP2 proteins. *Clinical Diagnostic and Laboratory Immunology* 9:1025–1031.

Macy, J.D., Cameron, G.A., Smith, P.C., Ferguson, T.A., & Compton, S.R. (2011) Detection and control of mouse parvovirus. *Journal of the American Association for Laboratory Animal Science* 50:516–522.

McKisic, M.D., Macy, J.D., Jr., Delano, M.L., Jacoby, R.O., Paturzo, F.X., & Smith, A.L. (1998) Mouse parvovirus infection potentiates allogeneic skin graft rejection and induces syngeneic graft rejection. *Transplantation* 65:1436–1446.

Ramairez, J.C., Fairen, A., & Almendral, J.M. (1996) Parvovirus minute virus of mice strain i multiplication and pathogenesis in the newborn mouse brain are restricted to proliferative areas and to migratory cerebellar young neurons. *Journal of Virology* 70:8109–8116.

Redig, A.J. & Besselsen, D.G. (2001) Detection of rodent parvoviruses by use of fluorogenic nuclease polymerase chain reaction assays. *Comparative Medicine* 51:326–331.

Segovia, J.C., Gallego, J.M., Bueren, J.A., & Almendral, J.M. (1999) Severe leukopenia and dysregulated erythropoiesis in SCID mice persistently infected with the parvovirus minute virus of mice. *Journal of Virology* 73:1774–1784.

Papillomavirus Infection

Handisurya, A., Day, P.M., Thompson, C.D., Bonelli, M., Lowy, D.R., & Schiller, J.T. (2014) Strain-specific properties and T cells regulate the susceptibility to papilloma induction by *Mus musculus* papillomavirus 1. *PLoS Pathogens* 10:e1004314.

Ingle, A., Ghim, S., Joh, J., Chepkoech, I., Bennett Jenson, A., & Sundberg, J.P. (2011) Novel laboratory mouse papillomavirus (MusPV) infection. *Veterinary Pathology* 48:500–505.

Joh, J., Jenson, A.B., King, W., Proctor, M., Ingle, A. Sundberg, J.P., & Ghim, S.J. (2011) Genomic analysis of the first laboratory mouse papillomavirus. *Journal of General Virology* 92:692–698.

Schulz, E., Gottschling, M., Ulrich, R.G., Richter, D., Stockfleth, E., & Nindl, I. (2012) Isolation of three novel rat and mouse papillomaviruses and their genomic characterization. *PLoS One* 7:e47164.

Polyoma Virus Infection

Berebbi, M., Dandolo, L., Hassoun, J., Bernard, A.M., & Blangy, D. (1988) Specific tissue targeting of polyomavirus oncogenicity in athymic nude mice. *Oncogene* 2:144–156.

Buffet, R.F. & Levinthal, J.D. (1962) Polyoma virus infection in mice. *Archives of Pathology* 74:513–526.

Carty, A.J., Franklin, C.L., Riley, L.K., & Besch-Williford, C. (2001) Diagnostic polymerase chain reaction assays for identification of murine polyomaviruses in biological samples. *Comparative Medicine* 51:145–149.

Dawe, C.J. (1979) Tumors of the salivary and lachrymal glands, nasal fossa and maxillary sinuses. In: *Pathology of Tumours in Laboratory Animals. II. Tumours of the Mouse* (ed. V.S. Turusov). IARC Scientific Publications, Lyon, France.

Dawe, C.J., Freund, R., Barncastle, J.P., Dubensky, T.W., Mandel, G., & Benjamin, T.L. (1987) Necrotizing arterial lesion in mice bearing tumors induced by polyoma virus. *Journal of Experimental Pathology* 3:177–201.

Demengeot, J., Jacquemier, J., Torrente, M., Blangy, D., & Berebbi, M. (1990) Pattern of polyomavirus replication from infection until tumor formation in the organs of athymic nu/nu mice. *Journal of Virology* 64:5633–5639.

Dubensky, T.W., Murphy, F.A., & Villarreal, L.P. (1984) Detection of DNA and RNA virus genomes in organ systems of whole mice: patterns of mouse organ infection by polyomavirus. *Journal of Virology.* 50:779–783.

Gross, L. (1953) A filterable agent recovered from AK leukemic extracts, causing salivary gland carcinomas in C3H mice. *Proceedings of the Society for Experimental Biology and Medicine* 83:414–421.

Lukacher, A.E., Ma, Y., Carroll, J.P., Abromson-Leeman, S.R., Laning, J.C., Dorf, M.E., & Benjamin, T.L. (1995) Susceptibility to tumors induced by polyoma virus is conferred by an endogenous mouse mammary tumor virus superantigen. *Journal of Experimental Medicine* 181:1683–1692.

McCance, D.J. & Mims, C.A. (1979) Reactivation of polyomavirus in kidneys of persistently infected mice during pregnancy. *Infection and Immunity* 25:998–1002.

McCance, D.J., Sebesteny, A., Griffin, B.E., Balkwill, F., Tilly, R., & Gregson, N.A. (1983) A paralytic disease in nude mice associated with polyoma virus infection. *Journal of General Virology* 64:57–67.

Rowe, W.P. (1961) The epidemiology of mouse polyoma virus infection. *Bacteriological Reviews.* 25:18–31.

Sebesteny, A., Tilly, R., Balkwill, F., & Trevan, D. (1980) Demyelination and wasting associated with polyomavirus infection in nude (nu/nu) mice. *Laboratory Animal Science* 14:337–345.

Stewart, S.E. (1960) The polyoma virus. *Advances in Virus Research* 7:61–90.

Szomolanyi-Tsuda, E., Dundon, P.L., Joris, L., Shultz, L.D., Woda, B.A., & Welsh, R.M. (1994) Acute, lethal, natural killer cell-resistant myeloproliferative disease induced by polyomavirus in severe combined immunodeficient mice. *American Journal of Pathology* 144:359–371.

Vandeputte, M., Eyssen, H., Sobis, H., & De Somer, P. (1974) Induction of polyoma tumors in athymic nude mice. *International Journal of Cancer* 14:445–450.

Wirth, J.J., Amalfitano, A., Gross, R., Oldstone, M.B., & Fluck, M.M. (1992) Organ- and age-specific replication of polyomavirus in mice. *Journal of Virology* 66:3278–3286.

K Virus Infection

Fisher, E.R. & Kilham, L. (1953) Pathology of a pneumotropic virus recovered from C3H mice carrying the Bittner milk agent. *Archives of Pathology* 55:14–19.

Greenlee, J.E. (1979) Pathogenesis of K virus infection in newborn mice. *Infection and Immunity* 26:705–713.

Greenlee, J.E. (1981) Effect of host age on experimental K virus infection in mice. *Infection and Immunity* 33:297–303.

Greenlee, J.E. (1986) Chronic infection of nude mice by murine K papovavirus. *Journal of General Virology* 67:1109–1114.

Greenlee, J.E., Phelps, R.C., & Stroop, W.G. (1991) The major site of murine K papovavirus persistence and reactivation is the renal tubular epithelium. *Microbial Pathogenesis* 11:237–247.

Greenlee, J.E., Clawson, S.H., Phelps, R.C., & Stroop, W.G. (1994) Distribution of K-papovavirus in infected newborn mice. *Journal of Comparative Pathology* 111:259–268.

Ikeda, K., Dorries, K., & ter Meulen, V. (1988) Morphological and immunohistochemical studies of the central nervous system involvement in papovavirus K infection in mice. *Acta Neuropathologica (Berlin)* 77:175–181.

Kilham, L. & Murphy, H.W. (1953) A pneumotropic virus isolated from C3H mice carrying the Bittner milk agent. *Proceedings of the Society for Experimental Biology and Medicine* 82:133–137.

Margolis, G., Jacobs, L.R., & Kilham, L. (1976) Oxygen tension and the selective tropism of K virus for mouse pulmonary endothelium. *American Review of Respiratory Disease* 114:4–51.

Mayer, M. & Dories, K. (1991) Nucleotide sequence and genome organization of the murine polyomavirus, Kilham strain. *Virology* 181:469–480.

Mokhtarian, F. & Shah, K.V. (1980) Role of antibody response in recovery from K papovavirus infection in mice. *Infection and Immunity* 29:1169–1179.

Mokhtarian, F. & Shah, K.V. (1983) Pathogenesis of K papovavirus infection in athymic nude mice. *Infection and Immunity* 41:434–436.

Poxvirus Infection

Allen, A.M., Clarke, G.L., Ganaway, J.R., Lock, A., & Werner, R.M. (1981) Pathology and diagnosis of mousepox. *Laboratory Animal Science* 31:599–608.

Bhatt, P.N. & Jacoby, R.O. (1987) Effect of vaccination on the clinical response, pathogenesis and transmission of mousepox. *Laboratory Animal Science* 37:610–614.

Bhatt, P.N. & Jacoby, R.O. (1987) Mousepox in inbred mice innately resistant or susceptible to lethal infection with ectromelia virus. I. Clinical responses. *Laboratory Animal Science* 37:11–15.

Bhatt, P.N. & Jacoby, R.O. (1987) Mousepox in inbred mice innately resistant or susceptible to lethal infection with ectromelia virus. III. Experimental transmission of infection and derivation of virus-free progeny from previously infected dams. *Laboratory Animal Science* 37:23–27.

Brownstein, D.G. & Gras, L. (1997) Differential pathogenesis of lethal mousepox in congenic DBA/2 mice implicates natural killer cell receptor NKR-PI in necrotizing hepatitis and the fifth component of complement in recruitment of circulating leukocytes to the spleen. *American Journal of Pathology* 150:1407–1420.

Dick, E.J., Jr., Kittell, C.L., Meyer, H., Farrar, P.L., Ropp, S.L., Esposito, J.J., Buller, R.M., Neubauer, H., Kang, Y.H., & McKee, A.E. (1996) Mousepox outbreak in a laboratory mouse colony. *Laboratory Animal Science* 46:602–611.

Esteban, D. & Buller, R. (2005) Ectromelia virus: the causative agent of mousepox. *Journal of General Virology* 86:2645–2659.

Fenner, F. (1949) Mouse pox (infectious ectromelia of mice): a review. *Journal of Immunology* 63:341–373.

Fenner, F. (1981) Mousepox (infectious ectromelia): past, present, and future. *Laboratory Animal Science* 31:553–559.

Jaboby, R.O. & Bhatt, P.N. (1987) Mousepox in inbred mice innately resistant or susceptible to lethal infection with ectromelia virus. II. Pathogenesis. *Laboratory Animal Science* 37:16–22.

Labelle, P., Hahn, N.E., Fraser, J.K., Kendall, L.V., Ziman, M., James, E., Shastri, N., & Griffey S.M. (2009) Mousepox detected in a research facility: case report and failure of mouse antibody production testing to identify Ectromelia virus in contaminated mouse serum. *Comparative Medicine* 59:180–186.

Lipman, N.S., Perkins, S., Nguyen, H., Pfeffer, M., & Meyer, H. (2000) Mousepox resulting from use of ectromelia virus-contaminated, imported mouse serum. *Comparative Medicine* 50:426–435.

Marchal, J. (1930) Infectious ectromelia: a hitherto undescribed virus disease of mice. *Journal of Pathology and Bacteriology* 33:713–718.

Wallace, G.W. & Buller, R.M.L. (1985) Kinetics of ectromelia virus (mousepox) transmission and clinical response in C57BL/6J, BALB/cByJ and AKR/J inbred mice. *Laboratory Animal Science* 35:41–46.

RNA Viral Infections

Arenavirus (LCMV) Infection

Borrow, P. & Oldstone, M. (1997) Lymphocytic choriomeningitis virus. In: *Viral Pathogenesis* (eds. N. Nathanson, R. Ahmed, F. Gonzalez-Scarano, D.E. Griffin, K.V. Holmes, F.A. Murphy, & H.L. Robinson,), pp. 593–627. Lippincott-Raven, Philadelphia, PA.

Dykewicz, C.A., Dato, V.M., Fisher-Hoch, S.P., Howarth, M.V., Perez-Oronoz, G.I., Ostroff, S.M., Gary, H., Jr., Schonberger, L.B., & McCormick, J.B. (1992) Lymphocytic choriomeningitis outbreak associated with nude mice in a research institute. *Journal of the American Veterinary Medical Association* 267:1349–1353.

Gossmann, J., Lohler, J., Utermohlen, O., & Lehmann-Grube, F. (1995) Murine hepatitis caused by lymphocytic choriomeningitis virus II. Cells involved in pathogenesis. *Laboratory Investigation* 72:559–570.

Homberger, F.R., Romano, T.P., Seller, P., Hansen, G.M., & Smith, A.L. (1995) Enzyme-linked immunosorbent assay for detection of antibody to lymphocytic choriomeningitis virus in mouse sera, with recombinant nucleoprotein as antigen. *Laboratory Animal Science* 45:493–496.

Lehmann-Grube, F. (1971) Lymphocytic choriomeningitis virus. *Virology Monographs* 10:1–173.

Lehmann-Grube, F. & Lohler, J. (1981) Immunopathologic alterations of lymphatic tissues of mice infected with lymphocytic choriomeningitis virus. II. Pathogenetic mechanisms. *Laboratory Investigation* 44:205–213.

Lehmann-Grube, F., Martinez Peralta, L., Bruns, M., & Lohler, J. (1983) Persistent infection of mice with the lymphocytic choriomeningitis virus. In: *Comprehensive Virology* (eds. H. Fraenkel-Conrat & R. Wagner), pp. 43–103. Plenum, New York.

Lilly, R.D. & Armstrong, C. (1945) Pathology of lymphocytic choriomeningitis in mice. *Archives of Pathology* 40:141–152.

Mims, C. (1966) Immunofluorescence study of the carrier state and mechanisms of vertical transmission in lymphocytic choriomeningitis virus infection in mice. *Journal of Pathology and Bacteriology* 91:395–402.

Oldstone, M. (2002) Biology and pathogenesis of lymphocytic choriomeningitis virus infection. *Current Topics in Microbiology and Immunology* 263:83–117.

Traub, E. (1936) The epidemiology of lymphocytic choriomeningitis in white mice. *Journal of Experimental Medicine* 64:183–200.

Arterivirus (LDV) Infection

Anderson, G.W., Even, C., Rowland, R.R., Palmer, G.A., Harty, J.T., & Plageman, P.G.W. (1995) C58 and AKR mice of all ages develop motor neuron disease after lactate dehydrogenase-elevating virus infection but only if antiviral immune responses are blocked by chemical or genetic means or as a result of old age. *Journal of Neurovirology* 1:244–252.

Anderson, G.W., Rowland, R.R., Palmer, G.A., Even, C., & Plageman, P.G.W. (1995) Lactate dehydrogenase-elevating virus replication persists in liver, spleen, lymph node, and testis tissues and results in accumulation of viral RNA in germinal centers, concomitant with polyclonal activation of B cells. *Journal of Virology* 69:5177–5185.

Carlson-Scholz, J.A. & Garg, R.A. (2011) Poliomyelitis in MuLV-infected ICR-SCID mice after injection of basement membrane matrix contaminated with lactate dehydrogenase-elevating virus. *Comparative Medicine* 61:404–411.

Chen, Z., Li, K., & Plageman, P.G.W. (2000) Neuropathogenicity and sensitivity to antibody neutralization of lactate dehydrogenase-elevating virus are determined by polylactosaminoglycan chains on the primary envelope glycoprotein. *Virology* 266:88–98.

Chen, Z. & Plageman, P.G.W. (1997) Detection of lactate dehydrogenase-elevating virus in transplantable mouse tumors by biological and RT-PCR assays and its removal from the tumor cells. *Journal of Virological Methods* 65:227–236.

Chen, Z., Li, K., Rowland, R.R., & Plagema, P.G.W. (1999) Selective antibody neutralization prevents neuropathogenic lactate dehydrogenase-elevating virus from causing paralytic disease in immunocompetent mice. *Journal of Neurovirology* 5:200–208.

Snodgrass, M.J., Lowery, D.S., & Hanna, M.G., Jr. (1972) Changes induced by lactic dehydrogenase virus in thymus and thymus-dependent areas of lymphatic tissue. *Journal of Immunology* 108:877–892.

Van den Broek, M.F., Sporri, R., Even, C., Plagemann, P.G., Hansler, E., Hengartner, H., & Zinkernagel, R.M. (1997) Lactate dehydrogenase-elevating virus (LDV): lifelong coexistence of virus and LDV-specific immunity. *Journal of Immunology* 159:1585–1588.

Wagner, A.M., Loganbill, J.K., & Besselsen, D.G. (2004) Detection of lactate dehydrogenase-elevating virus by use of a fluorogenic nuclease reverse transcriptase polymerase chain reaction. *Comparative Medicine* 54:288–292.

Zitterkopf, N.L., Haven, T.R., Huela, M., Bradley, D.S., & Cafruny, W.A. (2002) Transplacental lactate dehydrogenase-elevating virus (LDV) transmission: immune inhibition of umbilical cord infection, and correlation of fetal virus susceptibility with development of F4/80 antigen expression. *Placenta* 23:438–446.

Astrovirus Infection

Farkas, T., Fey, B., Keller, G., Martella, V., & Egyed, L. (2012) Molecular detection of novel astroviruses in wild and laboratory mice. *Virus Genes* 45:518–525.

Ng, T.F.F., Kondov, N.O., Hayashimoto, N., Uchida, R., Cha, Y., Beyer, A.I., Wong, W., Pesavento, P.A., Suemizu, H., Muench, M.O., & Delwart, E. (2013) Identification of an astrovirus commonly infecting laboratory mice in the US and Japan. *PLoS One* 8:e66937.

Yokoyama, C.C., Loh, J., Zhao, G., Stappenbeck, T.S., Wang, D., Huang, H.V., & Virgin, H.W. (2012) Adaptive immunity restricts replication of novel murine astroviruses. *Journal of Virology* 86:12262–12270.

Coronavirus (MHV) Infection

Bailey, O.T., Pappenheimer, A.M., Cheever, F.S., & Daniels, J.B. (1949) A murine virus (JHM) causing disseminated encephalomyelitis with extensive destruction of myelin. II. Pathology. *Journal of Experimental Medicine* 90:195–221.

Barthold, S.W. (1988) Olfactory neural pathway in mouse hepatitis virus nasoencephalitis. *Acta Neuropathologica* 76:502–506.

Barthold, S.W., Beck, D.S., & Smith, A.L. (1983) Enterotropic corononvirus (MHV) in mice: influence of host age and strain on infection and disease. *Laboratory Animal Science* 43:276–284.

Barthold, S.W. & Smith, A.L. (1987) Response of genetically susceptible and resistant mice to intranasal inoculation with mouse hepatitis virus. *Virus Research* 7:225–239.

Barthold, S.W. & Smith, A.L. (1989) Virus strain specificity of challenge immunity to coronavirus. *Archives of Virology* 104:187–196.

Barthold, S.W., Smith, A.L., Lord, P.F.S., Bhatt, P.N., & Jacoby, R.O. (1982) Epizootic coronaviral typhlocolitis in suckling mice. *Laboratory Animal Science* 32:376–383.

Barthold, S.W., Smith, A.L., & Povar, M.L. (1985) Enterotropic mouse hepatitis virus infection in nude mice. *Laboratory Animal Science* 35:613–618.

Biggers, D.C., Kraft, L.M., & Sprinz, H. (1964) Lethal intestinal virus in mice (LIVIM): an important new model for study of the response of the intestinal mucosa to injury. *American Journal of Pathology* 45:413–427.

Croy, B.A. & Percy, D.H. (1993) Viral hepatitis in *scid* mice. *Laboratory Animal Science* 43:193–194.

France, M.P., Smith, A.L., Stevenson, R., & Barthold, S.W. (1999) Granulomatous peritonitis and pleuritis in interferon gamma gene knockout mice naturally infected with mouse hepatitis virus. *Australian Veterinary Journal* 77:600–604.

Gustafsson, E., Blomqvist, G., Bellman, A., Homdahl, R., Mattson, A., & Mattson, R. (1996) Maternal antibodies protect immunoglobulin deficient mice from mouse hepatitis virus (MHV)-associated wasting syndrome. *American Journal of Reproductive Immunology* 36:33–39.

Homberger, F.R. & Barthold, S.W. (1992) Passively acquired challenge immunity to enterotropic coronavirus in mice. *Archives of Virology* 126:35–43.

Homberger, F.R., Barthold, S.W., & Smith, A.L. (1992) Duration and strain-specificity of immunity to enterotropic mouse hepatitis virus. *Laboratory Animal Science* 42:347–351.

Homberger, F.R., Smith, A.L., & Barthold, S.W. (1991) Detection of rodent coronaviruses in tissues and cell cultures using polymerase chain reaction. *Journal of Clinical Microbiology* 29:2789–2793.

Norovirus Infection

Hsu, C.C., Wobus, C.E., Steffen, E.K., Riley, L.K., & Livingston, R.S. (2005) Development of a microsphere-based serologic multiplexed fluorescent immunoassay and reverse transcriptase PCR assay to detect murine norovirus 1 infection in mice. *Clinical and Diagnostic Laboratory Immunology* 12:1145–1151.

Hsu, C.C., Riley, L.K., Wills, H.M., & Livingston, R.S. (2006) Persistent infection with and serologic cross-reactivity of three novel murine noroviruses. *Comparative Medicine* 56:247–251.

Karst, S.M., Wobus, C.E., Lay, M., Davidson, J., & Virgin, H.W., IV (2003) STAT1-dependent innate immunity to a Norwalk-like virus. *Science* 299:1575–1578.

Kelmenson, J.A., Pomerleau, D.P., Griffey, S.M., Zhang, W., Karolak, M.J., & Fahey, J.R. (2009) Kinetics of transmission, infectivity, and genome stability of two novel mouse norovirus isolates in breeding mice. *Comparative Medicine* 59:27–36.

Mumphrey, S.M., Changotra, H., Moore, T.N., Heimann-Nicols, E.R., Wobus, C.E., Reilly, M.J., Moghadamfalahi, M., Shukla, D., & Karst, S.M. (2007) Murine norovirus 1 infection is associated with histopathological changes in immunocompetent hosts, but clinical disease is prevented by STAT1-dependent interferon responses. *Journal of Virology* 81:3251–3263.

Thackray, L.B., Wobus, C.E., Chachu, K.A., Liu, B., Alegre, E.R., Henderson, K.S., Kelly, S.T., & Virgin, H.W., IV (2007) Murine noroviruses comprising a single genogroup exhibit biological diversity despite limited sequence divergence. *Journal of Virology* 81:10460–10473.

Ward, J.M., Wobus, C.E., Thackray, L.B., Erexson, C.R., Faucette, L.J., Belliot, G., Barron, E.L., Sosnovtsev, S.V., & Green, K.Y. (2006) Pathology of immunodeficient mice with naturally-occurring murine norovirus infection. *Toxicologic Pathology* 34:708–715.

Wobus, C.E., Karst, S.M., Thackray, L.B., Chang, K.O., Sosnovtsev, S.V., Belliot, G., Krug, A., Mackenzie, J.M., Green, K.Y., & Virgin, H.W. (2004) Replication of norovirus in cell culture reveals a tropism for dendritic cells and macrophages. *PLoS Biology* 2: e432.

Wobus, C.E., Thackray, L.B., & Virgin, H.W., Jr. (2006) Murine norovirus: a model system to study norovirus biology and pathogenesis. *Journal of Virology* 80:5104–5112.

Pneumonia Virus of Mice (PVM) and Sendai Virus Infection

Anh, D.B., Faisca, P., & Desmecht, D.J. (2006) Differential resistance/susceptibility patterns to pneumovirus infection among inbred mouse strains. *American Journal of Physiology. Lung, Cellular and Molecular Physiology* 291:L426–435.

Bray, M.V., Barthold, S.W., Sidman, C.L., Roths, J., & Smith, A.L. (1993) Exacerbation of *Pneumocystis carinii* pneumonia in immunodeficient (*scid*) mice by concurrent infection with pneumovirus. *Infection and Immunity* 61:1586–1588.

Brownstein, D.G. (1987) Resistance/susceptibility to lethal Sendai virus infection genetically linked to a mucociliary transport polymorphism. *Journal of Virology* 61:1670–1671.

Brownstein, D.G., Smith, A.L., & Johnson, E.A. (1981) Sendai virus infection in genetically resistant and susceptible mice. *American Journal of Pathology* 105:156–163.

Brownstein, D.G. & Winkler, S. (1986) Genetic resistance to lethal Sendai virus pneumonia: virus replication and interferon production in C57BL/6J and DBA/2J mice. *Laboratory Animal Science* 36:126–129.

Carthew, P. & Sparrow, S. (1980) A comparison in germ-free mice of the pathogenesis of Sendai virus and mouse pneumonia virus infections. *Journal of Pathology* 130:153–158.

Carthew, P. & Sparrow, S. (1980) Persistence of pneumonia virus of mice and Sendai virus in germ-free (nu/nu) mice. *British Journal of Pathology* 61:172–175.

Faisca, P. & Desmecht, D. (2006) Sendai virus, the mouse parainfluenza type 1: a longstanding pathogen that remains up-to-date. *Research in Veterinary Science* 82:115–125.

Itoh, T., Iwai, H., & Ueda, K. (1991) Comparative lung pathology of inbred strains of mice resistant and susceptible to Sendai virus infection. *Journal of Veterinary Medical Science* 53:275–279.

Jacoby, R.O., Bhatt, P.N., Barthold, S.W., & Brownstein, D.G. (1994) Sendai viral pneumonia in aged BALB/c mice. *Experimental Gerontology* 29:89–100.

Jakob, G. (1981) Interactions between Sendai virus and bacterial pathogens in the murine lung: a review. *Laboratory Animal Science* 31:170–177.

Percy, D.H., Auger, D.C., & Croy, B.A. (1994) Signs and lesions of experimental Sendai virus infection in two genetically distinct strains of SCID/bg mice. *Veterinary Pathology* 31:67–73.

Richter, C.B., Thigpen, J.E., Richter, C.S., & MacKenzie, J.M., Jr. (1988) Fatal pneumonia with terminal emaciation in nude mice caused by pneumonia virus of mice. *Laboratory Animal Science* 38:255–261.

Skiadopoulos, M.H., Surman, S.R., Riggs, J.M., Elkins, W.R., St Claire, M., Nishio, M., Garcin, D., Kolakofsky, D., Collins, P.L., & Murphy, B.R. (2002) Sendai virus, a murine parainfluenza virus type 1, replicates to a level similar to human PIV1 in the upper and lower respiratory tract of African green monkeys and chimpanzees. *Virology* 297:153–160.

Smith, A.L., Carrono, V.A., & Brownstein, D.G. (1984) Response of weanling random-bred mice to infection with pneumonia virus of mice (PVM). *Laboratory Animal Science* 34:35–37.

Wagner, A.M., Loganbill, J.K., & Besselsen, D.G. (2003) Detection of Sendai virus and pneumonia virus of mice by use of flurogenic nuclease reverse transcriptase polymerase chain reaction analysis. *Comparative Medicine* 53:173–177.

Weir, E.C., Brownstein, D.G., Smith, A.L., & Johnson, E.A. (1988) Respiratory disease and wasting in athymic mice infected with pneumonia virus of mice. *Laboratory Animal Science* 38:133–137.

Picornavirus (MEV) Infection

Abzug, M.J., Rotbart, H.A., & Levin, M.J. (1989) Demonstration of a barrier to transplacental passage of murine enteroviruses in late gestation. *Journal of Infectious Diseases* 159:761–765.

Brownstein, D., Bhatt, P., Ardito, R., Paturzo, F., & Johnson, E. (1989) Duration and patterns of transmission of Theiler's mouse encephalomyelitis virus infection. *Laboratory Animal Science* 39:299–301.

Gomez, R.M., Rinehart, J.E., Wollmann, R., & Roos, R.P. (1996) Theiler's mouse encephalomyelitis virus-induced cardiac and skeletal muscle disease. *Journal of Virology* 70:8926–8933.

Rozengurt, N. & Sanchez, S. (1992) Vacuolar neuronal degeneration in the ventral horns of SCID mice in naturally occurring Theiler's encephalomyelitis. *Journal of Comparative Pathology* 107:389–398.

Rozengurt, N. & Sanchez, S. (1993) A spontaneous outbreak of Theiler's encephalomyelitis in a colony of severe combined immunodeficient mice in the UK. *Laboratory Animals* 27:229–234.

Zurbriggen, A. & Fujinami, R.S. (1988) Theiler's virus infection in nude mice: viral RNA in vascular endothelial cells. *Journal of Virology* 62:3589–3596.

Reovirus Infection

Barthold, S.W., Smith, A.L., & Bhatt, P.N. (1993) Infectivity, disease patterns, and serologic profiles of reovirus serotypes 1, 2, and 3 in infant and weanling mice. *Laboratory Animal Science* 43:425–430.

Bennette, J.G., Bush, P.V., & Steele, R.D. (1967) Characteristics of a newborn runt disease induced by neonatal infection with an oncolytic strain of reovirus type 3 (REO3MH). I. Pathological investigations in rats and mice. *British Journal of Experimental Pathology* 48:251–266.

Bennette, J.G., Bush, P.V., & Steele, R.D. (1967) Characteristics of a newborn runt disease induced by neonatal infection with an oncolytic strain of reovirus type 3 (REO3MH). II. Immunological aspects of the disease in mice. *British Journal of Experimental Pathology* 48:267–284.

Branski, D., Lebenthal, E., Faden, H.S., Hatch, T.P., & Krasner, J. (1980) Reovirus type 3 infection in a suckling mouse: the effects on pancreatic structure and enzyme content. *Pediatric Research* 14:8–11.

George, A., Kost, S.I., Wizleben, C.L., Cebra, J.J., & Rubin, D.H. (1990) Reovirus-induced liver disease in severe combined immunodeficient (SCID) mice: a model for the study of viral infection, pathogenesis, and clearance. *Journal of Experimental Medicine* 171:929–934.

Papadimitriou, J.M. (1968) The biliary tract in acute murine reovirus 3 infection: light and electron microscopic study. *American Journal of Pathology* 52:595–611.

Papadimitriou, J.M. & Walters, M.N.-I. (1967) Studies on the exocrine pancreas. II. Ultrastructural investigation of reovirus pancreatitis. *American Journal of Pathology* 51:387–403.

Phillips, P.A., Keast, D., Papadimitriou, J.M., Walters, M.N., & Stanley, N.F. (1969) Chronic obstructive jaundice induced by reovirus type 3 in weanling mice. *Pathology* 1:193–203.

Stanley, N.F. (1974) The reovirus murine models. *Progress in Medical Virology* 18:257–272.

Uchiyma, A. & Besselsen, D.G. (2003) Detection of reovirus type 3 by use of flurogenic nuclease reverse transcriptase polymerase chain reaction. *Laboratory Animals* 37:352–359.

Walters, M.N., Leak, P.J., Joske, R.A., Stanley, N.F., & Perret, D.H. (1965) Murine infection with reovirus. 3. Pathology of infection with types 1 and 2. *British Journal of Experimental Pathology* 46:200–212.

Walters, M.N., Joske, R.A., Leak, P.J., & Stanley, N.F. (1963) Murine infection with reovirus. I. Pathology of the acute phase. *British Journal of Experimental Pathology* 44:427–436.

Rotavirus Infection

Blutt, S.E., Fenaux, M., Warfield, K.L., Greenberg, H.B., & Conner, M.E. (2006) Active viremia in rotavirus-infected mice. *Journal of Virology* 80:6702–6705.

Boshuizen, J.A., Reimerink, J.H., Korteland-van Male, A.M., van Ham, V.J., Koopmans, M.P., Buller, H.A., Dekker, J., & Einerhand, A.W. (2003) Changes in small intestinal homeostasis, morphology, and gene expression during rotavirus infection of infant mice. *Journal of Virology* 77:13005–13016.

Coelho, K.I.R., Bryden, A.S., Hall, C., & Flewett, T.H. (1981) Pathology of rotavirus infection in suckling mice: a study by conventional histology, immunofluorescence, and scanning electron microscopy. *Ultrastructural Pathology* 2:59–80.

Lundgren, O., Peregrin, A.T., Persson, K., Kordasti, S., Uhnoo, I., & Svensson, L. (2000) Role of enteric nervous system in the fluid and electrolyte secretion of rotavirus diarrhea. *Science* 287:491–495.

McNeal, M.M., Rae, M.N., & Ward, R.L. (1997) Evidence that resolution of rotavirus infection in mice is due to both CD4 and CD8 cell-dependent activities. *Journal of Virology* 71:8735–8742.

Riepenhoff-Talty, M., Dharakul, T., Kowalski, E., Michalak, S., & Ogra, P.L. (1987) Persistent rotavirus infection in mice with severe combined immunodeficiency. *Journal of Virology* 61:3345–3348.

Riepenhoff-Talty, M., Dharakul, T., Kowalski, E., Sherman, D., & Ogra, P.L. (1987) Rotavirus infection in mice: pathogenesis and immunity. *Advances in Experimental Biology and Medicine* 216:1015–1023.

Retrovirus Infection

Boeke, J.D. & Stoye, J.P. (1997) Retrotransposons, endogenous retroviruses, and the evolution of retroelements. In: *Retroviruses* (eds. J.M. Coffin, S.H. Huges, & H.E. Varmus), pp. 343–435. Cold Spring Harbor Press, New York.

Erianne, G.S., Wajchman, J., Yauch, R., Tsiagbe, V.K., Kim, B.S., & Ponzio, N.M. (2000) B cell lymphomas of C57L/J mice; the role of natural killer cells and T helper cells in lymphoma development and growth. *Leukemia Research* 24:705–718.

Gardner, M.B. (2008) Search for oncogenic retroviruses in wild mice and man: historical reflections. *Cancer Therapy* 6:285–302.

Gardner, M.B. & Rasheed, S. (1982) Retroviruses in feral mice. *International Review of Experimental Pathology* 23:209–267.

Pobezinskay, Y., Chervonsky, A.V., & Colovkina, T.V. (2004) Initial stages of mammary tumor virus infection are superantigen independent. *Journal of Immunology* 172:5582–5587.

Ribet, D., Dewannieux, M., & Heidmann, T. (2004) An active murine transposon family pair: retrotransposition of "master" MusD copies and ETn trans-mobilization. *Genetics Research* 14:2261–2267.

Rosenberg, N. & Jolicoeur, P. (1997) Retroviral pathogenesis. In: *Retroviruses* (eds. J.M. Coffin, S.H. Huges, & H.E. Varmus), pp. 475–585. Cold Spring Harbor Press, New York.

Taddesse-Heath, L., Chattopadhyay, S.K., Dillehay, D.L., Lander, M.R., Nagashfar, Z., Morse, H.C., III, & Hartley, J.W. (2000) Lymphomas and high-level expression of murine leukemia viruses in CFW mice. *Journal of Virology* 74:6832–6837.

Thomas, R.M., Haleem, K., Siddique, A.B., Simmons, W.J., Sen, N., Zhang, D.J., & Tsiagbe, V.K. (2003) Regulation of mouse mammary tumor virus env transcriptional activator initiated mammary tumor virus superantigen transcripts in lymphomas of SJL/J mice: role of Ikaros, demethylation, and chromatin structural change in the transcriptional activation of mammary tumor virus superantigen. *Journal of Immunology* 170:218–227.

Zhao, Y., Jacobs, C.P., Wang, L., & Hardies, S.C. (1999) MuERVC: a new family of murine retrovirus-related repetitive sequences and its relationship to previously known families. *Mammalian Genome* 10:477–481.

BACTERIAL INFECTIONS

Bacterial Enteric Infections
Brachyspira spp. Infection

Wild rodents, including house mice, have been shown to carry a wide variety of *Brachyspira* spp., including pathogenic porcine and avian *Brachyspira* spp., and mice are experimentally susceptible to infection. In addition to known *Brachyspira* spp., wild mice have also been found to carry slow-growing and weakly hemolytic spirochetes that represent a novel species within the genus *Brachyspira*. Infection among laboratory mice has not been reported, but the authors of this book have observed natural infection in NSG mice (Fig. 1.48). In addition to culture, *Brachyspira* organisms can be detected and speciated by PCR.

Citrobacter rodentium Infection: Transmissible Murine Colonic Hyperplasia

Citrobacter rodentium causes a syndrome in mice called transmissible murine colonic hyperplasia (TMCH). It has also been termed "hyperplastic colitis," "catarrhal enterocolitis," and "colitis cystica." Unlike most *Citrobacter* spp., pathogenic mouse isolates are nonflagellated and nonmotile. Isolates from different outbreaks possess similar sugar fermentation and other biochemical profiles, but minor differences exist. The causative agent was formerly classified as *Citrobacter freundii* but has been reclassified as *C. rodentium*. TMCH promotes the

evolution of preneoplastic and neoplastic change during chemical carcinogenesis and in *Apc*$^{+/Min}$ (Min) mice. *Citrobacter rodentium* has gained popularity as a model for the pathogenesis of attaching and effacing *E. coli*, as it possesses an analogous genetic pathogenicity island. Thus, there is increased potential for iatrogenic introduction of this pathogen to laboratory mouse populations.

Epizootiology and Pathogenesis

TMCH has been reported in laboratory mice in the United States, Europe, and Japan, but its prevalence in wild mice is unknown. *Citrobacter rodentium* appears to be highly species-specific in its host range. When present in a mouse population, it is associated with disease. The bacterium does not establish itself as permanent microflora and is not subclinically carried by mice. Its source of introduction into mouse colonies is presumably through contaminated food or bedding. The organism spreads slowly among mice, requiring direct contact or fecal contamination. Following oral inoculation, *C. rodentium* transiently colonizes the small intestine, and then selectively colonizes the cecum and colon within 4 days. The bacteria intimately attach in large numbers to surface mucosa of the descending colon, displacing other aerobic bacteria. Bacterial attachment is facilitated by a genetic pathogenicity island encoding bacterial intimin and type III secreted bacterial proteins, including the translocated intimin receptor (Tir). These proteins induce dissolution of the brush border, actin filament rearrangement, and pedestal formation by the plasma membrane (Fig. 1.49), similar to attaching and effacing enteropathogenic *E. coli* (EPEC) and enterohemorrhagic *E. coli* (EHEC). Through undefined mechanisms, bacterial colonization elicits an intense mucosal epithelial hyperplasia. The acquired immune response is important in clearance of infection but also contributes to

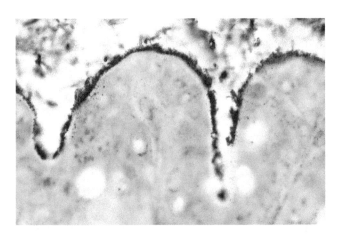

FIG. 1.48. Brachyspira *spp. infection of the intestine in a NSG mouse. Note the numerous bacteria attached to the brush border. (Warthin–Starry stain).*

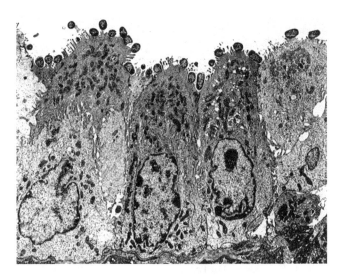

FIG. 1.49. *Electron micrograph of* Citrobacter rodentium *attached to colonic enterocytes. Note the intimate attachment of bacteria with disruption of the brush border. (Source: Johnson et al. 1979. Reproduced with permission from Elsevier.)*

inflammation and morbidity. As hyperplastic cells migrate to the surface, they displace infected cells, which are exfoliated from the surface. Peak hyperplastic response occurs within 2–3 weeks, at which point the causative agent may no longer be isolated from the colon. Clinical signs are most prominent at this interval. Young mice and certain mouse genotypes (C3H substrains, AKR, and FVB) tend to develop more severe disease with varying mortality due to secondary inflammatory and ulcerative lesions in the hyperplastic mucosa. DBA/2, BALB/c, B6, and NIH Swiss mice are susceptible to hyperplasia, but tend to develop less inflammation. In the ensuing weeks, lesions regress with a period of excessive goblet cell differentiation and development of cryptal cysts that can fill with mucin. By 2 months, the mucosa returns to normal. There is no known carrier state, and recovered mice are refractory to reinfection.

Studies have dissected the role of host immune response in controlling infection and in modulating the severity of disease, using a variety of GEMs with specific immune defects. Innate defenses, including beta defensins, IL-12, and IFN-gamma, affect early colonization and growth of the bacteria. Infection stimulates an acquired immune response, with recruitment of CD4 T cells into the mucosa, and the evolution of a Th1-polarized T-cell-dependent systemic antibody response. T-cell-dependent serum antibodies (IgM, IgG2c, or IgG2a), but not secretory IgA or IgM, are involved in clearance of infection and recovery, and this response does not require T- or B-cell responses in gut-associated lymphoid tissue. Effective immunity requires CD4 T cells and B cells but not CD8 T cells. The acquired immune response is necessary for clearance, but it is also a major factor in disease severity, since hyperplasia and inflammation are more severe in immunocompetent mice compared to *Rag-1* null mice. Mice devoid of B and T cells (*Rag-1* null), CD4 T cells, or B cells (*μMT* null) fail to clear infection and succumb from sepsis, with bacteremia arising from both *C. rodentium* and other gut bacteria.

Pathology

Affected mice may be runted and have sticky, unformed feces that smear the cage walls. Rectal prolapse often occurs (Fig. 1.50). Careful examination of the bowel will reveal a contracted, thickened, opaque, descending colon devoid of feces (Fig. 1.51). Lesions can extend into the transverse colon. The cecum is also frequently but variably involved. During the early stages of infection, the brush border of surface mucosa of affected bowel is heavily colonized by a carpet of intimately attached cocco-bacillary bacteria. As the lesion progresses, these infected cells are pushed aside by uninfected, hyperplastic epithelium, with retention of cells at the extrusion zones (Fig. 1.52). Inflammation and erosion can also occur, especially in infant mice or mice of certain genotypes or immune status, as discussed

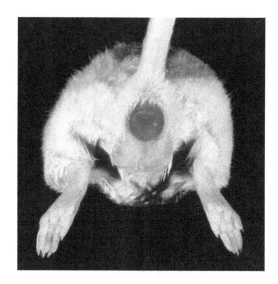

FIG. 1.50. *Rectal prolapse in a mouse with transmissible murine colonic hyperplasia due to* Citrobacter rodentium.

above. In mice that are incapable of mounting effective immunity, mortality occurs from bacteremia, with multifocal hepatitis and splenitis. As the hyperplasia regresses, cells can undergo differentiation into excessive numbers of goblet cells, and crypts can become distended with mucin and cellular debris (colitis cystica). Once regression is complete, the mucosa returns to normal. Secondary focal nonspecific ischemic necrosis and inflammation may arise in the liver during early infection.

Diagnosis

Infection is transient with no carrier state in immunocompetent mice. The causative agent is often absent when clinical signs are most apparent. Infection can be localized to the descending colon, and only a small percentage of mice in the population may be infected because of its low contagiousness. Isolation is enhanced

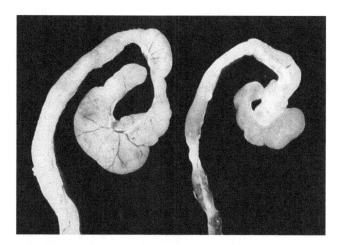

FIG. 1.51. *Cecum and colon of a mouse infected with* Citrobacter rodentium *(left) compared to a normal mouse (right). The infected bowel is contracted, opaque, and devoid of feces. (Source: Barthold et al. 1978. Reproduced with permission from SAGE Publications.)*

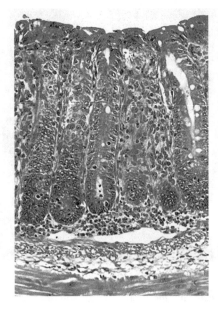

FIG. 1.52. *Descending colon from a mouse infected with* Citrobacter rodentium. *There is marked hyperplasia of the crypt epithelium with retention of cells on the surface and leukocytic infiltration in the lamina propria.*

by culturing feces or descending colon from multiple mice in the early stages of infection before clinical signs are evident. Citrobacter can be readily isolated on Mac-Conkey agar. Differential diagnoses include other agents that cause hyperplastic colitis, including *E. coli* and *Helicobacter* spp. Hyperplastic colitis has also been observed in nude mice chronically infected with enterotropic MHV. Rectal prolapse is frequently associated with TMCH, but can also occur spontaneously or in association with colitis of other causes.

Clostridium difficile *and* Clostridium perfringens: *Clostridial Enteropathy*

Clostridial enteropathy is typically associated with stressors or situations that induce intestinal dysbiosis, allowing opportunistic overgrowth. Clostridial enteropathy occurs sporadically in the mouse due to infection with toxigenic *C. difficile* and *C. perfringens.*

Epizootiology and Pathogenesis

Clostridium difficile causes enteropathy in many species, including the laboratory mouse. Toxigenic *C. difficile* produces two exotoxins known as *C. difficile* Toxin A (TcdA) and Toxin B (TcdB). *Clostridium perfringens* may produce one or more major exotoxins that are associated with disease in many species. Exotoxins define *C. perfringens* into 5 major types (A through E). Type A is most often associated with production of enterotoxin, but any type can produce enterotoxin. Natural disease in laboratory mice has been associated with *C. perfringens* nontype A, type A, type B, and type D. Anecdotal observations have associated outbreaks with high carbohydrate diets, inadequate normal microbial flora in

barrier-maintained pathogen-free colonies, reduced frequency of cage changing, and peak lactation.

Pathology

Enteropathy due to *C. difficile* has been common in mice from one commercial vendor. Lesions are similar to enteropathy associated with *C. perfringens* (below), and involve the small and/or large intestine. Clostrial enteropathy due to *C. perfringens* has been reported in mice ranging from 2 to 52 days of age and female mice of breeding age. Clinically affected mice have distended abdomens, soft feces, and sudden death. Both the small and large intestine may be dilated with gas and fluid, with mucosal hyperemia, petechiae, ulceration, and fibrinous pseudomembrane formation. Intestinal rupture and peritonitis may occur. In addition to inflammatory and hyperplastic changes in the mucosa of the small and/or large intestine (Fig. 1.53), multiple focal atypia were described in the duodenal mucosa of monocontaminated BALB/c mice, as well as atrial thrombosis and pulmonary inflammation. Intestinal lumina contain large numbers of rod-shaped Gram-positive bacteria. Affected mice have generalized lymphoid apoptosis and renal tubular vacuolation. In the recovery phase, the intestinal mucosa may be diffusely or segmentally hyperplastic. Disease outbreaks have been reported among cesarean rederived mice that had been associated with a limited bacterial flora, recently weaned clean conventional mice, and *C. perfringens*-contaminated axenic mice.

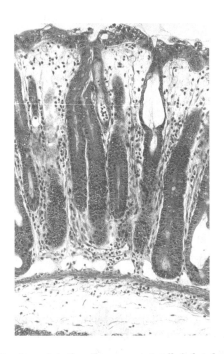

FIG. 1.53. *Large intestine of a mouse naturally infected with* Clostridium difficile. *There is moderate hyperplasia of crypts with marked edema and leukocytic infiltration of the mucosa and submucosa.*

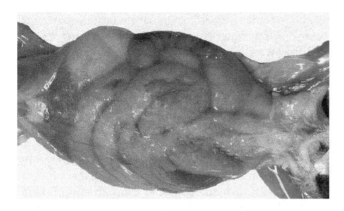

FIG. 1.54. *Postparturient lactating mouse with markedly dilated intestine filled with fluid and gas. The mouse has been skinned, and the intestine is visible through the unincised abdominal wall. This syndrome may be Clostridial in origin. (Source: Feinstein et al. 2008. Reproduced with permission from American Association for Laboratory Animal Science.)*

A spontaneous disease, which has been termed "paralysis of peristalsis in lactating mice," occurs in lactating dams of various genetic backgrounds, with mortality up to 40%. The syndrome is manifest as sudden death, usually during the second week of their first lactation. There may be fecal staining in the perineal region with distention of the abdomen. The stomach is usually slightly dilated and filled with watery fluid. The proximal small intestine is distended with fluid contents. Firm, conical fecal plugs may be present in the ileum and the tip of the cecum. Histological findings have been reported to be unremarkable, and pathogenic organisms were not recovered from the intestine or other tissues. More recently, similar syndromes have been described in which affected mice had segmental distention of the small intestine with fluid and gas (Fig. 1.54). Histology revealed widespread apoptosis of villus enterocytes, as well as surface epithelium in the large intestine. *Clostridium perfringens* A was incriminated in one report, in which mice had sudden death and necrohemorrhagic enteropathy. These syndromes are likely to be Clostridial in origin, with the common feature of peak lactation.

Diagnosis
A presumptive diagnosis can be based upon clinical history and intestinal lesions containing overgrowth of Gram-positive rods. Culture does not necessarily incriminate the bacterium, since they are often present without disease and may not be toxigenic. Although detection of exotoxins in the intestinal content is desirable, assays are generally not available, expensive, or insensitive due to lability of toxins. PCR can be used to speciate organisms and determine presence of toxin genes. Differential diagnoses include Tyzzer's disease and (in the recovery phase) causes of hyperplastic enteritides (*Citrobacter*, *Helicobacter*, *E. coli*, etc.).

Clostridium piliforme *Infection: Tyzzer's Disease*
Tyzzer's disease was first recognized and characterized by Ernest Tyzzer in 1917. He described an epizootic that decimated a colony of Japanese waltzing mice. The organism is now recognized to produce disease in a wide variety of other species, including rats, gerbils, hamsters, guinea pigs, and rabbits, but there is evidence for some degree of species specificity among different isolates. For decades, the causative agent was called *Bacillus piliformis*. However, based on 16S rRNA gene sequence analysis, it is now classified as *C. piliforme*. The organism is a spore-forming, Gram-negative, filamentous bacterium that can only be propagated in living cells.

Epizootiology and Pathogenesis
Infection occurs by ingestion of spores. Shed in the feces, spores can survive in contaminated bedding for at least 1 year, and in the natural environment for at least 5 years. Vertical transmission does not occur under natural conditions, although intrauterine transmission has been produced experimentally in mice inoculated intravenously. Based on serological assessment, up to 80% or more of clinically normal mice from known infected colonies may have detectable antibodies to the organism. Outbreaks of Tyzzer's disease in mice are usually characterized by low morbidity and high mortality in affected animals. Mouse strain, age, and immune status are factors in susceptibility to the disease. For example, DBA/2 mice are susceptible, and B6 mice are resistant to Tyzzer's disease. Depletion of NK cells in resistant adult B6 mice, but not DBA mice, rendered them more susceptible, and neutrophil depletion rendered both juvenile DBA and B6 mice more susceptible to disease. Macrophage depletion did not appear to influence susceptibility to disease. Infected DBA and B6 mice develop elevations in IL-12, and neutralization of IL-12 renders infected mice more susceptible to disease. Disease resistance also appears to be due, at least in part, to B-lymphocyte function. CBA/N and C3.CBA/N mice, which are B-cell-deficient, have been found to be more susceptible than immunocompetent or T-cell-deficient nude mice. T-cell-deficient nude mice were shown to be as resistant to the disease as immunocompetent mice. However, in one report of a spontaneous outbreak of Tyzzer's disease in a colony of nude mice, homozygous nude mice were particularly susceptible to high mortality compared with heterozygous mice. These apparent differences in nude mouse susceptibility may be related to the *C. piliforme* isolate, as the virulent isolate proved to be the first toxigenic isolate recovered from mice. In outbreaks of Tyzzer's disease, predisposing factors include overcrowding, poor sanitation, and experimental procedures that may compromise the immune response.

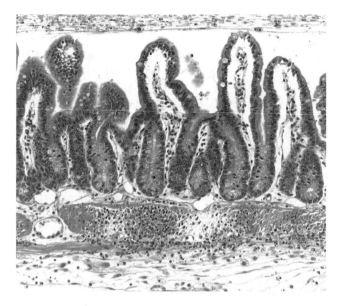

FIG. 1.55. *Small intestine of a mouse with acute Tyzzer's disease due to* Clostridium piliforme. *Villi are blunted and there is acute necrosis of the muscularis mucosae.*

Pathology

Infection is often subclinical, but sudden death and diarrhea may occur in immunodeficient mice. The primary lesion arises in the mucosa of the intestine, with grossly visible reddening of the ileum and cecum. Microscopically, foci of degeneration, inflammation, edema, and necrosis are evident in the intestinal mucosa and muscularis mucosae (Fig. 1.55). Clusters of organisms are apparent in enterocytes, but also in the smooth muscle and neurons of Auerbach's plexus. Lymphatic vessels and sinuses of mesenteric lymph nodes may contain cellular debris. Miliary pale foci or larger umbilicated foci are usually visible throughout the parenchyma of the liver (Fig. 1.56), and foci can be particularly large and umbilicated in immunodeficient mice. Lesions are characterized by multifocal coagulation to caseation hepatic necrosis, with polymorphonuclear leukocyte infiltration. Gray foci in the ventricular myocardium may

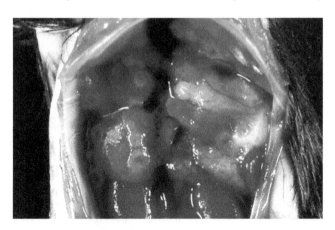

FIG. 1.56. *Liver of a mouse with Tyzzer's disease. Note the multiple pale umbilicated lesions on the capsular surface. (Source: R. Bunte. Duke University, Singapore. Reproduced with permission from R. Bunte.)*

also be present, with myocyte degeneration, myocarditis, and intracellular bacteria. In tissue sections stained with the Warthin–Starry, Giemsa, or PAS methods, typical intracytoplasmic bundles of bacilli are usually readily found in enterocytes, hepatocytes adjacent to necrotic foci, and myocardial cells (see Gerbil Chapter 4, "*Clostridium piliforme* Infection").

Diagnosis

The diagnosis of Tyzzer's disease can be confirmed by demonstration of the pathognomonic clusters of intracellular bacilli in tissue sections, using the appropriate stains. The typical bacilli may also be visualized in impression smears prepared from liver lesions and stained using the Giemsa method. Serologic assays are available and utilize whole bacterial lysates as antigen, but have proven to be inaccurate due to the antigenic diversity among *C. piliforme* isolates. *Clostridium piliforme* can be isolated by inoculation of embryonated hen's eggs, primary mouse or chick embryo cell cultures, primary mouse or chick liver cells, and several continuous cell lines. PCR amplification of *C. piliforme* in feces is an effective method of detection. The cortisone provocation test may be warranted to test for subclinical carrier animals. Differential diagnoses include diseases such as MHV infection, mousepox, salmonellosis, pseudomoniasis, corynebacteriosis, infections with *Helicobacter* spp., and Clostridial enteropathy.

Escherichia coli *Infection:* Coliform Typhlocolitis

A syndrome resembling *C. rodentium* and *Helicobacter* spp. colonic hyperplasia in immunodeficient mice has been associated with an atypical, non-lactose-fermenting *E. coli*.

Epizootiology and Pathogenesis

Large intestinal hyperplastic lesions have been observed primarily in young adult triple-deficient N:NIH(S)III (homozygous for *nu, xid, bg*) and to a lesser extent double-deficient mice. Other immunocompetent and partially deficient mice were infected without significant hyperplastic lesions. Bacteria were located in the gut lumen, attached to the surface, and within enterocytes. This syndrome has also been observed in SCID mice (Barthold, unpublished). These outbreaks are associated with an unusual non-lactose-fermenting *E. coli*, but its primary role as a pathogen remains to be determined. An outbreak of diarrhea and colonic mucosal hyperplasia was reported in DDY mice in Japan, which was associated with an atypical *E. coli* strain called mouse pathogenic *E. coli* (MPEC), but subsequent analysis has revealed that the MPEC agent was *C. rodentium*.

Pathology

Mice are depressed, with perianal fecal staining. Gross necropsy findings are limited to mild to moderate segmental thickening of colon or cecum (Fig. 1.57) and

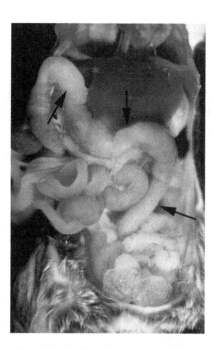

FIG. 1.57. *Hyperplastic colitis due to* Escherichia coli *infection in a SCID mouse. Note the segmental thickening of the colon (arrows), unlike the involvement of the descending colon in mice infected with* Citrobacter freundii *and diffuse involvement in mice infected with* Helicobacter *spp.*

occasional blood-tinged feces. Microscopic findings consist of mucosal hyperplasia in one or all segments of colon, with variable inflammation and erosion similar to *C. freundii*. Coliform bacteria are present in the gut lumen, attached to the surface, and within enterocytes of superficial mucosa of both small and large intestine.

Diagnosis

Segmental hyperplastic lesions in the colon and cecum of immunodeficient mice and isolation of atypical *E. coli* are required to confirm the diagnosis. The causative agent is non-lactose-fermenting, an unusual feature of *E. coli*. Differential diagnoses must include hyperplastic typhlocolitis caused by *C. rodentium* (which ferments lactose and is pathogenic in immunocompetent mice), *Helicobacter* spp., and enterotropic MHV in immunodeficient mice. Unlike *C. rodentium*, which invariably affects descending colon, *E. coli* lesions are segmental and usually affect other portions of the colon.

Helicobacter *spp. Infections*

Helicobacter spp. have emerged as a major group of gastrointestinal commensals with pathogenic potential in the laboratory mouse. Mice serve as hosts to several named species and additional novel isolates that are yet to be formally named. Named species include *H. hepaticus*, *H. bilis*, *H. muridarum*, *H. rodentium*, *H. typhlonius*, *H. ganmani*, *H. rappini*, *H. mastomyrinus*, *H. magdeburgensis*, and *H. pullorum*. In addition, *H. muricola* has been isolated from the cecum of Korean wild mice (*M.m. molossinus*), and other novel species are continually

being added to this list as they are isolated and characterized. *Helicobacter* spp. are microaerobic, curved to spiral rods with variable numbers of flagella. Each species has a somewhat distinctive electron microscopic appearance, which underscores their genetic (and antigenic) diversity. In the mouse, *Helicobacter* spp. occupy an enterohepatic niche and colonize the cecum and colon, with variable presence in the liver. Most immunocompetent mice develop minimal or no liver or intestinal lesions when infected with *Helicobacter* spp., but the pathogenic potential of these bacteria is manifest in a variety of immunodeficient types of mice. When disease occurs, typical lesions consist of hyperplastic typhlocolitis and hepatitis.

There is evidence that *H. bilis* infections in humans may be linked to gall bladder, biliary and liver disease, and associated cancers, and *H. pullorum* is a human pathogen. Aside from their direct pathogenic potential, particularly in immunodeficient mice, the association of *Helicobacter* spp. with promotion of hepatic neoplasia and the presence of invasive and dysplastic intestinal lesions in infected mice have led to claims that *Helicobacter* is a carcinogen. *Helicobacter hepaticus* (and probably other *Helicobacter* spp.) is associated with an increase in hepatocellular tumors in certain strains of infected mice, and has also been shown to promote experimental chemical hepatocarcinogenesis. *Helicobacter* typhlocolitis is extensively used as a model for human "inflammatory bowel disease" (IBD). *Helicobacter* typhlocolitis occurs in a variety of GEMs due to their various immunodeficiencies and is a classic example of "the disappearing phenotype syndrome" when GEM models are microbially rederived. The dysplastic and invasive nature of hyperplastic crypt epithelium, particularly when the mucosa is inflamed or eroded, may mimic neoplasia. These features, as well as proliferative kinetics (mitotic index and BUDR labeling patterns), lend credence to misinterpretation of lesions, with the use of terms like "carcinoma in situ" and "nonmetastatic colon cancer." Similar lesions have been shown to arise in the colon of mice infected with *C. rodentium* that are totally reversible upon recovery. Although claims of neoplasia may or may not be valid, it is incumbent upon a pathologist who is familiar with mouse biology and biologic characteristics of neoplasia to accurately assess the validity of these lesions as bonafide neoplasia.

Epizootiology and Pathogenesis

Natural outbreaks of hyperplastic typhlocolitis in immunodeficient mice have been associated with multiple species of *Helicobacter*, or (often) mixed infections. Observations by the authors have confirmed that most *Helicobacter* spp. of the mouse are capable of inducing proliferative typhlocolitis in immunodeficient mice, but some isolates may be nonpathogenic commensals. These agents appear to be widespread in conventional colonies of laboratory mice, but as awareness has arisen, there has been a concerted effort to eliminate *Helicobacter* spp. from both commercial and research laboratory settings. *Helicobacter hepaticus* and *H. rodentium* appear to be the most prevalent members of the group among laboratory mice.

Mice are likely exposed to infection through ingestion of contaminated feces, and *Helicobacter* spp. are readily transmitted by contaminated bedding. Colonization of the cecum with *H. hepaticus* has been associated with a significant decrease in the overall diversity of the cecal microflora. In B6 and A/JCr mice inoculated with *H. hepaticus*, the ceca were readily colonized with the organism. Although the ceca of B6 mice were more heavily colonized with *H. hepaticus*, significant lesions were, however, absent, and the inflammatory and immune responses were minimal compared with infected A/JCr mice. *Helicobacter* infections are persistent, with long-term fecal shedding of organisms. Transfer of neonatal mice from infected dams to *Helicobacter*-free foster dams has been found to be successful in eliminating the infection, providing the transfer occurred within the first 24 hours after birth. Cesarean rederivation and embryo transfer are effective means of eliminating infection. It is not safe to assume that infection is limited to intestine and liver in immunodeficient mice, as *H. hepaticus* has been documented to frequently contaminate transplantable human tumor xenografts when passaged through infected SCID mice. There is one report of transplacental infection of *H. hepaticus* in SCID/NCr mice.

In the liver, *H. hepaticus* and *H. bilis* localize and persist indefinitely within the bile canaliculi. Mouse genotype is pivotal in expression of hepatic disease when infected with *H. hepaticus*. A/JCr, SCID/NCr, BALB/cANCr, C3H/HeNCr, and SJL/NCr mice have been found to be susceptible to hepatitis, whereas B6 and B6C3F1 mice are hepatitis-resistant. A/J mice also develop an earlier onset and higher prevalence of hepatocellular tumors when infected with *H. hepaticus*. Studies indicate that multiple genes are involved in genetic susceptibility and resistance to liver disease. Hepatic lesions are more common in male A/JCr mice than females, and the incidence of lesions is increased in mice 6 months of age or older. Other *Helicobacter* spp. may also be associated with hepatitis. For example, *H. bilis* has been associated with hepatitis in outbred Swiss Webster mice.

The pathogenesis of hepatitis and hepatocellular tumors is unknown, but hepatotoxins or autoimmunity to heat shock protein 70 are suspected. Colonization of the liver leads to induction of apoptosis and cellular proliferation, which are linked to promotion of neoplasia. Pathogenesis of typhlocolitis, which has marked inflammatory and hyperplastic features, has been studied in SCID and nude mice as well as GEMs with selective immune deficiencies, including IL-2, IL-10, T-cell receptor (alpha, beta, delta), RAG, MHC class II, and other null mutations. It has been proposed that *Helicobacter* infection induces a highly Th1-polarized mucosal immune response, with production of IL-12, gamma interferon, and tumor necrosis factor (TNF) alpha in the lamina propria, resulting in expression of the epithelial mitogen, keratinocyte growth factor. Adoptive transfer of CD4 T cells expressing high levels of CD45RB into immunodeficient mice infected with *H. hepaticus* accelerates inflammation and hyperplasia, resulting in the conclusion that bowel disease is an immune-mediated disease that is directed against "normal" intestinal microflora.

Pathology

Infections in immunocompetent mice are usually inapparent. Clinical signs in immunodeficient mice include wasting (often complemented by pneumocystosis or other forms of pneumonia in immunodeficient mice) and mortality. Feces may be unformed, sticky, mucoid, or hemorrhagic. Rectal prolapse is a frequent, but nonspecific, sign of colitis in mice. The prolapsed mucosa is usually eroded and markedly inflamed and hyperplastic. These changes are nonspecific and due to the trauma of prolapse and may not be directly associated with *Helicobacter* spp. Thus, other areas of bowel should be examined to confirm the diagnosis. Segmental areas of cecum and colon are grossly thickened and opaque. Affected mucosa is thickened due to varying degrees of crypt hyperplasia, with markedly immature and mitotically active enterocytes occupying the entire crypt column. Typical *Helicobacter* organisms can be readily demonstrated within crypt lumina of the affected sections of gut, using Steiner or other silver staining methods (Fig. 1.58). In severely affected mucosa,

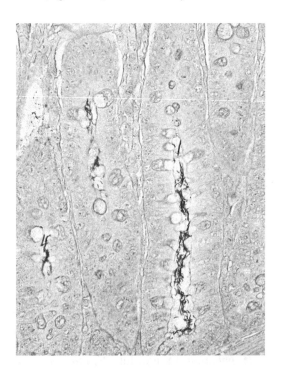

FIG. 1.58. *Colon from an immunodeficient mouse, depicting* Helicobacter *organisms within hyperplastic crypts (Steiner stain).*

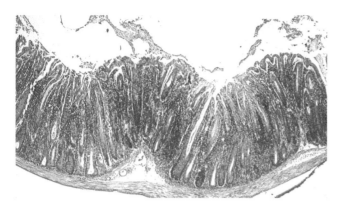

FIG. 1.59. *Colon from a MRL-lpr (immunodeficient) mouse chronically infected with* Helicobacter hepaticus. *There is marked mucosal hyperplasia, with mononuclear cell infiltration in the lamina propria.*

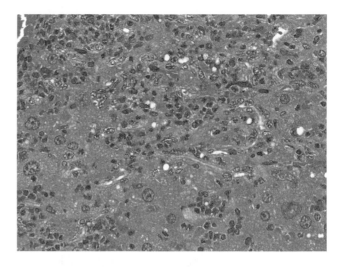

FIG. 1.61. *Liver from a mouse chronically infected with* Helicobacter hepaticus. *Note the hepatocytomegaly, polykarya, Ito cell proliferation, and leukocytic infiltration.*

especially mucosa that has been aggravated by erosion or rectal prolapse, there is often focal crypt dysplasia and invasion of hyperplastic crypts into the underlying submucosa, accompanied by cystic change with mucous retention. Depending upon the mouse genotype and stage of infection, there are varying degrees of mixed leukocytic infiltration in the lamina propria. In some strains, there may be marked lymphocytic infiltration (Fig. 1.59). Although there may be extensive lesions in the large intestine, hepatic lesions may be uncommon. An atypical enteric syndrome has been described in *H. muridarum*-infected mice with gastritis and gastric atrophy, but *Helicobacter* spp. are more typically associated with lower bowel disease in mice.

Hepatic lesions are quite variable. If present, they consist of randomly scattered grossly visible white foci up to 4 mm in diameter. Early lesions may be confined to one or more lobes of the liver, with focal necrosis and mixed leukocytic infiltrates (Fig. 1.60). Within a few months, there is marked hypertrophy and hyperplasia

of Kupffer, Ito, and oval cells, with increased mitotic activity among hepatocytes. There may be prominent bile ductule formation extending from the portal regions with apoptosis of individual hepatocytes. Cellular infiltrates consist primarily of lymphocytes and plasma cells (Fig. 1.61). In typical cases of chronic hepatitis, the elongated, helical microorganisms are best demonstrated within biliary canaliculi using the Steiner silver staining method (Fig. 1.62). Selected strains of mice, such as A/J mice, with *Helicobacter*-associated hepatitis develop foci of cellular alteration, including clear cell, vacuolated, and basophilic foci, with an increased incidence and earlier onset of hepatocellular tumors. C57L mice infected with *H. bilis* and fed a lithogenic diet develop a high frequency of gallstones.

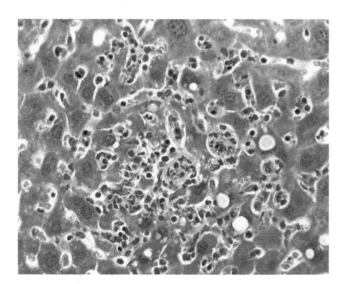

FIG. 1.60. *Liver from a mouse infected with* Helicobacter hepaticus *with focal necrotizing hepatitis.*

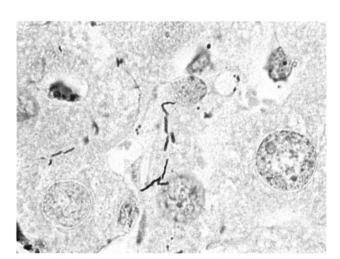

FIG. 1.62. *Liver from a mouse infected with* Helicobacter hepaticus *depicting characteristic* Helicobacter *organisms within bile canaliculi (Steiner stain).*

Diagnosis

Diagnosis is based upon the liver or intestinal lesions, but other etiologic agents must be considered. Definitive diagnosis requires culture, PCR, or demonstration of typical organisms within bile canaliculi or crypts using silver stains. The major challenge to serologic or molecular methods of diagnosis is the antigenic and genetic diversity among the various species of mouse *Helicobacter*. Major impediments to successful serology are the fact that there are no known or useful cross-species *Helicobacter* antigens. Furthermore, immunocompetent mice mount minimal antibody responses, and generally only late in infection. Relatively insensitive serologic assays are available that utilize species-specific membrane antigen extracts or recombinant proteins for detecting serum IgG and fecal IgA. PCR amplification of a conserved segment of 16S rRNA gene can be used to detect most *Helicobacter* spp., and embellished with restriction enzyme analysis to speciate *Helicobacter*. Multiplex species-specific PCR primers have also been developed for discrimination of several species. PCR is frequently used to test feces, but the authors have found that some species of mouse *Helicobacter* may not be consistently shed in feces, or only intermittently so. Optimal PCR detection (and culture) can be achieved by sampling cecal mucosa. Differential diagnosis of liver lesions includes infections with *Salmonella*, *Proteus*, *C. piliforme*, MHV, ectromelia virus, or nonspecific foci of hepatic necrosis and inflammation. Intestinal lesions must be differentiated from those induced by infection with *E. coli*, *C. rodentium*, enterotropic MHV, or the nonspecific lesions of rectal prolapse.

Lawsonia intracellularis *Infection*

Lawsonia intracellularis is emerging as a cause of intestinal disease in an expanding array of mammalian and avian species. It preferentially infects intestinal epithelial cells and induces proliferative enteritis, typhlitis, or colitis, depending upon host species. Natural infection occurs in wild mice, but has not been described in laboratory mice. The authors are aware of infection in pet mice, and laboratory mice are susceptible to infection and disease. Because *Lawsonia* has been documented in laboratory rats, hamsters, guinea pigs, and rabbits, as well as its relative lack of host specificity, it is wise to keep *Lawsonia* in mind as a possible pathogen in mice. Experimental inoculation of 129SvEv and 129-interferon-gamma receptor null mice resulted in hyperplastic inflammation in the ileum and colon. B6 mice were also susceptible. Interferon-gamma receptor null mice were more severely affected, and also developed intestinal hemorrhage. In another experimental study, there was differential susceptibility among a variety of mouse strains to rabbit- and pig-origin *L. intracelluaris*, suggesting some degree of biological specificity among isolates. Enterocytes become colonized by bacteria in the apical cytoplasm, typical of *Lawsonia* infections in other species (see Hamster Chapter 3 and Rabbit Chapter 6, "*Lawsonia intracellularis* infection"). Older mice tend to recover from infection, but the susceptibility and disease course following inoculation of infant mice has not been examined.

Salmonella enterica *Infection:* Salmonellosis

Salmonella, a member of the Enterobacteriaceae, continues to evoke unresolved debate over nomenclature. Among 2,500 serovars, DNA–DNA hybridization suggests that most serovars probably represent a single species, with the exception of *Salmonella bongori*. The Centers for Disease Control and Prevention recognizes only two species, *S. bongori* and *S. enterica*, which is divided into 6 subspecies. Pathogenic serovars belong to *S. enterica* spp. *enterica*. The *Salmonellae* of significance to the mouse are *S. enterica* spp. *enterica* serovar Typhimurium (aka *S. typhimurium*) and serovar Enteritidis (aka *S. enteritidis*). During the first half of the last century, sporadic outbreaks of salmonellosis were a relatively common occurrence in conventional colonies of mice. With improved quality control and husbandry, *Salmonella* infection of laboratory mice is now rare. Nevertheless, *Salmonella* is an extensively utilized experimental model system in mice, allowing opportunity for iatrogenic infections of mouse colonies. In addition, *Salmonella* infection of pet and fancy mice remains a zoonotic risk. Because *Salmonellae* have a broad host range, the danger of interspecies transmission, including zoonotic risk to humans, is an important consideration. Subclinical carrier animals pose a significant risk.

Epizootiology and Pathogenesis

Salmonella enterica serovars Enteritidis and Typhimurium are the most commonly identified natural serovars in mice, and *S. enterica* serovar Typhimurium is a commonly used experimental serovar. Infection is initiated by ingestion of contaminated feed or bedding, although conjunctival inoculation requires fewer organisms to establish an infection. Salmonellae exist intracellularly, stimulate their own uptake by enterocytes, and continue to survive and replicate in macrophages. Host susceptibility or resistance depends on a variety of factors, including age (weanlings are more susceptible than adult mice), gut microflora, strain of mice, virulence and dose of organism, route of inoculation, intercurrent infections, and manipulations that impair the immune response. Normal gut microflora create a natural microbial barrier to infection with *Salmonella*. Susceptibility to experimental infection is often enhanced by pretreatment with Streptomycin to abrogate the microbial barrier. B6, C3H/HeJ, C57BL/10ScCr, and BALB/c mice are highly susceptible, A/J and CBA/N are intermediate, and 129S6/SvEv are resistant. Resistance is mediated through several different factors, including the natural resistance-associated macrophage protein 1 (Nramp1) and TLR4, which explains the susceptibility of C3H/HeJ and C57BL/10ScCr mice. The intermediate susceptibility of CBA/N mice, which have a defect in humoral immunity, can be abrogated by passive transfer of *Salmonella* antiserum.

Following exposure by ingestion, the incubation period is usually 3–6 days. Organisms gain entry to mucosa via fimbrial attachment to M cells, followed by uptake through type III secretion systems that induce phagocytosis by enterocytes, and modification of the intracellular environment of macrophages to allow survival. Initial replication in enterocytes is followed by multiplication in gut-associated lymphoid tissue and then spread to the systemic circulation. In a small percentage of animals, there may be intermittent shedding of the organism in the feces for several months. The organism may also be harbored in the upper respiratory tract in carrier mice. *Salmonella* is readily killed by neutrophils, and neutrophil function is an important factor in resistance, but the bacterium has adapted to grow within macrophages, effectively evading clearance. In the liver, bacteria replicate intracellularly within macrophages, producing focal histiocytic granulomata as the hallmark lesion. Genetically susceptible mice die from massive bacterial proliferation and tissue destruction related to endotoxin.

Pathology

Clinical illness among naturally infected mice is rare, and persistently infected carrier mice are common. Clinical signs, when present, include diarrhea, anorexia, weight loss, conjunctivitis, and variable mortality. Gross findings may include splenomegaly, with multifocal pale miliary foci present on the liver. The alimentary tract is frequently essentially normal. In other cases, there may be ileal hyperemia, and scanty fluid contents may be present in the small and large intestine. Mesenteric lymph nodes can be enlarged and reddened. There may also be scant fibrinous peritoneal exudates. Microscopic changes include multifocal necrosis and venous thrombosis with leukocytic infiltration in the liver, spleen, Peyer's patches, and mesenteric lymph nodes. The hepatic lesions are typically granulomatous in nature (Fig. 1.63). In the terminal small intestine and cecum, there may be edema in the lamina propria and submucosa, with sloughing of enterocytes and leukocytic infiltration.

Diagnosis

Isolation and identification of the organism from sites such as liver, spleen, mesenteric lymph nodes, and intestine are essential and must accompany the standard macroscopic and histopathologic findings. Culture requires enrichment with Selenite F broth plus cysteine, followed by streaking on brilliant green agar. When screening a colony for possible *Salmonella* carriers, culturing of individual fecal samples is more sensitive than using pooled samples, and the highest rate of detection

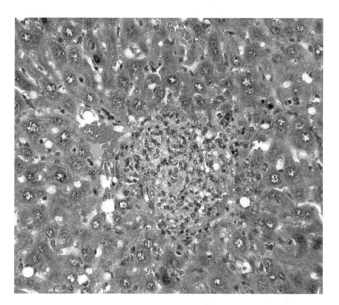

FIG. 1.63. *Liver from a mouse with salmonellosis. The circumscribed lesion consists of aggregations of histiocytes.*

among carriers is achieved by culturing mesenteric lymph node, since fecal shedding is intermittent. Differential diagnoses include Tyzzer's disease, coronaviral hepatitis, mousepox, *Helicobacter* hepatitis, and pseudomoniasis. Spontaneous mesenteric lymphadenopathy (mesenteric disease) can also occur in aging mice.

Segmented Filamentous Bacteria

Segmented filamentous bacteria (SFB) are Gram-positive spore-forming commensal organisms related to *Clostridium* spp. that typically populate the terminal small intestine of many species, including every species covered in this book. They attach end-on to enterocytes (Fig. 1.64), typified by actin polymerization similar to pedicle formation of other attaching and invasive intestinal bacteria. It remains unclear if SFBs from various

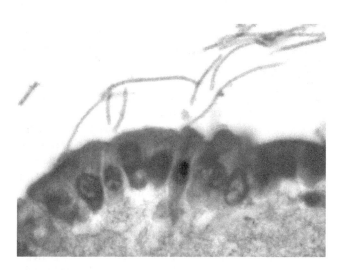

FIG. 1.64. *Ileal mucosa of a normal mouse, featuring segmented filamentous bacteria, with characteristic end-on attachment to the brush border.*

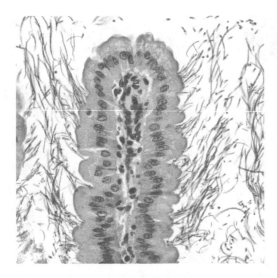

FIG. 1.65. *Ileal villus of an immunodeficient mouse with overgrowth of segmented filamentous bacteria. Note absence of inflammation or hyperplasia. (Source: C. Brayton.)*

hosts represent a single species, but cross-infection studies with ileal homogenates between mice and rats suggest host species specificity. In spite of the fact that SFB are members of the commensal gut microbiome, SFB are considered by some to be undesirable because they elicit physiological and immune responses. Normal maturation of intestinal mucosal proliferative kinetics and function is dependent upon acquisition of commensal gut microflora, including SFB. Overgrowth of SFB has been noted in some GEM (Fig. 1.65) without evidence of mucosal damage or inflammatory response.

Other Gram-Negative Bacterial Infections
Bordetella hinzii *Infection*
Mice in a number of university and research institute mouse colonies in Japan have been found to be infected with *B. hinzii*. The survey was prompted by an index C57BL/6 mouse with sneezing and histopathologic evidence of rhinitis, tracheitis, peribronchiolar lymphoid hyperplasia, and bronchopneumonia. Inoculation of ICR and NOD-SCID mice resulted in similar disease, with NOD-SCID mice developing interstitial pneumonia.

Burkholderia gladioli *Infection*
A single report of barrier-maintained mice with vestibular disorders due to otitis externa, media, and interna has been attributed to *B. gladioli*. Suppurative lesions in other organs also occurred sporadically. Affected mice were all immunodeficient strains. Acidification of water did not preclude infection.

Chlamydia *spp. Infection*
Chlamydiae are obligate intracellular bacteria whose classification and nomenclature are in flux. Current taxonomy features the family Chlamydiaeceae with two genera: *Chlamydophila*, which branches into 3

clusters, including *C. pneumoniae*, *C. pecorum*, and a third group that contains *C. psittaci*, *C. abortus*, *C. caviae*, and *C. felis*; and *Chlamydia*, which branches into two major groups of *C. suis* and a branch containing *C. trachomatis* and *C. muridarum*. There is a growing trend to return to the genus name *Chlamydia* for all chlamydiae. Mice have been shown to be naturally infected with *C. muridarum*, the mouse pneumonitis (MoPn) agent. The MoPn agent has also been referred to as the "Nigg Agent" after Clara Nigg, who discovered the agent following serial intranasal passage of human throat washings during attempts to isolate influenza virus. Natural infections with *C. psittaci* are also suspected, but incompletely confirmed. Mice are experimentally susceptible to both *C. trachomatis* and *C. psittaci* of human origin. Both mouse and human agents are used in laboratory mice as contemporary models for respiratory and genital chlamydiosis and thus can serve as potential iatrogenic sources of infection in mouse colonies.

Epizootiology and Pathogenesis
The prevalence of *C. muridarum* among wild and pet mice is unknown, and it is uncommon or absent in contemporary laboratory mouse populations. There are two widely studied MoPn agents, the Nigg and the Weiss strains. A closely related organism, SFPD, has been isolated from the intestine of hamsters. *Chlamydia muridarum* is closely related to, but genetically distinct from, *C. trachomatis* (bivars trachoma and lymphogranuloma venereum). The MoPn agent is generally believed to be transmitted by respiratory aerosols and/or by venereal transmission, but these routes are based upon experimental assumptions. In fact, contact exposure rarely results in transmission, with evidence for the intestine being the primary target with orofecal transmission. Immunocompetent animals develop transient infections, and infections are typically silent in naturally infected mice. Experimental lung infections are more severe in BALB compared to B6 mice. Immunity to the MoPn agent is dependent upon functional CD4 T cells. B-cell-deficient (Igh6 null) mice recover from infection, but T-cell-deficient RAG, SCID, MHC class II (CD4) null, but not beta-2 microglobulin (CD8) null mice, develop severe disease. Intravaginal inoculation of the MoPn agent results in infection of the exocervical epithelium, with ascending infection of the uterus and oviducts. C3H/HeN mice developed infections of longer duration than BALB/c or B6 mice. Chronic infection of the male genital tract has also been documented experimentally.

In addition, *C. psittaci* infects a wide range of mammals (and birds) and can experimentally cause respiratory and septicemic disease in mice. Documentation of natural infections of laboratory mice with *C. psittaci* is largely presumptive. In one case, intraperitoneal passage of mouse tissues resulted in splenomegaly, hepatomegaly, and serofibrinous peritonitis, and intranasal inoculation resulted in pneumonia following mouse passage.

In another, an agent was isolated following intranasal inoculation with lung tissue from enzootically infected mice, resulting in pulmonary disease. Speciation of the agents in these cases was presumed to be *C. psittaci*, based upon inaccurate methods (sulfadiazine resistance and glycogen staining). Experimental infection with *C. psittaci* is more severe in C3H, BALB/c, or A/J mice, compared to resistant B6 mice.

Pathology

Chlamydiae grow intracellularly, forming discernable elementary and reticulate bodies in the cytoplasm of infected cells. Naturally infected mice are subclinically infected. The pathology that has been described is related to mouse-passaged experimental inoculation. Intranasal inoculation results in suppurative rhinitis, pulmonary perivascular and peribronchiolar lymphocyte infiltration, and nonsuppurative interstitial pneumonia with atelectasis, which can have significant neutrophilic leukocyte infiltration with passage or high dose. Pulmonary lesions are manifest grossly as pinpoint, elevated gray foci on the pleural surfaces. Organisms grow within bronchiolar epithelium, type 1 alveolar cells, and macrophages, which can possess intracytoplasmic vesicles containing inclusions. The MoPn agent readily disseminates hematogenously and by lymphatics to multiple organs, regardless of route of inoculation, due to its tropism for macrophages. It frequently infects peritoneal macrophages. Genitourinary infections are characterized by nonspecific acute and chronic inflammation.

Diagnosis

Diagnosis can be made with impression smears, growth in cell culture, or embryonated chicken eggs. Accurate speciation can now be accomplished by DNA sequencing. Chlamydiae are Gram-negative but stain readily with Giemsa or Macchiavello staining methods.

Cilia-Associated Respiratory Bacillus Infection

Cilia-associated respiratory (CAR) bacilli are widespread and significant respiratory pathogens in rats, commonly infect rabbits, and probably infect mice at a higher rate than is currently recognized. The CAR bacillus is an unclassified, Gram-negative, motile, nonspore-forming bacterium that is closely related genetically with *Flexibacter* spp. and *Flavobacterium* spp. members of the gliding bacteria group. CAR bacilli possess considerable antigenic diversity among isolates from different host species, and the host range is generally restricted to the host of origin. CAR bacilli from various host species are sufficiently different that they may represent different genera. In breeding mouse populations, CAR bacillus is transmitted from infected dams to pups shortly after birth, and infection can be inefficiently transmitted among adult mice by direct contact, but airborne transmission to mice in adjacent cages does not appear to occur.

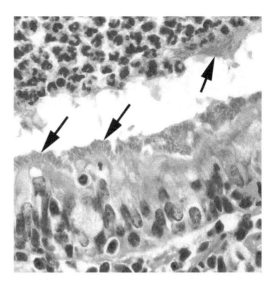

FIG. 1.66. *Respiratory mucosa of a mouse experimentally monoinfected with cilia-associated respiratory (CAR) bacillus. Note rafts of bacteria (arrows) on the epithelial brush border and within the exudate.*

Experimental, and probably natural, infections may be inapparent with no discernable lesions. The organism has been associated with chronic respiratory disease in conventional B6 and B6 obese mutant mice dying with the disease. Chronic suppurative cranioventral bronchopneumonia with marked peribronchiolar infiltration with lymphocytes and plasma cells and luminal neutrophilic exudation were evident microscopically. Warthin–Starry silver impregnation staining revealed typical filamentous CAR bacilli among cilia. Although disease can be experimentally induced by CAR bacillus monoinfection (Fig. 1.66), natural outbreaks of disease in mice seem to be associated with viral infections, including Sendai virus and PVM. Chronic respiratory disease and seroconversion have been produced in BALB/c mice inoculated intranasally with the CAR bacillus, but B6 mice developed less severe lesions and lower antibody responses.

Diagnosis is achieved by silver staining of respiratory tissue to reveal characteristic organisms among cilia of the respiratory epithelium. Organisms can be grown in cell cultures, cell culture medium, and embryonated hens' eggs. Serologic assays utilize bacterial lysates, which are prone to considerable nonspecificity due to cross-reactivity with other bacteria. PCR can be utilized to detect mild or subclinical infections in rodents and can be applied to nasal, oral, and tracheal swabs, with the oral cavity being the most suitable noninvasive site for detecting early infection.

Coxiella burnetii *Infection*

Q fever, caused by *Coxiella burnetii*, is an important zoonotic disease in humans that is usually acquired through contact with ruminants. *Coxiella burnetii* infection has been documented in C.B-17-*scid/beige* mice that received fetal bovine xenografts. Mice developed multifocal necrotizing hepatitis with Kupffer cell hyperplasia, Ito cell hyperplasia, and sinusoidal neutrophil and macrophage infiltration. Basophilic cytoplasmic inclusions (organisms) were present in Kupffer cells and macrophages. Other organs were also variably infected.

Klebsiella *spp. Infection*

Klebsiellae are commensal Enterobacteriae of the gastrointestinal tract, but may become opportunistic pathogens. Disease in mice has been associated with *Klebsiella oxytoca* and *K. pneumoniae*. *Klebsiella oxytoca* has been associated with suppurative female reproductive tract lesions in a large population of aging B6C3F mice. Other organisms isolated from affected mice included *K. pneumoniae*, *E. coli*, *Enterobacter*, and others. Aged mice had suppurative endometritis in association with cystic endometrial hyperplasia, salpingitis, and perioophoritis and/or peritonitis, often resulting in the formation of abscesses and adhesions (Fig. 1.67). *Klebsiella oxytoca* has also been associated with a wide range of opportunistic infections in a number of different strains of mice of all ages from a large commercial supplier of mice, including perianal dermatitis, preputial abscesses, otitis, tooth infections, urogenital infections, pneumonia, and bacteremic disease. Higher morbidity has been observed in immunodeficient female breeder NSG mice, which were prone to development of acute and chronic ascending urinary tract infections. *Klebsiella pneumoniae* has been associated with bacteremic disease in mice with cervical

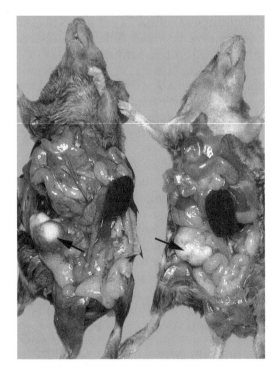

FIG. 1.67. *Female mice with abscesses (arrows) involving the abdominal viscera associated with chronic* Klebsiella oxytoca *infection. (Source: T.R. Schoeb, University of Alabama, Tuscaloosa, Alabama. Reproduced with permission from T.R. Schoeb.)*

lymphadenopathy, liver and kidney abscesses, empyema, pneumonia, ventricular endo- and myocarditis, and thrombosis. Diagnosis is based on isolation of the agent in association with lesions that are not necessarily specific for *Klebsiella*.

Leptospira *spp. Infection: Leptospirosis*

Leptospirae defy attempts at logical nomenclature and classification. Prior to 1989, the genus *Leptospira* was divided into two species, *Leptospira interrogans*, which contained all pathogenic strains, and *Leptospira biflexa*, which contained saphrophytic strains. These were divided into over 200 *L. interrogans* and 60 *L. biflexa* serovars, and serovars were clustered into related serogroups. Genome analysis has resulted in an alternative classification scheme, with nearly 20 genomospecies, but these groups do not correlate in any way with former species, serovar, or pathogenicity. Thus, the serological classification still prevails. Individual serotypes tend to prefer a single maintenance host, but may infect many different host species. Mice can be infected with a number of *Leptospira* serotypes, but *Leptospira ballum* is the most common. Leptospirosis is a zoonotic disease and is the most geographically widespread zoonotic disease in the world. Human infections have been acquired from both pet and laboratory mice infected with *L. ballum*. Clinical manifestations of leptospirosis in humans are highly varied, including the most severe icteric form of infection, Weil's disease, characterized by renal and liver failures. Humans can become infected when handling subclinically infected mice, and infection is usually acquired through abraded skin and conjunctiva.

Pathology

Infection of wild mice is frequent, but disease is typically silent. Infection of laboratory mice appears to be rare, but testing for this bacterium is seldom performed. Mice do not become clinically ill when naturally infected and develop persistent infections with intermittent shedding of organisms in the urine throughout life. Lesions are absent in naturally acquired infections, but mice are experimentally susceptible to disease. Experimental inoculation of C3H/He mice with *L. interrogans* serovar Icterohaemorrhagiae results in pulmonary fibrinoid vasculitis, thrombosis, and hemorrhage, as well as renal tubular necrosis and interstitial nephritis. T-cell deficiency (CD4 and CD8) increased susceptibility to disease. Infection of C3H/HeJ and C3H-*scid* mice with *L. interrogans* serovar Copenhageni results in lethal disease, characterized by discohesion of hepatic cords, hyperplasia of Kuppfer cells and macrophages, focal hepatic necrosis, interstitial nephritis, and tubular damage, with spirochetes visible in the renal interstitium.

Diagnosis

Leptospirae can be isolated by kidney culture, which should be performed on serial 10-fold dilutions of tissue homogenates because growth inhibition can occur in undiluted samples. PCR can be used for detection of *Leptospira* in tissues and urine and is more sensitive than culture. Serology is also possible; however, mice infected as neonates may become persistently infected but never seroconvert. Under natural conditions, this phenomenon is common.

Mycoplasma spp. Infections

Mycoplasmae are pleomorphic organisms that lack a cell wall and are enclosed by a single limiting membrane. Despite their lack of a cell wall, they are genetically related to several Gram-positive bacteria (*Streptococcus, Lactobacillus, Clostridium,* etc.). Their lack of a cell wall places them within the class Mollicutes. Mice are host to several *Mycoplasma* species, which cluster into two groups, the "pneumoniae" and "hemotropic" groups. With the exception of *Mycoplasma pulmonis*, members of the pneumoniae group are marginally pathogenic or nonpathogenic and inhabit not only the respiratory tract but also the genital tract. Sequence analysis of the 16S rRNA genes has revealed that the genera *Eperythrozoon* and *Hemobartonella*, previously considered Rickettsiae, are hemotropic mycoplasmas (often referred to as hemoplasmas) that infect erythrocytes. These include *Mycoplasma coccoides* (formerly *Eperythrozoon coccoides*) and *Mycoplasma haemomuris* (formerly *Hemobartonella muris*).

Respiratory and Genital Mycoplasmosis

Laboratory mice are host to several *Mycoplasma* species within the pneumoniae group, including *M. pulmonis, M. arthritidis, M. neurolyticum, M. collis,* and *M. muris*. An unclassified *Mycoplasma*, the "gray lung" agent, appears to be distantly related to *M. pulmonis* (84% homology) and more closely related to *M. hominis* (94% homology). The name *M. ravipulmonis* (ravi, gray; pulmonis, lung) has been proposed. *Mycoplasma pulmonis, M. arthritidis,* and *M. neurolyticum* inhabit the upper respiratory tract, and *M. collis* and *M. muris* inhabit the genital tract. Only *M. pulmonis* is a significant natural pathogen that produces respiratory and genital tract disease in mice and rats. *Mycoplasma arthritidis* may cause respiratory disease following intranasal inoculation, but under natural conditions, it is generally nonpathogenic. It is problematic primarily because it can cause seroconversion to *M. pulmonis*. *Mycoplasma arthritidis* may induce arthritis when inoculated intravenously, thereby earning its name, but *M. pulmonis* can induce arthritis naturally or following either intravenous or intranasal inoculation. *Mycoplasma neurolyticum* is the causative agent of "rolling disease," a term used to denote the neurologic signs associated with the exotoxin that follows experimental intracerebral inoculation of the organism in mice. Spontaneous outbreaks of conjunctivitis have been associated with *M. neurolyticum* infection in young mice, but the organism is nonpathogenic under most

conditions and is exceedingly rare or nonexistent among laboratory mice.

Epizootiology and Pathogenesis

Prior to and during the 1960s, infections with *M. pulmonis* were widespread among colonies of laboratory mice. With improvements in management practices, there has been a marked reduction in the prevalence of infected colonies of mice. Exposure occurs by aerosol transmission, but infection may also be venereally transmitted. Newborn animals become infected during the first few weeks of life from contact with infected mothers. Transplacental transmission can occur in rats and is likely, but not documented, in immunodeficient mice with disseminated infections. *Mycoplasma* has the potential of being transmitted through cesarean transfer, embryo transfer, or in vitro fertilization.

Compared with the laboratory rat, mice are relatively resistant to disease, and experimental disease severity is closely linked to inoculum dose. Susceptibility to disease depends upon the strain or isolate of *M. pulmonis*, but also on the genetic strain of mouse. Genetic resistance is complex and does not appear to be *H-2* linked. C57BR, B6, and B10 mice are resistant, whereas C57L, SJL, BALB, A/J, C3H/HeJ, C3H/HeN, C3HeB, SWR, AKR, CBA/N, C58, and DBA/2 mice have been shown to be variably susceptible. Most experimental studies have compared disease between susceptible C3H and resistant B6 mice, and female mice have been found to develop more severe disease. Chronic suppurative arthritis has been produced in immunocompetent mice inoculated intravenously with *M. pulmonis*. Athymic nude, thymectomized, CBA/N (X-linked immunodeficient), and SCID mice inoculated intranasally with *M. pulmonis* develop significantly less severe respiratory disease compared to immunocompetent mice, but have disseminated infection with severe polyarthritis. Spontaneous cases of *M. pulmonis* associated arthritis have not been reported in mice, but the potential for this manifestation is real with the increased use of immunodeficient mice.

Mycoplasma pulmonis colonizes the apical cell membranes of respiratory epithelium and interferes with mucociliary clearance. Mycoplasmosis is exacerbated by viral infections, particularly Sendai virus, by other bacteria, including *Pasteurella pneumotropica*, and by environmental ammonia levels. These cofactors probably play a significant role in driving subclinical mycoplasmal infections into overt disease. *Mycoplasma pulmonis* is mitogenic for B cells, which contributes to the pathology (peribronchiolar lymphoplasmacytic infiltrates) observed in the lungs. CAR bacillus has similar mechanisms of altered mucociliary clearance and B-cell mitogenesis, thereby causing similar disease. Coinfection with CAR bacillus in cases of mycoplasmosis is common. The acquired immune response is important in limiting hematogenous dissemination of the infection, but contributes little to elimination of infection or resolution of disease (for additional information, see Rat Chapter 2, "*M. pulmonis* infection").

Pathology

Infection is often subclinical or mild in mice. In natural outbreaks of disease, affected mice may exhibit weight loss, dyspnea, and a characteristic "chattering" sound. Mice with otitis may display head tilt, circling, or vestibular signs. Mucopurulent exudate may be present in the nasal passages, tympanic bullae, trachea, and major airways. In advanced cases, anteroventral gray-purple areas of atelectasis, bronchiolectasis, bronchopneumonia, and raised yellow-tan nodules with abscessation may be evident on gross examination (Fig. 1.68). On microscopic examination, suppurative rhinitis, with neutrophil and lymphocyte infiltration and hyperplasia of submucosal glands, are characteristic findings. In the respiratory epithelium of the nasal passages and major airways, there may be loss of cilia and flattening of epithelial lining cells. In association with the chronic suppurative process, syncytia may be present in affected nasal mucosa and larynx (Fig. 1.69). Suppurative otitis media (Fig. 1.70) is frequently found, with extension to otitis interna and meningitis in some cases. In the lower respiratory tract, lesions vary from discrete peribronchiolar and perivascular lymphocytic and plasma cell infiltration to chronic suppurative bronchiolitis and alveolitis, with mobilization of alveolar macrophages. In advanced cases, there may be squamous metaplasia of respiratory epithelium, bronchiolectasis, and abscessation, with obliteration of the normal architecture. Mice do not develop the intense peribronchiolar lymphocytic infiltrates and severe bronchiolectasis that are common features of respiratory mycoplasmosis in the rat.

Although more common in the rat, chronic suppurative oophoritis, perioophoritis, salpingitis, and

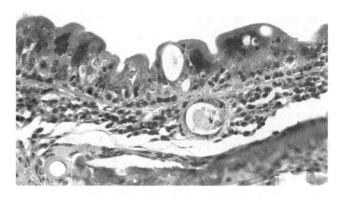

FIG. 1.69.   *Larynx from a mouse with chronic* Mycoplasma pulmonis *infection. Multinucleated giant cells are present in the respiratory epithelium. This is a common feature of the disease in this species that is not seen in rats.*

endometritis are readily induced experimentally in mice and have been reported to occur in naturally infected mice. Isolation from the vagina and uterus of naturally infected mice and mice in contact with experimentally infected mice has also been documented. Disseminated infection in SCID mice has been shown to result in suppurative splenitis, pericarditis, myocarditis, atrioventricular valvulitis, and polyarthritis. Although arthritis has not been described naturally, it is readily induced experimentally in B-cell-deficient, SCID, and C3H/HeN mice.

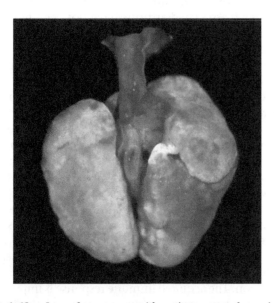

FIG. 1.68.   *Lungs from a mouse with respiratory mycoplasmosis. Note the multiple pale raised bronchiolectatic lesions.*

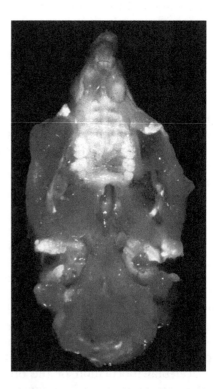

FIG. 1.70.   *Bilateral chronic suppurative otitis media due to* Mycoplasma pulmonis *infection. Note the presence of exudate in the opened tympanic bullae.*

Diagnosis

Gross and microscopic lesions are characteristic. Histological assessment should include a search for syncytia in the upper respiratory tract, a characteristic of mycoplasmosis in mice. Staining procedures such as the Warthin–Starry method should be performed on tissue sections of major airways to determine if there is coinfection with CAR bacillus. Serology, based upon whole bacterial lysate antigen, is widely used for detecting infection in mouse populations. Some infected mice, such as B6 mice or young mice, may have relatively low antibody titers to *M. pulmonis*, and seroconversion to *M. pulmonis* may occur in mice infected with *M. arthritidis*. For culture, nasopharyngeal flushing and tracheobronchial lavages with *Mycoplasma* broth or phosphate-buffered saline are recommended procedures, but cultures are often negative in affected animals and have been supplanted by PCR assays. The respiratory tract should also be cultured for bacteria such as *P. pneumotropica* and serum should be tested for antibody to other respiratory pathogens. Differential diagnoses include bronchopneumonia associated with CAR bacillus, as well as primary infections with Sendai virus and secondary bacterial infections. Otitis media and genital tract inflammation can be caused by a variety of other opportunistic bacteria.

Hemotropic Mycoplasma *Infections*

Mycoplasma (Eperythrozoon) coccoides is naturally transmitted by the louse *Polyplax serrata*, but both the infection and the vector are essentially nonexistent in laboratory mice. The organism is not transmitted transovarially and is not transmitted by other mouse arthropods. With Giemsa and Romanowsky stains, the organism can be found attached to erythrocytes as well as free in the plasma of peripheral blood. In early infection, a high level of parasitemia occurs within a few days, with clinical signs ranging from inapparent to severe anemia and death. Splenomegaly is a prominent feature of this infection, and this organ plays a central role in clearance of the parasite from the blood. Although infection is persistent, mice eventually recover. Wild mice may also be infected with a related hemotropic *Mycoplasma*, *M. haemomuris* (previously *Hemobartonella muris*), which typically infects rats.

Pasteurella pneumotropica *Infection*

Pasteurella pneumotropica frequently infects mice, often without clinical disease. It is associated with a number of lesions in mice as an opportunistic pathogen, but its true nature as a primary pathogen is questionable. However, with the increased use of GEM and immunocompromised mice, the incidence of clinical disease is on the increase. The bacterium acquired its name (*pneumotropica*) because it produced severe pulmonary disease following serial passage and intranasal inoculation. It is not primarily pneumotropic, and colonizes the respiratory, enteric, and genital tracts of clinically normal mice.

Although mice are experimentally susceptible to *Pasteurella multocida*, naturally occurring disease due to *P. multocida* is rare in mice.

Epizootiology and Pathogenesis

Pasteurella pneumotropica is a ubiquitous commensal bacterium in nearly all, if not all, wild mice, and is common among laboratory mouse populations. Elimination of *P. pneumotropica* from a mouse population allows some other Gram-negative bacterium, such as *K. oxytoca*, to fill its opportunistic niche. Infection is typically inapparent, but the bacterium has a propensity to complicate or cause disease in tissues that have been perturbed by other factors. *Pasteurella pneumotropica* is shed from upper respiratory secretions and feces and is spread by direct contact. The vagina and uterus are often colonized without disease, and thus it is transmitted from dam to pups during or shortly after birth. Fetuses can also be infected in utero, which may explain why *P. pneumotropica* is a frequent agent in failure of cesarean rederivation. Seroconversion normally occurs only in mice with overt disease.

Pathology

Disease associated with *P. pneumotropica* is varied, including conjunctivitis, panophthalmitis, dacryoadenitis, periorbital abscessation, rhinitis, otitis (externa, media, and interna), and cervical lymphadenitis. It is also associated with suppurative lesions and abscesses of preputial glands, bulbourethral glands, and muscles. In addition, necrotizing dermatitis, subcutaneous abscesses, mastitis, metritis, and ascending urinary tract infections may occur. Reproductive disorders attributed to *P. pneumotropica* have included abortions and infertility. Immunocompromised and some genetically altered mice are especially susceptible to disease. Severe suppurative bronchopneumonia has been documented in B-cell-deficient mice coinfected with *Pneumocystis murina*. *P. pneumotropica* has also been associated with respiratory disease in immunocompetent mice, primarily in association with *Mycoplasma* or Sendai virus infections.

Diagnosis

Culture of the organism from lesions, with subsequent identification, is required. In live animals, oral swabs or fecal culture appear to be sites of choice for sample collection. Although most strains will grow in conventional media (e.g., blood agar plates), NAD growth factor-requiring strains of *P. pneumotropica* have been identified, as have closely related Pasteurellaceae, including *Actinobacillus muris* and *Haemophilus influenzaemurium*. *Pasteurella ureae* may also cause abortion, metritis, and stillbirths and can be discriminated from *P. pneumotropica* biochemically as indole negative and mannitol positive. PCR assay and DNA extraction are other techniques used to identify the organism. In screening mouse colonies for *P. pneumotropica*, serology is not particularly helpful, since subclinically infected mice are normally seronegative. Differential diagnoses include infections from other pyogenic organisms. The primary cause for *P. pneumotropica* opportunism should be sought, such as predilection for conjunctivitis in BALB mice, fighting injuries, and respiratory tract infections due to *M. pulmonis*, *Pneumocystis*, and Sendai virus.

Proteus mirabilis *Infection*

Proteus mirabilis is a ubiquitous bacterium in the environment and can be isolated from the upper respiratory tract and feces of normal mice. Opportunistic infection resulting in disease has been observed in both immunocompetent and immunodeficient laboratory mice. Based upon the pattern of histologic lesions, infection of internal organs is likely to be hematogenous. Along with *P. aeruginosa*, *P. mirabilis* is known to cause mortality in irradiated mice.

Suppurative pyelonephritis has been reported in male MM mice that are prone to development of diabetes, and nephritis has also been found in male C3H/HeJ mice. In SCID and SCID-beige mice, splenomegaly and multifocal hepatic lesions are typical macroscopic findings. In some cases, fibrinopurulent exudate may be present in the peritoneal cavity (Fig. 1.71). On microscopic examination, there are multifocal areas of coagulation necrosis in the subcapsular regions of the liver and around central veins, with minimal to moderate infiltration with neutrophils. Septic thrombi may be present in vessels of tissues such as liver, intestinal serosa, and pancreas. Pulmonary lesions, when present, are characterized by serous flooding of alveoli and mobilization of

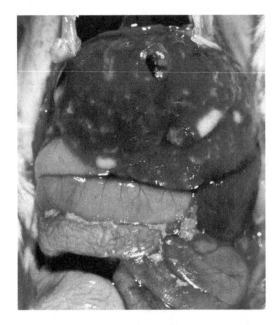

FIG. 1.71.   *Abdominal viscera of a SCID mouse with naturally occurring* Proteus mirabilis *septicemia. Note the irregular focal to coalescing hepatic lesions and the fibrinous exudate in the peritoneal cavity.*

alveolar macrophages. Lung infection has also been found in NADPH oxidase deficient B6.129S6-*Cybb^{tm1Din}*/J mice. In addition to the presence of histological lesions consistent with bacterial sepsis, the recovery of large numbers of *P. mirabilis* from sites such as lung, liver, peritoneal cavity, and kidney will serve to confirm the diagnosis.

Pseudomonas aeruginosa *Infection*

Pseudomonas aeruginosa is a nonspore-forming rod that is widespread in warm, moist environments, including water bottles and sipper tubes, which play a major role in mouse infections. It does not establish itself as part of the mouse microflora, but is frequently isolated from the oropharynx and feces of mice. It is associated with high mortality among mice that are rendered neutropenic or lymphopenic.

Epizootiology and Pathogenesis

Pseudomonas aeruginosa readily grows in water bottle sipper tubes, thereby facilitating cross-contamination among mice within a cage. Following procedures that impair granulocyte production and/or immune function, including X-irradiation, cyclophosphamide treatment, or cortisone treatment, bacteremia is initiated when organisms penetrate nasal and oral mucous membranes. Following treatment with cyclophosphamide, bacteria are detectable at the nasal squamocolumnar junction and gingival epithelium, followed by invasion of regional lymph nodes and subsequent systemic disease. Invasion of *P. aeruginosa* from the intestinal tract, particularly the cecum and colon, is another means of systemic infections. In one study, coinvasion with group B streptococci from the oral cavity may have facilitated the invasion of *Pseudomonas* into the systemic circulation. Similarly, disease with mortality in a colony of SCID mice was attributed to concurrent infections with enterococci and *P. aeruginosa*. There is mouse strain-related variation in susceptibility to experimental *P. aeruginosa* infections of the respiratory tract, with B6 and DBA/2 mice being susceptible, and BALB/c mice being relatively resistant. The increased susceptibility of some strains of mice was attributed to their inability to recruit large numbers of neutrophils and to a defect in tumor necrosis factor alpha production.

Pathology

Clinical signs may include listlessness, anorexia, conjunctivitis, nasal discharge, subcutaneous edema around the head, and acute death. Microscopic changes include necrosis of epithelium at sites of invasion in the upper respiratory tract and gingival tissues, with ulceration, and necrosis of the regional lymph nodes. Vasculitis, thrombosis, necrosis, and hemorrhage may occur in other organs, such as spleen and liver. Pseudomonas may also be associated with otitis media in mice that have not been rendered neutropenic, including C3H mice and Swiss Webster mice. MyD88-deficient mice have been reported to develop chronic suppurative lesions.

Diagnosis
Culture of the organism confirms the diagnosis. A history of experimental procedures that impair the immune response and/or leukocyte function usually precedes the onset of outbreaks of systemic disease, in which *P. aeruginosa* may be recovered from internal organs and blood. Differential diagnoses include postimmunosuppression deaths due to other opportunistic bacteria such as *P. mirabilis*, *Enterobacter cloacae*, *K. oxytoca*, and *Enterococcus* spp., which have also been shown to cause mortality in irradiated mice.

Streptobacillus moniliformis Infection
Streptobacillus moniliformis is a commensal organism that inhabits the nasopharynx of wild, pet, and occasionally laboratory rats. When introduced to laboratory mouse populations, it may result in high morbidity and mortality. In humans, it is the cause of rat bite fever, transmitted by direct contact or bites, and Haverhill fever, transmitted through contaminated food and water. Rat bite fever, usually acquired through contact with pet rats, is a serious, and sometimes fatal, zoonotic disease.

Epizootiology and Pathogenesis
Although *S. moniliformis* is generally associated with wild rats, natural infection in wild mice with polyarthritis has been documented. Exposure of laboratory mouse populations to infected rats is generally the source of infection. Once infection has been introduced to a mouse population, infection can spread rapidly with high mortality. Following oral inoculation, *S. moniliformis* can be isolated from submaxillary and cervical lymph nodes within 48 hours, with subsequent bacteremia and development of cervical lymphadenitis. A large number of organisms can be isolated from the blood during this stage. Bacteremia is cleared over the course of weeks, with persistence of infection in joints. Studies in rats have revealed that the organism preferentially localizes to metaphyseal capillaries, with subsequent evolution of arthritis. In experimental studies, B6 mice appeared to be uniquely susceptible to severe illness, whereas BALB/c, C3H/He, CBF1, and B6D2F1 mice were more resistant and DBA/2 intermediate in susceptibility. Although generally considered rare in laboratory mice, several outbreaks of streptobacillosis have been documented in the 1990s.

Pathology
Clinical signs during the acute bacteremic stage of infection include conjunctivitis, cervical lymphadenitis, diarrhea, hemoglobinuria, cyanosis, anemia, weight loss, and high mortality. There are disseminated foci of necrosis and inflammation in liver, spleen, and lymph nodes, with petechial and ecchymotic hemorrhages on serosal surfaces. Suppurative embolic interstitial nephritis with prominent bacterial colonies may be evident. In one outbreak, teat dermatitis with formation of brown crusts was found in breeding female mice. Some mice, particularly those that survive the acute phase, can develop suppurative polyarthritis, osteomyelitis, cervical abscesses, and subcutaneous abscesses. Arthritis frequently involves the feet and tail. Mice may exhibit limb or tail swelling, spinal involvement, posterior paresis, kyphosis, and priapism. Fetal infection with abortion or resorption has also been seen in infected mouse colonies.

Diagnosis
Definitive diagnosis of streptobacillosis is made by isolation from infected tissues, using blood agar. Large numbers of bacteria are present in blood and tissues during the acute bacteremic phase and in abscesses and joints during the chronic phase of infection. Organisms are nonmotile and highly pleomorphic, forming long filamentous forms under ideal growth conditions. Both serology and PCR can supplement diagnostic efforts, but neither method is generally applied to routine diagnostics because of the rarity of infections. Differential diagnoses must include other forms of bacteremic disease, such as pseudomoniasis, corynebacterial, staphylococcal, and streptococcal infections, as well as arthritis caused by *Mycoplasma* and *C. kutscheri*.

Other Gram-Positive Bacterial Infections
Aerococcus viridans Infection
Aerococcus viridans is a facultative anaerobic bacterium that is present in the environment and may be isolated from human skin. It is a known opportunistic pathogen in immunosuppressed humans. It has been associated with an outbreak of septicemia in immunodeficient NOD/SCID mice in Denmark. The mice developed pulmonary and hepatic abscesses and peritonitis following xenotransplantation of human tissues. Affected animals had weight loss, dyspnea, and distended abdomens. A similar syndrome has been noted by the authors in a U.S. colony of immunodeficient NSG mice, underscoring the propensity of this otherwise commensal organism to be an opportunistic pathogen. Infection was characterized by massive overgrowth of the bacteria (Fig. 1.72), with variable degrees of inflammation, which may be negligible in some tissues.

Corynebacterium bovis Infection: Coryneform Hyperkeratosis; Scaly Skin Disease
An organism initially identified as *C. pseudodiphtheriticum* was associated with scaling dermatitis in nude mice. The agent has subsequently been classified as *C. bovis*. The disease is characterized by weight loss and diffuse hyperkeratotic dermatitis in athymic nude mice. Bovine isolates of *C. bovis* can cause experimental disease in nude mice, but most natural mouse isolates are represented by a single HAC strain of *C. bovis*.

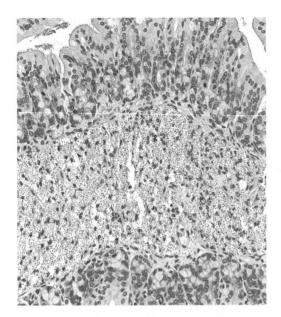

FIG. 1.72. *Proximal colon from an NSG mouse with disseminated* Aerococcus viridans *infection. Note the numerous pinpoint cocci expanding the submucosa.*

Epidemiology and Pathogenesis

Corynebacterium bovis is lipophilic and grows in keratin. Environmental contamination with infected keratin flakes is a likely means of transmission and persistence. The organism may be transmitted by topical application to the skin, by direct contact with infected mice, and by contaminated environment, such as cage lids, and inner surfaces of cages. Infections are usually transient in immunocompetent hirsute animals. B6, BALB/c, DBA/2, C3H/HeN, and Swiss mice develop low-level, transient infections. Haired SCID mice are susceptible to infection and develop mild scaly dermatitis, and immunocompetent hairless mice are susceptible to disease, but disease is typically associated with the combination of immunodeficiency and hairlessness in nude mice. Nude mice are persistently infected, but disease manifestations can be ephemeral, with bouts of resolution and recrudescence. This pattern of disease has been suggested to be associated with patterns of the hair growth cycle. In infected colonies of nude mice, the morbidity is frequently high, but mortality usually occurs only in suckling mice. Skin lesions are often transient or mild in older animals, with smaller numbers of bacteria present.

Pathology

Affected mice have a diffuse, scaling dermatitis (Fig. 1.73). Microscopically, there is marked epidermal hyperplasia, orthokeratotic hyperkeratosis, and a sparse mononuclear and polymorphonuclear cell infiltrate in the underlying dermis (Fig. 1.74). Gram-positive coryneform rods can be demonstrated in the keratin layers (Fig. 1.75). In haired SCID and other immunodeficient mice, lesions, when present, consist of areas of alopecia with scaling dermatitis on the back, flanks, neck, and cheeks. Examination of the

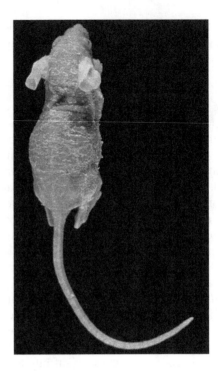

FIG. 1.73. *Nude mouse with* Corynebacterium bovis *hyperkeratosis. (Source: C. Richter, Gettysburg, PA. Reproduced with permission from C. Richter.)*

external ear canals of these mice enhances the opportunity to visualize bacteria within keratinized epithelium.

Diagnosis

Corynebacterium bovis can be isolated from the oral cavity, skin, and heart blood of infected mice. Definitive diagnosis can be achieved by culture or PCR of skin swabs or feces. Cultures should be held for up to 7 days, since *C. bovis* is slow growing. Differential diagnoses include hyperkeratosis associated with low ambient humidity. A similar syndrome of hyperkeratosis has been found to be associated with *Staphylococcus xylosus*.

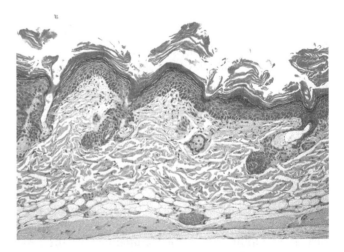

FIG. 1.74. *Skin from an athymic mouse with chronic* Corynebacterium bovis *infection. There is a marked epidermal hyperplasia and hyperkeratosis.*

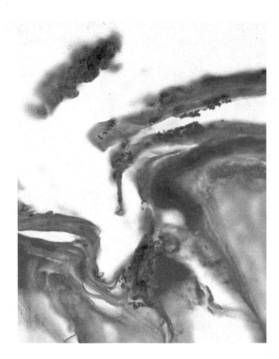

FIG. 1.75.   *Gram-positive* Corynebacterium bovis *within keratinized layer of an athymic mouse.*

There have been anecdotal reports of similar lesions in athymic mice associated with heavy infections of *Proteus* or other opportunistic bacteria on the skin.

Corynebacterium kutscheri *Infection: Pseudotuberculosis*

Corynebacterium kutscheri is a diphtheroid bacillus that causes a syndrome in mice and rats termed "pseudo-tuberculosis." This was one of the first infectious disease syndromes to be recognized in laboratory mice and rats in 1894 by D. Kutscher. Once quite common in these species, it is now rare. However, it remains a significant pathogen that occasionally infects colonies of mice and rats.

Epizootiology and Pathogenesis

Infection is usually subclinical, with sporadic hematogenous dissemination following entry through oral or enteric mucosa, from which the organisms spread to regional lymph nodes and to other internal organs. The organism may persist as a subclinical infection for long periods with no detectable circulating antibodies. The usual sites for the colonization of *C. kutscheri* in mice are the oral cavity, cecum, and colon. Clinical manifestations of the disease usually occur in conjunction with predisposing factors that compromise the immune response. Variation in susceptibility to *C. kutscheri* among strains of mice has been attributed to mononuclear phagocyte function. BALB/c-*nude*, A/J, CBA/N, MPS, and BALB/cCr mice were found to be most susceptible, C3H/He mice intermediate, and C57BL/6Cr, B10. BR/SgSn, ddY, and ICR mice resistant to colonization and disease induction. Male mice appear to harbor higher numbers of bacteria and a higher carrier rate.

Pathology

Infection is most often subclinical, but disease may arise as outbreaks or intermittent morbidity in enzootically infected colonies. Cervical and mesenteric lymph nodes of carrier animals may be enlarged (reactive) but without abscessation. Raised, gray-white nodules up to 1 cm in diameter may be present in liver, kidney, and lungs and, to a lesser extent, in other tissues, including subcutis. Suppurative and erosive arthritis may also be present, particularly in the carpal/metacarpal or tarsal/metatarsal joints, with marked swelling and erythema. Conjunctivitis has also been described. Microscopically, lesions feature coagulation to caseation necrosis, with peripheral aggregations of leukocytes, dominated by neutrophils. Suppurative thrombosis and embolization involving the pulmonary or mesenteric and portal vessels may be evident. Prominent colonies of Gram-positive bacilli are evident, particularly in the junctional areas between necrotic centers and peripheral reactive zones (see Rat Chapter 2, "*Corynebacterium kutscheri* Infection").

Diagnosis

Characteristic bacterial colonies, with "Chinese letter configurations" among less dense colonies, are readily evident within suppurative lesions and are best visualized in tissue sections stained with Gram stains. The distribution and nature of the lesions consistent with pseudotuberculosis require culture and identification of *C. kutscheri*. Differential diagnoses include other disseminated chronic bacterial infections that induce abscesses, including *Staphylococcus* and *Streptococcus*, and arthritis associated with *Mycoplasma* or *Streptobacillus*. Culture of oropharyngeal washes, cervical lymph nodes, mesenteric lymph nodes, and cecum is useful for detecting carrier animals, and culture of feces has been shown to be a useful noninvasive screening method.

Other Corynebacterium *spp.-Associated Disease*

Keratoconjunctivitis with ulcerative keratitis has been reported in aged B6 mice infected with *Corynebacterium* spp. Older mice inoculated in the conjunctival sac with the organism developed the typical lesions, but younger mice were resistant to the disease. *Corynebacterium hoffmani* can be a frequent isolate from BALB/c mice with conjunctivitis. It is likely that ocular infection is predisposed by microophthalmia (B6) or entropion (BALB/c) in these strains. *Corynebacterium mastitidis* has been associated with suppurative preputial gland adenitis.

Staphylococcus *spp. Infections*

Coagulase-negative staphylococci are commensal and opportunistic pathogenic bacteria that commonly inhabit the skin, nasopharynx, and intestine. In the mouse, disease has been associated with *Staphylococcus aureus* and *S. xylosus*. *Staphylococcus epidermidis* and other species may be isolated from skin and mucous membranes, but have yet to be incriminated as pathogens in mice. *Staphylococcus* spp. are associated with several relatively distinct but overlapping common syndromes in mice:

Chronic suppurative inflammation. *Staphylococcus aureus* is often associated with chronic suppurative inflammation of skin adnexae, conjunctiva, periorbital tissue, preputial glands, and regional lymph nodes. Euthymic mice, as well as urokinase plasminogen activator-deficient mice, may develop suppurative conjunctivitis, ophthalmitis, and periocular abscessation, with involvement of regional lymph nodes. Ocular lesions tend to occur in strains of mice that are prone to development of conjunctivitis or with ocular defects, such as BALB and B6 mice. Preputial gland inflammation and abscesses are sporadically common in male mice. Occasionally, deep visceral abscesses may also be found. Lymphadenitis and abscesses have botryomycotic-like features, characterized by necrotizing suppurative inflammation with a central core of necrotic neutrophils and colonies of Gram-positive bacteria surrounded by bright eosinophilic amorphous to fibrillar Splendore-Hoeppli material (Fig. 1.76). The authors have also observed botryomycotic abscesses involving bone and extending into the nasal cavity associated with foreign body periodontitis.

Furunculosis. Distorted vibrissal hair shaft growth and impaired T-cell function predispose athymic nude mice to staphylococcal furunculosis of the muzzle (Fig. 1.77). These mice frequently have suppurative lymphadenitis of the regional lymph nodes. Microscopic findings are similar to those described above with botryomycotic features.

Ulcerative dermatitis. An important form of staphylococcal disease is ulcerative dermatitis in association with *S. aureus* or *S. xylosus*. Staphylococci produce an array of biologically active proteins, including

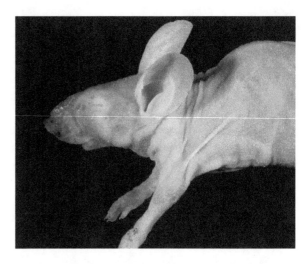

FIG. 1.77.   *Muzzle furunculosis in a nude mouse associated with* Staphylococcus aureus *infection.*

hemolysins, nucleases, proteases, lipases, hyaluronidase, and collagenase, and many produce exotoxins, including exfoliative toxins, leukocidin, and several superantigens, particularly enterotoxin A, enterotoxin B, enterotoxin C, and toxic shock syndrome toxin-1. This armamentarium is important in understanding the pathogenesis of staphylococcal ulcerative dermatitis in mice (and rats), which is characterized by superficial colonization of bacteria on the surface of the skin, with underlying burn-like features.

Ulcerative dermatitis is quite common in young and aged B6, BALB/c, DBA/2, and C3H/He mice and their hybrids, as well as other strains and stocks of mice. Disease prevalence is linked to other predisposing factors, including behavioral idiosyncrasies and ectoparasite hypersensitivity. For example, B6 mice are prone to trichotillomania and frequently suffer from ulcerative dermatitis (Fig. 1.78). Superficial excoriation of the skin is followed by colonization with *Staphylococcus*, pruritus, and then development of progressive necrotizing

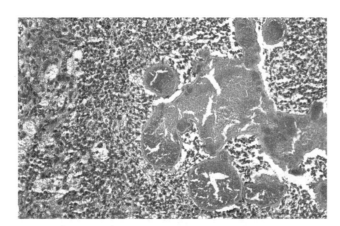

FIG. 1.76.   *Cervical lymph node, illustrating the botryomycotic inflammatory response due to* Staphylococcus aureus *infection. There are bacterial colonies and central aggregates of eosinophilic material consistent with a Splendore-Hoeppli reaction.*

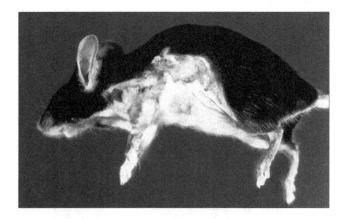

FIG. 1.78.   *Ulcerative dermatitis in a B6 mouse associated with* Staphylococcus aureus *infection. Note that the ventral abdomen is bald due to trichotillomania, with ulcerative dermatitis on the side.*

dermatitis. The syndrome has been well studied in hairless DS-Nh mice infected with *S. aureus*. DS-Nh mice normally manifest excessive scratching behavior. When they are housed in a conventional environment, they develop erythema, excoriation, and erosion around their head and neck. When first introduced to the environment, the mice become colonized with several *Staphylococcus* species, but *S. aureus* gradually becomes the dominant skin commensal over time, with selection for *S. aureus* types that produce enterotoxin C. Lesions do not develop in mice maintained under *Staphylococcus*-free barrier conditions. A similar syndrome is associated with *S. xylosus* in athymic nude mice and B6-*Nos2^{tm1Lau}* (NOS2) mice, which have defective inducible NO synthase. NOS2 mice have less severe disease compared to nude mice, which develop more severe disease with mortality. Notably, skin lesions do not appear to be extensive enough in nude mice to explain the high mortality, suggesting that the mice are succumbing to systemic toxic events. Immunocompetent SJL mice (which are NK cell-deficient) have also been reported to develop necrotic dermatitis on their tails in association with *S. xylosus*. Severe ulcerative conjunctivitis and dermatitis, with extensive facial and neck involvement, occur in CD18 (leukocyte integrin) null mice on B6 and 129 mixed background. The *Staphylococcus* isolate was not speciated, but lesions contained prominent colonies of staphylococcal-type bacteria in the superficial exudate, consistent with better characterized forms of this disease.

Staphylococcal ulcerative dermatitis is characterized by focal small to large chronic ulcerative lesions, often around the head and neck, but also on the trunk or base of the tail. In the tail form of disease, gangrene and sloughing of the tail may occur. Apparently, the location of the skin lesions is associated with the initiating cause of excoriation (ectoparasites, grooming, fighting, etc.). Regardless of location, the microscopic appearance of these lesions is similar (Fig. 1.79), with prominent colonies of Gram-positive organisms in the superficial exudate, and acute coagulative necrosis of the underlying

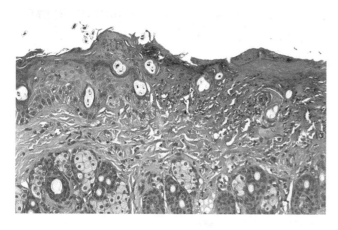

FIG. 1.79. *Skin from a mouse with ulcerative dermatitis. Note the coagulation necrosis of the epidermis and dermis with the presence of bacterial colonies on the surface.*

epidermis and dermis, which can extend to the subcutis and panniculus carnosis. The lesions are reminiscent of 1st, 2nd, or 3rd degree burns, which implicate the toxins elaborated by the *Staphylococcus* colonizing the surface of the lesions. Varying degrees of leukocytic infiltration and granulation are also present. The chronic lesions of Staphyloccal disease result in acceleration of multi-systemic amyloidosis and splenomegaly, with marked extramedullary myelopoiesis in liver and spleen. Plasmacytosis is present in regional lymph nodes. Scaly skin disease in nude mice, similar to the disease caused by *C. bovis*, has been associated with *S. xylosus*. However, lesions were more inflammatory and included foci of epidermal ulceration and pustule formation.

Diagnosis
An etiologic diagnosis requires isolation and speciation, but factors that predispose to susceptibility should be investigated, including immune status, strain-related behavior patterns, ectoparasitism, and ectoparasite-related hypersensitivity. Differential diagnoses include abscessation due to other bacterial infections and streptococcal necrotizing dermatitis. Amputation of the tail secondary to *Staphylococcus*-related dry gangrene must be differentiated from mousepox and tail lesions in mice infected with *Mycobacterium chelonae*.

Streptococcus and Enterococcus *Infections*
Streptococci are commensal and pathogenic bacteria that colonize the nose, mouth, intestine, genital tract, and skin. Pathogenic streptococci produce beta hemolysin and polysaccharide surface antigens that can be differentiated serologically into Lancefield groups. Pathogenic streptococci in mice belong to Lancefield groups A, B, C, and G. Genetic analysis has resulted in reclassification of Lancefield group D streptococci into the genus *Enterococcus*. Like staphylococci, pathogenic streptococci elaborate an array of extracellular proteins that facilitate adherence, invasion, and tissue destruction for the release of nutrients. Among these products are pyogenic and superantigen exotoxins. In addition, bacteremic disease can occur in immunodeficient or irradiated mice infected with alpha hemolytic *Streptococcus* or *Enterococcus* spp. that would otherwise be considered nonpathogenic.

Systemic streptococcal infections can occur as a cause of sporadic disease or outbreaks of disease in both immunocompetent and immunocompromised mice. Group A *Streptococcus* has been isolated from bacteremic Swiss mice that were inoculated with sterile endotoxin. The mice were found to carry *Streptococcus* in their pharynges, and affected animals had cervical lymphadenitis, with bacteria isolated from multiple organs. Group B *Streptococcus* has been associated with meningoencephalitis, ependymitis, and periventriculitis in nude mice. Infection of the brain was presumed to arise by extension from the nose, where bacteria were isolated from subclinical carriers. Group B *S. agalactiae* has been associated with an epizootic in a barrier colony of DBA/2 mice, which had ascending pyelonephritis with subsequent bacteremia resulting in suppurative lesions in a variety of organs, including heart, kidneys, spleen, and liver, and less commonly in uterus, thorax, lymph nodes, and lungs. DBA/2 and B6D2F1 or D2B6F1 hybrid mice were susceptible, whereas C3H, NOD, and B6 mice in the same colony were not infected. Experimental inoculation of DBA and Swiss mice confirmed the unique susceptibility of DBA/2 mice. Group C *Streptococcus equisimilis* (*S. dysgalactiae* subsp. *equisimilis*) has been associated with subcutaneous, hepatic, and abdominal abscesses in ICR Swiss mice. The bacteria also colonized the nasopharynx and intestine. An outbreak of an untyped beta-hemolytic *Streptococcus* involved conventional C3H3 mice. The mice were bacteremic, with colonies of bacteria associated with endocarditis, mural thrombi, gastric mucosal necrosis, and renal cortical necrosis. Alpha hemolytic *Enterococcus durans*, in concert with *P. aeruginosa*, has been shown to cause bacteremic disease in SCID mice, and was most commonly problematic in pregnant and lactating animals. Bacteria were isolated from various organs and middle ear. The mice developed focal pericarditis and thickened hepatic capsules, with multifocal nonsuppurative hepatitis.

Systemic disease due to alpha hemolytic *S. viridans* has been noted in irradiated SCID and SCID-beige mice. Mice were severely ill, with splenomegaly and pulmonary congestion. Massive numbers of Gram-positive bacteria were present in vessel lumina, with virtually no host response, particularly in glomerular capillaries (Fig. 1.80). A similar syndrome has been seen by the authors in irradiated SCID mice infected with *E. faecalis*.

An alternative form of streptococcal disease in mice is ulcerative dermatitis, which resembles the syndrome associated with *Staphylococcus*. Group G *Streptococcus* has been incriminated in an epizootic of necrotizing dermatitis. Ulcerative lesions were present on the dorsal

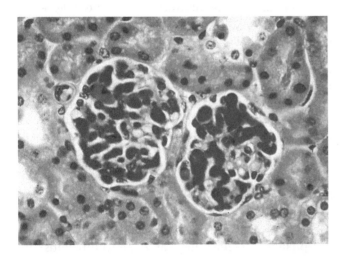

FIG. 1.80. *Kidney from an irradiated SCID/beige mouse with disseminated alpha-hemolytic streptococcal infection. Numerous bacterial colonies are present in glomerular vessels.*

thoracic or lumbar regions, with progressive spread to the shoulder and pelvic regions. Underlying tissue had vasculitis and thrombosis, with bacterial invasion of subcutaneous tissue. The bacterium was isolated from the oropharynx and spleens of many of the mice.

Acid-Fast Bacterial Infections

Mycobacterium spp. Infections

Although laboratory mice are susceptible to experimental infections with *Mycobacteria*, naturally occurring infections are rare. An outbreak of *M. avium-intracellulare* infection in B6 mice, but not C3H/HeN or B6C3F1, has been documented. The authors have observed similar outbreaks. *Mycobacterium avium-intracellulare* complex organisms can be isolated from soil, water, and sawdust, which was the presumed origin of the infection in mice. Infected mice were subclinical. At necropsy, there were a few subpleural 1–5-mm diameter tan-colored masses in lung. Microscopic findings consisted of focal accumulations of epithelioid cells, foamy macrophages, and lymphocytes in alveolar spaces and septa, with variable amounts of necrosis and neutrophilic leukocyte infiltration. Many of the mice had microgranulomas with occasional Langhans-type giant cells in liver parenchyma and mesenteric lymph nodes. Large numbers of acid-fast bacilli were visualized in some lesions. There has been a rise in interest in using the mouse as a model for nontuberculous mycobacterial infections because of their importance in AIDS patients. B6 mice have emerged as the preferred susceptible mouse strain for such studies. It is now known that B6 and BALB/c mice carry a susceptibility (*Bcg^s*) allele, and DBA/2 and C3H/He carry a resistance (*Bcg^r*) allele that is a determinant of phagocytic host defense mechanisms that control intracellular pathogen infections. Definitive diagnosis can be made by demonstrating acid-fast organisms in granulomas and isolation of *Mycobacterium*. Differential diagnoses for pulmonary granulomas should include *M. pulmonis* and *C. kutscheri* infections, as well as lesions associated with the administration of Freund's adjuvant.

Another form of mycobacterial infection has been reported, which involved tail infections with *M. chelonae* in several types of immunocompromised mice, including RAG1, T-cell receptor, and *Fas^lpr* null mice, as well as thymectomized mice. Lesions consisted of focal granulomata and osteomyelitis of the tail, resulting in grossly apparent nodular swellings.

BIBLIOGRAPHY FOR BACTERIAL INFECTIONS

See "General References for Infectious Diseases"

Bacterial Enteric Infections

Brachyspira spp. Infection

Backhans, A., Johansson, K.-E., & Fellstrom, C. (2010) Phenotypic and molecular characterization of *Brachyspira* spp. isolated from wild rodents. *Environmental Microbiology Reports* 2:720–727.

Citrobacter rodentium Infection

Barthold, S.W. & Beck, D. (1980) Modification of early dimethyl-hydrazine carcinogenesis by colonic mucosal hyperplasia. *Cancer Research* 40:4451–4455.

Barthold, S.W., Coleman, G.L., Jocaby, R.O., Livestone, E.M., & Jonas, A.M. (1978) Transmissible murine colonic hyperplasia. *Veterinary Pathology* 15:223–236.

Barthold, S.W., Osbaldiston, G.W., & Jonas, A.M. (1977) Dietary, bacterial, and host genetic interactions in the pathogenesis of transmissible murine colonic hyperplasia. *Laboratory Animal Science* 27:938–945.

Bry, L. & Brenner, M.B. (2004) Critical role of T cell-dependent serum antibody, but not the gut-associated lymphoid tissue, for surviving acute mucosal infection with *Citrobacter rodentium*, an attaching and effacing pathogen. *Journal of Immunology* 172:433–441.

Bry, L., Brigl, M., & Brenner, M.B. (2006) CD4+-T-cell effector functions and costimulatory requirements essential for surviving mucosal inflammation with *Citrobacter rodentium*. *Infection and Immunity* 74:673–681.

Higgens, L.M., Frankel, G., Connerton, I., Goncalves, N.S., Dougan, G., & MacDonald, T.T. (1999) Role of bacterial intimin in colonic hyperplasia and inflammation. *Science* 285:588–591.

Higgins, L.M., Frankel, G., Douce, G., Dougan, G., & MacDonald, T.T. (1999) *Citrobacter rodentium* infection in mice elicits a mucosal Th1 cytokine response and lesions similar to those in murine inflammatory bowel disease. *Infection and Immunity* 67:3031–3039.

Johnson, E. & Barthold, S.W. (1979) Ultrastructure of transmissible murine colonic hyperplasia. *American Journal of Pathology* 97:291–314.

Newman, J.V., Kosaka, T., Sheppard, B.J., Fox, J.G., & Schauer, D.B. (2001) Bacterial infection promotes colon tumorigenesis in Apc (Min/+) mice. *Journal of Infectious Diseases* 184:227–230.

Raczynski, A.R., Muthupalani, S., Schlieper, K., Fox, J.G., Tannenbaum, S.R., & Schauer, D.B. (2012) Enteric infection with *Citrobacter rodentium* induces coagulative liver necrosis and hepatic inflammation prior to peak infection and colonic disease. *PLoS One* 7:e33099.

Simmons, C.P., Clare, S., Ghaem-Maghami, M., Uren, T.K., Rankin, J., Huett, A., Goldin, R., Lewis, D.J., MacDonald, T.T., Strugnell, R.A., Frankel, G., & Dougan, G. (2003) Central role for B lymphocytes and CD4+ T cells in immunity to infection by the attaching and effacing pathogen *Citrobacter rodentium*. *Infection and Immunity* 71:5077–5086.

Vallance, B.A., Deng, W., Knodler, L.A., & Findlay, B.B. (2002) Mice lacking T and B lymphocytes develop transient colitis and crypt hyperplasia yet suffer impaired bacterial clearance during *Citrobacter rodentium* infection. *Infection and Immunity* 70:2070–2081.

Clostridium difficle and Clostridium perfringens Infections

Clapp, H.W. & Graham, W.R. (1970) An experience with *Clostridium perfringens* in cesarean derived barrier sustained mice. *Laboratory Animal Care* 20:1081–1086.

Feinstein, R.E., Morris, W.E., Waldermason, A.H., Hedenqvist, P., & Lindberg, R. (2008) Fatal acute intestinal pseudoobstruction in mice. *Journal of the American Association for Laboratory Animal Science* 47:58–63.

Krugner-Higby, L., Girard, I., Welter, J., Gendron, A., Rhodes, J.S., & Garland, T., Jr. (2006) Clostridial enteropathy in lactating outbred Swiss-derived (ICR) mice. *Journal of the American Association for Laboratory Animal Science* 45:80–87.

Kunstyr, I. (1986) Paresis of peristalsis and ileus lead to death in lactating mice. *Laboratory Animals* 20:32–35.

Matsushita, S. & Matsumoto, T. (1986) Spontaneous necrotic enteritis in young RFM/Ms mice. *Laboratory Animals* 20:114–117.

Rollman, C., Olshan, K., & Hammer, J. (1998) Abdominal distension in lactating mice: paresis (paralysis) of peristalsis in lactating mice. *Laboratory Animals* 27 (1): 19–20.

Sanchez, S. & Rozengurt, N. (1994) Lesions caused by *Clostridium perfringens* in germ-free mice. *Laboratory Animal Science* 44:397

Clostridium piliforme Infection

Franklin, C.L., Motzel, S.L., Besch-Williford, C.L., Hook, R.R., Jr., & Riley, L.K. (1994) Tyzzer's infection: host specificity of *Clostridium piliforme* isolates. *Laboratory Animal Science* 44:568–572.

Fries, A.S. (1978) Demonstration of antibodies to *Bacillus piliformis* in SPF colonies and experimental transplacental infection by *Bacillus piliformis* in mice. *Laboratory Animals* 12:23–26.

Furukawa, T., Furumoto, K., Fujieda, M., & Okada, E. (2002) Detection by PCR of the Tyzzer's disease organism (*Clostridium piliforme*) in feces. *Experimental Animals* 51:513–516.

Livingston, R.S., Franklin, C.L., Besch-Williford, C.L., Hook, R.R., Jr., & Riley, L.K. (1996) A novel presentation of *Clostridium piliforme* infection (Tyzzer's disease) in nude mice. *Laboratory Animal Science* 46:21–25.

Motzel, S.L. & Riley, L.K. (1991) Detection of serum antibodies to *Bacillus piliformis* in mice and rats using an enzyme-linked immunoabsorbent assay. *Laboratory Animal Science* 41:26–30.

Tsuchitani, M., Umemura, T., Narama, I., & Yanabe, M. (1983) Naturally occurring Tyzzer's disease in a clean mouse colony: high mortality with coincidental cardiac lesions. *Journal of Comparative Pathology* 93:499–507.

Tyzzer, E.E. (1917) A fatal disease of the Japanese waltzing mouse caused by a spore-bearing bacillus (*Bacillus piliformis* N.sp.). *Journal of Medical Research* 37:307–338.

Van Andel, R.A., Hook, R.R., Jr., Franklin, C.L., Besch-Williford, C.L., & Riley, L.K. (1998) Interleukin-12 has a role in mediating resistance of murine strains to Tyzzer's disease. *Infection and Immunity* 66:4942–4946.

Van Andel, R.A., Hook, R.R., Jr., Franklin, C.L., Besch-Williford, C.L., van Roojen, N., & Riley, L.K. (1997) Effects of neutrophil, natural killer cell, and macrophage depletion on murine *Clostridium piliforme* infection. *Infection and Immunity* 65:2725–2731.

Waggie, K.S., Hansen, C.T., Ganaway, J.R., & Spenser, T.S. (1981) A study of mouse strain susceptibility to *Bacillus piliformis* (Tyzzer's disease): the association of B-cell function and resistance. *Laboratory Animal Science* 31:139–142.

Escherichia coli Infection

Waggie, K.S., Hansen, C.T., Moore, T.D., Bukowski, M.A., & Allen, A.M. (1988) Cecocolitis in immunodeficient mice associated with an enteroinvasive lactose negative *E. coli*. *Laboratory Animal Science* 38:389–393.

Luperchio, S.A., Newman, J.V., Dangler, C.A., Schrenzel, M.D., Brenner, D.J., Steigerwalt, A.G., & Schauer, D.B. (2000) *Citrobacter rodentium*, the causative agent of transmissible murine colonic hyperplasia, exhibits clonality: synonymy of *C. rodentium* and mouse-pathogenic *Escherichia coli*. *Journal of Clinical Microbiology* 38:4343–4350.

Helicobacter spp. Infections

Boutin, S.R., Shen, Z., Roesch, P.L., Stiefel, S.M., Sanderson, A.E., Multari, H.M., Pridhoko, E.A., Smith, J.C., Taylor, N.S., Lohmiller, J.J., Dewhirst, F.E., Klein, H.J., & Fox, J.G. (2010) *Helicobacter pullorum* outbreak in C57BL/6NTac and C3H/HeNTac barrier-maintained mice. *Journal of Clinical Microbiology* 48:1908–1910.

Cahill, R.J., Foltz, C.J., Fox, J.G., Dangler, C.A., Powrie, F., & Schauer, D.B. (1997) Inflammatory bowel disease: an immunity-mediated condition triggered by bacterial infection with *Helicobacter hepaticus*. *Infection and Immunity* 65:3126–3131.

Diwan, B.A., Ward, J.M., Ramljak, D., & Anderson, L.M. (1997) Promotion of *Helicobacter hepaticus*-induced hepatitis of hepatic tumors initiated by *N*-nitrosodimethylamine in male A/JCr mice. *Toxicologic Pathology* 25:597–605.

Eaton, K.A., Opp, J.S., Gray, B.M., Bergin, I.L., & Young, V.B. (2011) Ulcerative typhlocolitis associated with *Helicobacter mastomyrinus* in telomerase-deficient mice. *Veterinary Pathology* 48:713–725.

Feng, S., Ku, K., Hodzic, E., Lorenzana, E., Freet, K., & Barthold, S.W. (2005) Differential detection of five mouse helicobacters with multiplex polymerase chain reaction. *Clinical and Diagnostic Laboratory Immunology* 12:531–536.

Fox, J.G., Rogers, A.B., Whary, M.T., Taylor, N.S., Xu, S., Feng, Y., & Keys, S. (2004) *Helicobacter bilis*-associated hepatitis in outbred mice. *Comparative Medicine* 54:571–577.

Franklin, C.L., Riley, L.K., Livingston, R.S., Beckwith, C.S., Besch-Williford, C.L., & Hook, R.R., Jr. (1998) Enterohepatic lesions in SCID mice infected with *Helicobacter bilis*. *Laboratory Animal Science* 48:334–339.

Franklin, C.L., Riley, L.K., Livingston, R.S., Beckwith, C.S., Hook, R.R., Jr., & Besch-Williford, C.L. (1999) Enteric lesions in SCID mice infected with "*Helicobacter typhlonicus*," a novel urease-negative *Helicobacter* species. *Laboratory Animal Science* 49:496–505.

Goto, K., Ishihara, K.I., Kuzuoka, A., Ohnishi, Y., & Itoh, T. (2001) Contamination of transplantable human tumor-bearing lines by *Helicobacter hepaticus* and its elimination. *Journal of Clinical Microbiology* 39:3703–3704.

Kuehl, C.J., Wood, H.D., Marsh, T.L., Schmidt, T.M., & Young, V.B. (2005) Colonization of the cecal mucosa by *Helicobacter hepaticus* impacts on the diversity of the indigenous microbiota. *Infection and Immunity* 73:6952–6961.

Li, X., Fox, J.G., Whary, M.T., Yan, L., Shames, B., & Zhao, Z. (1998) SCID/NCr mice naturally infected with *Helicobacter hepaticus* develop progressive hepatitis, proliferative typhlitis, and colitis. *Infection and Immunity* 66:5477–5484.

Riley, L.K., Franklin, C.L., Hook, R.R., Jr., & Besch-Williford, C. (1996) Identification of murine helicobacters by PCR and restriction enzyme analysis. *Journal of Clinical Microbiology* 34:942–946.

Singletary, K.B., Kloster, C.A., & Baker, D.G. (2003) Optimal age at fostering for derivation of *Helicobacter hepaticus*-free mice. *Comparative Medicine* 53:259–264.

Ward, J.M., Anver, M.R., Haines, D.C., & Benveniste, R.R. (1994) Chronic active hepatitis in mice caused by *Helicobacter hepaticus*. *American Journal of Pathology* 145:959–968.

Ward, J.M., Anver, M.R., Haines, D.C., Melhorn, J.M., Gorelick, P., Yan, L., & Fox, J.G. (1996) Inflammatory large bowel disease in immunodeficient mice naturally infected with *Helicobacter hepaticus*. *Laboratory Animal Science* 46:15–20.

Ward, J.M. Benveniste, R.E., Fox, C.H., Battles, J.K., Gonda, M.A., & Tully, J.G. (1996) Autoimmunity in chronic active *Helicobacter* hepatitis of mice: serum antibodies and expression of heat shock protein 70 in liver. *American Journal of Pathology* 148:509–517.

Ward, J.M., Fox, J.G., Anver, M.R., Haines, D.C., George, C.V., Collins, M.J., Jr., Gorelick, P.L., Nagashima, K., Gonada, M.A., Gilden, R.V., Tully, J.G., Russell, R.J., Benveniste, R.E., Paster, B.J., Dewhirst, F.E., Donovan, J.C., Anderson, L.M., & Rice, J.M. (1994) Chronic active hepatitis and associated liver tumors in mice caused by a persistent bacterial infection with a novel *Helicobacter* species. *Journal of the National Cancer Institute* 86:1222–1227.

Whary, M.T., Cline, J., King, A., Ge, Z., Shen, Z., Sheppard, B., & Fox, J.G. (2001) Long-term colonization levels of *Helicobacter hepaticus* in the cecum of hepatitis-prone A/JCr mice are significantly lower than those in hepatitis-resistant C57BL/6 mice. *Comparative Medicine* 51:413–417.

Whary, M.T., Cline, J.H., King, A.E., Hewes, K.M., Chojnacky, D., Salvarrey, A., & Fox, J.G. (2000) Monitoring sentinel mice for *Helicobacter hepaticus*, *H. rodentium*, and *H. bilis* by use of polymerase chain reaction analysis and serologic testing. *Comparative Medicine* 50:436–443.

Whary, M.T. & Fox, J.G. (2004) Natural and experimental *Helicobacter* infections. *Comparative Medicine* 54:125–158.

Won, Y.S., Yoon, J.H., Lee, C.H., Kim, B.H., Hyun, B.H., & Choi, Y.K. (2002) *Helicobacter muricola* sp. nov., a novel *Helicobacter* species isolated from the ceca and feces of Korean wild mouse (*Mus musculus molossinus*). *FEMS Microbiology Letters* 209:45–51.

Lawsonia intracellularis Infection

Lawson, G.H.K. & Gebbert, C.J. (2000) Proliferative enteropathy. *Journal of Comparative Pathology* 122:77–100.

Murakata, K., Sato, A., Yoshiya, M., Kim, S., Watarai, M., Omata, Y., & Furuoka, H. (2008) Infection of different strains of mice with *Lawsonia intracellularis* derived from rabbit or porcine proliferative enteropathy. *Journal of Comparative Pathology* 139:8–15.

Smith, D.G.E., Mitchell, S.C., Nash, T., & Rhind, S. (2000) Gamma interferon influences intestinal epithelial hyperplasia caused by *Lawsonia intracellularis* infection in mice. *Infection and Immunity* 68:6737–6743.

Salmonella enterica Infection

Caseboldt, D.B. & Schoeb, T.R. (1988) An outbreak in mice of salmonellosis caused by *Salmonella enteritidis* serotype *enteritidis*. *Laboratory Animal Science* 38:190–192.

Clark, M.A., Hirst, B.H., & Jepson, M.A. (1998) Inoculum composition and *Salmonella* pathogenicity island 1 regulate M-cell invasion and epithelial destruction by *Salmonella typhimurium*. *Infection and Immunity* 66:724–731.

Khan, S.A., Everest, P., Servos, S., Foxwell, N., Zahringer, U., Brade, H., Rietschel, E.T., Dougan, G., Charles, I.G., & Maskell, D.J. (1998) A lethal role for lipid A in *Salmonella* infections. *Molecular Microbiology* 29:571–579.

Lam-Yuk-Tseung, S. & Gros, P. (2003) Genetic control of susceptibility to bacterial infections in mouse models. *Cellular Microbiology* 5:299–313.

Moncure, C.W., Guo, Y.N., Xu, H.R., & Hsu, H.S. (1998) Comparative histopathology in mouse typhoid among genetically diverse mice. *International Journal of Experimental Pathology* 79:183–192.

Richter-Dahlfors, A., Buchan, A.M., & Finlay, B.B. (1997) Murine salmonellosis studied by confocal microscopy: *Salmonella typhimurium* resides intracellularly inside macrophages and exerts a cytotoxic effect on phagocytes in vivo. *Journal of Experimental Medicine* 186:569–580.

Tannock, G.W. & Smith, J.M.B. (1971) A *Salmonella* carrier state involving the upper respiratory tract of mice. *Journal of Infectious Diseases* 123:502–506.

Vassiloyanakopoulos, A.P., Okamoto, S., & Fierer, J. (1998) The crucial role of polymorphonuclear leukocytes in resistance to *Salmonella dublin* infections in genetically susceptible and resistant mice. *Proceedings of the National Academy of Sciences of the United States of America* 95:7676–7681.

Segmented Filamentous Bacteria

Blumershine, R.V. & Savage, D.C. (1997) Filamentous microbes indigenous to the murine small bowel: a scanning-electron microscopic study of their morphology and attachment to the epithelium. *Microbial Ecology* 4:95–103.

Caselli, M., Holton, J., Boldrini, P., Vaira, D., & Calo, G. (2010) Morphology of segmented filamentous bacteria and their patterns of contact with the follicle-associated epithelium of the mouse terminal ileum: implications for the relationship with the immune system. *Gut Microbes* 1:367–372.

Ericsson, A.C., Hagan, C.E., Davis, D.J., & Franklin, C.L. (2014) Segmented filamentous bacteria: commensal microbes with potential effects on research. *Comparative Medicine* 64:90–98.

Jepson, M.A., Clark, M.A., Simmons, N.L., & Hirst, B.H. (1993) Actin-accumulation at sites of attachment of indigenous apathogenic segmented filamentous bacteria to mouse ileal epithelial cells. *Infection and Immunity* 61:4001–4004.

Koopman, J.P., Stadhouders, A.M., Kenkis, H.M., & De Boer, H. (1987) The attachment of filamentous segmented microorganisms to the distal ileum wall of the mouse: a scanning- and transmission-electron-microscopy study. *Laboratory Animals* 21:48–52.

Tannock, G.W., Miller, J.R., & Savage, D.C. (1984) Host specificity of filamentous, segmented microorganisms adherent to the small bowel epithelium in mice and rats. *Applied Environmental Microbiology* 47:441–442.

Other Gram-Negative Bacterial Infections

Bordetella hinzii Infection

Hayashimoto, N,. Morita, H., Yasuda, M., Ishida, T., Kameda, S., Takakura, A., & Itoh, T. (2011) Prevalence of *Bordetella hinzii* in mice in experimental facilities in Japan. *Research in Veterinary Science* 93:624–626.

Hayashimoto, N., Yasuda, M., Goto, K., Takakura, A., & Itoh, T. (2008) Study of a *Bordetella hinzii* isolated from a laboratory mouse. *Comparative Medicine* 58:440–446.

Burkholderia gladioli Infection

Foley, P.L., LiPuma, J.J., & Feldman, S.H. (2004) Outbreak of otitis media caused by *Burkholderia gladioli* infection in immunocompromised mice. *Comparative Medicine* 54:93–99.

Chlamydia spp. Infection

Ata, F.A., Stephenson, E.H., & Storz, J. (1971) Inapparent respiratory infection of inbred Swiss mice with sulfadiazine-resistant, iodine-negative chlamydia. *Infection and Immunity* 4:506–507.

Bai, H., Yang, J., Qiu, H., Wang, S., Fan, Y., Han, X., Xie, S., & Yang, X. (2005) Intranasal inoculation of *Chlamydia trachomatis* mouse pneumonitis agent induces significant neutrophil infiltration which is not efficient in controlling the infection in mice. *Immunology* 114:246–254.

Gogalak, F.M. (1953) The histopathology of murine pneumonitis infection and the growth of the virus in mouse lung. *Journal of General Microbiology* 15:292–304.

Karr, H.V. (1943) Study of a latent pneumotropic virus of mice. *Journal of Infectious Diseases* 72:108–116.

Kaukoranta-Tolvanen, S.S., Laurila, A.L., Saikku, P., Leinonen, M., Liesirova, L., & Laitinen, K. (1993) Experimental infection of *Chlamydia pneumoniae* in mice. *Microbial Pathogenesis* 15:293–302.

Masson, N.D., Toseland, C.D., & Beale, A.S. (1995) Relevance of *Chlamydia pneumoniae* murine pneumonitis model to evaluation of antimicrobial agents. *Antimicrobial Agents and Chemotherapy* 39:1959–1964.

Moazed, T.C., Kuo, C.C., Grayston, J.T., & Campbell, L.A. (1998) Evidence of systemic dissemination of *Chlamydia pneumoniae* via macrophages in the mouse. *Journal of Infectious Diseases* 177:1322–1325.

Nigg, C. (1942) Unidentified virus which produces pneumonia and systemic infection in mice. *Science* 95:49–50.

Nigg, C. & Eaton, M.D. (1944) Isolation from normal mice of a pneumotropic virus which forms elementary bodies. *Journal of Experimental Medicine* 79:496–510.

Yang, X. & Brunham, R.C. (1998) Gene knockout B cell-deficient mice demonstrate that B cells play an important role in the initiation of T cell responses to *Chlamydia trachomatis* (mouse pneumonitis) lung infection. *Journal of Immunology* 161:1439–1446.

Yang, X., Hayglass, K.T., & Brunham, R.C. (1998) Different roles are played by alpha beta and gamma delta T cells in acquired immunity to *Chlamydia trachomatis* pulmonary infection. *Immunology* 94:469–475.

Yang, Z.P., Kuo, C.C., & Grayson, J.T. (1995) Systemic dissemination of *Chlamydia pneumoniae* following intranasal inoculation in mice. *Journal of Infectious Diseases* 171:736–738.

Cilia-Associated Respiratory Bacillus (CAR) Infection

Cundiff, D.D., Besch-Williford, C.L., Hook, R.R., Jr., Franklin, C.L., & Riley, L.K. (1994) Characterization of cilia-associated respiratory bacillus isolates from rats and rabbits. *Laboratory Animal Science* 44:305–312.

Franklin, C.L., Pletz, J.D., Riley, L.K., Livingston, B.A., Hook, R.R., Jr., & Besch-Williford, C.L. (1999) Detection of cilia-associated respiratory (CAR) bacillus in nasal-swab specimens from infected rats by use of polymerase chain reaction. *Laboratory Animal Science* 49:114–117.

Goto, K., Nozu, R., Takakura, A., Matsushita, S., & Itoh, T. (1995) Detection of cilia-associated respiratory bacillus in experimentally and naturally infected mice and rats by the polymerase chain reaction. *Experimental Animals* 44:333–336.

Griffith, J.W., White, W.J., Danneman, P.J., & Lang, C.U. (1988) Cilia-associated respiratory (CAR) bacillus infection in obese mice. *Veterinary Pathology* 25:72–76.

Hook, R.R., Jr., Franklin, C.L., Riley, L.K., Livingston, B.A., & Besch-Williford, C.L. (1998) Antigenic analyses of cilia-associated respiratory (CAR) bacillus isolates by use of monoclonal antibodies. *Laboratory Animal Science* 48:234–239.

Kendall, L.K., Riley, L.K., Hook, R.R., Jr., Besch-Williford, C.L., & Franklin, C.L. (2000) Antibody and cytokine responses to the cilium-associated respiratory bacillus in BALB/c and C57BL/6 mice. *Infection and Immunity* 68:4961–4967.

Kendall, L.V., Riley, L.K., Hook, R.R., Jr., Besch-Williford, C.L., & Franklin, C.L. (2002) Characterization of lymphocyte subsets in the bronchiolar lymph nodes of BALB/c mice infected with cilia-associated respiratory bacillus. *Comparative Medicine* 52:322–327.

Matsushita, S., Joshima, H. Matsumoto, T., & Fukutsu, K. (1989) Transmission experiments of cilia-associated respiratory bacillus in mice, rabbits and guinea pigs. *Laboratory Animals* 23:96–102.

Schoeb, T.R., Dybvig, K., Davidson, M.K., & Davis, J.K. (1993) Cultivation of cilia-associated respiratory bacillus in artificial medium and determination of the 16S rRNA gene sequence. *Journal of Clinical Microbiology* 31:2751–2757.

Shoji-Darkye, Y., Itoh, T., & Kagiyama, N. (1992) Pathogenesis of CAR bacillus in rabbits, guinea pigs, Syrian hamsters, and mice. *Laboratory Animal Science* 41:567–571.

Coxiella burnetii Infection

Criley, J.M., Carty, A.J., Besch-Williford, C.L., & Franklin, C.L. (2001) *Coxiella burnetii* infection of C. B-17-scid-bg mice xenotransplanted with fetal bovine tissue. *Comparative Medicine* 51:357–360.

Klebsiella spp. Infections

Bleich, A., Kirsch, P., Sahly, H., Fahey, J., Smoczek, A., Hedrich, H.J., & Sundberg, J.P. (2008) *Klebsiella oxytoca*: opportunistic infections in laboratory rodents. *Laboratory Animals* 42:369–375.

Bolister, N.J., Johnson, H.E., & Wathes, C.M. (1992) The ability of airborne *Klebsiella pneumoniae* to colonize mouse lungs. *Epidemiology and Infection* 109:121–131.

Davis, J.K., Gaertner, D.J., Cox, N.R., Lindsey, J.R., Cassell, G.H., Davidson, M.K., Kervin, K.C., & Rao, G.N. (1987) The role of *Klebsiella oxytoca* in utero-ovarian infection of B6C3F1 mice. *Laboratory Animal Science* 37:159–166.

Flamm, H. (1957) *Klebsiella* enzootic in a mouse strain. *Schweizerische Zeitschrift fur Pathologie und Bakteriologie* 20:23–27.

Foreman, O., Kavirayani, A.M., Griffey, S.M., Reader, R., & Schultz, L.D. (2011) Opportunistic bacterial infections in breeding colonies of the NSG mouse strain. *Veterinary Pathology* 48:495–499.

Rao, G.N., Hickman, R.L., Seilkop, S.K., & Boorman, G.A. (1987) Utero-ovarian infection in aged B6C3F1 mice. *Laboratory Animal Science* 37:153–158.

Schneemilch, H.D. (1976) A naturally acquired infection of laboratory mice with *Klebsiella* capsule type 6. *Laboratory Animals* 10:305–310.

Leptospira spp. Infection

Birnbaum, S., Shenberg, E., & Torten, M. (1972) The influence of maternal antibodies on the epidemiology of leptospiral carrier state in mice. *American Journal of Epidemiology* 96:313–317.

Friedmann, C.T., Spiegel, E.L., Aaron, E., & McIntyre, R. (1973) Leptospirosis ballum contracted from pet mice. *California Medicine* 118:51–52.

Levett, P.N. (2001) Leptospirosis. *Clinical Microbiology Reviews* 14:296–326.

Nally, J.E., Fishbein, M.C., Blanco, D.R., & Lovett, M.A. (2005) Lethal infection of C3H/HeJ and C3H/SCID mice with an isolate of *Leptospira interrogans* serovar copenhageni. *Infection and Immunity* 73:7014–7017.

Pereira, M.M., Andrade, J., Marchevsky, R.S., & Ribeiro dos Santos, R. (1998) Morphological characterization of lung and kidney lesions in C3H/HeJ mice infected with *Leptospira interrogans* serovar *icterohaemorrhagiae*: defect of CD4+ and CD8+ T-cells are prognosticators of the disease progression. *Experimental Toxicologic Pathology* 50:191–198.

Stoenner, H.G. (1957) The laboratory diagnosis of leptospirosis. *Veterinary Medicine* 52:540–542.

Stoenner, H.G. & Maclean, D. (1958) Leptospirosis (ballum) contracted from Swiss albino mice. *Archives of Internal Medicine* 101:706–710.

Mycoplasma spp. Infection

Andrewes, C.H. & Glover, R.E. (1946) Grey lung virus: an agent pathogenic for mice and other rodents. *British Journal of Experimental Pathology* 26:379–387.

Baker, H.J., Cassell, G.H., & Lindsey, J.R. (1971) Research complications due to *Hemobartonella* and *Eperythrozoon* infections in experimental animals. *American Journal of Pathology* 64:625–656.

Banerjee, A.K., Angulo, A.F., Polak-Vogelzang, A.A., & Kershof, A.M. (1985) Naturally occurring genital mycoplasmosis in mice. *Laboratory Animals* 19:275–276.

Berkenkamp, S.D. & Wescott, R.B. (1988) Arthropod transmission of *Eperythrozoon coccoides* in mice. *Laboratory Animal Science* 38:398–401.

Cartner, S.C., Lindsey, J.R., Gibbs-Erwin, J., Cassell, G.H., & Simecka, J.W. (1998) Roles of innate and adaptive immunity in respiratory mycoplasmosis. *Infection and Immunity* 66:3485–3491.

Cartner, S.C., Simecka, J.W., Lindsey, J.R., Cassell, G.H., & Davis, J.K. (1995) Chronic respiratory mycoplasmosis in C3H/HeN and C57BL/6N mice: lesion severity and antibody response. *Infection and Immunity* 63:4138–4142.

Evengard, B.K., Sandstedt, K., Bolske, G., Feinstein, R., Riesenfelt-Orn, I., & Smith, C.L. (1994) Intranasal inoculation of *Mycoplasma pulmonis* in mice with severe combined immunodeficiency (SCID) causes a wasting disease with grave arthritis. *Clinical and Experimental Immunology* 98:388–394.

Hill, A.C. & Stalley, G.P. (1991) *Mycoplasma pulmonis* infection with regard to embryo freezing and hysterectomy derivation. *Laboratory Animal Science* 41:563–566.

Jones, H.P., Tabor, L., Sun, X., Woolard, M.D., & Simecka, J.W. (2002) Depletion of CD8+ T cells exacerbates CD4+ Th cell-associated inflammatory lesions during murine *Mycoplasma* respiratory disease. *Journal of Immunology* 168:3493–3501.

Kishima, M., Kuniyasu, C., & Eguchi, M. (1989) Cell-mediated and humoral immune responses in mice during experimental infection with *Mycoplasma pulmonis*. *Laboratory Animals* 23:138–142.

Neimark, H., Mitchelmore, D., & Leach, R.H. (1998) An approach to characterizing uncultivated prokaryotes: the Grey Lung agent and proposal of a *Candidatus* taxon for the organism, "*Candidatus* Mycoplasma ravipulmonis." *International Journal of Systematic Bacteriology* 48:389–394.

Niven, J.S.F. (1950) The histology of "grey lung virus" lesions in mice and cotton rats. *British Journal of Experimental Pathology* 31:759–778.

Saito, M., Nakayama, K., Suzuki, E., Kinoshita, K., & Imaizumi, K. (1981) Synergistic effect of Sendai virus on *Mycoplasma pulmonis* infection in mice. *Japanese Journal of Veterinary Research* 43:43–50.

Sandstedt, K., Berglof, A. Feinstein, R., Bolske, G., Evemgard, B., & Smith, C.L. (1997) Differential susceptibility to *Mycoplasma pulmonis* intranasal infection in X-linked immunodeficient (xid), severe combined immunodeficient (scid), and immunocompetent mice. *Clinical and Experimental Immunology* 108:490–496.

Yancey, A.L., Watson, H.L., Cartner, S.C., & Simecka, J.W. (2001) Gender is a major factor determining the severity of *Mycoplasma* respiratory disease in mice. *Infection and Immunity* 69:2865–2871.

Pasteurella pneumotropica Infection

Ackerman, J.I. & Fox, J.G. (1981) Isolation of *Pasteurella ureae* from reproductive tracts of congenic mice. *Journal of Clinical Microbiology* 13:1049–1053.

Artwohl, J.E., Flynn, J.C., Bunte, R.M., Angen, O., & Herold, K.C. (2000) Outbreak of *Pasteurella pneumotropica* in a closed colony of STOCK-Cd28^tm1Mak mice. *Contemporary Topics in Laboratory Animal Science* 39:39–41.

Boot, R., Thuis, H., & Teppema (1993) Colonization and antibody response in mice and rats experimentally infected with Pasteurellaceae from different rodent species. *Laboratory Animals* 28:130–137.

Brennan, P.C., Fritz, T.E., & Flynn, R.J. (1969) Role of *Pasteurella pneumotropica* and *Mycoplasma pulmonis* in murine pneumonia. *Journal of Bacteriology* 97:337–349.

Macy, J.D., Weir, E.C., Compton, S.R., Schlomchik, M.J., & Brownstein, D.G. (2000) Dual infection with *Pneumocystis carinii* and *Pasteurella pneumotropica* in B cell-deficient mice: diagnosis and therapy. *Comparative Medicine* 50:49–55.

Needham, J.R. & Cooper, J.E. (1975) An eye infection in laboratory mice associated with *Pasteurella pneumotropica*. *Laboratory Animals* 9:197–200.

Scharmann, W. & Heller, A. (2001) Survival and transmissibility of *Pasteurella pneumotropica*. *Laboratory Animals* 35:163–166.

Wagner, J.E., Garrison, R.G., Johnson, D.R., & McGuire, T.J. (1969) Spontaneous conjunctivitis and dacryoadenitis of mice. *Journal of the American Veterinary Medical Association* 155:1211–1217.

Ward, G.E., Moffatt, R., & Olfert, E. (1978) Abortion in mice associated with *Pasteurella pneumotropica*. *Journal of Clinical Microbiology* 8:177–180.

Weisbroth, S.H., Scher, S., & Boman, I. (1969) *Pasteurella pneumotropica* abscess syndrome in a mouse colony. *Journal of the American Veterinary Medical Association* 155:1206–1210.

Proteus mirabilis Infection

Bingel, S.A. (2002) Pathology of a mouse model of X-linked chronic granulomatous disease. *Contemporary Topics in Laboratory Animal Science* 41:33–38.

Jones, J.B., Estes, P.C., & Jordan, A.E. (1972) *Proteus mirabilis* infection in a mouse colony. *Journal of the American Veterinary Medical Association* 161:661–664.

Maronpot, R.R. & Peterson, L.G. (1981) Spontaneous *Proteus* nephritis among male C3H/HeJ mice. *Laboratory Animal Science* 21:697–700.

Scott, R.A.W. (1989) Fatal *Proteus mirabilis* infection in a colony of SCID-beige immunodeficient mice. *Laboratory Animal Science* 39:470–471.

Scott, R.A.W., Croy, B.A., & Percy, D.H. (1991) Diagnostic exercise: hepatitis in SCID-beige mice. *Laboratory Animal Science* 41:166–168.

Taylor, D.M. (1988) A shift from acute to chronic spontaneous pyelonephritis in male MM mice associated with a change in the causal micro-organisms. *Laboratory Animals* 22:27–34.

Wensinck, F. (1961) The origin of endogenous *Proteus mirabilis* bacteremia in irradiated mice. *Journal of Pathologic Bacteriology* 81:395–401.

Pseudomonas aeruginosa Infection

Brownstein, D.G. (1978) Pathogenesis of bacteremia due to *Pseudomonas aeruginosa* in cyclophosphamide-treated mice and potentiation of virulence of endogenous streptococci. *Journal of Infectious Diseases* 137:795–801.

Dietrich, H.M., Khaschabi, D., & Albini, B. (1996) Isolation of *Enterococcus durans* and *Pseudomonas aeruginosa* in a scid mouse colony. *Laboratory Animals* 30:102–107.

Ediger, R.D., Rabstein, M.M., & Olson, L.D. (1971) Circling in mice caused by *Pseudomonas aeruginosa*. *Laboratory Animal Science* 21:845–848.

Furuya, N., Hirakata, Y., Tomono, K., Matsumoto, T., Tateda, K., Kaku, M., & Yamaguchi, K. (1993) Mortality rates amongst mice with endogenous septicemia caused by *Pseudomonas aeruginosa* isolates from various clinical sources. *Journal of Medical Microbiology* 39:141–146.

Kohn, D.F. & MacKenzie, W.F. (1980) Inner ear disease characterized by rolling in C3H mice. *Journal of the American Veterinary Medical Association* 177:815–817.

Matsumoto, T. (1980) Early deaths after irradiation of mice contaminated by *Enterobacter cloacae*. *Laboratory Animals* 14:247–249.

Morissette, C., Francoeur, C., Darmond-Zwaig, C., & Gervais, F. (1996) Lung phagocyte bacterial function in strains of mice resistant and susceptible to *Pseudomonas aeruginosa*. *Infection and Immunity* 64:4984–4992.

Olson, L.D. & Ediger, R.D. (1972) Histopathologic study of the heads of circling mice infected with *Pseudomonas aeruginosa*. *Laboratory Animal Science* 22:522–527.

Pier, G.B., Meluleni, G., & Neuger, E. (1992) A murine model of chronic mucosal colonization by *Pseudomonas aeruginosa*. *Infection and Immunity* 60:4768–4776.

Villano, J.S., Rong, F., & Cooper, T.K. (2014) Bacterial infections in *Myd88*-deficient mice. *Comparative Medicine* 64:110–114.

Streptobacillus moniliformis Infection

Anderson, L.C., Leary, S.L., & Manning, P.G. (1983) Rat-bite fever in animal research laboratory personnel. *Laboratory Animal Science* 33:292–294.

Boot, R., Oosterhuis, A., & Thuis, H.C. (2002) PCR for the detection of *Streptobacillus moniliformis*. *Laboratory Animals* 36:200–208.

Boot, R., Oosterhuis, A., & Thuis, H.C. (1993) An enzyme-linked immunosorbent assay (ELISA) for monitoring rodent colonies for *Streptobacillus moniliformis* antibodies. *Laboratory Animals* 27:350–357.

Feundt, E.A. (1959) Arthritis caused by *Streptobacillus moniliformis* and pleuropneumonia-like organisms in small rodents. *Laboratory Investigation* 8:1358–1375.

Glastonbury, J.R.W., Morton, J.G., & Matthews, L.M. (1996) *Streptobacillus moniliformis* infection in Swiss white mice. *Journal of Veterinary Diagnostic Investigation* 8:202–209.

Kaspareit-Rittinghausen, J., Wullenweber, M., Deerberg, F., & Farouq, M. (1990) Pathological changes in *Streptobacillus moniliformis* infection of C57BL/6J mice. *Berliner und Munchener tierztliche Wochenschrift* 103:84–87.

Savage, N.L., Joiner, G.N., & Florey, D.W. (1981) Clinical, microbiological, and histological manifestations of *Streptobacillus moniliformis*-induced arthritis in mice. *Infection and Immunity* 34:605–609.

Sawicki, L., Bruce, H.M., & Andrews, C.H. (1962) *Streptobacillus moniliformis* infection as a probable cause of arrested pregnancy and abortion in laboratory mice. *British Journal of Experimental Pathology* 43:194–197.

Taylor, J.D., Stephens, C.P., Duncan, R.G., & Singleton, G.R. (1994) Polyarthritis in wild mice (*Mus musculus*) caused by *Streptobacillus moniliformis*. *Australian Veterinary Journal* 71:143–145.

Wullenweber, M., Kaspareit-Rittinghausen, J., & Farouq, M. (1990) *Streptobacillus moniliformis* epizootic in barrier-maintained C57BL/6J mice and susceptibility to infection of different strains of mice. *Laboratory Animal Science* 90:608–612.

Other Gram-Positive Bacterial Infections

Aerococcus viridans Infection

Dagnaes-Hansen, F., Kilian, M., & Fuursted, K. (2004) Septicemia associated with an *Aerococcus viridans* infection in immunodeficient mice. *Laboratory Animals* 38:321–325.

Corynebacterium bovis Infection

Clifford, C.B., Walton, B.J., Reed, T.H., Coyle, M.B., White, W.J., & Amyx, H.L. (1995) Hyperkeratosis in athymic nude mice caused by a coryneform bacterium: microbiology, transmission, clinical signs, and pathology. *Laboratory Animal Science* 45:131–139.

Dole, V.S., Henderson, K.S., Fister, R.D., Pietrowski, M.T., Maldonado, G., & Clifford, C.B. (2013) Pathogenicity and genetic variation of 3 strains of *Corynebacterium bovis* in immunodeficient mice. *Journal of the American Association for Laboratory Animal Science* 52:458–466.

Duga, S., Gobbi, A., Asselta, R., Crippa, L., Tenchini, M.L., Simonic, T., & Scanziani, E. (1998) Analysis of the 16S rRNA gene sequence of the coryneform bacterium associated with hyperkeratotic dermatitis of athymic nude mice and development of a PCR-based detection assay. *Molecular and Cellular Probes* 12:191–199.

Gobbi, A., Crippa, L., & Scanziani, E. (1999) *Corynebacterium bovis* infection in immunocompetent hirsute mice. *Laboratory Animal Science* 39:209–211.

Scanziani, E., Gobbi, A., Crippa, L., Giusti, A.M., Giavazzi, R., Cavalletti, E., & Luini, M. (1997) Outbreaks of hyperkeratotic dermatitis of athymic mice in northern Italy. *Laboratory Animals* 31:206–211.

Scanziani, E., Gobbi, A., Crippa, L., Giusti, A.M., Pesenti, E., Cavalletti, E., & Luini, M. (1998) Hyperkeratosis-associated coryneform infection in severe combined immunodeficient mice. *Laboratory Animals* 32:330–336.

Corynebacterium kutscheri Infection

Amao, H., Komukai, Y., Sugiyama, M., Saito, T.R., Takahashi, K.W., & Saito, M. (1993) Differences in susceptibility of mice among various strains to oral infection with *Corynebacterium kutscheri*. *Jikken Dobutsu* 42:539–545.

Amao, H., Komukai, Y., Sugiyama, M., Takahashi, K.W., Sawada, T., & Saito, M. (1995) Natural habitats of *Corynebacterium kutscheri* in subclinically infected ICGN and DBA/2 strains of mice. *Laboratory Animal Science* 45:6–10.

Amao, H., Moriguchi, N., Komukai, Y., Kawasumi, H., Takahashi, K., & Sawada, T. (2008) Detection of *Corynebacterium kutscheri* in the faeces of subclinically infected mice. *Laboratory Animals* 42:376–382.

Komukai, Y,. Amao, H., Goto, N., Kusajima, Y., Sawada, T., Saito, M., & Takahashi, K.W. (1999) Sex differences in susceptibility of ICR mice to oral infection with *Corynebacterium kutscheri*. *Experimental Animals* 48:37–42.

Other *Corynebacterium* spp. Infections

McWilliams, T.S., Waggie, K.S., Luzarraga, M.B., French, A.W., & Adams, R.J. (1993) *Corynebacterium* species-associated keratoconjunctivitis in aged male C57BL/6J mice. *Laboratory Animal Science* 43:509–512.

Radaelli, E., Manarolla, G., Pisoni, G., Balloi, A., Aresu, L., Sparaciari, P., Maggi, A., Caniatti, M., & Scanziani, E. (2010) Suppurative adenitis of preputial glands associated with *Corynebacterium mastitidis* infection in mice. *Journal of the American Association for Laboratory Animal Science* 49:69–74.

***Staphylococcus* spp. Infections**

Bradfield, J.F., Wagner, J.E., Boivin, G.P., Steffen, E.K., & Russell, R.J. (1993) Epizootic of fatal dermatitis in athymic nude mice due to *Stapylococcus xylosus*. *Laboratory Animal Science* 43:111–113.

Haraguchi, M., Hino, M., Tanaka, H., & Maru, M. (1997) Naturally occurring dermatitis associated with *Staphylococcus aureus* in DS-Nh mice. *Experimental Animals* 46:225–229.

Hikita, I., Yoshioka, T., Mizoguchi, T., Tsukahara, K., Tsuru, K., Nagai, H., Hirasawa, T., Tsuruta, Y., Suzuki, R., Ichihashi, M., & Horikawa, T. (2002) Characterization of dermatitis arising spontaneously in DS-Nh mice maintained under conventional conditions: another possible model for atopic dermatitis. *Journal of Dermatological Science* 30:142–153.

McBride, D.F., Stark, D.M., & Walberg, J.A. (1981) An outbreak of staphylococcal furunculosis in nude mice. *Laboratory Animal Science* 31:270–272.

Scharffetter-Kochanek, K., Lu, H., Norman, K., van Nood, N., Munoz, F., Grabbe, S., McArthur, M., Lorenzo, I., Kaplan, S., Ley, K., Smith, C.W., Montgomery, C.A., Rich, S., & Beaudet, A.L. (2006) Spontaneous skin ulceration and defective T cell function in CD18 null mice. *Journal of Experimental Medicine* 188:119–131.

Shapiro, R.L., Duquette, J.G., Nunes, I., Roses, D.F., Harris, M.N., Wilson, E.L., & Rifkin, D.B. (1997) Urokinase-type plasminogen activator-deficient mice are predisposed to staphylococcal botryomycosis, pleuritis, and effacement of lymphoid follicles. *American Journal of Pathology* 150:359–369.

Thornton, V.B., Davis, J.A., St Clair, M.B., & Cole, M.N. (2003) Inoculation of *Staphylococcus xylosus* in SJL/J mice to determine pathogenicity. *Contemporary Topics in Laboratory Animal Science* 42:49–52.

Wardrip, C.L., Artwohl, J.E., Bunte, R.M., & Bennett, B.T. (1994) Diagnostic exercise: head and neck swelling in A/JCr mice. *Laboratory Animal Science* 44:280–282.

Won, Y.S., Kwon, H.J., Oh, G.T., Kim, B.H., Lee, C.H., Park, Y.H., Hyun, B.H., & Choi, Y.K. (2002) Identification of *Staphylococcus xylosus* isolated from C57BL/6J-*Nos2^{tm1Lau}* mice with dermatitis. *Microbiology and Immunology* 46:629–632.

Yoshioka, T., Hikita, I., Matsutani, T., Yoshida, R., Asakawa, M., Toyosaki-Maeda, T., Hirasawa, T., Suzuki, R., Arimura, A., & Horikawa, T. (2003) DS-Nh as an experimental model of atopic dermatitis induced by *Staphylococcus aureus* producing staphylococcal enterotoxin C. *Immunology* 108:562–569.

***Streptococcus* spp. Infections**

Dietrich, H.M., Khaschabi, D., & Albini, B. (1996) Isolation of *Enterococcus durans* and *Pseudomonas aeruginosa* in a scid mouse colony. *Laboratory Animals* 30:102–107.

Duignan, P.J. & Percy, D.H. (1992) Diagnostic exercise: unexplained deaths in recently acquired C3H3 mice. *Laboratory Animal Science* 42:610–611.

Geistfield, J.G. & Weisbroth, S.H. (1993) An epizootic of beta hemolytic group B type V streptococcus in DBA and DBA hybrid mice. *Laboratory Animal Science* 43:387–388.

Geistfield, J.G., Weisbroth, S.H., Jansen, E.A., & Kumpfmiller, D. (1998) Epizootic of group B *Streptococcus agalactiae* serotype V in DBA/2 mice. *Laboratory Animal Science* 48:29–33.

Greenstein, G., Drozdowicz, C.K., Nebiar, F., & Bozik, R. (1994) Isolation of *Streptococcus equisimilis* from abscesses detected in specific-pathogen-free mice. *Laboratory Animal Science* 44:374–376.

Hook, E.W., Wagner, R.R., & Lancefield, R.C. (1960) An epizootic in Swiss mice caused by a group A streptococcus, newly designated type 50. *American Journal of Hygiene* 72:111–119.

Morris, T.H. (1992) Sudden death in young mice. *Laboratory Animals* 21:15–17.

Percy, D.H. & Barta, J.R. (1993) Spontaneous and experimental infections in SCID and SCID/beige mice. *Laboratory Animal Science* 43:127–132.

Schenkman, D.I., Rahija, R.J., Klingenberger, K.L., Elliott, J.A., & Richter, C.B. (1994) Outbreak of group B streptococcal meningoencephalitis in athymic mice. *Laboratory Animal Science* 44:639–641.

Stewart, D.D., Buck, G.E., McConnell, E.E., & Amster, R.L. (1975) An epizootic of necrotic dermatitis in laboratory mice caused by Lancefield group G streptococci. *Laboratory Animal Science* 25:296–302.

***Mycobacterium* spp. Infections**

Mahler, M. & Jelinek, F. (2000) Granulomatous inflammation in the tails of mice associated with *Mycobacterium chelonae* infection. *Laboratory Animals* 34:212–216.

Stokes, R.W., Orme, I.M., & Collins, F.M. (1986) Role of mononuclear phagocytes in expression of resistance and susceptibility to *Mycobacterium avium* infection in mice. *Infection and Immunity* 54:811–819.

Waggie, K.S., Wagner, J.E., & Lentsch, R.H. (1983) Experimental murine infections with a *Mycobacterium avium*–intracellulare complex organism isolated from mice. *Laboratory Animal Science* 33:254–257.

Waggie, K.S., Wagner, J.E., & Lentsch, R.H. (1983) A naturally occurring outbreak of *Mycobacterium avium*–intracellulare infections in C57BL/6N mice. *Laboratory Animal Science* 33:249–253.

Xu, D.L., Goto, Y., Amoako, K.K., Nagatomo, T., Fujita, T., & Shinjo, T. (1996) Establishment of Bcg^r congenic mice and their susceptibility/resistance to mycobacterial infection. *Veterinary Microbiology* 50:73–79.

FUNGAL INFECTIONS

Dermatophytosis

Trichophyton mentagrophytes is the predominant dermatophyte among mice, although other dermatophytes, including *Microsporum canis*, have been isolated. Both are nonselective in their host range and can infect other laboratory animals and humans. Two varieties of *T. mentagrophytes* have been recovered from mice: *T. mentagrophytes* var. *quinckeanum* and *T. mentagrophytes* var. *mentagrophytes*. Dermatophytosis was once common among laboratory mice. Lesions attributed to *T. mentagrophytes* include alopecia and focal crusts, particularly on the head, but the majority of infections are subclinical. Subclinical carriers have been shown to occur in high prevalence in some mouse populations. It is now rare except in pet mice, but its true prevalence in laboratory mouse colonies is unclear, since the great majority of infections are subclinical, especially among adult mice. The most severe manifestation, favus, is usually associated with *T. mentagrophytes* var. *quinckeanum*. Favus is characterized by dull yellow, cuplike crusts on the muzzle, head, ears, face, tail, and extremities. These crusts are composed of epithelial debris, exudate, mycelia, and masses of arthrospores, with underlying dermatitis. Hair invasion has not been observed in mouse favus. Other predisposing factors probably play a role in the manifestation of favus.

Systemic and Pulmonary Mycoses

Systemic mycosis is rare in immunocompetent mice, but is rising in importance among GEMs. A single case of *Cryptococcus neoformans*, a single case as well as outbreaks of *Candida tropicalis*, and a single case of *Actinomyces* sp. (presumptive, based upon morphology) have been reported in immunocompetent mice. Fungal hyphae may be found incidentally in microscopic sections of the nasal passages of mice, associated with chronic inflammation. Contaminated bedding is a possible source for a variety of fungal agents, including *C. albicans* and *Aspergillus fumigatus*. Spontaneous fungal infections posed a significant risk to B6.129S6-*Cybb*^{tm1Din} mice, which have defective NADPH oxidase. Chronic granulomatous disease, particularly in the lungs, was associated with *Paecilomyces* sp., *Aspergillus fumigatus*, *Rhizopus* sp., and *Candida guilliermondii*. Likewise, B6-*p47*(phox) null mice, which are also defective in NADPH oxidase, have been reported to develop pyogranulomata in lung, liver, lymph nodes, salivary gland, and skin, from which *Trichosporon beigelii* was cultured. Mice that lack NADPH oxidase function through null mutation of *gp91*(phox) developed pulmonary infections with *Paecilomyces variotii*. Another colony of *p47* phox null mice with a concomitant gamma interferon mutation was found to develop granulomatous pneumonia in association with *Aspergillus terreus*. Interferon regulatory factor (IRF-1) null mice have been found to develop granulomatous gastritis, with fungal hyphae consistent with *Zygomycetes* sp.

Gastric Candidiasis

Candida pintolopesii (formerly *Torulopsis pintolopesii*) is a yeast that inhabits the surface mucosa of the glandular stomach of normal mice and rats (Fig. 1.81). The yeast *Candida albicans* is frequently present as a member of the normal flora of the alimentary tract in laboratory rodents. When microscopic examination of the murine stomach reveals scattered pseudohyphae in the keratinized epithelium of the forestomach, it is usually regarded as an incidental finding. However, there have been reports of extensive gastric candidiasis with mortality in immunocompromised mice. These mice have thickening of the squamous portion of the stomach with necrotic debris adherent to the surface forming a

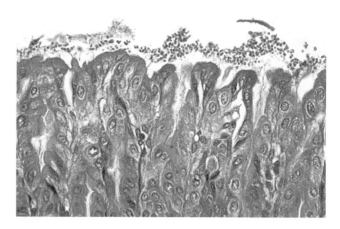

FIG. 1.81. Candida pintolopesii *yeast forms populating the surface of the glandular stomach of a normal mouse.*

pseudomembrane. There is marked epithelial hyperplasia with hyperkeratosis and leukocytic infiltration. The typical filamentous structures with pseudohyphae formation are readily visualized with PAS or silver stains. T-cell-deficient mice are particularly at risk.

Encephalitozoon cuniculi Infection: Microsporidiosis

Although rare in contemporary mouse colonies, *Encephalitozoon cuniculi* was common in laboratory mice in the 1950s and 1960s. It is likely to be common in pet and fancy mice. This agent infects a wide variety of species, including humans. Natural infection in mice has been associated with granulomatous hepatitis, interstitial nephritis, and meningoencephalitis, as well as ascites in cortisonized animals. Immunodeficient mice develop ascites and chronic wasting. In immunodeficient mice, organisms are readily apparent in brain, heart, lungs, liver, spleen, adrenals, kidneys, pancreas, intestine, and serosa. Spores are Gram-positive, which facilitates diagnosis (see rabbit Chapter 6, "Encephalitozoon cuniculi infection"). Additional microsporidia that are infectious to humans have been detected in feces of wild mice, including *Enterocytozoon bieneusi* and *E. hellem*, underscoring the lack of species specificity of these agents, and the potential risk to immunosuppressed humans in contact with wild, pet, and laboratory mice.

Pneumocystis murina Infection: Pneumocystosis

Pulmonary pneumocystosis is a common finding in immunodeficient strains of mice, and may be a life-limiting disease in these strains. It may also occur to a lesser degree in aging immunocompetent mice. Although it was once thought that pneumocystosis in the mouse was due to *Pneumocystis carinii*, it is now known that there are many host-specific *Pneumocystis* species. Pneumocystosis in the mouse is due to infection with mouse-specific *P. murina*.

Epizootiology and Pathogenesis

Nonfilamentous yeast-like trophic forms adhere to type I pneumocytes with clusters of developmental stages extending into the alveolar lumen. These forms have abundant thin filopodia. Asci (cysts) are also present, and contain eight ascospores. *Pneumocystis murina* isolated from laboratory and wild mice are genetically similar. Normally, infection is subclinical and probably transient in immunocompetent mice. Immunosuppression of subclinically infected mice may result in development of *Pneumocystis* pneumonia and more efficient transmission to contact animals. Spontaneous enzootics of *Pneumocystis* pneumonia are now common in a variety of immunodeficient strains of mice. Superimposed viral infection can exacerbate disease, and superimposed bacterial infections, such as *Pasteurella pneumotropica*, may result in suppurative bronchopneumonia. Immunocompromised mice subclinically infected with *P. murina* inoculated with PVM developed severe respiratory tract lesions attributed to the dual infection.

Pathology

Clinical signs of pneumocystosis in immunodeficient mice include dyspnea, wasting, hunched posture, and dry, scaly skin. Lungs collapse poorly and have a rubbery consistency, with pale, patchy areas of consolidation (Fig. 1.82). Microscopic examination reveals interstitial pneumonitis, with proteinaceous exudation into the alveolar lumina. There is marked thickening of alveolar septa and infiltration with mononuclear leukocytes (Fig. 1.83). Finely vacuolated, eosinophilic material containing punctate cyst forms and alveolar macrophages

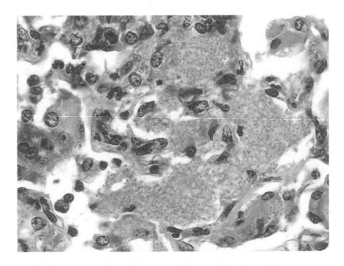

FIG. 1.83. *Lung from an athymic mouse with spontaneous* Pneumocystis murina *pneumonia. Alveolar septa are hypercellular, with mononuclear cell infiltration. Foamy proteinaceous exudate containing punctate P. murina cyst forms is present in alveoli.*

are scattered in affected alveoli. In tissue sections stained with the PAS or methenamine silver procedures, numerous rounded and irregularly shaped 3–5 μm cyst forms are present in affected areas (Fig. 1.84). Electron microscopy reveals numerous trophic forms with long filapodia intermixed with thicker walled asci. The quality of the pneumonia associated with *Pneumocystis* in immunodeficient mice can be quite variable, depending upon the immune deficiency. Some types of mice may have very few visible cysts or alveolar exudation, with principally an interstitial pneumonia. Extrapulmonary infection of other tissues, including bone marrow, heart, liver, and spleen, may be encountered in SCID mice. Aged immunocompetent mice may develop focal areas of alveolar pneumocystosis as an incidental finding.

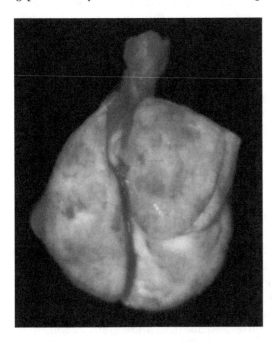

FIG. 1.82. *Lungs from an immunodeficient mouse with* Pneumocystis murina *pneumonia. The lungs are pale, fleshy, and collapse poorly, typical gross findings with this disease.*

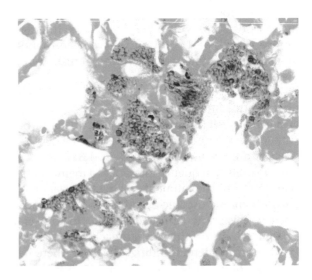

FIG. 1.84. *Lung from a mouse with* Pneumocystis murina *pneumonia. Large numbers of cyst forms are present in alveoli (methenamine silver stain).*

Diagnosis

A history of experimental procedures leading to immunosuppression or disease in genetically immunodeficient mice is a critical predisposing factor. Organisms may be demonstrated in the typical foamy alveolar exudate, using methenamine silver or PAS stains. Differential diagnoses for chronic progressive pneumonia in immunodeficient mice include viral pneumonitis due to Sendai virus and PVM and pulmonary edema secondary to congestive heart failure. Coinfections with respiratory viruses or *Pasteurella pneumotropica* are known to aggravate pulmonary pneumocystosis. PCR can be used to screen for *P. murina* infection, but it is important to test young mice, as infection is transient in immunocompetent animals.

BIBLIOGRAPHY FOR FUNGAL INFECTIONS

See "General References for Infectious Diseases"

Dermatophytosis

Booth, B.H. (1952) Mouse ringworm. *Archives of Dermatology and Syphilology* 66:65–69.

Cetin, E.T., Tahsinoglu, M., & Volkan, S. (1965) Epizootic of *Trichophyton mentagrophytes* (interdigitale) in white mice. *Pathologia et Microbiologia* 28:839–846.

Dolan, M.M., Kligman, A.M., Koylinski, P.G., & Motsavage, M.A. (1958) Ringworm epizootics in laboratory mice and rats: experimental and accidental transmission of infection. *Journal of Investigative Dermatology* 30:23–25.

Mackenzie, D.W.R. (1961) *Trichophyton mentagrophytes* in mice: infections of humans and incidence amongst laboratory animals. *Sabouradia* 1:178–182.

Papini, R., Gazzano, A., & Mancianti, F. (1997) Survey of dermatophytes isolated from the coats of laboratory animals in Italy. *Laboratory Animal Science* 47:75–77.

Systemic, Pulmonary, and Gastric Mycotic Infections

Austwick, P.K. (1974) Apparently spontaneous *Candida tropicalis* infection of a mouse. *Laboratory Animals* 8:133–136.

Bingel, S.A. (2002) Pathology of a mouse model of X-linked chronic granulomatous disease. *Contemporary Topics in Laboratory Animal Science* 41:33–38.

Dixon, D., Goelz, M.F., Locklear, J., Myers, P.H., & Thigpen, J.E. (1993) Diagnostic exercise: gastritis in athymic nude mice. *Laboratory Animal Science* 43:497–499.

France, M.P. & Muir, D. (2000) An outbreak of pulmonary mycosis in respiratory burst-deficient (gp91(phox−/−)) mice with concurrent acidophilic macrophage pneumonia. *Journal of Comparative Pathology* 123:190–194.

Goetz, M.E. & Taylor, D.O. (1967) A naturally occurring outbreak of *Candida tropicalis* infection in a laboratory mouse colony. *American Journal of Pathology* 50:361–369.

Lacy, S.H., Gardner, D.J., Olson, L.C., Ding, L., Holland, S.M., & Bryant, M.A. (2003) Disseminated trichosporonosis in a murine model of chronic granulomatous disease. *Comparative Medicine* 53:303–308.

Mayeux, P., Dupepe, L., Dunn, K., Balsamo, J., & Domer, J. (1995) Massive fungal contamination in animal care facilities traced to bedding supply. *Applied Environmental Microbiology* 61:2297–2301.

Mullink, J.W. (1968) A case of actinomycosis in a male NZW mouse. *Zeitschrift für Versuchstierkunde* 10:225–227.

Sacquet, E., Drouhet, E., & Valee, A. (1959) Un cas spontane de cryptococcose (*Cryptococcus neoformans*) chez la souris. *Annales de l'Institut Pasteur, Paris* 97:252–253.

Savage, D.C. & Dubos, R. (1967) Localization of indigenous yeast in the murine stomach. *Journal of Bacteriology* 94:1811–1816.

Encephalitozoon cuniculi Infection

Al-Sadi, H.I. & Al-Mahmood, S.S. (2014) Pathology of experimental *Encephalitozoon cuniculi* in immunocompetent and immunosuppressed mice in Iraq. *Pathology Research International* 2014: e857036.

Didier, E.S., Varner, P.W., Didier, P.J., Aldras, A.M., Millichamp, N.J., Murphey-Corb, M., Bohm, R., & Shadduck, J.A. (1994) Experimental microsporidiosis in immunocompetent and immunodeficient mice and monkeys. *Folia Parasitiligica* 41:1–11.

El-Naas, A., Viera, R., Valeria, L., Monica, H., & Stefkovic, M. (1998) Murine encephalitozoonosis and kidney lesions in some Slovak laboratory animal breeding centers. *Helminthologia* 35:107–110.

Innes, J.R.M., Zeman, A., Frenkel, J.K., & Borner, G. (1962) Occult endemic encephalitozoonosis of the central nervous system of mice (Swiss–Bagg–O'Grady strain). *Journal of Neuropathology and Experimental Neurology* 21:519–533.

Lallo, M.A. & Bondan, E.F. (2005) Experimental meningoencephalomyelitis by *Encephalitozoon cuniculi* in cyclophosphamide-immunosuppressed mice. *Arquivos de Neuro-Psisquiatria* 63:246–251.

Liu, J.J., Greeley, E.H., & Shadduck, J.A. (1988) Murine encephalitozoonosis: the effect of age and mode of transmission on occurrence of infection. *Laboratory Animal Science* 38:675–679.

Niederkorn, J.Y., Shadduck, J.A., & Schmidt, E.C. (1981) Susceptibility of selected inbred strains of mice to *Encephalitozoon cuniculi*. *Journal of Infectious Diseases* 144:249–253.

Sak, B., Kvac, M., Kvetonova, D., Albrecht, T., & Pialek, J. (2011) The first report on natural *Enterocytozoon bienusi* and *Encephalitozoon* spp. infections in wild East-European house mice (*Mus musculus musculus*) and West-European house mice (*M.m. domesticus*) in a hybrid zone across the Czech Republic–Germany border. *Veterinary Parasitology* 178:246–250.

Pneumocystis murina Infection

Bray, M.V., Barthold, S.W., Sidman, C.L., Roths, J., & Smith, A.L. (1993) Exacerbation of *Pneumocystis carinii* pneumonia in immunodeficient (scid) mice by concurrent infection with a pneumovirus. *Infection and Immunity* 61:1586–1588.

Chabe, M., Aliouat-Denis, C.M., Delhaes, L., Aliouat, el M., Viscogliosi, E., & Dei-Cas, E. (2011) *Pneumocystis*: from a doubtful unique entity to a group of highly diversified fungal species. *FEMS Yeast Research* 11:2–17.

Macy, J.D., Weir, E.C., Compton, S.R., Shlomchik, M.J., & Brownstein, D.G. (2000) Dual infection with *Pneumocystis carinii* and *Pasteurella pneumotropica* in B cell-deficient mice: diagnosis and therapy. *Comparative Medicine* 50:49–55.

Powles, M.A., McFadden, D.C., Pittarelli, L.A., & Schmatz, D.M. (1992) Mouse model for *Pneumocystis carinii* pneumonia that uses natural transmission to initiate infection. *Infection and Immunity* 60:1397–1400.

Soulez, B., Palluault, F., Cesbron, J.Y., Dei-Cas, E., Capron, A., & Camus, D. (1991) Introduction of *Pneumocystis carinii* in a colony of scid mice. *Journal of Protozoology* 38:123S–125S.

Walzer, P.D., Powell, R.D., Jr., & Yoneda, K. (1979) Experimental *Pneumocystis carinii* pneumonia in different strains of cortisonized mice. *Infection and Immunity* 24:939–947.

Walzer, P.D., Kim, C.K., Linke, M.J., Pogue, C.L., Huerkamp, M.J., Chrisp, C.E., Lerro, A.V., Wixson, S.K., Hall, E., & Shultz, L.D. (1989) Outbreaks of *Pneumocystis carinii* pneumonia in colonies of immunodeficient mice. *Infection and Immunity* 57:62–70.

Weir, E.C., Brownstein, D.G., & Barthold, S.W. (1986) Spontaneous wasting disease in nude mice associated with *Pneumocystis carinii* infection. *Laboratory Animal Science* 36:140–144.

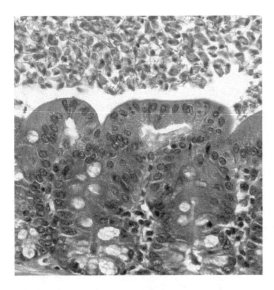

FIG. 1.85.   *Cecum from a transgenic mouse with overgrowth of* Tritrichomonas muris *within the lumen. Note the absence of inflammation.*

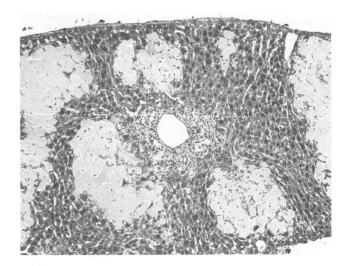

FIG. 1.86.   *Liver from an athymic mouse with chronic cryptosporidiosis. There are multiple foci of acute coagulation necrosis with chronic cholangitis and peribiliary fibrosis.*

PARASITIC DISEASES

Protozoal Infections

Mice may be host to several marginally pathogenic intestinal protozoa, including several species of *Eimeria*, *Cryptosporidium muris*, *C. parvum*, *C. tyzzeri*, *Giardia muris*, and *S. muris*. Under some circumstances, they may become opportunistic pathogens. *Tritrichomonas muris*, *Tritrichomonas minuta*, *Trichomonas wenyoni*, *Octomitus pulcher*, *Chilomastix bettencourti*, *Entamoeba muris*, and others inhabit the intestine of laboratory mice but are not pathogens. Impressive numbers of *T. muris* and/or *T. minuta* may be present in the intestinal lumen, with no lesions (Fig. 1.85). Other coccidians, including *Klossiella muris* and *Sarcocystis muris*, are rare in laboratory mice. Wild mice are frequent intermediate hosts for *Toxoplasma gondii*, but *Toxoplasma* infections in laboratory mice are essentially nonexistent, since it requires cats as the definitive host. Nevertheless, it is important to expect the unexpected in mouse pathology, as *Sarcocystis muris*, which also requires cats as the definitive host, has appeared in recent decades among laboratory mice.

Cryptosporidium *spp. Infection: Cryptosporidiosis*

Ernest Tyzzer initially named the genus *Cryptosporidium* when describing two morphologically distinct species, *C. muris* that infects the gastric mucosa and *C. parvum* that infects the small intestinal epithelium in the mouse. Based upon similar morphology, Cryptosporidium of other host species were often considered *C. parvum*, but genetic analysis has revealed far more complexity within the group. It is now apparent that the previously

named *C. parvum* in the mouse includes at least three morphologically similar and genetically related species: *C. tyzzeri* (formerly mouse genotype I), mouse genotype II, and *C. parvum*, which vary in host specificity and natural host range. *Cryptosporidium muris* is more distantly related to the *C. parvum* cluster. *C. muris* is relatively nonpathogenic and occurs primarily within glands of the gastric mucosa of mice. Similarly, members of the *C. parvum* group of mouse cryptosporidium are marginally pathogenic inhabitants of the small intestine, but heavy infections may cause blunting and fusion of villi, crypt proliferation, and lymphocytic infiltration of the lamina propri. Mice are also susceptible to the bovine genotype of *C. parvum*. The prevalence of infection with these various species is not known. Suckling mice are particularly at risk, and intestinal microflora play a role in resistance. Infection may also ascend the biliary tract in nude and SCID mice, resulting in chronic cholangiohepatitis with focal hepatic coagulative necrosis (Fig. 1.86). SCID and athymic nude mice are unable to clear infections with *C. muris* and *C. parvum*, whereas immunocompetent mice develop transient infections. A number of recent publications have claimed that *C. parvum*, but not *C. muris*, infection of SCID mice treated with dexamethasone results in development of neoplasia in the stomach, duodenum, and ileocecal region. Heavy infection is associated with mucosal hyperplasia and foci of dysplasia, but claims of neoplasia are overstated. The possibility of zoonotic risk to humans and the potential danger to immunocompromised mice is significant.

Eimeria *spp. Infection: Intestinal Coccidiosis*

Mice are host to 18 species of *Eimeria*, of which *Eimeria falciformis*, *Eimeria vermiformis*, *Eimeria papillata*, and *Eimeria ferrisi* are the most significant as pathogens. Intestinal coccidiosis rarely occurs in well-managed

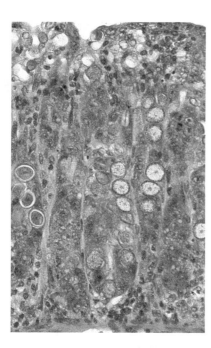

FIG. 1.87.   *Colon from a young wild mouse with intestinal coccidiosis. There are multiple developmental stages of the parasite with associated hyperplastic and inflammatory change.*

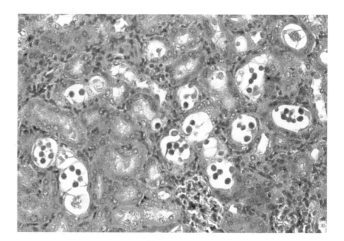

FIG. 1.88.   *Kidney from a mouse with renal coccidiosis due to* Klossiella muris. *Large numbers of sporocysts are present in epithelial cells of renal tubules.*

facilities. Intestinal coccidiosis is very common among pet and wild mice, where it causes marked typhlocolitis (Fig. 1.87) and runting in juvenile animals. Oocysts can be found in the mucosa of older mice without discernible lesions.

Giardia muris *Infection: Giardiasis*

Giardia muris is a flagellate that normally resides in the lumen of the duodenum. Mice, hamsters, rats, and other rodents are natural hosts. Based upon some surveys, infection is quite prevalent among laboratory mice. In the naturally occurring disease, trophozoites proliferate in the small intestine and adhere to the microvilli of enterocytes near the base of villi by means of concave sucking disks. Organisms also wedge in furrows on the epithelial surface and lodge in mucus overlying intestinal epithelium. Giardia infects both young and adult mice, and duration of infection is dependent upon mouse strain and immunodeficiency. Following experimental inoculation, B6, B10, C3H/He, and athymic nude mice had prolonged infections, whereas BALB/c mice recovered from infection rapidly. In heavy infections, animals have a rough hair coat and distended abdomen, usually with no evidence of diarrhea. At necropsy, the small intestine is usually distended with yellow to white watery contents. Microscopic examination of tissue sections of the small intestine reveals pear-shaped trophozoites with a broadly rounded anterior sucking disk. There may be a reduction in the crypt: villus ratio, with increased numbers of leukocytes in the lamina propria. Invasion of the lamina propria with organisms may occur in immunocompromised mice.

Diagnosis can be achieved by identification of organisms in histologic sections, visualization of typical motile forms in wet mounts of intestinal contents, or identification of cysts in feces.

Klossiella muris *Infection: Renal Coccidiosis*

Klossiella muris is rarely observed in laboratory mice, but is quite common in wild mice. Infection occurs by the ingestion of sporocysts, with hematogenous spread to glomerular capillaries and schizogony. Gametogeny and sporogony occur in epithelial cells lining convoluted tubules. On microscopic examination, lesions are usually confined to the convoluted tubules. Sporocysts appear as eosinophilic spherical structures within the cytoplasm of epithelial cells, with minimal inflammatory response (Fig. 1.88). There have been anecdotal reports of transmission of *K. muris* to guinea pigs, but guinea pigs have own *Klossiella* (*K. cobayae*). *Klossiella* has been observed in albino laboratory rats, but the agent was not speciated.

Sarcocystis muris *Infection*

Cats are the definitive host for *S. muris*, and mice serve as the only intermediate host for this coccidian parasite. Infection of mice occurs through ingestion of oocyts in cat feces, but can also be sustained within a mouse population through cannibalism. *Sarcocystis* organisms have been observed in the diaphragm, heart, and skeletal muscle of naturally infected laboratory mice, possibly exposed through contamination by cat-owning technicians rather than food contamination. The authors are also aware of *S. muris* in skeletal muscle of mice maintained for toxicology studies. It has been found that SCID mice can also serve as definitive hosts for *S. muris*, with fecal shedding of oocysts.

Spironucleus muris *Infection: Spironucleosis*

Spironucleus (formerly *Hexamita*) *muris* is a flagellated protozoan that is frequently present in the alimentary tract of clinically normal mice, rats, and hamsters. Inter-species transmission has been demonstrated between hamsters and mice but not to rats. Infection seldom results in clinical disease (spironucleosis), except in young mice, and generally in association with predisposing factors. Mice become infected by ingestion of trophozoites or cysts. The organism colonizes the small intestine, primarily in the crypts and intervillus spaces of the duodenum. Clinical manifestations are usually associated with immunosuppression, immunodeficiency in GEMs, enteric viral infections (MHV), or environmental stress. Animals 3–6 weeks of age are particularly at risk.

Clinical signs of spironucleosis include depression, weight loss, dehydration, hunched posture, diarrhea, and mortality rates of up to 50% in young animals. The small intestine is distended with dark red to brown watery contents and gas. In tissue sections of small intestine examined microscopically from animals with the acute form of the disease, there may be edema of the lamina propria, with mild leukocytic infiltration. Crypts and intervillus spaces are distended with elongated, pear-shaped trophozoites (Figs. 1.89 and 1.90). Organisms may also be present between enterocytes and within the lamina propria. In the chronic form of the disease, the cellular infiltrate consists primarily of lymphocytes and plasma cells. Scattered duodenal crypts may be markedly dilated and contain leukocytes and cellular debris. The trophozoites stain well with the PAS stain, while the organism is poorly delineated in H & E-stained preparations. Trophozoites with fast straight or zigzag movements can be visualized microscopically on direct wet mount smears prepared from small intestine. Typical banded "Easter egg" cysts are present in the

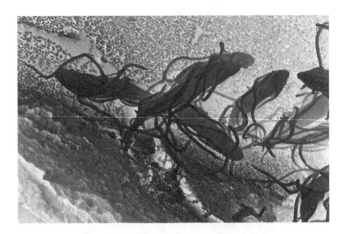

FIG. 1.90. *Scanning electron micrograph of* Spironucleus muris *trophozoites on the duodenal mucosal surface.*

intestinal contents. PCR assay of feces is a highly sensitive method for detecting infection.

Helminth Infestations

Wild, and probably pet mice, may serve as hosts to numerous helminth species, but laboratory mice have a limited repertoire of helminth parasitisms, most notably pinworms and tapeworms.

Pinworm Infestations

Syphacia obvelata and *Aspiculuris tetraptera* are extremely common pinworms in the laboratory mouse, and coinfections are common. In unique circumstances, mice can also be infested with the rat pinworm, *Syphacia muris*.

Epizootiology

Pinworms are difficult to control in mouse facilities due to the high degree of environmental resistance of eggs, the propensity of eggs to drift in air and dust, and their ability to contaminate cage surfaces and the hands of technicians. Pinworms are often the first break in rederived mouse colonies. The life cycle of *Syphacia* is direct and is completed in approximately 12–15 days. Following ingestion of eggs, larvae emerge and migrate to the cecum and ascending colon. They develop into adults and mate, and females then migrate to the perianal region for egg deposition. Eggs become infective within a few hours. The life cycle of *A. tetraptera* is also direct and takes approximately 23–25 days. Adults live in the colon. Mature females lay eggs in the descending colon, which are then passed in the feces. Eggs require incubation at room temperature for 6–7 days in order to become infective and can survive for weeks outside the host. Most mouse pinworm infestations are subclinical. Young mice are particularly susceptible to pinworm infestation, and athymic nude mice have increased susceptibility. Enteric lesions are generally absent, but mucosal invasion with colitis can be noted on occasion in immunodeficient mice. Although mice are susceptible

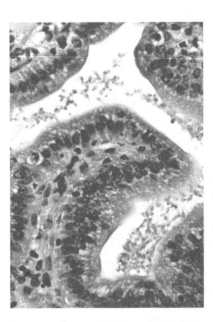

FIG. 1.89. *Spironucleosis (*Spironucleus muris *infection) in a young mouse with diarrhea. Large numbers of trophozoites are present on the duodenal mucosal surface.*

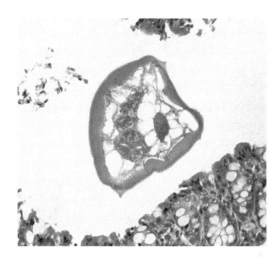

FIG. 1.91.   *Pinworm in the ascending colon of an adult mouse. Note the characteristic lateral alae.*

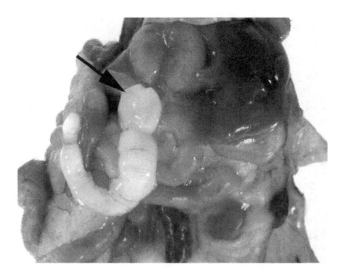

FIG. 1.92.   *Laboratory mouse with* Cysticercus fasciolaris *infestation of the liver. The lesion has been opened. Note the scolex (arrow) and identifiable segments of the parasite.*

to experimental infection with *S. muris*, natural infection is rare. However, natural infection in B6;129-STAT6 null mice with *S. muris* was found to result in massive parasite loads, whereas other mice in the facility, including other immune effector null strains, were not infected. Clinical signs associated with heavy infestations include rectal prolapse, intussusception, fecal impaction, and diarrhea.

Diagnosis

Adult worms are readily visible in the cecum and colon at necropsy. These nematodes are also frequently found in tissue sections of cecum and colon, which have distinctive lateral alae (Fig. 1.91). Cellophane tape applied to the perianal region may be utilized for collection of *Syphacia* eggs for microscopic identification, but fecal flotation is the best means for identifying ova. Ova can be readily differentiated: *Aspiculuris* ova are bilaterally symmetrical, while *Syphacia* ova are banana-shaped. Fecal PCR is now used as a screening method for pinworm infestation.

Tapeworm Infestations

Wild, pet, and laboratory rodents can be infested with 3 separate species of adult tapeworm, including *Rodentolepis* (formerly *Hymenolepis*) *nana* (dwarf tapeworm), *Hymenolepis diminuta*, and *Rodentolepis microstoma*. Laboratory mice have also been found to be infested with the intermediate stage of the cat tapeworm, *Taenia taeniaformis*. All are rare in laboratory mice.

Epizootiology

A variety of species of laboratory animals are susceptible to infection with the dwarf tapeworm, including mice, rats, and hamsters. Its wide host range also includes humans. Husbandry conditions have essentially eliminated *H. diminuta* and *R. microstoma* and have greatly reduced the prevalence of *R. nana* in laboratory mouse populations. These tapeworms all utilize arthropods

(flour beetles, fleas, moths, etc.) as intermediate hosts, but *R. nana* can also have a direct life cycle in which onchospheres penetrate the mucosa and develop into the cysticercoid stage, subsequently emerging into the lumen as adults. The entire life cycle can occur in the intestine within 20–30 days. Thus, superinfections can occur in the absence of an intermediate host. Immunity develops to these worms, with reduction of parasite numbers over time in immunocompetent mice. In addition, *R. microstoma* can have a direct life cycle in immunodeficient nude and NOD-*scid*, NOD-*scid*-IL-2R gamma null mice. Clinical signs associated with heavy infestations include poor weight gains and diarrhea.

Mice may serve as the intermediate host for the cat tapeworm, *Taenia taeniaformis*. The larval strobilocercus form, *Cysticercus fasciolaris*, consists of a scolex and segments within a cyst and thus resembles an adult tapeworm (Fig. 1.92). The liver is the most frequent location for strobilocerci. The source of the parasite is usually via feed contaminated with cat feces. While cysticercosis should be nonexistent in laboratory mice, the authors have seen infected laboratory mice on multiple occasions.

Pathology

Rodentolepis nana adults are threadlike worms in the small intestine. Microscopic findings include the presence of cysticeri within the lamina propria and adults with prominent serrated edges in the lumen. Occasionally, cysticeri can be found in the mesenteric lymph nodes. *Hymenolepis diminuta* adults are much larger, and intermediate forms do not appear in the mucosa. *Rodentolepis microstoma* adults are the size of *H. diminuta* and often exist within the biliary or pancreatic ducts, inciting inflammatory and atrophic changes in the pancreas and cholangitis. The strobilocerci of *T. taeniaeformis* are most often embedded in the liver

Diagnosis

Adult tapeworms can be identified grossly. *Rodentolepis nana* is typically threadlike (1 mm wide), while the other species are much larger (4 mm wide). The *R. nana* scolex possesses hooks, and the ova have polar filaments, while those of *H. diminuta* do not (figures of *R. nana* and *H. diminuta* are shown in Hamster Chapter 3).

Ectoparasitic Infestations
Fur Mite Infestations: Acariasis

Laboratory mice are commonly infested with mixed populations of fur mites, including *Myobia musculi*, *Radfordia affinis*, *Myocoptes musculinis*, and less commonly *Radfordia ensifera* (the rat fur mite) and *Trichoecius romboutsi*. *Myobia musculi* is the most clinically significant mouse mite because of its association with hypersensitivity of the host. *Trichoecius romboutsi* closely resembles *Myocoptes*, and its actual prevalence is therefore unknown.

Epizootiology, Life Cycles, and Pathogenesis

Myobia musculi mites prefer to live in the fur of the head, neck, and shoulder regions. *Myobia* eggs are laid on hair shafts adjacent to the epidermis. Larvae hatch in 7–8 days, and egg-laying adults evolve as early as 16 days after the eggs are laid. *Myobia* mites feed on skin secretions and interstitial fluid, but apparently not on blood. This intimate feeding pattern is unique to *Myobia*, resulting in immune sensitization of the host. Transmission is by direct transfer of adult mites. Adults migrate to suckling mice from infested mothers at around 1 week of age, which corresponds with the appearance of pelage on the young mice. The presence of hair shafts is critical for successful colonization. Nude mice are resistant to experimental infection. In newly infested mice, mite populations increase for the first 8–10 weeks, but host immunity diminishes the populations to a point of equilibrium. This state of equilibrium persists for months to years, with cyclic variations corresponding to waves of egg hatches. Factors recognized to influence parasite load include strain of mouse, age, self-grooming, and mutual grooming. Impairment of grooming function by procedures such as hind toe amputation or Elizabethan collars result in increased parasite load.

Adverse effects of *Myobia* infestation are highly varied and often difficult to prove with certainty. *Myobia* can sensitize the host, resulting in pruritis, with evolution of severe ulcerative lesions from secondary bacterial infections (*Staphylococcus* and *Streptococcus*). These lesions typically arise around the head and neck region. Sensitivity is genetically associated, and strains such as B6 are highly prone to hypersensitivity dermatitis. Lesion susceptibility is affected by non-H-2 linked haplotypes shared by all B6 background strains. Cutaneous allergy due to mite infestation may also occur in other strains, including BALB/c mice and atopic hypersensitivity-prone NC/Jic mice. The hypersensitivity

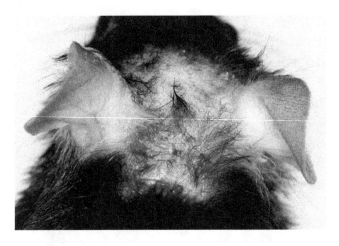

FIG. 1.93. *Ulcerative dermatitis with denuding of hair associated with acariasis and secondary staphylococcal infection. Pruritus associated with acariasis may lead to self-inflicted skin abrasions with superimposed bacterial infection.*

component was confirmed by the histopathologic findings and the markedly elevated serum IgE levels present in affected mice. Manifestations of acariasis range from ruffled fur and alopecia on the head, eyelids, neck, or shoulder regions to severe ulcerative dermatitis with marked pruritis, occasionally resulting in traumatic amputation of the ear pinnae. Self-trauma is an important factor in the development of these lesions (Fig. 1.93). Other adverse effects include reduced life span, weight loss, and infertility.

Radfordia affinis is also common among mice, but its life cycle is not well studied. It does not induce overt disease like *Myobia* and often exists in mixed infestations. Mice may also be infested with the closely related *R. ensifera*, the rat fur mite, and rats are susceptible to *R. affinis*. *Myocoptes musculinis* is the most common of the mouse fur mites and usually exists as a mixed infestation with *Myobia*. In mixed or heavy infestations, *Myocoptes* will inhabit other areas of the body. *Myocoptes* is a surface dweller and feeds upon material in the superficial epidermis. Transmission occurs by close contact, and mites can be transferred within 1 week of birth to newborns. In mixed infestations, *Myobia* tends to dominate the head and shoulder pelage, and *Myocoptes* may be found primarily in the inguinal, ventral abdomen, and back. Clinical signs are usually mild, including patchy hair loss, erythema, and mild pruritis. However, severe pruritis with ulcerative dermatitis has been observed in BALB/c mice infected with *M. musculinus* only (with the caveat that mixed infestations are common and often overlooked).

Pathology

Microscopic examination of fur mite-induced skin lesions will reveal mild epidermal hyperplasia and hyperkeratosis, with variable dermal infiltrates of mononuclear leukocytes and mast cells. In ulcerated lesions, exudation and secondary bacterial colonization (see

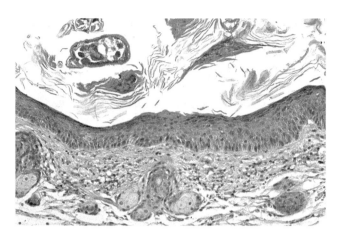

FIG. 1.94. *Skin from a mouse with acariasis. There is epidermal hyperplasia, with mononuclear cell infiltration in the dermis. A mite is present on the surface of the lesion.*

sections in this chapter on staphylococcal and streptococcal infections) are often present, with underlying fibrovascular proliferation, mixed leukocyte infiltration, and hyperplasia of the adjacent intact epidermis. Mites may be present on the surface of the lesions, particularly in early, mild lesions (Fig. 1.94).

Diagnosis
Fur mites can be demonstrated by placing the mouse or a portion of the skinned pelt (head and shoulder regions) in a Petri dish for one or more hours. The mites will climb up the hair shafts and can then be visualized under a dissecting microscope, collected, and identified under a light or stereoscopic microscope. Skin scrapings or cellophane tape applied to the hair can then be placed on a glass slide for microscopic evaluation. A number of points are important to consider in the diagnosis of acariasis. The number of mites will be greatest in young mice, before immune-mediated equilibrium has occurred. For this reason, the number of mites on mice with severe hypersensitivity-induced lesions may be exceedingly few. Infestations are usually mixed, so identification of a single mite will not reflect the true population. Finally, *Myobia* is the most clinically significant, but clinical signs are variable, depending on host factors. One does not have to be a sophisticated acarologist to identify mouse fur mites. A few distinguishing features allow simple speciation. *Myobia* and *Radfordia* are remarkably similar in morphology, with slightly elongated bodies possessing bulges between their legs. If the second pair of legs is carefully examined, *Myobia* has a single terminal tarsal claw, while *Radfordia* has two tarsal claws of unequal length. Myocoptes is oval, with heavily chitinized, pigmented third and fourth legs and suckers on its tarsi. Differential diagnoses for fur mite infestation includes pediculosis, trauma, bacterial dermatitis, dermatophytosis, hair chewing, and mechanically induced muzzle alopecia. PCR is increasingly used as an effective detection method, including testing feces for mite DNA.

Follicle Mite Infestations
Mice are susceptible to infestation with *Demodex musculi*. Reports of infestation are rare, but possibly underrecognized. *Demodex musculi* infestation has been reported in transgenic mice lacking mature T cells and NK cells. Mites were located in the superficial dermis of the dorsal thorax, at the opening of hair follicles, with no inflammatory reaction. Infestation of immunocompetent mice was documented, but they harbored very few mites. Contact transmission of the mites to SCID mice was readily accomplished. Diagnosis can be achieved by examination of plucked hair or skin sections. The authors are aware of additional accounts of Demodex in various types of transgenic mice in both the eastern and western United States. Older accounts of *Demodex* infestations in *M. musculus* include observations of mites in the tongue (unknown species) and preputial and clitoral glands (*D. flagellarus*).

Psorergates simplex was once common among laboratory mice but is now rare. It remains common in wild and pet mice. This small mite inhabits hair follicles, inciting the formation of comedones containing mites (Fig. 1.95) in the skin of the head, shoulders, and lumbar areas, and, less commonly, elsewhere. These can best be observed as white nodules on the subcutaneous side of the dermis when the skin is reflected from the head and

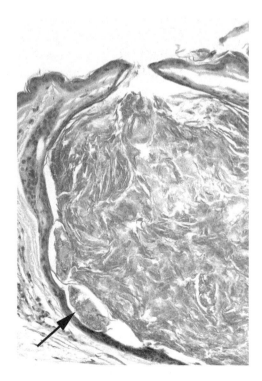

FIG. 1.95. *Skin from the head of a wild mouse infested with* Psorergates simplex. *Note the mites at the periphery (arrow) of a cystic follicle filled with keratin.*

neck. The life cycle of this mite is not known, but all of its life stages can be found within a single hair follicle.

Ornithonyssus bacoti *Infestation*

Ornithonyssus bacoti, or tropical rat mite, is a blood-sucking mesostigmate mite that infests wild rats, as well as other species. It is nonselective in its host range. It inhabits its host only to feed and then hides in nearby niches. It causes intense pruritis, and its presence in a rodent population is often first manifest on human handlers. Its complete life cycle can occur within 2 weeks, allowing massive infestation to occur within a short period of time. Because of its nonselective nature, *Ornithonyssus* has been found in laboratory mouse colonies.

Louse Infestation: Pediculosis

Polyplax serrata is a relatively common louse of wild mice, and at one time it infested laboratory mice throughout the world. It is now essentially nonexistent in laboratory mouse colonies, although the authors have found them on mice raised for reptile food under less than ideal conditions. Eggs attach to the base of hair shafts and hatch through an operculum at their top. Stage I nymphs can be found over the entire body, but the later 4 stages tend to prefer the anterior dorsum of the body. Eggs hatch within 5–6 days, and nymphs develop into adults within 1 week. Transmission is by direct contact. Host immunity appears to develop, as parasite numbers diminish with time. Heavy infestations can result in anemia and debilitation. Bites are pruritic, resulting in intense scratching and dermatitis. Polyplax once played a significant role as a vector of *Mycoplasma* (*Eperythrozoon*) *coccoides*.

BIBLIOGRAPHY FOR PARASITIC DISEASES

Protozoal Infections

See "General Reference for Infectious Diseases"

Cryptosporidium spp. Infection

Benamrouz, S., Conseil, V., Creusy, C., Calderon, E., Dei-Cas, E., & Certad, G. (2012) Parasites and malignancies, a review, with emphasis on digestive cancer induced by *Cryptosporidium parvum* (Alveolata: Apicomplexa). *Parasite* 19:101–115.

Current, W.L. & Reese, N.C. (1986) A comparison of endogenous development of three isolates of *Cryptosporidium* in suckling mice. *Journal of Protozoology* 33:98–108.

Harp, J.A.W., Chen, W., & Harmsen, A.G. (1992) Resistance of combined immunodeficient mice to infection with *Cryptosporidium parvum*: the importance of intestinal microflora. *Infection and Immunity* 60:3509–3512.

Kuhls, T.L., Greenfield, R.A., Mosier, D.A., Crawford, D.L., & Joyce, W.A. (1992) Cryptosporidiosis in adult and neonatal mice with severe combined immunodeficiency. *Journal of Comparative Pathology* 113:399–410.

McDonald, V., Deer, R., Uni, S., Iseki, M., & Bancroft, G.J. (1992) Immune responses to *Cryptosporidium muris* and *Cryptosporidium parvum* in adult immunocompetent and immunocompromised (nude and SCID) mice. *Infection and Immunity* 60:3325–3331.

Mead, J.R., Arrowood, M.J., Sidwell, R.W., & Healey, M.C. (1991) Chronic *Cryptosporidium parvum* infections in congenitally immunodeficient SCID and nude mice. *Journal of Infectious Diseases* 163:1297–1304.

Ren, X., Zhao, J., Zhang, L., Ning, C., Jian, F., Wang, R., Lv, C., Wang, Q., Arrowood, M.J., & Xiao, L. (2012) *Cryptosporidium tyzzeri* n. sp. (Apicomplexa: Cryptosporidiidae) in domestic mice (*Mus musculus*). *Experimental Parasitology* 130:274–281.

Tyzzer, E. (1910) An extracellular coccidium, *Cryptosporidium muris* (gen. & sp. nov.) of the gastric glands of the common mouse. *Journal of Medical Research* 18:487–509.

Tyzzer, E. (1912) *Cryptosporidium parvum* (sp. nov.), a coccidium found in the small intestine of the common mouse. *Archiv fur Protistenkunde* 26:394–412.

Eimeria spp. Infections

Blagburn, B.L. & Todd, K.S., Jr. (1984) Pathological changes and immunity associated with experimental *Eimeria vermiformis* infections in *Mus musculus*. *Journal of Protozoology* 31:556–561.

Levine, N.D. & Ivens, V. (1990) *The Coccidan Parasites of Rodents*. CRC Press, Boca Raton, FL.

Mesfin, G.M., Bellamy, J.E.C., & Stockdale, P.H.G. (1978) The pathological changes caused by *Eimeria flaciformis* var *pragensis* in mice. *Canadian Journal of Comparative Medicine* 42:496–510.

Giardia muris Infection

Csiza, C.K. & Abelseth, M.K. (1973) An epizootic of protozoan enteritis in a closed mouse colony. *Laboratory Animal Science* 23:858–861.

MacDonald, T.T. & Ferguson, A. (1978) Small intestinal epithelial cell kinetics and protozoal infection in mice. *Gastroenterology* 74:496–500.

Owen, R.L., Nemanic, P.C., & Stevens, D.P. (1979) Ultrastructural observations on giardiasis in a murine model. I. Intestinal distribution, attachment, and relationship to the immune system of *Giardia muris*. *Gastroenterology* 76:757–769.

Roberts-Thompson, I.C. & Mitchell, G.F. (1978) Giardiasis in mice. I. Prolonged infections in certain mouse strains and hypothymic (nude) mice. *Gastroenterology* 75:42–46.

Venkatesan, P., Finch, R.G., & Wakelin, D. (1997) A comparison of mucosal inflammatory responses to *Giardia muris* in resistant B10 and susceptible BALB/c mice. *Parasite Immunology* 19:137–143.

Klossiella muris Infection

Hartig, V.F. & Hebold, G. (1970) Das Vorkommen von Klossiellen in der Niere der Weissen Ratte. *Experimental Pathology* 4:367–377.

Otto, H. (1957) Kidney lesions in mice with *Klossiella muris* infection. *Frankfurter Zeitschrift fur Pathologie* 68:41–48.

Yang, Y.H. & Grice, H.C. (1964) *Klossiella muris* parasitism in laboratory mice. *Canadian Journal of Comparative Medicine* 28:63–66.

Sarcocystis muris Infection

Koudela, B,. Modry, D., Svobodova, M., Votypka, J., & Hudcovic, T. (1999) The severe combined immunodeficient mouse as a definitive host for *Sarcocystis muris*. *Parasitology Research* 85:737–742.

Tillman, T., Kamino, K., & Mohr, U. (1999) *Sarcocystis muris*: a rare case in laboratory mice. *Laboratory Animals* 33:390–392.

Spironucleus muris Infection

Boorman, G.A., Lina, P.H., Zurcher, C., & Nieuwerkerk, H.T. (1973) *Hexamita* and *Giardia* as a cause of mortality in congenitally thymus-less (nude) mice. *Clinical and Experimental Immunology* 15:623–627.

Flatt, R.E., Halvorsen, J.A., & Kemp, R.L. (1978) Hexamitiasis in a laboratory mouse colony. *Laboratory Animal Science* 28:62–65.

Jackson, G.A., Livingston, R.S., Riley, L.K., Livingston, B.A., & Franklin, C.L. (2013) Development of a PCR assay for the detection of *Spironucleus muris*. *Journal of the American Association for Laboratory Animal Science* 52:165–170.

Kunstyr, I., Ammerpohl, E., & Meyer, B. (1977) Experimental spironucleosis (hexamitiasis) in the nude mouse as a model for immunologic and pharmacologic studies. *Laboratory Animal Science* 27:782–788.

Meshorer, A. (1969) Hexamitiasis in laboratory mice. *Laboratory Animal Care* 19:33–37.

Sebesteny, A. (1979) Transmission of *Spironucleus* and *Giardia* spp. and some non-pathogenic intestinal protozoa from infested hamsters to mice. *Laboratory Animals* 13:189–191.

Shagemann, G., Bohnet, W., Kunstyr, I., & Friedhoff, K.T. (1990) Host specificity of cloned *Spironucleus muris* in laboratory rodents. *Laboratory Animals* 24:234–239.

Van Kruinigen, H.J., Knibbs, D.R., & Burke, C.N. (1978) Hexamitiasis in laboratory mice. *Journal of the American Veterinary Medical Association* 173:1202–1204.

Helminth Infestations

Andreassen, J., Ito, A., Ito, M., Nakao, M., & Nakaya, K. (2004) *Hymenolepis microstoma*: direct life cycle in immunodeficient mice. *Journal of Helminthology* 78:1–5.

Balk, M.W. & Jones, S.R. (1970) Hepatic cysticercosis in a mouse colony. *Journal of the American Veterinary Medical Association* 157:678–679.

Franklin, C.L. (2006) Microbial considerations in genetically engineered mouse research. *ILAR Journal* 47:141–155.

Jacobson, R.H. & Reed, N.D. (1974) The thymus dependency of resistance to pinworm infections in mice. *Journal of Parasitology* 60:976–979.

Lytvynets, A., Langrova, I., Lachout, J., & Vadlejch, J. (2013) Detection of pinworm eggs in the dust of laboratory animals breeding facility, in the cages and on the hands of the technicians. *Laboratory Animals* 47:71–73.

Parel, J.D., Galula, J.U., & Ooi, H.K. (2008) Characterization of rDNA sequences from *Syphacia obvelata*, *Syphacia muris*, and *Aspiculuris tetraptera* and development of a PCR-based method for identification. *Veterinary Parasitology* 153:379–383.

Ectoparasite Infestations

Bukva V. (1985) *Demodex flagellarus* sp. n. (Acari: Demodicidae) from the preputial and clitoral glands of the house mouse, *Mus musculus*. *Folia Parasitologica* 32:73–81.

Csiza, C.K. & McMartin, D.N. (1976) Apparent acaridal dermatitis in a C57BL/6Nya mouse colony. *Laboratory Animal Science* 26:781–787.

Dawson, D.D., Whitmore, S.P., & Bresnahan, J.F. (1986) Genetic control of susceptibility to mite-associated ulcerative dermatitis. *Laboratory Animal Science* 36:262–267.

French, A.W. (1987) Elimination of *Ornithonyssus bacoti* in a colony of aging mice. *Laboratory Animal Science* 37:670–672.

Friedman, S. & Weisbroth, S.H. (1975) The parasitic ecology of the rodent mite, *Myobia musculi*. II. Genetic factors. *Laboratory Animal Science* 25:440–445.

Hill, L.R., Kille, P.S., Weiss, D.A., Craig, T.M., & Coghlan, L.G. (1999) *Demodex musculi* in the skin of transgenic mice. *Contemporary Topics in Laboratory Animal Science* 38:13–18.

Hirst, S. (1917) Remarks on certain species of the genus *Demodex*, Owen (the Demodex of man, the horse, dog, rat and mouse). *Annals and Magazine Natural History* 20:233–235.

Jungmann, P., Guénet, J.L., Cazenave, P.A., Coutinho, A., & Huerre, M. (1996) Murine acariasis. I. Pathological and clinical evidence suggesting cutaneous allergy and wasting syndrome in BALB/c mouse. *Research in Immunology* 147:27–38.

Morita, E., Kaneko, S., Hiragun, T., Shindo, H., Tanaka, T., Furudawa, T., Nobukiyo, A., & Yamamoto, S. (1999) Fur mites induce dermatitis associated with IgE hyperproduction in an inbred strain of mice, NC/Kuj. *Journal of Dermatological Science* 19:37–43.

Tuzdil, N. (1957) Das vorkommen von Demodex in der zunge einer maus. *Zeitschrift fur Tropenmedizin und Parasitologie* 8:274–278.

Weisbroth, S.H., Friedman, S., Powell, M., & Scher, S. (1974) The parasitic ecology of the rodent mite *Myobia musculi*. I. Grooming factors. *Laboratory Animal Science* 24:510–516.

Weisbroth, S.H., Friedman, S., & Scher, S. (1976) The parasitic ecology of the rodent mite *Myobia musculi*. III. Lesions in certain host strains. *Laboratory Animal Science* 26:725–735.

Weiss, E.E., Evans, K.D., & Griffey, S.M. (2012) Comparison of a fur-mite PCR assay and the tape test for initial and posttreatment diagnosis during a natural infection. *Journal of the American Association for Laboratory Animal Science* 51:574–578.

BEHAVIORAL DISORDERS

Behavior and behavioral aberrations are significant contributors to disease in the laboratory mouse. Both optimal management of mouse populations and effective behavioral testing can be facilitated by knowledge of mouse behavior, including behavior of mice in their natural environment (reviewed in Brown et al. 2000; Bailey et al. 2006; Dixon 2004; Latham and Mason 2004; Van Loo et al. 2003). In-depth discussion of mouse behavior is beyond the scope of this text, but several issues need to be emphasized for the pathologist. Mice live in structured communal groups, known as demes, composed of a despotic dominant male, subordinant males, and a hierarchy of dominant to subordinant females. Mice will strive to achieve this social order when placed within the artificial confines of a cage environment. There are marked differences in behavior among mouse strains. B6, B10, C57L, and C57BR mice have high levels of open-field locomotion and low anxiety, compared to DBA/2, CBA, AKR, and LP mice, which are intermediate. DBA/1, BALB/c, and A/J mice exhibit low locomotor activity and high levels of emotional reactivity. Normal behavior patterns may be disrupted in specific strains of mice with retinal degeneration (C3H, FVB, SJL, and many outbred Swiss mice), late-onset deafness (B6 and BALB mice), hippocampal and corpus callosum defects (129 and BALB mice), hydrocephalus (B6 mice), pituitary adenomas (FVB mice), seizures (DBA/2 and FVB mice), and numerous other anomalies.

Infertility

The pathologist may be called upon to investigate infertility in breeding mouse populations. In the absence of discernable lesions, a behavioral basis of the problem should be explored. The reproductive cycle in the mouse is highly volatile and sensitive to changes in light cycle, noise, stress, and other factors. Despite being maintained in controlled environments for many generations, mice have seasonal variations in fertility and fecundity, which may be more apparent in some strains of mice. In addition, sudden changes in light cycle can induce long-term anestrus. The behavior and reproductive cycles of mice are significantly influenced by olfactory pheromone cues. Altered estrous cycles, fetal resorption, and anestrus, as well as maternal cannibalism, can result from pheromone-driven responses. The most common cause of unexplained infertility in a mouse colony is the introduction of foreign adult males to the room. Known as the Bruce effect, it results in termination of early pregnancy among females. Foreign males may also stimulate maternal cannibalism. Anestrus may be induced among females in the absence of males or by a dominant breeding female within a deme. The presence of males or male urine will synchronize estrus and accelerate onset of puberty among females (Whitten effect). In addition, breeding performance varies markedly among different strains of mice. B6 mice have high copulatory behavior, DBA/2 and AKR intermediate, and BALB/c and A/J mice have low libido, which may influence breeding efficiency and fertility. Inbred mice have smaller litters than outbred mice.

Male Aggression

Adult male mice that are cohoused in a cage will fight unless reared as siblings or peers from infancy. Aggressive behavior is especially high among DBA, Swiss (CD-1, SJL, FVB), and BALB/c male mice. Female aggression is less of a problem but varies with reproductive state and strain. The olfactory cues of a stable environment are drastically destabilized with cage changing, which is notorious for stimulating aggressive behavior among its occupants. Fight wounds can be diffuse (Fig. 1.96) but are often oriented around the tail and external genitalia. Severe trauma to the penis can result in obstructive uropathy.

Stereotypy

Stereotypic behavior occurs commonly among caged mice, but is often overlooked because of their nocturnal activity patterns. Individual mice may display bar-mouthing, jumping, circling, somersaulting, route-tracing, and other forms of repetitive functionless behavior. Mice presented to necropsy may continue to manifest these signs. In some surveys, stereotypies occurred in nearly 100% of ICR Swiss mice and 80% of B6 mice. Some of these activities, such as compulsive circling, must be differentiated from vestibular disease.

Barbering and Trichotillomania

Another form of abnormal repetitive behavior is impulsive/compulsive behavior, which is frequently manifest among mice as hair plucking or barbering. It is also known as the Dalilah effect or trichotillomania. The driving forces behind this abnormal behavior are highly complex, including dominance, genetic background, social learning, diet, and boredom. It is more common among females, but both sexes can be involved. B6 and A2G strains are especially prone to this disorder. Patterns of hair loss vary and seem to be dependent upon the "style" preferences of the barber, which is usually only a single mouse within a cage. A common manifestation is loss of vibrissae and facial hair (Fig. 1.97). Muzzle alopecia must be differentiated from hair loss due to abrasion on cage feeding devices. Hair plucking can be self-directed, with hair loss on the ventral abdomen. Another common pattern is dorsal alopecia in B6 mice when the barber is conspecific (Fig. 1.98). In addition, cutaneous excoriation, inflammation, and terminal gangrene of the tail have been found to be manifestations of social interactions among weaning-age male and female C3H mice. As healing occurs, small pale scars are visible on the tails of the pigmented mice. This entity is related

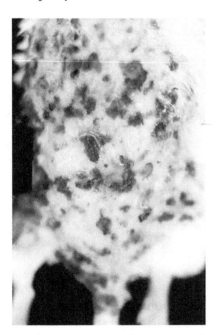

FIG. 1.96. *Multifocal cutaneous excoriations on the dorsal lumbar region of a pugilistic male BALB/c mouse.*

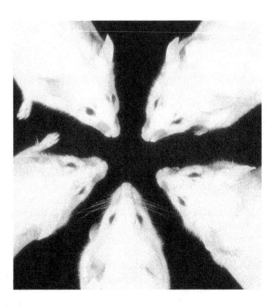

FIG. 1.97. *Mice illustrating barbering of vibrissae. Note the culprit with the intact vibrissae (bottom center).*

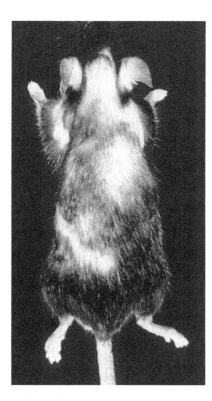

FIG. 1.98. *Dorsal alopecia in a B6 mouse due to conspecific hair plucking.*

to high cage population densities. Collectively, these behavioral vices are not only disfiguring to the pelage but are also a major initiator of ulcerative dermatitis (see *Staphylococcus* "*Staphylococcus* spp. infections"). Finally, barbering can also occur in which the hair is clipped rather than plucked. Typically, there is a well-defined, clipped edge to the affected fur.

Penis Self-Mutilation

B6 mice have been reported to self-mutilate their penis, ranging from damage to the distal penis to complete amputation. This was observed in 8.5% of harem breeder males and may be related to the high level of copulatory behavior in this mouse strain and its tendency toward impulsive/compulsive disorders. The affected mice were noted to be hyperactive and constantly chasing and mounting the females in the cage. This syndrome, like pugilistic trauma to the penis, can lead to obstructive uropathy.

BIBLIOGRAPHY FOR BEHAVIORAL DISORDERS

Bailey, K.R., Rustay, N.R., & Crawley, J.N. (2006) Behavioral phenotyping of transgenic and knockout mice: practical concerns and potential pitfalls. *ILAR Journal* 47:124–131.

Brown, R.E., Stanford, L., & Schellinck, H.M. (2000) Developing standardized behavioral tests for knockout and mutant mice. *ILAR Journal* 41(3), 163–174.

Dixon, A.K. (2004) The social behaviour of mice and its sensory control. In: *The Laboratory Mouse*, The Handbook of Experimental Animals (eds. H.J. Hedrich & G. Bullock), pp. 287–300. Elsevier, San Diego, CA.

Garner, J.P. (2005) Stereotypies and other abnormal repetitive behaviors: potential impact on validity, reliability, and replicability of scientific outcomes. *ILAR Journal* 46:106–117.

Garner, J.P. & Mason, G.J. (2002) Evidence for a relationship between cage stereotypies and behavioural disinhibition in laboratory rodents. *Behavioural Brain Research* 136:83–92.

Garner, J.P., Weisker, S.M., Dufour, B., & Mench, J.A. (2004) Barbering (fur and whisker trimming) by laboratory mice as a model for human trichotillomania and obsessive-compulsive disorders. *Comparative Medicine* 54:216–224.

Hong, C.C. & Ediger, R.D. (1978) Self-mutilation of the penis in C57BL/6N mice. *Laboratory Animals* 12:55–57.

Koopman, J.P., Van der Logt, J.T., Mullink, J.W., Heesen, F.W., Stadhouders, A.M., Kennis, H.M., & Van der Gulden, W.J. (1984) Tail lesions in C3H/He mice. *Laboratory Animals* 18:106–109.

Latham, N. & Mason, G. (2004) From house mouse to mouse house: the behavioral biology of free-living *Mus musculus* and its implications in the laboratory. *Applied Animal Behaviour Science* 86:261–289.

Les, E.P. (1972) A disease related to cage population density: tail lesions of C3H/HeJ mice. *Laboratory Animal Science* 22:56–60.

Long, S.Y. (1972) Hair-nibbling and whisker-trimming as indicators of social hierarchy in mice. *Animal Behavior* 20:10–12.

Sarna, J.R., Dyck, R.H., & Whishaw, I.Q. (2000) The Dalila effect: C57BL6 mice barber whiskers by plucking. *Behavioural Brain Research* 108:39–45.

Strozik, E. & Festing, M.F.W. (1981) Whisker trimming in mice. *Laboratory Animals* 15:309–312.

Thornburg, L.P., Stowe, H.D., & Pick, J.R. (1973) The pathogenesis of the alopecia due to hair-chewing in mice. *Laboratory Animal Science* 23:843–850.

Van Loo, P.L.P., Zutpehn, L.F.M., & Baumans, V. (2003) Male management: coping with aggression problems in male laboratory mice. *Laboratory Animals* 37:300–313.

Whary, M.T., Baumgarth, N., & Fox, J.G. (2015) Biology and diseases of mice. In: *Laboratory Animal Medicine*, 2nd edn, pp. 1–280. Academic Press, New York.

AGING, DEGENERATIVE, AND MISCELLANEOUS DISORDERS

Multisystemic Disorders
Dehydration

Mice require relatively large volumes of drinking water and easily become dehydrated. Hydration can be evaluated at necropsy by skin plasticity, "stickiness" of tissues, pale and contracted spleens, vascular hypovolemia, or elevated hematocrit. Thorough anamnesis will often reveal failure of watering devices. Even if water bottles are full, sipper tubes can become obstructed, or if new, they can contain metal filings that interfere with water flow. Dehydration can also occur when water bottle sipper tubes are too high for young mice to reach or if newly arrived mice are unaccustomed to automatic watering devices. Dehydration frequently accompanies other diseases that preclude drinking, such as hydrocephalus. A consistent microscopic finding in dehydrated mice is massive thymic apoptosis (stress reaction).

Hypothermia and Hyperthermia

Although mice are highly adaptable to living in different climates, they are inefficiently homeothermic and cannot tolerate sudden and extreme changes in environmental temperature. In a stabile environment, core body temperature will normally fluctuate several degrees in a day, depending upon activity. Hypothermia and hyperthermia are all too common occurrences during shipping, when crates are moved from one environment to another. Water bottle accidents cause high mortality within a cage from hypothermia. All of these factors can result in high mortality with few, if any, discernible lesions. As in dehydration, massive lymphocytic apoptosis in the thymus is a hallmark lesion.

Amyloidosis and Amyloid-Like Nasal Deposition

Amyloid (from the Greek amylon, "starch") was so named by Virchow because it stained with iodine similar to that seen with cellulose. Amyloidosis is an important disease of laboratory mice, both as a spontaneously occurring, life-limiting disease and as an experimentally induced disease.

Amyloid is a chemically diverse family of insoluble proteins that are deposited in tissues but have in common a biophysical polymerized conformation known as the beta-pleated sheet. There are 2 types of amyloid in the mouse: AA and AapoAII. AA amyloid is associated with an increase in serum precursor apoSAA, which is induced in hepatocytes and elevated in blood in response to cytokines produced during inflammatory and neoplastic diseases. Local tissue injury elicits a complex of events in which macrophages release monokines, including interleukin 1 and tumor necrosis factor, which in turn stimulate apoSAA synthesis in liver. AA fibril formation and deposition involves partial degradation of apoSAA by macrophages. AA amyloidosis can be induced by repeated injections of casein and other inflammatory stimuli, thereby earning the name "secondary amyloidosis." The spleen, liver, intestine, and kidney are the most common sites for AA amyloid deposition. Experimental secondary amyloidosis can be readily induced in a variety of laboratory mouse strains with casein injections. The order of susceptibility (in decreasing order) among common mouse strains is CBA, B6, outbred Swiss, C3H/He, BALB/c, and SWR. A/J mice are resistant. The second type of amyloid is AapoAII amyloid, which is also known as "primary" or "senile amyloid." AapoAII amyloid consists primarily of apoAII proteins without degradation. The precursor apoAII is also produced by the liver. Mouse strains that are prone to AapoAII amyloidosis include A/J and SJL. AapoAII amyloid deposition tends to be less severe in spleen and liver (compared to AA amyloidosis), with more deposition in adrenals, intestine, heart, lungs, thyroid, parathyroid, ovaries, and testes. In addition, a number of localized forms of amyloidosis occur, such as in endocrine tumors, ovaries, and the brain (in Alzheimer's disease), each with differing composition.

Spontaneous amyloidosis is a common event in many strains of aging mice. It is difficult to distinguish between primary and secondary amyloidosis in spontaneous cases, since amyloid deposits are typically mixed, and patterns of tissue deposition may vary with mouse strain. Amyloidosis tends to occur at high prevalence and early onset in A, SJL, and outbred Swiss mice (mostly AapoII amyloid); high prevalence but late onset in B6 and B10 mice (mixed amyloid); and is extremely rare in BALB, C3H, and DBA mice. Unlike Syrian hamsters, there does not appear to be a clear sex-related predisposition in most strains of mice, although it can be more common in males that are prone to fighting. The prevalence of spontaneous amyloidosis is significantly affected by stress, ectoparasitism, and chronic inflammatory conditions, such as ulcerative dermatitis, preputial adenitis, cervical lymphadenitis, conjunctivitis, and pyometra, among others. Individually housed SPF mice have a lower prevalence of amyloid compared to group housed mice. Localized forms of amyloidosis can also be found in mice. Tumor-associated amyloid can be found in pulmonary adenomas of A and BALB mice, and localized deposition in the corpora lutea is common in CBA and DBA mice, even though BALB and DBA mice are refractory to other forms of amyloidosis.

Amyloid has a characteristic hypocellular eosinophilic appearance in H & E-stained sections, and can be stained positively with Congo Red, Oil Red O, Alcian Blue, and Thioflavine T. Staining intensity may vary considerably. When stained with Congo Red and subjected to polarized light, amyloid is birefringent. Amyloid deposition occurs in renal glomeruli (Fig. 1.99), renal interstitium, lamina propria of the intestine (Fig. 1.100), myocardium, nasal submucosa, parotid salivary gland, thyroid gland, parathyroid gland, adrenal cortex, perifollicular areas of the spleen, pulmonary alveolar septa, periportal regions of the liver, tongue, testes, ovary, myometrium, aorta, pancreas, skin, and other tissues. Intestinal deposition may be segmental in distribution.

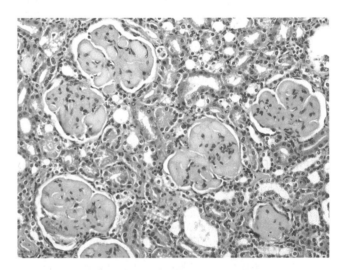

FIG. 1.99. *Kidney from a mouse with renal amyloidosis, characterized by obliteration of the glomerular architecture by deposition of amyloid.*

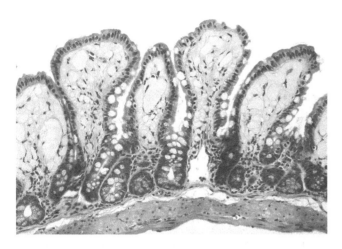

FIG. 1.100. *Ileum from a mouse with intestinal amyloidosis. There is marked deposition of amorphous amyloid in the lamina propria.*

Amyloidosis is often associated with cardiac atrial thrombosis with left- or right-sided congestive heart failure. The mechanism for this association is unknown but is probably related to renal disease. Mice with amyloid deposition in the renal medullary interstitium can develop papillary necrosis. Healed lesions give the illusion of hydronephrosis.

A common site of amyloid-like deposition is the nasal submucosa, particularly above the vomeronasal organs (Fig. 1.101). This material is not amyloid, as it does not stain with Congo Red, is Trichrome-positive, and PAS-positive after diastase treatment. Ultrastructurally, it consists of amorphous material and collagen. It is believed to be composed of complex carbohydrate that is secreted by nasal epithelium.

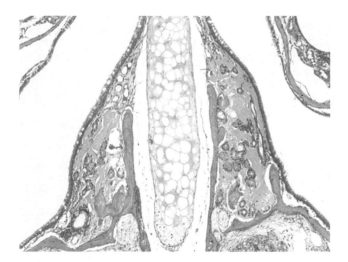

FIG. 1.101. *Cross section through the nose of a mouse with deposition of amyloid-like material around submucosal glands. Although this material looks like amyloid in H&E stained sections, it is believed to be composed of complex carbohydrate originating from nasal glands.*

Soft Tissue Calcification: Cardiac Calcinosis/ Myocardial Calcification

Spontaneous mineralization/calcification of the heart and other soft tissues is a common if not universal finding in BALB/c, C3H, and DBA mice. Lesions arise in mice as early as 3 weeks of age and increase with age. Epicardial mineralization, accompanied by varying degrees of fibrosis, is found on the right ventricular free wall in BALB/c mice. In contrast, C3H mice do not develop epicardial mineralization, but rather develop foci of degeneration and mineralization throughout the myocardium of both ventricular walls and the interventricular septum. C3H mice also develop skeletal myofiber mineralization, particularly in axial muscles. DBA mice are especially prone to soft tissue mineralization. They develop both epicardial and myocardial mineralization, and dystrophic mineralization may also be found in aorta, testes, tongue, muscle, cornea, kidney, stomach, small intestine, and ovary. In the tongue, calcified nodules may form polypoid lesions. Dystrophic mineralization of the superficial corneal stroma is a common finding in DBA, C3H, and BALB (including C.B.-17-*scid*) mice. A variety of factors have been implicated in this condition, including environment, diet, concomitant disease, and elevated levels of corticosteroids. Female mice appear to be particularly at risk. The mineralization appears to be dystrophic in nature, since there is no evidence of elevated serum calcium levels in affected mice.

There may be chalky linear streaks evident on the heart, particularly on the epicardium of the right ventricular free wall (Fig. 1.102). In young mice, these lesions are composed predominantly of mineral, but as mice age, they become enveloped in fibrous connective tissue

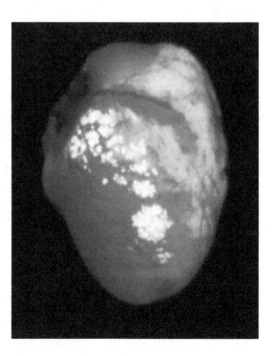

FIG. 1.102. *Heart of a BALB/c mouse, depicting epicardial mineral deposition on the surface of the right ventricular free wall.*

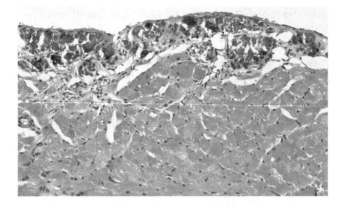

FIG. 1.103. *Epicardial mineralization in a DBA mouse, illustrating deposition of mineral and fibrosis.*

(Fig. 1.103). Myocardial lesions are present in the right and left ventricles, interventricular septum, and atria. Changes vary from single mineralized fibers to extensive linear calcification. In recent lesions, there may be interstitial edema. In lesions interpreted to be of some duration, there may be concurrent fibrosis and mononuclear cell infiltration. Foci of calcification in the tongue, when present, are often concentrated in the longitudinal musculature adjacent to the lamina propria, frequently with concurrent granulomatous inflammatory response and polyp formation. Lesions may be distributed anywhere along the tongue from the apex to the root of the tongue. Ulceration of the epithelium overlying affected areas is an infrequent finding. Foci of calcification, when present in the aorta, are characterized by mineralization of the elastic lamina and smooth muscle of the vessel wall. Corneal lesions are characterized by calcium deposition in the superficial layers of the corneal stroma. As lesions progress, deposits may become large aggregates of mineralized material, with stromal scarring, often leading to loss of overlying corneal epithelium and secondary ophthalmitis.

Acidophilic Macrophage Pneumonia/ Epithelial Hyalinosis

Acidophilic macrophage pneumonia (AMP) is characterized by focal to diffuse accumulation of acidophilic crystals within macrophages, alveolar spaces, and airways. This condition is widespread among many strains of mice, and the authors have noted it in wild mice as well. It tends to be most evident in older animals. Some strains, such as B6, 129 (particularly 129S4/SvJae), and Swiss mice, tend to have a higher prevalence and earlier onset of this lesion, and it can cause mortality in severely affected mice, particularly in B6-motheaten (*Ptpn6^{me}*) mice and various types of immunodeficient GEMs on the B6 or 129 background. Grossly, there is lobar to diffuse tan to red discoloration of the lungs, which do not collapse. Microscopically, macrophages have abundant cytoplasm packed with large numbers of needle to rhomboid-shaped eosinophilic crystals (Fig. 1.104).

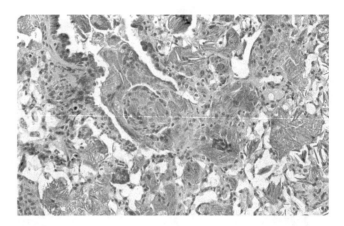

FIG. 1.104. *Terminal airway of an aged B6 mouse with acidophilic macrophage pneumonia. Hyaline, eosinophilic crystals are present within alveolar macrophages and alveolar spaces with multinucleate giant cell formation.*

They are present in alveolar spaces, alveolar ducts, terminal airways, and bronchiolar glands. Crystal-bearing multinucleated giant cells and granulocytes are frequently scattered within affected areas of the lung. The crystalline material is complex and has been shown to contain iron, alpha-1 antitrypsin, immunoglobulin, and breakdown products of granulocytes. Based on ultrastructural studies, the crystals resemble Charcot-Leyden crystals, which are unique to humans and nonhuman primates in association with eosinophil-related diseases. AMP crystals are composed predominantly of Ym1 chitinase. Any disease process that impairs normal clearance (pulmonary tumors, Pneumocystosis, or other chronic pneumonias) can predispose to AMP. AMP may be very extensive, leading to dyspnea in some mice.

Although AMP is the most overt manifestation of this condition, "hyalinosis" of olfactory, nasal respiratory, middle ear, trachea, lung, stomach, gall bladder, bile duct, and pancreatic duct epithelium is part of the syndrome. Hyaline eosinophilic material fills the cytoplasm of affected epithelium, with blebbing of material from their apical surfaces (Fig. 1.105). Square to

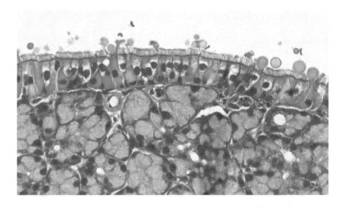

FIG. 1.105. *Nasal epithelium from a B6 mouse, depicting hyaline eosinophilic material in the cytoplasm of respiratory epithelium and blebbing from the apical surfaces.*

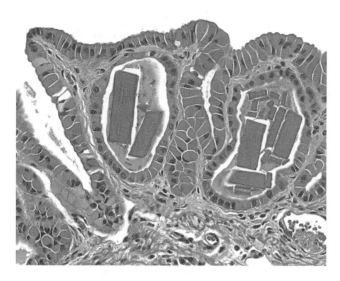

FIG. 1.106. *Gall bladder of a B6 mouse with hyaline eosinophilic material in biliary epithelial cells and crystals within mucosal glands.*

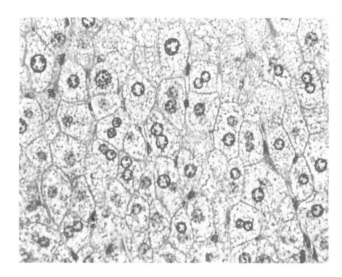

FIG. 1.107. *Liver from a case of Reye's-like syndrome in a BALB/cByJ mouse. Hepatocytes are distended with microvesicles and compress sinusoidal spaces.*

rhomboid extracellular crystals may accumulate in glands of these tissues (Fig. 1.106). As in the lung, the hyaline material is composed of Ym1 and Ym2 chitinase. These changes may lead to thickening of the bile ducts and gall bladder, with dilatation and thickened, opaque walls.

Reye's-Like Syndrome

Reye's-like syndrome, an important cause of morbidity and mortality among human infants and children, is characterized as hepatoencephalopathy and fatty degeneration of viscera. Antecedent viral infections and aspirin therapy are precipitating factors in humans. Outbreaks of Reye's-like syndrome, although rare, occur with high morbidity and mortality. The natural disease has been principally associated with BALB/cByJ mice, but similar findings have been reported in infant C3H-*H-2^O* mice. Precipitating factors have not been defined but may be linked to enterotropic MHV or other infections. Experimental infection of C.B-17-*scid* mice with mouse adenovirus (MAdV-1) can induce the syndrome. Reye's-like syndrome in mice, as in humans, is characterized by a rapidly deteriorating encephalopathy secondary to hepatic dysfunction with hyperammonemia. The metabolic defect is unknown, but mitochondrial swelling with dysfunction in hepatocytes is the primary lesion. Affected mice become precipitously stuporous and comatose with hyperventilation. Death occurs in most cases within 6-18 hours after onset, but some mice regain consciousness.

Livers are swollen, greasy, and pale, and kidneys are swollen, with pale cortices. Intestines can be fluid- and gas-filled, with empty ceca. Microscopic findings include marked microvesicular fatty change and swelling of hepatocytes, with sinusoidal hypoperfusion (Fig. 1.107). Ultrastructural changes include disruption of mitochondrial cristae and cytoplasmic vacuolation filled with lipid. Moderate numbers of fat vacuoles are also present in renal proximal convoluted tubular epithelium. Neurologic lesions consist of swelling of protoplasmic astrocyte nuclei (Alzheimer type II astrocytes) in the neocortex, corpus striatum, hippocampus, and thalamus. The hepatic pathology must be differentiated from hepatocellular fatty change that is common in BALB/c mice, which normally possess a moderate degree of this change.

Graft Versus Host Diseases

Although graft versus host disease (GVHD) is not a naturally occurring syndrome in laboratory mice, the mouse has been used extensively to study various elements of acute and chronic GVHD, and the reader is referred to recent reviews (Anderson & Bluestone 2005; Schroeder & DiPersio 2011). GVHD has become important with xenotransplantation of human stem cell and T cells into NOD/SCID, NSG and other immunodeficient mice, so mouse pathologists are often involved in examining such mice. Acute GVHD is primarily mediated through the CD8+ T-cell alloreactivity, resulting in acute disease with infiltration of lymphocytes into skin, liver, intestine, lungs, and kidneys. Chronic GVHD is primarily mediated through CD4+ T-cell alloreactivity, with B-cell expansion, lymphadenopathy, splenomegaly, biliary damage, scleroderma, and autoantibody production, resulting in glomerulonephritis.

Disorders of Skin
Mechanical Muzzle Alopecia

Hair loss in the muzzle region occurs occasionally in laboratory mice due to mechanical denuding from improperly constructed openings for feeders or watering devices. This must be differentiated from barbering.

Alopecia Areata in C3H Mice

Aging C3H mice develop irregular, diffuse alopecia of the ventral and dorsal trunk, which closely mimics human alopecia areata. Hair loss increases with age, particularly after 6 months of age, in both males and females. Microscopic examination of affected skin reveals densely packed anagen follicles with dystrophic hair formation, "melanin incontinence," interfollicular epidermal thickening, and perifollicular mononuclear leukocyte infiltrates.

Alopecia of B6 Mice

This extremely common multifactorial syndrome in B6 mice is fundamentally a behavioral disorder. It is influenced by husbandry factors, such as premature weaning and diet. The alopecia is associated with barbering or trichotillomania but becomes secondarily inflammatory in character. B6 mice are prone to *Myobia* hypersensitivity dermatitis, which can significantly contribute to the syndrome. Immune complex vasculitis and primary follicular dystrophy have been proposed as underlying factors. These factors collectively predispose B6 mice to necrotizing dermatitis, which is driven by opportunistic infection with *Staphylococcus* and *Streptococcus*. Ulcerative dermatitis is a major life-limiting disease, with mice succumbing prematurely to systemic amyloidosis and atrial thrombosis. See sections on Staphylococcus, Streptococcus, ectoparasitism, behavioral disorders, amyloidosis, and atrial thrombosis.

Clown Mouse Syndrome

This rare syndrome is seen among weaning-age mice, in which one or the entire litter may be affected. Typically, mice are runted and have general alopecia, with varying amounts of normal-appearing hair on the head, neck, and thorax (Fig. 1.108). There is also often hyperkeratosis of the affected hairless skin. Affected mice have ongoing severe systemic disease or have recovered, resulting in temporary cessation of normal hair growth cycling. Hair growth cycles extend from head to tail, so that regrowth appears first around the head and progresses posteriorly. Thus, the amount of hair varies and may extend over the neck and thorax in some animals. Clown mouse syndrome has especially been associated with both natural and experimental mouse hepatitis virus infection.

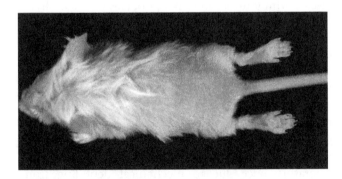

FIG. 1.108. *Clown mouse syndrome in a young mouse due to arrested hair growth following mouse hepatitis virus infection.*

Ear Gangrene and Notching

Erosive inflammation and necrosis of the edges of the ear pinnae, with formation of notches in healed lesions, has been described in Swiss mice, but the authors have observed the lesion frequently in C3H mice as well. The etiology of this disorder is not known, but it is assumed to be environmental. Lesions begin as erythema, progress to erosions with serous exudation, and eventually develop into necrosis of the ear. Histopathology reveals hyperkeratosis and underlying chronic inflammation. Severely affected mice may develop ulcerative dermatitis of the neck and shoulders.

Auricular Chondritis

Both mice and rats are prone to development of bilateral thickening of the ear pinnae (Fig. 1.109) due to underlying chronic granulomatous inflammation and degeneration of cartilage. Lesions may be diffuse or nodular in appearance. Lesions are associated with metal identification tags, which are believed to stimulate an autoimmune chondritis. The autoimmune basis is underscored by the development of similar lesions in the contralateral, untagged ear, and induction of the lesion by immunization with type II collagen. Lesions may stimulate formation of squamous cell carcinomas.

Ringtail

Low ambient humidity is associated with "ringtail," or annular constrictions of the tail and occasionally digits in infant mice, resulting in edema of the distal extremity and dry gangrene. Hairless strains of mice are prone to skin problems as adults, which may be manifest as

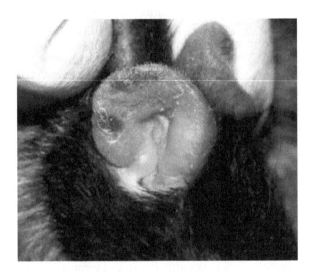

FIG. 1.109. *Auricular chondrosis in a B6 mouse. This inflammatory syndrome is believed to have an autoimmune basis, can be experimentally induced by collagen immunization, and often arises naturally in response to ear tags. (Source: Buckner, J.H., David, C.S. & Bradley, D.S. (2006) Mice expressing HLA-DQ6alpha8beta transgene develop polychondritis spontaneously. Arthritis Research and Therapy 8:R134. Reproduced under the Creative Commons License http://creativecommons.org/licenses/by/4.0/)*

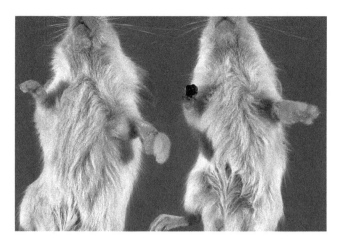

FIG. 1.110. *Edema and gangrene of digits and feet of suckling mice associated with inadvertent winding of cotton fibers around digits and limbs. (Source: Percy et al. 1994. Reproduced with permission from American Association for Laboratory Animal Science.)*

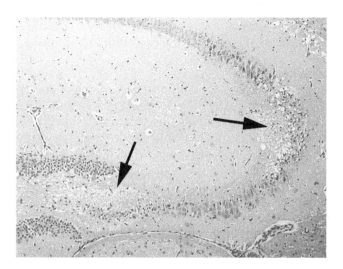

FIG. 1.111. *Post-ictal neuronal necrosis (arrows) in the hippocampus of an FVB mouse.*

inflammation and gangrene without the classic ringtail antecedent stage. The nature of the predisposing factors and the precise pathogenesis of ringtail have yet to be resolved but are thought to be related to low (less than 40%) relative humidity and high (greater than 80°F) temperature. Lesions must be differentiated from behavior-related dermatitis of the tail.

Sloughing of Extremities Due to Cotton Nesting Material

Necrosis and sloughing of digits and feet in suckling mice have been associated with infarction due to the wrapping of absorbent cotton (cotton wool) nesting material around one or more legs or digits (Fig. 1.110).

Frostbite

Rarely, mice may develop gangrene of their limbs due to frostbite. Nude mice are especially prone to this syndrome, which is associated with cold exposure of shipping boxes during air transportation.

Mammary Hyperplasia

Virgin female FVB/N mice develop mammary gland lobuloalveolar hyperplasia, with secretory product in alveoli and ducts. These changes increase with age and are correlated with the presence of proliferative lesions of prolactin-secreting cells in the pars distalis of the pituitary. In addition, FVB/N mice are prone to a high incidence of pituitary adenomas and mammary tumors in aged multiparous females. Persistent mammary hyperplasia, without involution, is especially prominent in multiparous FVB/N females and may be present in the absence of pituitary changes.

Disorders of the Central Nervous System and Sensory Organs
Seizures

Several strains of mice, particularly DBA/2 mice, but also SJL, LP, and FVB mice, are prone to audiogenic

(high-frequency) seizures. Susceptibility in DBA mice wanes with age. B6, C3H, and BALB/c mice tend to be resistant, but some BALB mice may be susceptible at old (>400 days) age. Seizures progress after a short latency period following sound stimulation. Mice manifest an explosive bout of frenzied running, followed by clonic seizures with violent kicking movements. A tonic phase ensues with rigid extension of limbs and flattening of ear pinnae. During this phase, respiratory arrest may occur. Individual mice may not progress through all phases. Other forms of sensory stimulation, including alteration of equilibrium, can induce seizures in some mice, such as EL mice. Some populations of FVB mice are highly prone to audiogenic seizures, which have been elicited by tattooing, hair clipping, and fire alarms. Seizures often occur at night, resulting in unexplained deaths. Seizures are characterized by facial grimace, chewing automatism, whole-body tics, ptyalism, and clonic convulsions. At necropsy, there is neuronal necrosis in the cerebral cortex, hippocampus, and thalamus, especially in the organized pyramidal cell layers of the hippocampus (Fig. 1.111). Mice that have endured multiple convulsive events may have generalized gliosis. Acute coagulation necrosis of centrilobular hepatocytes may also be present in some mice. Other common observations at necropsy include enlarged and flaccid urinary bladders, distended gall bladders, enlarged adrenals, and increased brain weights. A general consequence of seizures in male mice may be ejaculation, retention of urethral plugs, and obstructive uropathy.

Hypocallosity

Forebrain commissure defects, with aplasia of the corpus callosum, are common (up to 70%) in BALB/c, 129 (including 129/J, 129/Sv, 1229/ReJ, and 129/Ola), and some other less common strains of mice. This feature makes the affected animals poor candidates for learning behavior research, and hypocallosity has been mistaken as a "phenotype" in GEMs derived from 129 ES cells.

Hydrocephalus

Internal hydrocephalus is relatively common among C57BL mouse strains. It becomes clinically significant at weaning, when mice are unable to independently eat and drink. Mice present with domed skulls and are usually runted and dehydrated. Recently, it has been found that high levels of Cre recombinase expression in neuronal precursor cells can lead to reduced neuronal proliferation and apoptosis, with defects in ependymal lining, lamination of the cortex, microencephaly, and communicating hydrocephalus. This phenomenon was noted in 3 different nestin-Cre transgenic lines of mice.

Central Nervous System Miscellany

Vacuolation of the white matter is a common fixation artifact in mouse brains. Artifactual vacuoles can be differentiated from antemortem vacuolation by their distinct outlines, lack of cellular debris, and lack of gliosis. Multilaminated mineralized concretions are common in the thalamus of old mice. Developmental midline malformations are relatively common, including hamartomas, choristomas, teratomas, epithelial inclusion cysts, and adipose tissue (lipomas). A number of other artifacts and lesions have been described.

Cochlear Degeneration

Age-related hearing loss is common in many strains of inbred mice. Its basis is genetically complex, with different mutant genes, modifier genes, and pathogenesis, depending upon mouse strain. At least 8 mapped loci and a mitochondrial variant are known to contribute to age-related hearing loss in mice. A survey of 80 inbred mouse strains has revealed 18 strains that have significantly elevated auditory-evoked brain stem response thresholds by 3 months of age, including 129P1/ReJ, A/J, DBA/2, and NOD/Lt mice, and others that have elevated thresholds at older ages, including B6 and BALB/c mice. High-frequency losses occur first, with cochlear hair cell loss progressing from the base to the apex. Outer hair cells are affected before inner hair cells, and ganglion cells degenerate as a consequence of hair cell loss.

Vestibular Syndrome

A significant manifestation of polyarteritis (see "Polyarteritis") is vestibular syndrome. Head tilt, circling, and more severe manifestations of vestibular disease are common clinical signs. This syndrome occurs in a number of mouse strains in the absence of detectable viral and bacterial causes of otitis. The internal and middle ear structures are normal, but careful examination of surrounding tissues will reveal active necrotizing and/or inflammatory changes in medium-sized arteries (Fig. 1.112). It is typically found with concomitant involvement of arteries in other tissue, particularly

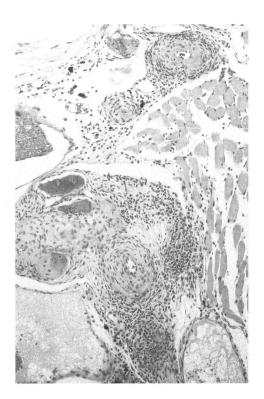

FIG. 1.112. *Chronic arteritis near the middle and inner ear. Arteritis occurs in multiple organs in adult mice with polyarteritis, but involvement of vessels in the head may result in vestibular signs.*

coronary arteries. Other causes of vestibular syndrome include otitis, neoplasia, and spontaneous unilateral brainstem infarction, which has been reported to occur in Swiss mice.

Corneal Opacity

Corneal opacities have been observed in a variety of strains of mice. Opacities are characterized by acute to chronic inflammatory changes of the corneal epithelium and anterior corneal stroma, including acute keratitis with corneal erosion to ulceration, vascularization of the corneal stroma, and mineralization of corneal basement membranes. In some cases, the problem can be alleviated by more frequent cage cleaning, and it has been concluded that an environmental factor, such as ammonia, may play a role in the development of the disease.

Blepharitis and Conjunctivitis

Several common inbred strains of mice are prone to develop blepharitis and blepharoconjunctivitis, including 129P3/J, A/HeJ, BALB/cJ, BALB/cByJ, and CBA/J mice. Suppurative conjunctivitis with ulcerations at the mucocutaneous junction has been observed in 129, BALB, and other strains of mice. Abscessation of the meibomian glands may also occur. A variety of bacteria have been isolated from affected conjunctivae, including *Corynebacterium*, coagulase-negative *Staphylococcus*, and *P. pneumotropica*. These are likely to be opportunistic infections, and the specific etiopathogenesis is unknown. C57BL mice are also prone to develop blepharoconjunctivitis in association with microphthalmia, and mutant mice that have premature opening of eyelids are prone to eye trauma and blepharoconjunctivitis.

Microphthalmia and Anophthalmia
This syndrome is relatively common and unique to various types of C57BL mouse, with females more prone to lesions than males. Mice usually have asymmetric microphthalmia or anophthalmia, most often involving the right eye.

Retinal Degeneration
Homozygosity of the *Pde6b^rd1* allele is common among both inbred and outbred mice, resulting in retinal degeneration and blindness at an early age. Retinal degeneration is a strain characteristic of several common inbred strains of mice, including C3H/He, CBA, FVB, SJL, SWR, and others. It also occurs in most outbred Swiss and non-Swiss albino stocks and may be observed in some populations of wild mice. A study examined the prevalence of this lesion among outbred albino mice and found retinal degeneration to be very common, but there was marked variation in prevalence, depending upon the mouse stock. Notably, retinal degeneration was not found in Crl:CD-1(ICR)BR, HsdWin:CFW1, and Hsd:NSA(CF-1) mice. NIH Swiss and Black Swiss mice are also affected. Mice are born with normal-appearing retinas and develop normal photoreceptors that rapidly undergo apoptosis, beginning in the third wk of life. Affected mice become totally blind. Microscopic changes include absence or degeneration of the rods, outer nuclear layer, and outer plexiform layer (Fig. 1.113). Active

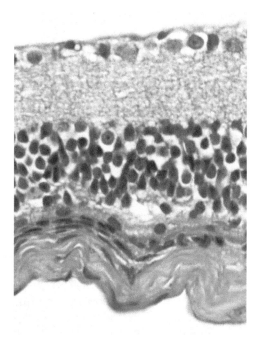

FIG. 1.113. *Retinal degeneration in a C3H mouse that is homozygous for the rd1 (rodless retina) allele. There is loss of the outer plexiform and bipolar cell layers.*

degenerative changes can be encountered in young mice, but the lesion evolves rapidly within a few weeks of weaning. Unaware investigators have often been duped by blind mice that fail to perform normally in behavioral studies.

Disorders of the Cardiovascular and Respiratory Systems
Polyarteritis
Inflammatory lesions of small and medium-sized arteries are common in many strains of laboratory mice. The character of the lesions varies and may include fibrinoid degeneration and necrosis of the tunica media and inflammation associated with neutrophilic and/or mononuclear leukocytes. There may be thickening and fibrosis of the vascular wall. The distribution of affected vessels is quite variable but most often involves arteries of the tongue, head, pancreas, heart, kidneys, mesentery, urinary bladder, uterus, testes, and gastrointestinal tract, among others. Lesions tend to be segmental, feature different stages of acute to chronic inflammation, and involve multiple vessels. The etiology of polyarteritis is not known, but immune complexes have been demonstrated within affected vessels. It is common in mice that are prone to autoimmune disease, including MRL and NZB mice. Polyarteritis is usually an incidental finding, but it can be associated with segmental infarction of the kidneys with scarring. It may also have vestibular manifestations when vessels of the head are involved (see "Vestibular Syndrome").

Atrial Thrombosis and Heart Failure
Thrombosis of the auricle is a frequent finding in mice, which may manifest as left- or right-sided heart failure (Fig. 1.114). The left auricle is most frequently affected. Atrial thrombosis typically involves organizing thrombi in the auricle, but the process may extend into the ventricles, cardiac vessels, and pulmonary veins. This syndrome is typically precipitated by multisystemic amyloidosis, but it is also relatively common in BALB/c mice, which are not prone to amyloidosis. Left heart failure due to atrial thrombosis is the most common cause of noninfectious dyspnea in mice.

Perivascular Lymphoid Infiltrates
Mild to severe infiltrates of lymphoid cells may arise in the adventitia of pulmonary vessels, with extension into adjacent alveolar septa. This is invariably in response to antigenic stimuli, such as a prior virus infection. They should not be present in pathogen-free mice. They also frequently appear in older mice with perivascular mononuclear cell infiltrates in salivary glands, kidneys, and other organs. These infiltrates seem to be antecedent to lymphoproliferative disorders.

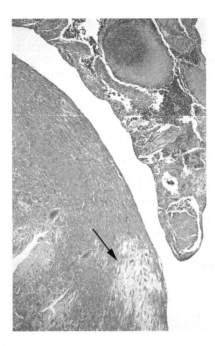

FIG. 1.114. *Heart of a mouse with auricular thrombosis. Note the organizing thrombus within the auricular lumen and the patch of amyloid infiltration in the myocardium (arrow). Auricular thrombosis is often associated with renal disease, including amyloidosis.*

Pulmonary Histiocytosis/Lipoproteinosis/ Alveolar Proteinosis

Focal accumulations of foamy lipid-laden macrophages are occasionally observed in the peripheral (particularly subplural) regions in the lung of aging mice of all types. Some of the macrophages may contain cholesterol crystalloid material. These changes can follow focal pulmonary hemorrhage, and hemoglobin crystals may also be present in the area. These lesions are rare in SPF mice. Alveolar lipoproteinosis is another more severe condition, in which there is progressive intra-alveolar accumulation of granular pale eosinophilic phospholipid (surfactant), with hypertrophy and vacuolation of type II pneumocytes, and mobilization of scattered macrophages with vacuolated cytoplasm. Experimental manipulations (e.g., inhalation of toxic aerosols) are frequently used to produce lesions of this type. To add to the confusion of this complex, there appears to be considerable overlap in the interpretation and terminology affixed to these changes, and they may overlap with acidophilic macrophage pneumonia.

Alveolar Hemorrhage

Regardless of the cause of death, acute extravasation of blood into alveolar spaces is a common agonal finding in mice. It must be differentiated from congestive heart failure and other causes.

Freund's Adjuvant Pulmonary Granulomata

Focal histiocytic granulomata can be found in the lungs of mice that have been immunized with Freund's adjuvant, regardless of the site of immunization (Fig. 1.115).

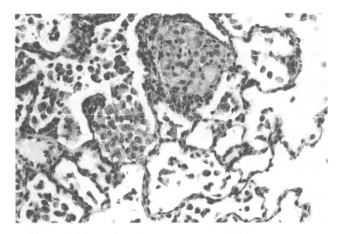

FIG. 1.115. *Lung from a mouse immunized subcutaneously with Freund's adjuvant. Note the focal granulomatous inflammatory response with prominent epithelioid cells.*

Aspiration Pneumonia

Mice are obligate nasal breathers, but aspiration pneumonia is common following accidental inhalation of foreign material. This event can occur under a number of circumstances but especially when shipping crates containing wood shavings are handled roughly in transit. Foreign plant material can be readily identified in airways.

Disorders of the Gastrointestinal System
Malocclusion

Malocclusion due to improperly aligned upper and lower incisor teeth may result in marked overgrowth, particularly of the lower incisors. This condition has a hereditary basis and is relatively common among B6 mice.

Foreign Body Periondontitis: Hair Tooth

A commonly encountered lesion in a variety of mouse strains is inflammation and erosion of the gingival sulci of the cheek teeth, with impaction of hair and food particles (Fig. 1.116). These lesions give rise to secondary suppurative bacterial infections that may extend into the tooth root and surrounding tissues of the head. The syndrome may be associated with excessive barbering or trichotillomania.

Cleft Lip/Palate

Congenital cleft lip and cleft palate are common in A strain mice and may be accompanied by premature eyelid opening in that strain. A/WySn mice are particularly prone to this disorder. These malformations appear to be genetically complex in inheritance, but A/WySn mice have an IAP retrotransposon integration in the region of *Wnt9b* that is suspected to be a major determinant of susceptibility. Cleft palates are often blamed for mortality among mutant mice derived from chemical mutagenesis, transgenesis, and targeted mutagenesis. Because these lesions are obvious, they tend to be

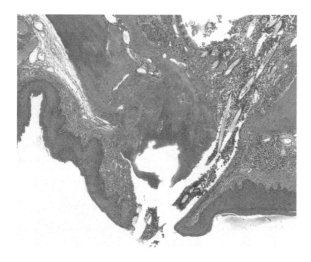

FIG. 1.116. *Periodontal inflammation associated with impaction of hair shafts in the gingival sulci. Inflammation often extends into the adjacent structures of the head.*

blamed for other causes of embryonic and postnatal mortality.

Megaesophagus

Dilatation of the esophagus has been reported in inbred Swiss ICRC/HiCri mice. These mice have smooth muscle in the abdominal segment of the esophagus, in contrast to the normal configuration of smooth muscle in the lowermost portion, adjacent to the stomach. In addition, the mice have aplasia of the myenteric plexus, with fibrosis. The condition was most severe in older mice. A similar syndrome has been observed among aging 129S4/SvJae mice, with significant mortality associated with esophageal impaction. There are now a number of mutant mice that develop megaesophagus, which are revealing a number of pathogenetic mechanisms underlying this complex disease.

Gastric Mucosal Hyperplasia

Diffuse mucosal hyperplasia of the glandular mucosa of the stomach has been observed periodically in immunodeficient mice. Its etiology is not known.

Liver Disorders

A progressive increase in ploidy (polyploidy) occurs in hepatocyte nuclei with age. The number of chromosomes may increase to ploidy values of 16 or 32. Thus, karyomegaly, anisokaryosis, polykarya, and cytomegaly are common incidental findings (Fig. 1.5). Intranuclear cytoplasmic invaginations are also common and can be recognized as delineated eosinophilic structures within the nucleus (Fig. 1.6). Eosinophilic cytoplasmic inclusions, composed of secretory material in dilated endoplasmic reticulum of hepatocytes, are also common, especially in B6 mice (Fig. 1.117). They are most frequently observed in hepatocytes of older mice and transgenic mice. A multitude of these features are

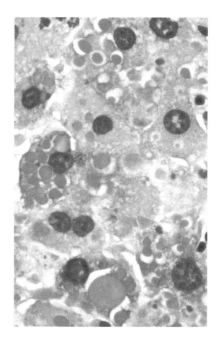

FIG. 1.117. *Liver from an aged B6 mouse with eosinophilic cytoplasmic inclusions in hepatocytes.*

present at all ages but increase with age and disease and may be particularly extreme in some GEMs (Fig. 1.118). Hepatocellular fatty change is a normal finding in BALB mice, and the livers of these mice are typically paler than in other strains. One or more foci of hepatic coagulation necrosis in the absence of an infectious agent may be observed as incidental findings in many strains of mice. They are probably ischemic in origin. Epithelial hyalinosis and crystals are a frequent incidental finding in the biliary and gall bladder epithelium of B6 and 129 mice. Bile ductular proliferation is a common incidental finding in all laboratory rodents and lagomorphs. Proliferation of Kupffer cells and Ito cells can occur under a variety of circumstances but should signal inquiry into the presence of *Helicobacter*.

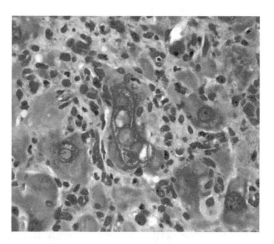

FIG. 1.118. *Liver from an aged transgenic mouse with cytomegaly, polykarya, megalokarya, intranuclear cytoplasmic invagination, and oval cell hyperplasia.*

Mesenteric Disease

Mesenteric lymph nodes of aged mice may become enlarged and filled with blood. This lesion occurs sporadically in various mouse strains, appearing more frequently in C3H mice. Its etiology is unknown. Mesenteric lymph nodes are grossly enlarged and appear bright red. Microscopically, lymphoid tissue is often atrophic, and medullary sinuses are filled with blood. Differential diagnoses must include various causes of mesenteric lymphadenomegaly, including *Salmonella*. This is an incidental finding and of no clinical significance.

Disorders of the Endocrine System

Epithelial cysts are common in the thyroid and pituitary in many strains of mice. Thyroid cysts are often lined by ciliated cells. A high prevalence of virgin inbred FVB/NCr mice have been reported to develop prolactin-secreting foci of hyperplasia and adenomas of the pituitary pars distalis. These lesions are associated with lobulo-alveolar hyperplasia of mammary tissue in virgin females and spontaneous mammary tumors in aged multiparous females.

Disorders of the Urogenital Systems
Glomerulonephritis/Glomerulopathy

Glomerular disease is common in mice. Glomeruli are a frequent site of amyloid deposition in multisystemic amyloidosis (see "Amyloidosis"). Membranoproliferative glomerulonephritis develops in a number of inbred strains of mice. Mice with naturally occurring auto-immune disease, such as the (NZB x NZW) hybrid, usually have extensive glomerular lesions by the time they reach 12 or more months of age. Lesions are also relatively common in certain strains of older mice, such as AKR, BALB/c, B6, CBA, and 129/SvTer mice. There are a variety of other factors that may be involved, including viruses (e.g., LCMV and retroviruses), bacteria or bacterial products, and the deposition of antigen–antibody complexes on glomerular basement membranes. In addition, the glomeruli of aged mice often have non-specific basement membrane thickening, which has been termed "glomerular hyalinosis." This tends to be part of "chronic progressive nephropathy." These forms of glomerular disease often overlap. Glomerular disease may be associated with coagulopathy, which may result in atrial thrombosis. Indeed, several erroneous reports of cardiomyopathy with heart failure in GEMs are actually related to this association.

In mice with glomerulonephritis, there may be marked pitting of the cortical surfaces in advanced cases, and small cysts may be evident on the cut surface. Microscopic changes are characterized by thickening of glomerular basement membranes with deposition of PAS-positive material that does not stain for amyloid. There may be proliferation of mesangial cells and, in advanced cases, obliteration of the normal architecture

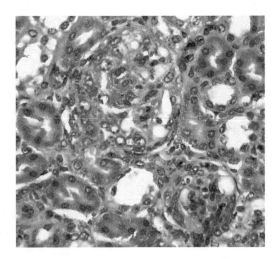

FIG. 1.119.   *Kidney of a mouse with severe glomerulonephritis.*

of affected glomeruli (Fig. 1.119). Focal to diffuse mononuclear cell infiltration and varying degrees of fibrosis in the interstitial regions are other changes that commonly occur.

Chronic Nephropathy

A syndrome resembling chronic progressive nephropathy (CPN) in aged rats occurs in aged mice. It is also referred to as interstitial nephritis or chronic nephritis. CPN has been specifically described in B6C3F1 mice but occurs commonly in other strains. The pathogenesis is not known, but it features glomerular hyalinosis, glomerulosclerosis, tubular degeneration, regeneration, interstitial inflammation, and dilated tubules with protein-rich fluid in their lumina (Figs. 1.120). Advanced cases have irregular pitting of the renal cortices and uremic syndrome. Anemia and ascites may be present in advanced cases, but metastatic calcification of tissues is usually not a feature of renal disease in the mouse.

Hydronephrosis

Unilateral or bilateral hydronephrosis is a relatively common finding in laboratory mice. It is usually

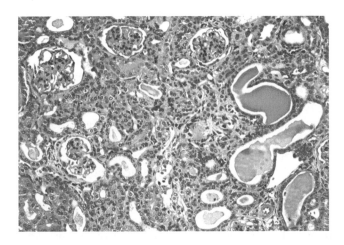

FIG. 1.120.   *Chronic nephropathy in an aged mouse.*

regarded as an incidental finding, particularly if only one kidney is involved. Hydronephrosis can occur in high prevalence among certain strains or lines of mice or be secondary to urinary obstruction or pyelonephritis.

Renal Infarction

Wedge-shaped infarcts of the kidney with scarring are a common finding in aged mice and are presumed to be the aftermath of arteritis of the interlobular arteries.

Polycystic Disease

Certain strains of mice, such as BALB/c mice, are prone to congenital cysts of varying size in the kidneys. In some cases, these cysts are quite large and impinge on renal function, resulting in mortality at an early age.

Renal Tubular Hyaline Bodies

Hyaline eosinophilic bodies in the cytoplasm of renal tubules may be observed in association with histiocytic sarcomas involving distant tissue sites (Fig. 1.121).

Inclusion Body Nephritis

Over the course of 40 years, the authors have encountered multiple sporadic incidents and referrals in which renal tubules have epithelial nuclei with marginated chromatin and prominent, homogeneous eosinophilic inclusions. This is typically accompanied by adjacent interstitial infiltrates of lymphocytes in immunocompetent mice (Fig. 1.122). Ultrastructurally, the inclusions contain flocculent electron-lucent material. Numerous inclusions without interstitial infiltrates have been noted in globally immunodeficient Rag1 null mice (C. Brayton, unpublished). The inclusions are reminiscent of virus inclusions, but affected mice are negative for polyoma virus, K virus, and adenovirus.

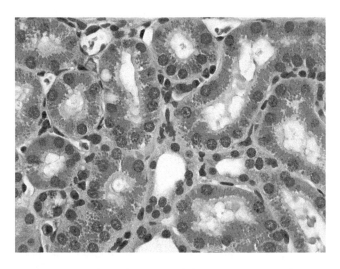

FIG. 1.121. *Kidney of a mouse with histocytic sarcoma in distant tissues. Renal tubular cells are filled with eosinophilic hyaline bodies.*

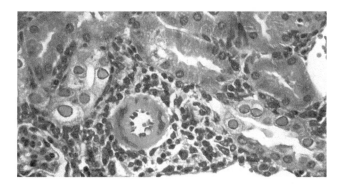

FIG. 1.122. *Inclusion body nephritis in a mouse. Note the prominent intranuclear inclusions within tubular epithelium and interstitial infiltration of lymphocytes.*

Chloroform Toxicity

Adult male mice of certain genotypes such as DBA and C3H are exquisitely sensitive to development of renal tubular necrosis and mineralization when exposed to chloroform fumes, with high mortality. One factor associated with the sex-related susceptibility appears to be the increased renal binding of chloroform in males, compared with females. Castration of males will eliminate their susceptibility to chloroform nephrotoxicity. Severely affected mice develop swollen, pale kidneys. Microscopic changes are characterized by coagulation necrosis of renal tubules, particularly the proximal convoluted tubules. Surviving mice have residual nephrocalcinosis. "Outbreaks" of mortality, with selective deaths among male mice of sensitive genotypes, have been described.

NSAIDS-Associated Nephropathy

The authors have observed renal tubular degeneration associated with an overdose and/or prolonged treatment with Banamine. Initially, there are foci of tubular degeneration with mineralization, particularly at the corticomedullary junction. In surviving mice, changes may progress to chronic nephropathy. Affected kidneys are pale, with irregular cortical outlines. On microscopic examination, there is degeneration and atrophy of renal tubules in both the cortex and medulla, with relative sparing of glomeruli.

Mucometra/Hydrometra

Mucometra has been observed in a variety of strains, including BALB/c, B6, and DBA. It is most commonly encountered among large groups of presumably pregnant mice in which a few never whelp. The abdomen is often distended. One or both uterine horns are dilated (Fig. 1.123). Some mice have congenital imperforate lower reproductive tracts or persistent vaginal septa, while in others the cause cannot be determined. Mice with an imperforate vagina frequently present with bilobed distention in the perineal region, resembling a scrotum. Imperforate vagina with mucometra or hydrometra appears to be inherited as a complex recessive

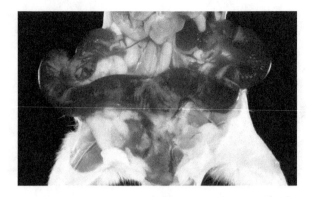

FIG. 1.123. *Congenital mucometra in a young adult mouse. The uterine horns are distended with mucoid material.*

genetic defect. Differential diagnoses include pyometra (which may occur secondary to mucometra), retained fetuses, and neoplasia. The uterus of mice (and rats) normally contains a small amount of fluid during certain stages of the estrous cycle.

Cystic Endometrial Hyperplasia

Cystic endometrial hyperplasia of endometrial glands is frequent in aged female mice. It may be associated with secondary bacterial pyometras (e.g., *K. oxytoca*).

Adenomyosis

Adenomyosis may be encountered as a relatively rare incidental finding in female mice. There is glandular invasion of the myometrium, often extending to the serosa (Fig. 1.124). It must be differentiated from neoplasia.

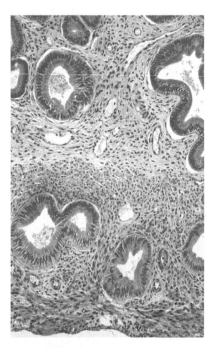

FIG. 1.124. *Uterus of a mouse with adenomyosis. Note invasion of uterine glands into the myometrium.*

Murine Urologic Syndrome (MUS)

Male mice are prone to obstructive uropathy that is associated with retention of ejaculated coagulum in the uretha. Acutely affected mice may be found dead. In acute cases, the urinary bladder is usually markedly distended with clear yellow urine. Dull white, firm, proteinaceous plugs are often evident in the neck of the urinary bladder and proximal urethra. In subacute and chronic forms of the syndrome, clinical signs may vary from dribbling of urine and wetting of the perineal region to cellulitis with ulceration of the preputial area. Paraphimosis is a variable finding. In chronic cases, the bladder may be distended with cloudy urine and/or calculi. The vesicular glands are sometimes distended with inspissated material, and there may be some evidence of hydronephrosis. It seems to be particularly common in older male B6C3F1 and ICR mice. On microscopic examination of acute cases, amorphous eosinophilic material containing spermatozoa may be present in the proximal urethra, with mild to minimal inflammatory response. In chronic obstruction, there may be varying manifestations of inflammatory response, such as prostatitis, cystitis, urethritis, and balanoposthitis. Differential diagnoses include bacterial cystitis and pyelonephritis, as well as agonal ejaculation at death, which must be differentiated from antemortem urinary obstruction. Careful microscopic examination for evidence of urethral inflammation near the coagulum is warranted. Urinary obstruction can occur as a result of fighting injuries or self-induced trauma to the external genitalia, as well as in male mice following seizures.

Bulbourethral Gland Cysts

The bulbourethral glands are small pear-shaped structures located at the base of the penis and embedded in the skeletal muscle. Secretions of these glands contribute to the formation of the copulatory plug. Cystic glands present as unilateral or bilateral swellings in the perineal region. Bacterial infection of these glands may also occur. Bacteria isolated from suppurative lesions include *S. aureus* and *P. pneumotropica*. Impaired reproductive performance has been associated with cystic bulbourethral glands.

Seminal Vesicular Dilatation and Atrophy

Aged male B6 mice may develop unilateral or bilateral dilatation or contraction (atrophy) of their seminal vesicles (Fig. 1.125). The dilated vesicles may result in marked abdominal distention. There may often be contraction of one and dilatation of the other.

Pseudocanalization and Megalokaryocytosis of Male Reproductive Epithelium

The epithelium lining the epididymis and vas deferens of aged male mice frequently has cells with large, polyploid nuclei. In addition, the epithelial lining may contain open spaces between cells that suggest canalization.

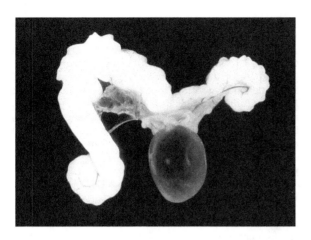

FIG. 1.125. *Seminal vesicles and urinary bladder of an aged male B6 mouse. There is marked enlargement of one seminal vesicle in contrast to the normal contralateral vesicle.*

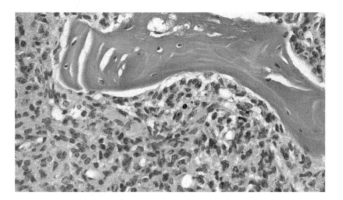

FIG. 1.126. *Vertebra from an aged female mouse with fibro-osseous hyperplasia. There is marked infiltration of the bone marrow by fusiform mesenchymal cells, with displacement of hematopoietic elements.*

Disorders of the Musculoskeletal System
Muscular Dystrophy
Muscular dystrophy in humans has promulgated the development of a number of GEM models, but two important natural mutations arose in inbred strains of mice. A and SJL mice have retroelement (Etn) insertional mutations in the *dysferlin* gene and both develop progressive degenerative changes in proximal skeletal muscle groups with age. C57BL/10ScSn mice have an X chromosome mutation (*mdx* allele) in the *dystrophin* gene, similar to Duchenne's muscular dystrophy in humans. This allele has been crossed onto other mouse models, and the gene has been targeted for the creation of additional models. The naturally occurring mutations are mentioned because they arose in relatively common inbred strains of mice, and in the case of A and SJL mice, they are characteristics of the parental strains.

Fibro-Osseous Lesions in Aged Mice
Fibro-osseous lesions arise commonly in the sternebrae, vertebrae, femurs, and other bones in a number of strains of mice. They arise most frequently in females, and they are age-related. Female B6C3F1 mice appear to be especially prone (100% at 110 week of age) to this lesion, when compared to B6 and CD-1 mice. Early changes have been detected as early as 32 weeks of age, but the proliferative lesions are more common (and more evident) in mice examined at 50 or more weeks of age. Estrogens have been presumed to play a role in development of these lesions. Mice have been shown to be particularly responsive to estrogen that can alter the microenviroment of bone. However, they also arise in ovariectomized females and castrated males, suggesting that other factors are involved. Similar changes have been produced in selected strains of mice treated with estrogens or a prostaglandin E_1 analogue. In affected bones, there is partial to complete replacement of bone marrow by fibroblast-like cells in an eosinophilic matrix (Fig. 1.126). There is displacement of the

hematopoietic elements of the marrow, and osteoblasts are present around bony spicules within the medullary cavity. In some cases, there is extension into the periosteal region, but there is no evidence of malignant transformation. Differential diagnosis includes histiocytic sarcomas with intramedullary involvement, which typically consist of a more anaplastic population of cells, including prominent multinucleated giant cells. We have observed a number of osteosarcomas arising from the vertebrae and long bones of $p53^{+/-}$ heterozygotes on the B6C3F1 background, but we have not seen any convincing evidence of progression of fibro-osseous lesions to osteosarcomas.

Spinal Fracture and Posterior Paresis
Mice are commonly the victim of cage lid closure, when they are inadvertently crushed while attempting to climb out of the cage. Rushed husbandry and inattentive technicians in large mouse colonies are factors that contribute to this lesion. Clinical signs must be differentiated from viral encephalomyelitis or demyelination and other factors that may physically impinge upon the spinal cord.

Vertebral Disk Degeneration
Although often not examined, aged mice develop a number of degenerative lesions of their intervertebral disk annulus fibrosus, including matrix degradation, protrusion into the spinal canal, cartilaginous proliferative lesions, and ossification, as well as eosinophilic change in the nucleus pulposus.

Osteoarthritis and Osteopenia
Degenerative joint disease arises in the aged mouse, which may be particularly evident in the knee joints, with degenerative changes in cartilage. Mice develop osteopenia with age, which varies by strain and gender of mice, with females more affected than males.

Lateral Femoral Triangle Hernias

FVB/NHsd mice, and their transgenic derivative strains, have been found to be prone to development of unilateral or bilateral hernias of the femoral triangle region. Female mice developed these lesions more frequently than male mice.

BIBLIOGRAPHY FOR AGING, DEGENERATIVE, AND MISCELLANEOUS DISORDERS

See "General References on Diseases of Mice"

Amyloidosis and Amyloid-Like Nasal Deposition

Conner, M.W., Conner, B.H., Fox, J.G., & Rogers, A. (1983) Spontaneous amyloidosis in outbred CD-1 mice. *Survey and Synthesis of Pathology Research* 1:67–78.

Doi, T., Kotani, Y., Kokoshima, H., Kanno, T., Wako, Y., & Tsuchitani, M. (2007) Eosinophilic substance is "not amyloid" in the mouse nasal septum. *Veterinary Pathology* 44:796–802.

Frith, C.H. & Chandra, M. (1991) Incidence, distribution, and morphology of amyloidosis in Charles Rivers CD-1 mice. *Toxicologic Pathology* 19:123–127.

Lipman, R.D., Gaillard, E.T., Harrison, D.E., & Bronson, R.T. (1993) Husbandry factors and the prevalence of age-related amyloidosis in mice. *Laboratory Animal Science* 43:439–444.

Soft Tissue Mineralization

Brownstein, D.G. (1983) Genetics of dystrophic epicardial mineralization in DBA/2 mice. *Laboratory Animal Science* 33:247–248.

Imaoka, K., Honjo, K., Doi, K., & Mitsuoka, T. (1986) Development of spontaneous tongue calcification and polypoid lesions in DBA/2NCrJ mice. *Laboratory Animals* 20:1–4.

Meador, V.P., Tyler, R.D., & Plunkett, M.L. (1992) Epicardial and corneal mineralization in clinically normal severe combined immunodeficiency (SCID) mice. *Veterinary Pathology* 29:247–249.

Vargas, K.J., Stephens, L.C., Clifford, C.B., Gray, K.N., & Price, R.E. (1996) Dystrophic cardiac calcinosis in C3H/HeN mice. *Laboratory Animal Science* 46:572–575.

Yamate, J., Tajima, M., Maruyama, Y., & Kudow, S. (1987) Observations on soft tissue calcification in DBA/2NCrj mice in comparison with CRJ:CD-1 mice. *Laboratory Animals* 21:289–298.

Acidophilic Macrophage Pneumonia/Epithelial Hyalinosis

Giannetti, N., Moyse, E., Ducray, A., Bondier, J.R., Jourdan, F., Propper, A., & Kastner, A. (2004) Accumulation of Ym1/2 protein in the mouse olfactory epithelium during regeneration and aging. *Neuroscience* 123:907–917.

Guo, L., Johnson, R.S., & Schuh, J.C.L. (2000) Biochemical characterization of endogenously formed eosinophilic crystals in the lungs of mice. *Journal of Biological Chemistry* 275:8032–8037.

Harbord, M., Novelli, M., Canas, B., Power, D., Davis, C., Godovac-Zimmermann, J., Roes, J., & Segal, A.W. (2002) Ym1 is a neutrophil granule protein that crystallizes in p47phox-deficient mice. *Journal of Biological Chemistry* 277:5468–5475.

Hoenerhoff, M.J., Starost, M.F., & Ward, J.M. (2006) Eosinophilic crystalline pneumonia as a major cause of death in 129S4/SvJae mice. *Veterinary Pathology* 43:682–688.

Murray, A.B. & Luz, A. (1990) Acidophilic macrophage pneumonia in laboratory mice. *Veterinary Pathology* 27:274–281.

Nio, J., Fujimoto, W., Konno, A., Kon, Y., Owashi, M., & Iwanaga, T. (2004) Cellular expression of murine Ym1 and Ym2, chitinase family proteins, as revealed by in situ hybridization and immunohistochemistry. *Histochemistry and Cell Biology* 121:473–482.

Ward, J.M. (1978) Pulmonary pathology of the motheaten mouse. *Veterinary Pathology* 15:170–178.

Ward, J.M., Yoon, M., Anver, M.R., Haines, D.C., Kudo, G., Gonzalez, F.J., & Kimura, S. (2001) Hyalinosis and Ym1/Ym2 gene expression in the stomach and respiratory tract of 129S4/SvJae and wild-type and CYP1A2-null B6, 129 mice. *American Journal of Pathology* 158:323–332.

Yang, Y.H. & Campbell, J.S. (1964) Crystalline excrements in bronchitis and cholecystitis of mice. *American Journal of Pathology* 45:337–345.

Reye's-Like Syndrome

Brownstein, D.G., Johnson, E.A., & Smith, A.L. (1984) Spontaneous Reye's-like syndrome in BALB/cByJ mice. *Laboratory Investigation* 51:386–395.

Koizumi, T., Nikaido, H., Hayakawa, J., Nonomura, A., & Yoneda, T. (1988) Infantile disease with microvesicular fatty infiltration of viscera spontaneously occurring in the C3H-H-2(0) strain of mouse with similarities to Reye's syndrome. *Laboratory Animals* 22:83–87.

Pirofski, L., Horwitz, M.S., Scharff, M.D., & Factor, S.M. (1991) Murine adenovirus infection of SCID mice induces hepatic lesions that resemble human Reye syndrome. *Proceedings of the National Academy of Sciences of the United States of America* 88:4358–4362.

Graft Versus Host Diseases

Anderson, M.S. & Bluestone, J.A. (2005) The NOD mouse: a model of immune dysregulation. *Annual Reviews in Immunology* 23:447–485.

Schroeder, M.A. & DiPersio, J.F. (2011) Mouse models of graft-versus-host disease: advances and limitations. *Disease Models and Mechanisms* 4:318–333.

Disorders of Skin

Andrews, A.G., Dysko, R.C., Spilman, S.C., Kunkel, R.G., Brammer, D.W., & Johnson, K.J. (1994) Immune complex vasculitis with secondary ulcerative dermatitis in aged C57BL/6NNia mice. *Veterinary Pathology* 31:293–300.

Baron, B.W., Langan, G., Huo, D., Baron, J.M., & Montag, A. (2005) Squamous cell carcinomas of the skin at ear tag sites in aged FVB/N mice. *Comparative Medicine* 55:231–235.

Bell, J.F., Moore, G.J., Clifford, C.M., & Raymond, G.H. (1970) Dry gangrene of the ear in white mice. *Laboratory Animals* 4:245–254.

Kitagaki, M. & Hirota, M. (2007) Auricular chondritis caused by metal ear tagging in C57BL/6 mice. *Veterinary Pathology* 44:458–466.

Lamoureux, J.L., Buckner, J.H., David, C.S., & Bradley, D.S. (2006) Mice expressing HLA-DQ6alpha8beta transgene develop polychondritis spontaneously. *Arthritis Research and Therapy* 8:R134.

Lawson, G. (2010) Etiopathogenesis of mandibulofacial and maxillofacial abscesses in mice. *Comparative Medicine* 60:200–204.

Litterst, C.L. (1974) Mechanically self-induced muzzle alopecia in mice. *Laboratory Animal Science* 24:806–809.

Nieto, A.I., Shyamala, G., Galvez, J.J., Thordarson, G., Wakefield, L.M., & Cardiff, R.D. (2003) Persistent mammary hyperplasia in FVB/N mice. *Comparative Medicine* 53:433–438.

Percy, D.H., Greenword, J.D., Blake, B., Copps, J.S., & Croy, B.A. (1994) Diagnostic exercise: sloughing of limb extremities in immunocompromised suckling mice. *Contemporary Topics in Laboratory Animal Science* 33:66–67.

Rowson, K.E.K. & Michaels, L. (1980) Injury to young mice caused by cottonwool used as nesting material. *Laboratory Animals* 14:187.

Slattum, M.M., Stein, S., Singleton, W.L., & Decelle, T. (1998) Progressive necrotizing dermatitis of the pinna in outbred mice: an institutional survey. *Laboratory Animal Science* 48:95–98.

Stowe, H.D., Wagner, J.L., & Pick, J.R. (1971) A debilitating fatal murine dermatitis. *Laboratory Animal Science* 21:892–897.

Sundberg, J.P., Cordy, W.R., & King, L.E., Jr. (1994) Alopecia areata in aging C3H/HeJ mice. *Journal of Investigative Dermatology* 102:847–857.

Sundberg, J.P., Taylor, D., Lorch, G., Miller, J., Silva, K.A., Sundberg, B.A., Roopenian, D., Sperling, L., Ong, D., King, L.E., & Everts, H. (2011) Primary follicular dystrophy with scarring dermatitis in C57BL/6 mouse substrains resembles central centrifugal cicatricial alopecia in humans. *Veterinary Pathology* 48:513–524.

Witt, W.M. (1989) An idiopathic dermatitis in C57BL/6N mice effectively modulated by dietary restriction. *Laboratory Animal Science* 39:470.

Disorders of the Central Nervous System and Sensory Organs

Clapcote, S.J., Lazar, N.L., Bechard, A.R., Wood, G.A., & Roder, J.C. (2005) NIH Swiss and Black Swiss mice have retinal degeneration and performance deficits in cognitive tests. *Comparative Medicine* 55:310–316.

Fuller, J.L. & Sjursen, F.H. (1967) Audiogenic seizures in eleven mouse strains. *Journal of Heredity* 58:135–140.

Goelz, M.F., Mahler, J., Harry, J., Myers, P., Clark, J., Thigpen, J.E., & Forsythe, D.B. (1998) Neuropathologic findings associated with seizures in FVB mice. *Laboratory Animal Science* 48:34–37.

Hulcrantz, M. & Li, H.S. (1993) Inner ear morphology in CBA/Ca and C57BL/6 mice in relationship to noise, age and phenotype. *European Archives of Oto-Rhino-Laryngology* 250:257–264.

Johnson, K.R., Zheng, Q.Y., & Noben-Trauth, K. (2006) Strain background effects and genetic modifiers of hearing in mice. *Brain Research* 1091:79–88.

Livy, D.J. & Wahlsten, D. (1991) Tests of genetic allelism between four inbred mouse strains with absent corpus collosum. *Journal of Heredity* 82:459–464.

Livy, D.V. & Wahlsten, D. (1997) Retarded formation of the hippocampal commisure in embryos from mouse strains lacking a corpus callosum. *Hippocampus* 7:2–14.

Serfilippi, L.M., Pullman, D.R.S., Gruebbel, M.M., Kern, T.J., & Spainhour, C.B. (2004) Assessment of retinal degeneration in outbred albino mice. *Comparative Medicine* 54:69–76.

Seyfried, T.N., Glaser, G.H., Yu, R.K., & Palayoor, S.T. (1986) Inherited convulsive disorders in mice. *Advances in Neurology* 44:115–133.

Sidman, R.L. & Green, M.C. (1965) Retinal degeneration in the mouse: location of the RD locus in linkage group XVIII. *Journal of Heredity* 56:23–29.

Smith, R.S., Roderick, T.H., & Sundberg, J.P. (1994) Microphthalmia and associated abnormalities in inbred black mice. *Laboratory Animal Science* 44:551–560.

Southard, T. & Brayton, C.F. (2011) Spontaneous unilateral brainstem infarction in Swiss mice. *Veterinary Pathology* 48:726–729.

Sundberg, J.P., Brown, K.S., Bates, R., Cunliffe-Beamer, T.L., & Bedigian, H. (1991) Suppurative conjunctivitis and ulcerative blepharitis in 129/J mice. *Laboratory Animal Science* 41:516–518.

Todorova, M.T., Dangler, C.A., Drage, M.G., Sheppard, B.J., Fox, J.G., & Seyfried, T.N. (2003) Sexual dysfunction and sudden death in epileptic male EL mice: inheritance and prevention with ketogenic diet. *Epilepsia* 44:25–31.

Van Winkle, T.J. & Balk, M.W. (1986) Spontaneous corneal opacities in laboratory mice. *Laboratory Animal Science* 36:248–255.

Wahlsten, D., Crabbe, J.C., & Dudek, B.C. (2001) Behavioral testing of standard inbred and 5Ht(1B) knockout mice: implications of absent corpus collosum. *Behavioral Research* 125:23–32.

Disorders of the Cardiovascular and Respiratory Systems

Good, M.E. & Whitaker, M.S. (1989) Idiopathic cardiomyopathy in C3H/Bd mice. *Laboratory Animal Science* 39:137–141.

Hewicker, M. & Trautwein, G. (1987) Sequential study of vasculitis in MRL mice. *Laboratory Animals* 21:335–341.

Maeda, N., Doi, K., & Mitsuoka, T. (1986) Development of heart and aortic lesions in DBA/2NCrj mice. *Laboratory Animals* 20:5–8.

Mathiesen P.W., Qasim, F.J., Esnault, V.L., & Oliveira, D.B. (1993) Animal models of systemic vasculitis. *Journal of Autoimmunity* 6:251–264.

Hook, G.E. (1991) Alveolar proteinosis and phospholipidosis of the lungs. *Toxicologic Pathology* 19:482–513.

Disorders of the Gastrointestinal System

Diehl, S.R. & Erickson, R.P. (1997) Genome scan for teratogen-induced clefting susceptibility loci in the mouse: evidence of both allelic and locus heterogeneity distinguishing cleft lip and cleft palate. *Proceedings of the National Academy of Sciences of the United States of America* 94:5231–5236.

Juriloff, D.M., Harris, M.J., Dewell, S.L., Brown, C.J., Mager, D.L., Gagnier, L., & Mah, D.G. (2005) Investigation of the genomic region that contains the *clf1* mutation, a causal gene in multifactorial cleft lip and palate in mice. *Birth Defects Research A: Clinical and Molecular Teratology* 73:103–113.

Kalter, H. (1979) The history of the A family of inbred mice and the biology of its congenital malformations. *Teratology* 20:213–232.

Goyal, R.K. & Chaudhury, A. (2010) Pathogenesis of achalasia: lessons from mutant mice. *Gastroenterology* 139:1086–1090.

Hollander, C.F., van Bezooijen, C.F., & Solleveld, H.A. (1987) Anatomy, function, and aging in the mouse liver. *Archives of Toxicology* 10: (Suppl.) 244–250.

Randelia, H.P., Panicker, K.N., & Lalitha, V.S. (1990) Mega-esophagus in the mouse: histochemical and ultrastructural studies. *Laboratory Animals* 24:78–86.

Disorders of the Endocrine System

Dunn, T.B. (1970) Normal and pathologic anatomy of the adrenal gland of the mouse, including neoplasms. *Journal of the National Cancer Institute* 44:1323–1389.

Wakefield, L.M., Thordarson, G., Nieto, A.I., Shyamala, G., Galvez, J.J., Anver, M.R., & Cardiff, R.D. (2003) Spontaneous pituitary abnormalities and mammary hyperplasia in FVB/NCr mice: implications for mouse modeling. *Comparative Medicine* 53:424–432.

Disorders of the Genitourinary Systems

Baze, W.B., Steinbach, T.J., Fleetwood, M.L., Blanchard, T.W., Barnhart, K.F., & McArthur, M.J. (2006) Karyomegaly and intra-nuclear inclusions in the renal tubules of sentinel ICR mice (*Mus musculus*). *Comparative Medicine* 56:435–438.

Cunliffe-Beamer, T.L. & Feldman, D.B. (1976) Vaginal septa in mice: incidence, inheritance, and effect on reproduction performance. *Laboratory Animal Science* 26:895–898.

Hill, L.R., Coghlan, L.G., & Baze, W.B. (2001) Perineal swelling in two strains of mice. *Contemporary Topics in Laboratory Animal Science* 41:51–53.

Myles, M.H., Foltz, C.J., Shinpock, S.G., Olszewski, R.E., & Franklin, C.L. (2002) Infertility in CFW/R1 mice associated with cystic dilatation of the bulbourethral gland. *Comparative Medicine* 52:273–276.

Sundberg, J.P. & Brown, K.S. (1994) Imperforate vagina and mucometra in inbred laboratory mice. *Laboratory Animal Science* 44:380–382.

Disorders of the Musculoskeletal System

Albassam, M.A., Wojcinski, Z.W., Barsoum, N.J., & Smith, G.S. (1991) Spontaneous fibro-osseous proliferative lesions in the sternums and femurs of B6C3F1 mice. *Veterinary Pathology* 28:381–388.

Allamand, V. & Cambell, K.P. (2000) Animal models for muscular dystrophy: valuable tools for the development of therapies. *Human Molecular Genetics* 9:2459–2467.

Bulfield, G., Siller, W.B., Wight, P.A.L., & Moore, K.J. (1984) X chromosome-linked muscular dystrophy (mdx) in the mouse. *Proceedings of the National Academy of Sciences of the United States of America* 81:1189–1192.

Dangain, J. & Vrbova, G. (1984) Muscle development in (mdx) mutant mice. *Muscle and Nerve* 7:700–704.

Gervais, F. & Attia, M.A. (2005) Fibro-osseous proliferation in the sternums and femurs of female B6C3F1, C57black, and CD-1 mice: a comparative study. *Deutsche Tierarztliche Wochenschrift* 112:323–326.

Paquet, M., Penney, J., & Boerboom, D. (2008) Lateral femoral hernias in a line of FVB/NHsd mice: a new confounding lesion linked to genetic background? *Comparative Medicine* 58:395–398.

Rittinghausen, S., Kohler, M., Kamino, K., Dasenbrock, C., & Mohr, U. (1997) Spontaneous myelofibrosis in castrated and ovariectomized NMRI mice. *Experimental Toxicologic Pathology* 49:351–353.

Sass, B. & Montali, R.J. (1980) Spontaneous fibro-osseous lesions in aging female mice. *Laboratory Animal Science* 30:907–909.

Silberberg, M. & Silberberg, R. (1962) Osteoarthritis and osteoporosis in senile mice. *Gerontologia* 6:91–101.

Vainzof, M., Ayub-Guerrieri, D., Onofre, P.C., Martins, P.C., Lopes, V.F., Zilberztajn, D., Maia, L.S., Sell, K., & Yamamoto, L.U. (2008) Animal models for genetic neuromuscular diseases. *Journal of Molecular Neuroscience* 34:241–248.

Yamasaki, K. (1996) Vertebral disk changes in B6C3F$_1$ mice. *Laboratory Animal Science* 46:576–578.

NEOPLASMS

The very origins of the laboratory mouse were promulgated by an interest in the genetic basis of cancer, and this interest has accelerated with GEMs. Many of the common inbred strains of mice were originally developed because of their propensity to develop tumors, such as mammary tumors in C3H/He mice, testicular teratomas in 129/Sv mice, multicentric lymphomas in BALB/c mice, and thymic lymphomas in AKR mice. Perchance, some strains that were not selectively bred for cancer also happen to be prone to cancer, such as DBA mice with hepatocellular neoplasia. Others were bred for their predisposition to one type of tumor but unexpectedly develop a high prevalence of other types of tumors, such as A strain mice, which were selectively bred for mammary tumors but also develop pulmonary adenomas. Other strains were developed for their longevity and low tumor prevalence, such as B6 mice. Regardless, the genetic homozygosity of mice and the presence of retroviral elements in their genome make neoplasia a common cause of morbidity in many strains. This text covers only the major neoplastic disorders of common strains of mice and does not attempt to describe and document all types of spontaneous or induced neoplasia in laboratory mice. There are several excellent references for "wallpaper matching" naturally occurring mouse neoplasms with published images (see "General References on Diseases of Mice").

There are several features about the mouse that may reflect upon interpretation of neoplasia. Mouse tumors tend to grow by blunt expansion, rather than by invasive infiltration, but this does not mean that they do not display malignant properties. For example, most human pathologists would tend to deem spontaneous mouse mammary tumors as morphologically benign, yet nearly 60% metastasize to the lung. When tumors are metastatic in the mouse, the most common site of metastasis is the lung, which differs from other species, including humans. True metastasis must be differentiated from tumor embolization. The pathologist can assist with this distinction by careful examination for the presence of endothelial cells surrounding the suspect metastatic masses within the lumina of blood vessels. These emboli may behave differently from truly invasive metastases. Pulmonary adenomas, which are common in mice, are often misconstrued as metastases of other epithelial tumors. In addition, mouse epithelium of tubular organs, including neoplastic epithelium, is prone to herniation, which can be misconstrued as malignant behavior. This is especially common in hyperplastic epithelium of the colon, particularly when mice are infected with *C. rodentium*, *Helicobacter* spp., *Cryptosporidium parvum*, or when the mucosa is perturbed by rectal prolapse. These stimuli induce marked mucosal hyperplasia and dysplasia with frequent crypt herniation into underlying tissues. As the hyperplastic stimulus wanes within the herniated epithelium, mucinous differentiation tends to occur, with the formation of mucin-filled cysts, erosion of lining epithelium, crypt suppuration, crypt effacement, inflammation, and fibrosis. This process (colitis cystica) may be erroneously diagnosed as mucinous adenocarcinomas. Proof of neoplasia is autonomous growth and metastasis, which are seldom proven experimentally in these models.

Genetic engineering, particularly the integration of onco-transgenes, has resulted in the expression of novel tumor phenotypes that do not occur as spontaneous tumors in mice. The failures of the mouse as a model of human cancer are increasingly being resolved by genomic manipulation. GEM neoplasms that mimic not only human tumor morphology but also human tumor biology are being increasingly studied. The raison d'etre of the laboratory mouse is to model human disease. Thus, nomenclature of mouse neoplasia continues to evolve in an effort to align mouse neoplasia with that of the human. Organ-site consensus reports have been published by the National Cancer Institute's Mouse Models of Human Cancer Consortium (MMHCC). These reports are intended to facilitate communication among pathologists about mouse models of human disease. These reports generally agree with, but somewhat modify, the World Health Organization (WHO) classification and nomenclature.

Signature GEM Phenotypes: Molecular Pathology of Neoplasia

The microscopic appearance of spontaneous epithelial tumors of the mouse seldom resembles human cancers. In contrast, GEM tumors are often quite different from spontaneous mouse tumors and may more closely mimic the human condition. It is becoming increasingly apparent that oncogenic transgenes induce "signature phenotypes" in GEMs that can be recognized among tumors derived from multiple tissue types. For example, tumors arising in a single organ, such as mammary gland, display different but consistent morphology depending upon the signal transduction pathway that is affected. These signature phenotypes cluster with genes that share common signal transduction pathways. Age, sex, immune status, strain background, and tissue-specific promoters may modify biology of GEM tumors, but seldom affect the signature phenotype. Furthermore, signature phenotypes span not only a single tissue but can be recognized in a variety of tumors arising in other organs. The field of "molecular pathology" is highly informative and needs the expertise of mouse pathologists who are aware of this evolving concept.

Lymphoid Neoplasia

Tumors of lymphoid and nonlymphoid hematopoietic lineages are a major cause of morbidity and mortality among laboratory mice. The overall prevalence among all mouse strains is estimated to be 1–2%, but thymic lymphoma may occur in virtually 100% in some strains, such as AKR and C58 mice, by 12 months of age (Fig. 1.44). SCID mice also develop a high incidence of thymic lymphomas (Fig. 1.127). In contrast, BALB/c mice develop a high incidence of multicentric lymphomas (Fig. 1.45). The mouse is prone to these entities because of its inbred nature, which provides the requisite combinations of endogenous retroelements that are a consequence of the mosaic origins of the laboratory mouse genome and selective inbreeding for tumor phenotypes (see "Retroelements and Retrovirus Infections"). Furthermore, the mouse is unique because of the persistence and proliferative nature of the thymus into adult life, resulting in vulnerability to T-cell tumors. The mouse spleen also provides a unique milieu for evolution of neoplasia. It is a major hematopoietic organ throughout life, and it functions as the major secondary lymphoid compartment (in contrast to humans), with very active marginal zones.

The classification of mouse lymphomas has been in continuous flux but seems to be resolving with the use of immunological markers and more precise comparison with human disease. There is not much point in reviewing the various classification and nomenclature schemes that have been proposed in the past. The MMHCC consensus classification (Morse et al. 2002) generally agrees with but builds upon the WHO classification (Mohr 2001). The reader is encouraged to seek more detailed information regarding these types of neoplasms and their differential immunologic markers. Many of them rarely occur as spontaneous diseases in laboratory mice. Those that are most likely to be encountered in common laboratory mice are discussed below.

Small B-Cell Lyphoma/Leukemia

These neoplasms occur sporadically in a number of strains of aged mice. They arise multisystemically, with infiltration of numerous organs, including lung and kidney, and often have a leukemic phase. They are composed of small round cells with scant cytoplasm, condensed chromatin, and a sIg+/B220+/CD19+ immunophenotype.

Splenic Marginal Zone Lymphoma

This form of lymphoma occurs in low incidence (1–2%) among most inbred strains of mice. They may be supplanted by follicular lymphomas and have therefore been largely overlooked until recently. They are common in NFS.N mice that are congenic for ecotropic proviruses contributed by AKR and C58 mice, and NZB mice. These lymphomas arise in the marginal zones of the splenic white pulp. Early lesions are often multicentric in the spleen, with extension from the marginal zone into the white and red pulp as the disease progresses. The spleens become enlarged, with occasional involvement of splenic lymph nodes, but disease in other tissues is generally not present. They consist of medium, uniform cells with abundant, grayish to pale eosinophilic cytoplasm, round to ovoid nuclei containing stippled or vesicular chromatin, and a sIgM+/B220+/CD19+ immunophenotype.

Follicular B-Cell Lymphoma

These lymphomas are the most common spontaneous lymphoma among many inbred strains of mice. They

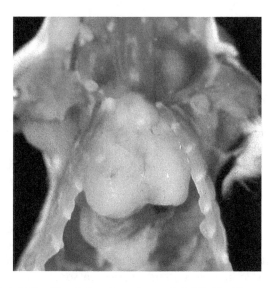

FIG. 1.127. *Thymic lymphoma in an adult C.B-17-scid mouse. These neoplasms are relatively common in SCID mice.*

involve the spleen, Peyer's patches, and mesenteric lymph nodes. The tumors arise in follicles of the splenic white pulp, with a nodular appearance that can be seen as white mottling or nodules at necropsy. Microscopically, neoplastic cells are small to large, with scant cytoplasm and large, vesicular, irregularly folded to cleaved nuclei, and poorly delineated cytoplasmic boundaries. They typically are low grade, with cell populations resembling germinal center cells (large centroblasts or immunoblasts, and small centrocytes), as well as concurrent infiltration of other cell types, including significant numbers of T cells. Less than half of the cells are centroblasts or immunoblasts. Their immunophenotype is sIgM+/B220+/CD19+.

Diffuse Large B-Cell Lymphoma

These tumors are also common among inbred strains of mice and resemble follicular B-cell lymphomas. Gross enlargement of the spleen and abdominal lymph nodes is seen. They may also arise in the mediastinum with thymic enlargement. DLBCLs arise from centroblasts in the splenic white pulp. Cells are medium-sized and have scant cytoplasm with round vesicular nuclei. Nucleoli are prominent, often multiple, and typically adherent to the nuclear membrane. Mitotic activity is high. Over half of the cells are centroblasts, and less than 10% are immunoblasts. The immunophenotype is sIgM+/B220+/CD19+.

Histiocyte-Associated Diffuse Large B-Cell Lymphoma

This form of lymphoma has a variable incidence among inbred strains of mice. It is a diffuse large B-cell lymphoma but features sheets of pink, fusiform to round, vacuolated histiocytes with large numbers of lymphocytes. Greater than half of the cells are histiocytes, which are not considered to be neoplastic. They frequently involve liver. Spleens are nodular, and lymph node involvement tends to be diffuse. It may be difficult to differentiate these neoplasms from histiocytic sarcomas because of their large populations of histiocytes.

Burkitt-Like (Lymphoblastic) Lymphoma

"Lymphoblastic" is less anthropomorphic, not associated with herpesvirus, and is unique to the mouse, but the MMHCC lists these tumors as "Burkitt-Like" as a comparative feature to human disease. These tumors arise frequently in some inbred strains of mice, especially in aged animals. Typically, there is generalized lymphadenopathy, splenomegaly, and sometimes thymic involvement. The tumors are composed of medium-sized, uniform lymphoblastic cells with round to ovoid nuclei, fine chromatin, and single or several small central nucleoli. Mitotic activity is high, and there is sometimes a "starry sky" appearance. Their immunophenotype is sIgM+/B220+/CD19+.

Plasmacytoma

This type of B-cell neoplasm is rare among most strains of laboratory mice but is notable because it can be readily induced with pristane in some strains of mice, such as BALB/c, NZB, or F1 crossed mice, or by infection with acutely transforming retroviruses. It may be common in some types of GEMs. Cells resemble plasma cells with eccentric nuclei, marginated chromatin, and moderate amounts of cytoplasm. Pristane-induced tumors arise in the peritoneum following intraperitoneal injection. Their immunophenotype is cytIg+/CD43+/CD138+.

Precursor T-Cell Lymphoblastic Lymphoma

These tumors are typically CD3+, CD4-/CD8-, TCR+, cytTdT+ thymic lymphomas that are common in some inbred strains of mice, such as AKR and C58. Some may be CD4+/CD-, CD4-/CD8+, or CD4+/CD8+. They also arise frequently in SCID mice and are commonly induced by irradiation and chemicals. Affected mice have enlarged thymuses, which may be associated with dyspnea, with variable involvement of spleen and lymph nodes. Cells are medium-sized and uniform with scant cytoplasm, round nuclei, and fine chromatin. Nucleoli are small, prominent, and multiple. Mitotic activity is high.

Small T-Cell Lymphoma

These lymphomas occur rarely in inbred mice and tend to arise in aged mice. They resemble small B-cell lymphomas and cause splenomegaly and lymphadenomegaly but not thymic involvement. Their immunophenotype is CD3+/TCR+/CD4+ or CD8+/cytoTdT+.

Nonlymphoid Hematopoietic Neoplasms

The most significant spontaneous nonlymphoid hematopoietic neoplasm among common inbred mice is histiocytic sarcoma. Other forms of nonlymphoid hematopoietic tumors occur sporadically, or not at all, except under experimental circumstances or in GEMs (see Kogan 2002 for details on the MMHCC consensus classification/nomenclature for this group of tumors).

Histiocytic Sarcoma

Neoplasms of histiocytic origin are especially common in certain strains of laboratory mice, particularly in aged B6 and SJL mice. Neoplasms of this type have been produced experimentally using retroviruses or carcinogens in intact or thymectomized mice. Based on immunohistochemistry, these neoplasms arise from mononuclear phagocytic cells, such as Kupffer cells and tissue macrophages. Gross findings may include marked enlargement of the spleen, with nodular involvement of other tissues, such as liver, uterus, vagina, kidney, lung, and ovaries. In some cases, only 1 organ (e.g., uterine wall) may be involved. On microscopic examination, there are circumscribed nodular to

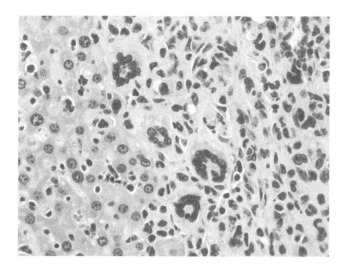

FIG. 1.128. *Histiocytic sarcoma infiltrating the liver. The tumor consists of neoplastic histiocytes and multinucleated giant cells.*

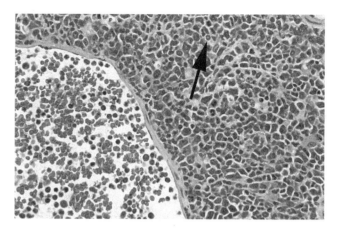

FIG. 1.129. *Liver from a mouse with myeloid leukemia. Note the spectrum of differentiation, including some cells with doughnut-shaped nuclei (arrow), and the presence of neoplastic cells within the blood of the hepatic vein.*

multifocal infiltrates in tissues such as liver, spleen, lymph nodes, intestine, bone marrow, female reproductive tract, and lung. Neoplastic infiltrates consist of large histiocytic cells with irregular basophilic nuclei, fibrillar, eosinophilic cytoplasm, and indistinct cytoplasmic outlines. Neoplasms may vary in composition, from elongated fibrillar cells forming pallisading patterns to rounded cell types. Large nuclei and multinucleated giant cells are a common finding (Fig. 1.128). The neoplastic cells tend to be particularly elongated in those arising in the uterine wall, and thus have on occasion been diagnosed as malignant Schwannomas. Erythrophagocytosis may be associated with the neoplastic infiltrates, particularly in the liver. Occasionally tumors of this type involve a solitary lymph node or multiple ones. They consist of a prominent stromal component interspersed within a dense population of well-differentiated lymphocytes. They may be difficult to differentiate from histiocyte-associated diffuse large B-cell lymphomas.

Myeloid Leukemia

Spontaneous myeloid (granulocytic) leukemias are occasionally observed in some strains of older laboratory mice. They have been associated with retroviral infections and may be produced experimentally with chemical carcinogens or irradiation. The neoplastic process usually originates in the spleen, with subsequent involvement of a variety of tissues, including bone marrow, liver, lung, adrenal, and kidney. Clinically, animals are anemic and depressed, and peripheral leukocyte counts may approach 200,000/mm^3. Mice usually have marked splenomegaly, with variable involvement of liver, kidneys, and other organs. There is massive infiltration of the splenic red pulp with malignant myeloid cells, with sparing of the splenic follicles. Diffuse infiltration of the bone marrow commonly occurs. Focal to diffuse infiltration of lung, liver, kidney,

and adrenal may also occur (Fig. 1.129). Myeloid cells have large, vesicular nuclei that vary in shape with round, indented, and ring forms. Marked extramedullary myelopoiesis in the spleen and liver has been misconstrued as myeloid leukemia by the uninformed.

Mammary Neoplasia

There is great variation in the incidence of mammary tumors among different strains of mice. For example, the incidence of mammary tumors in the BALB/c strain is low, whereas up to 100% of C3H females develop mammary tumors by the time they reach 9 months of age (Fig. 1.46). Endogenous (as well as exogenous) mammary tumor viruses (MMTVs) play an important role in mouse mammary neoplasia. Chemical carcinogens and hormones also influence the incidence of mammary tumors in laboratory mice. Prolactin, progesterone, and estrogens may all play a role in the development of hormone-responsive mammary tumors. Multiparous FVB mice are prone to development of mammary tumors, which may be related to their pituitary prolactin secretion dynamics. Stress due to conditions such as intensive breeding or overcrowding has been found to have a significant influence on the incidence of mammary neoplasia in C3H/He mice.

Spontaneous mouse mammary tumors were originally classified under a scheme developed by Thelma Dunn, using letter designations (A, B, C, AB, L, P, Y, etc.). Subsequently, a tissue-based system (alveolar, ductal, myoepithelial) was used, but both of these schemes were not effective at defining the new types of tumors that are arising in GEMs and relate poorly to human disease. The MMHCC consensus classification uses glandular, acinar, cribriform, papillary, solid, squamous, fibroadenoma, adenomyoepithelioma, adenosquamous, and NOS.

Mammary neoplasia in the mouse is related to insertional mutagenesis by MMTVs. MMTVs are either exogenous or endogenous (see "Retroelements and Retrovirus Infections") but induce similar lesions, although endogenous viruses tend to induce low-grade lesions that arise later in life. Unless purposely introduced and maintained in mouse populations, exogenous MMTVs are not encountered in laboratory mice. Thus, the viruses of significance for induction of spontaneous mammary neoplasia are the endogenous replication-competent MMTVs that are present in a relatively few strains of mice, including C3H, BALB/c, and GR, among others. Other strains of mice that do not harbor replication-competent MMTV may be susceptible to experimental infection with MMTV, but B6 mice are remarkably resistant. The earliest discernable microscopic lesions are focal and multifocal hyperplasias within the terminal ductule or alveolar buds. Two types of lesions arise in MMTV-infected mice. Hyperplastic alveolar nodules (HANs) resemble prelactating mammary gland but stand out from the background of the nonlactating gland as nodules. Plaques are circumscribed ductal proliferations that appear during pregnancy and regress on parturition. As either of these lesions evolve and become autonomous of hormonal influences, some progress into mammary intraepithelial neoplasias (MINs) (high- or low-grade), adenomas, or carcinomas.

Mammary tumors are often multicentric and multinodular in character, well circumscribed, and easily separated from surrounding tissue. The tissue is usually grayish white and soft but may contain blood-filled cysts and areas of necrosis. Tumors with squamous features may contain flaky white material, and others may contain milky secretory product. Despite their circumscribed noninvasive nature, pulmonary metastases are common. There are a variety of patterns seen histologically, which may vary with the strain background of the mouse and the MMTV strain. However, multiple patterns of tumor may arise in a single strain of mouse.

Mammary tumors that are induced in GEMs with onco-transgenes under control of mammary gland promoters, such as MMTV-LTR or whey acidic protein (WAP), follow predictable behaviors (signature pathology). Most notably, those that are induced by *Wnt-1* resemble naturally occurring, MMTV-induced tumors. Spontaneous mammary tumors arise from activation of either *Wnt-1*, *Notch4*, or *Fgf3* proto-oncogenes (which are all members of the *Wnt-1* signal transduction pathway) through integration of the MMTV provirus. *Wnt-1* or *Fgf* transgenic mice will develop the full range of tumors that arise spontaneously and often in the same mouse. Other GEMs have tumors of unique phenotype, but they, too, fall within discernable phenotypic (signature) categories that do not resemble MMTV-induced tumors.

Pulmonary Neoplasia

Primary pulmonary adenomas and adenocarcinomas are among the most common tumors found in mice. A strain mice are highly susceptible, with tumors arising by 3–4 months of age and reaching 100% prevalence by 18–24 months. Pulmonary tumors are also common in somewhat less susceptible strains, such as outbred Swiss, FVB, BALB/c, 129, and B6;129 hybrids. The uniquely high susceptibility of A strain mice is related to their K-ras allele, with activation of K-ras in the tumors. The onset and prevalence of pulmonary tumors can be enhanced with viral infections, such as Sendai virus, or chemical carcinogens. Most spontaneous pulmonary tumors are believed to originate from type II pneumocytes or a common precursor cell for type II and Clara cells. Most GEM models for pulmonary neoplasia develop pulmonary tumors that resemble spontaneous or chemically induced tumors. The recent MMHCC consensus classification has attempted to align mouse pulmonary tumors with those that arise in humans. For this reason, the terms "bronchioloalveolar" or "alveolar/bronchiolar" that have been used for mouse tumors in the past have been dropped. Spontaneous or carcinogen-induced tumors are now simply diagnosed as pulmonary adenomas or carcinomas with appropriate qualifications (solid, papillary, or mixed). Other types of tumors are included in the new classification, such as papilloma, squamous cell carcinoma, adenosquamous carcinoma, neuroendocrine carcinoma, and others, but these are rarely encountered as spontaneous tumors in the mouse.

Pulmonary tumors are often encountered as incidental findings, but those that grow expansively can result in clinical signs of dyspnea. They appear as circumscribed, firm to resilient, pearl-gray nodules located in the subpleural regions or deep within the parenchyma of the lung. Tumors may be large, with bulging contours (Fig. 1.130). There may be evidence of pleural invasion, with seeding of the visceral and parietal pleura. On microscopic examination, adenomas display compression of

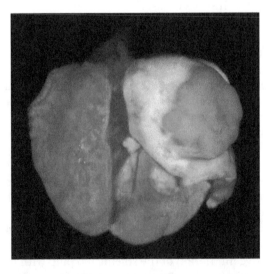

FIG. 1.130.   *Pulmonary adenoma in an aged laboratory mouse. There is a large, raised, circumscribed mass in the cranial region of the right lung.*

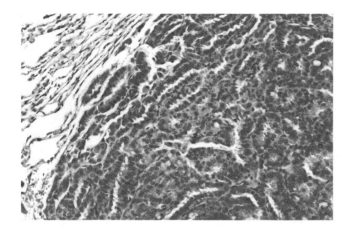

FIG. 1.131. *Pulmonary adenoma. Cuboidal epithelial cells are lining alveolar septa. There is a distinct line of demarcation between the tumor and the adjacent compressed normal lung tissue.*

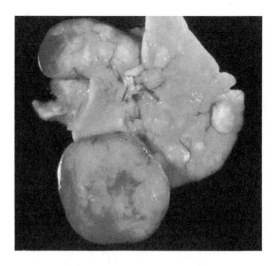

FIG. 1.132. *Hepatocellular tumors in a DBA mouse. Note the multicentric nodules of varying size.*

the adjacent structures (Fig. 1.131). They are composed of closely packed cuboidal to columnar cells lining remnants of alveolar septa, with a sparse stroma of collagenous tissue. Tumor cells are relatively uniform in size, with round, hyperchromatic nuclei and acidophilic cytoplasm. Cells are nonciliated, and mitotic figures are rare. Those that are adjacent or protruding into bronchioles may consist of tubular to papillary patterns composed of columnar epithelial cells with convoluted to folded basal nuclei. There is compression of the adjacent alveolar structures. Pulmonary carcinomas tend to invade the adjacent parenchyma, including the pleura; frequently form papillary structures; and consist of large, pleomorphic epithelial cells with irregular, polygonal, hyperchromatic nuclei. There may be extensive invasion of the adjacent pleural surface and occasionally extension into the intercostal muscles. Occasionally, pulmonary tumors are encountered with mucinous differentiation. Differential diagnoses include metastatic tumors from sites such as mammary gland, liver or Harderian gland, and focal alveolar epithelial cell hyperplasia, as seen occasionally in older mice.

Hepatocellular Neoplasia

Spontaneous hepatic neoplasms in the mouse include hepatocellular adenomas and carcinomas, hepatoblastoma, cholangioma, cholangiocarcinoma, cholangiohepatocellular (mixed) carcinoma, hemangioma, hemangiosarcoma, and histiocytic sarcoma. Rarely, Ito cell tumors may also be encountered. The most common hepatocellular tumors are adenomas and carcinomas, which arise more frequently in aged males than females. Some strains of mice, such as A and DBA, are especially prone to hepatocellular tumors (Fig. 1.132), and infection with *Helicobacter* spp. has been associated with an earlier onset and higher prevalence among A strain mice. Foci of cellular alteration, including clear cell foci, basophilic cell foci, and eosinophilic cell foci, are generally

considered to be antecedent to hepatocellular neoplasia. Primary hepatic tumors readily occur in mice treated with a variety of hepatocarcinogens.

Hepatocellular tumors may vary from single to multiple, circumscribed, raised, moderately firm, gray to tan nodules to large, poorly delineated, pale to dark red fleshy masses. Hepatocellular tumors are composed of two major histological types: trabecular (Fig. 1.133) or solid (Fig. 1.134), but other patterns may arise, including adenoid. Cellular morphology may be well differentiated to poorly differentiated, and the degree of differentiation does not predict metastatic potential. Well-differentiated hepatocellular adenomas may be difficult to distinguish from adjacent tissue. Most hepatocellular tumors are well circumscribed and not encapsulated, but some

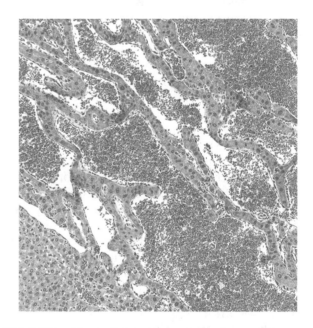

FIG. 1.133. *Hepatocellular carcinoma, trabecular type. The neoplasm consists of cords of neoplastic hepatocytes growing in a trabecular pattern.*

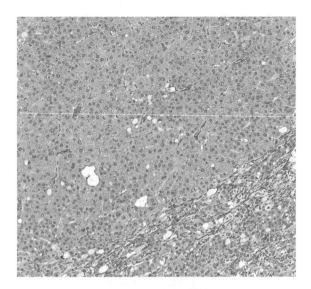

FIG. 1.134. *Hepatocellular carcinoma, solid type. The adjacent liver parenchyma (lower right) is compressed by the tumor.*

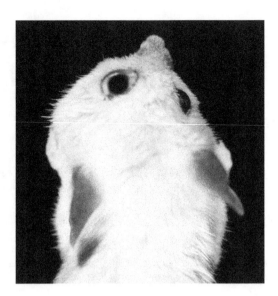

FIG. 1.135. *Mouse with retrobulbar Harderian gland adenocarcinoma resulting in facial distortion and periocular porphyrin staining.*

may be locally infiltrative. Anisokaryosis, karyomegaly, and cytomegaly are frequently prominent. A rare variant is hepatoblastoma, which has characteristic organoid structures arranged around vascular channels or forming rows and rosettes. Cholangiomas and cholangiocarcinomas are also rare. Hemangiomas and hemangiosarcomas are somewhat more common and may arise as primary liver neoplasms. The liver is frequently involved in multisystemic lymphoreticular neoplasms and may occasionally be the site of metastatic dissemination of other tumor types.

Harderian Gland Neoplasia

Naturally occurring tumors of the Harderian lacrimal gland are slow-growing neoplasms and appear late in life. The incidence of Harderian gland tumors can be increased with irradiation or the administration of chemical carcinogens. At necropsy, there may be protrusion of the eye on the affected side, accompanied by porphyrin staining of the periocular hair (Fig. 1.135). These tumors typically consist of a lobulated, resilient, light tan to white mass in the retro-orbital space. Microscopically, the tumors are usually papillary cystadenomas or solid adenomas and are composed of relatively well-differentiated epithelial cells with vacuolated cytoplasm. Harderian gland adenocarcinomas may also occur (Fig. 1.136) and tend to be highly invasive, with blunt infiltration of bone and other structures of the head. They tend to be less well differentiated and may metastasize to other sites, such as lung.

Myoepitheliomas

Myoepitheliomas arise infrequently in most strains of mice but are relatively more common in some strains, such as BALB/c and BALB/cBy mice, especially females.

They most frequently arise from submaxillary and parotid salivary glands but may also be associated with mammary, preputial, and Harderian glands. These tumors can become very large, with cystic chambers containing mucinoid fluid (Fig. 1.137). Microscopically, tumors are composed of large, pleomorphic spindle cells with epithelial and mesenchymal features (Fig. 1.138). Cystic areas form as a result of necrosis. Metastasis to the lung may occur with large tumors. A curious feature is concomitant myeloid hyperplasia of bone marrow and spleen, apparently related to a secretory product of the tumor.

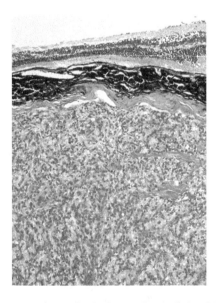

FIG. 1.136. *Harderian gland adenocarcinoma depicted in Figure 1.135. The neoplasm consists of poorly differentiated fusiform to cuboidal epithelial cells, with compression of the adjacent sclera and retina.*

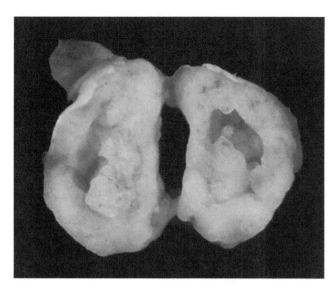

FIG. 1.137. *Parotid salivary gland myoepithelioma of a mouse. The tumor has been bisected to demonstrate the cystic center that contained necrotic cellular debris and mucinous material.*

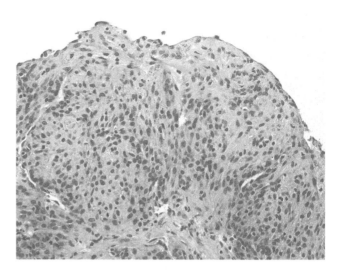

FIG. 1.138. *Myoepithelioma, demonstrating the morphology of the epithelioid/spindle-shaped neoplastic cells lining the cystic center.*

Neoplasia of the Reproductive System

Neoplasms of the female reproductive tract that arise in aged mice include papillary cystadenomas of the ovary, ovarian tubular adenomas, granulosa cell, and thecal cell tumors. Dysgerminomas are exceedingly rare. In p53$^{+/-}$ mice, malignant granulosa cell tumors with metastases have been noted occasionally. Vascular tumors (hemangiomas and hemangiosarcomas) occur in both the ovary and uterus. Uterine endometrial stromal tumors, adenocarcinomas, and leiomyosarcomas of uterine wall are other neoplasms encountered in this species. The uterus may also be a primary site for development of histocytic sarcomas. Ovarian teratomas are rare, except in LT/Sv mice. Neoplasms of the male reproductive tract are relatively rare, except in GEMs. Occasionally, sebaceosquamous adenomas and carcinomas may arise from preputial glands of both males and females, and tumors may also arise in other accessory sex glands.

Teratomas: Embryonal Carcinomas/Teratocarcinomas

Teratomas of the testis (Fig. 1.139) are frequent in 129/Sv-ter+ mice (currently named 129S4/SvJae, and other lines derived from Stevens), with up to 10% of mice affected by 3 weeks of age. Up to 94% of older ter+/+ homozygous mice may have testicular teratomas, with up to 75% with bilateral involvement. Extragonadal teratomas arise in the perigenital region or midline of chimeras derived from 129 embryonic stem cells. Teratomas characteristically contain tissue elements derived from ectoderm, mesoderm, and endoderm (Fig. 1.140).

Mesenchymal Neoplasms
Rhabdomyosarcomas

Rhabdomyosarcomas are generally uncommon, but arise more frequently in some strains of mice. A strain mice, which carry a mutation in the dysferlin gene which results in development muscular dystrophy, also develop a very high frequency (>70%) of rhabdomyosarcomas at greater than 20 months of age. Tumors are pleomorphic and arise from the axial and proximal appendicular skeleton. It has been proposed that regeneration of skeletal muscle due to the dysferlin mutation has a promoting effect upon tumor development, since muscles that are most affected by muscular dystrophy are most prone to neoplasia. Aside from A strain mice, BALB mice are more prone to development of rhabdomyosarcomas than other strains of mice. Quadriceps muscle is the most frequent site for these tumors in BALB mice (Fig. 1.141).

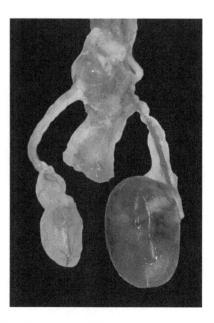

FIG. 1.139. *Enlarged testis (right) in a 129 mouse due to growth of a teratoma. (Source: A. Haertel, Davis, CA. Reproduced with permission from A. Haertel.)*

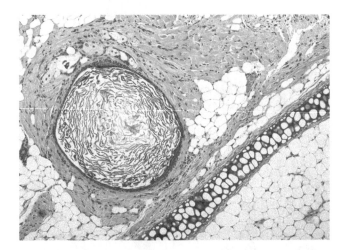

FIG. 1.140. *Testicular teratoma from a mouse. This field illustrates the presence of well-differentiated cartilage, adipose tissue, muscle, an epithelial lined cyst filled with keratin, and adjacent sebaceous glands.*

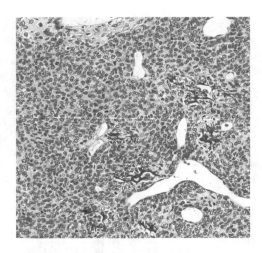

FIG. 1.142. *Femoral osteosarcoma. The tumor is highly cellular with sparse osteoid formation.*

Osteomas and Osteosarcomas

Primary bone tumors are relatively rare in nonmanipulated strains of laboratory mice. Exceptions are outbred OF-1 and CF-1 mice, which develop benign, frequently multicentric osteomas in up to 30% of the mice. A relatively high incidence (7%) of osteosarcomas has been noted to develop in NOD and NOD-derived substrains of mice (Fig. 1.142). Tumors arise primarily in the appendicular skeleton, and particularly the femur. Bone tumors are also relatively common in *Trp53* null heterozygous mice. Rare osteosarcomas arise sporadically in other strains of mice, and have been noted to arise from spinal vertebrae, sternebrae, or long bones. Possible sites for metastatic spread include lung, liver, spleen, and kidney. The lumbosacral region appears to be the most common site for primary tumors arising from the vertebral column. Tumors at this site frequently impinge on the spinal cord, resulting in a clinical presentation of posterior paresis or paralysis. In advanced cases, changes in the adjacent spinal cord are consistent with Wallerian degeneration. Natural infection of nude mice with polyoma virus has been associated with vertebral bone tumors and posterior paresis.

Other Mesenchymal Tumors

Mesenchymal tumors can be readily induced by carcinogens and viruses, such as Moloney murine sarcoma virus. Soft tissue sarcomas are common in some GEMs, especially *Trp53* homozygous and heterozygous null mice, with tumor prevalence partially determined by mouse strain background. Sarcomas can be readily induced in nearly 80% of *Trp53* heterozygous mice following subcutaneous implantation of transponders or plastic foreign bodies.

Endocrine Neoplasms

Pituitary gland adenomas are relatively common in B6 and Swiss mice (Fig. 1.143). FVB/N mice are particularly prone to development of these tumors. Most pituitary

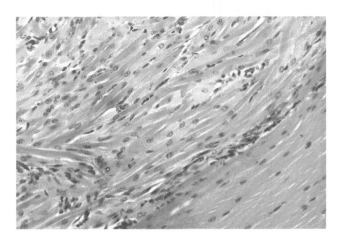

FIG. 1.141. *Rhabdomyosarcoma arising from the quadriceps muscle (lower right) of a BALB mouse. The tumor is composed of disorganized neoplastic myocytes (strap cells).*

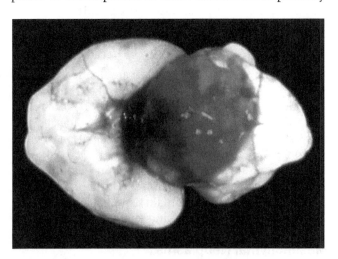

FIG. 1.143. *Pituitary adenoma in a Swiss mouse. These tumors grow by expansion and are typically red because of sinusoids filled with blood.*

adenomas produce prolactin and arise more frequently in females. Tumor cell growth patterns may be solid, sinusoidal, or cystic, with the latter two types appearing quite bloody. These tumors grow expansively, with compression of the overlying brain. Carcinomas are less common and are more anaplastic and invasive. Adrenocortical adenomas, pheochromocytomas, pancreatic islet tumors, follicular cell adenomas of the thyroid gland, and other endocrine types of tumor occur sporadically in laboratory mice and are usually represented in "lists" of tumors arising in aged mice.

Other Neoplasms

A myriad of different tumor types have been reported in laboratory mice and a variety of GEMs. It is beyond the scope of this summary to include descriptions of all the spontaneous, genetically induced, and chemically induced neoplasms that occur in this species. The reader is encouraged to seek further information in the General References cited below.

BIBLIOGRAPHY FOR NEOPLASMS

See "General References on Diseases of Mice"

General References on Neoplasia

Boivin, G.P., Washington, K., Yang, K., Ward, J.M., Pretlow, T.P., Russell, R., Besselsen, D.G., Godfrey, V.L., Dove, W.F., Pitot, H.C., Halberg, R.B., Itzkowitz, S.H., Groden, J., & Coffey, R.J. (2003) Pathology of mouse models of intestinal cancer: consensus report and recommendations. *Gastroenterology* 124:762–777.

Cardiff, R.D., Munn, R.J., & Galvez, J.J. (2007) The tumor pathology of genetically engineered mice: a new approach to molecular pathology. In: *The Mouse in Biomedical Research: Diseases*, Vol. 2, 2nd edn (eds. J.G. Fox, S.W. Barthold, M.T. Davisson, C.E. Newcomer, F.W. Quimby, & Smith), pp. 581–622. Academic Press, New York.

Holland, E.C. (2004) *Mouse Models of Human Cancer*. Wiley-Liss, Hoboken, NJ.

Hruban, R.H., Adsay, N.V., Albores-Saavedra, J., Anver, M.R., Biankin, A.V., Boivin, G.P., Furth, E.E., Furukawa, T., Klein, A., Klimstra, D.S., Kloopel, G., Lauwers, G.Y., Longnecker, D.S., Luttges, J., Maitra, A., Offerhaus, G.J., Perez-Gallego, L., Redston, M., & Tuveson, D.A. (2006) Pathology of genetically engineered mouse models of pancreatic exocrine cancer: consensus report and recommendations. *Cancer Research* 66:95–106.

Ittman, M., Huang, J., Radaelli, E., Martin, P., Signoretti, S., Sullivan, R., Simons, B.W., Ward, J.M., Robinson, B.D., Chu, G.C., Loda, M., Thomas, G., Borowsky, A., & Cardiff, R.D. (2001) Animal models of human prostate cancer: the consensus report of the New York meeting of the mouse models of human cancer consortium prostate pathology committee. *Cancer Research* 73:2718–2736.

Mohr, U. (2001) *International Classification of Rodent Tumors: The Mouse*. WHO/Springer, New York.

Percy, D.H. & Jonas, A.M. (1971) Incidence of spontaneous tumors in CD®-1 HaM/ICR mice. *Journal of the National Cancer Institute* 46:1045–1065.

Son, W.-C. & Gopinath, C. (2004) Early occurrence of spontaneous tumors in CD-1 mice and Sprague-Dawley rats. *Toxicologic Pathology* 32:371–374.

Weiss, W.A., Israel, M., Cobbs, C., Holland, E., James, C.D., Louis, D.N., Marks, C., McClatchey, A.I., Roberts, T., Van Dyke, T., Wetmore, C., Chiu, I.M., Giovannini, M., Guha, A., Higgins, R.J., Marino, S., Radovanovic, I., Reilly, K., & Aldape, K. (2002) Neuropathology of genetically engineered mice: consensus report and recommendations from an international forum. *Oncogene* 21:7453–7463.

Lymphoid and Nonlymphoid Hematopoietic Neoplasia

Frederickson, T.N. & Harris, A.W. (2000) *Atlas of Mouse Hematopathology*. Harwood Academic, Amsterdam.

Fredrickson, T.N., Lennert, K., Chattopadhyay, S.K., Morse, H.C., 3rd, & Hartley, J.W. (1999) Splenic marginal zone lymphomas of mice. *American Journal of Pathology* 154:805–812.

Frith, C.H. (1985) *A Color Atlas of Hematopoietic Pathology of Mice*. Toxicology Pathology Associates, Little Rock, AR.

Hao, X., Fredrickson, T.N., Chattopadhyay, S.K., Han, W., Qi, C.F., Wang, Z., Ward, J.M., Hartley, J.W., & Morse, H.C., III (2010) The histopathologic and molecular basis for the diagnosis of histiocytic sarcoma and histiocyte-associated lymphoma in mice. *Veterinary Pathology* 47:434–445.

Hori, M., Xiang, S., Qi, C.F., Chattopadhyay, S.K., Fredrickson, T.N., Hartley, J.W., Kovalchuk, A.L., Bornkamm, G.W., Janz, S., Copeland, N.G., Jenkins, N.A., Ward, J.M., & Morse, H.C., 3rd (2001) Non-Hodgkin lymphomas of mice. *Blood Cells, Molecules and Diseases* 27:217–222.

Kogan, S.C., Ward, J.M., Anver, M.R., Berman, J.J., Brayton, C., Cardiff, R.D., Carter, J.S., de Coronado, S., Downing, J.R., Fredrickson, T.N., Haines, D.C., Harris, A.W., Harris, N.L., Hiai, H., Jaffe, E.S., MacLennan, I.C., Pandolfi, P.P., Pattengale, P.K., Perkins, A.S., Simpson, R.M., Tuttle, M.S., Wong, J.F., & Morse, H.C., 3rd (2002) Bethesda proposals for classification of non-lymphoid hematopoeitic neoplasms in mice. *Blood* 100:238–245.

Morse H.C., 3rd, Anver, M.R., Fredrickson, T.N., Haines, D.C., Harris, A.W., Harris, N.L., Jaffe, E.S., Kogan, S.C., MacLennan, I.C., Pattengale, P.K., & Ward, J.M. (2002) Bethesda proposals for classification of lymphoid neoplasms in mice. *Blood* 100:246–258.

Pattengale, P.K. & Frith, C.H. (1983) Immunomorphologic classification of spontaneous lymphoid cell neoplasms occurring in female BALB/c mice. *Journal of the National Cancer Institute* 70:169–179.

Taddesse-Heath, L., Chattopadhyay, S.K., Dillehay, D.L., Lander, M.R., Nagashfar, Z., Morse, H.C., 3rd, & Hartley, J.W. (2000) Lymphomas and high-level expression of murine leukemia viruses in CFW mice. *Journal of Virology* 74:6832–6837.

Ward, J.M. & Sheldon, W. (1993) Expression of mononuclear phagocyte antigens in histiocytic sarcoma of mice. *Veterinary Pathology* 30:560–565.

Ward, J.M. (2006) Lymphomas and leukemias in mice. *Experimental and Toxicologic Pathology* 57:377–381.

Mammary Neoplasia

Cardiff, R.D., Anver, M.R., Gusterson, B.A., Hennighausen, L., Jensen, R.A., Merino, M.J., Rehm, S., Russo, J., Tavassoli, F.A., Wakefield, L.M., Ward, J.M., & Green, J.E. (2000) The mammary pathology of genetically engineered mice: the consensus report and recommendations from the Annapolis meeting. *Oncogene* 19:968–988.

Dunn, T.B. (1953) Morphology of mammary tumors in mice. In: *The Pathophysiology of Cancer* (ed. F. Homburger;), pp. 38–84. Hoeber, New York.

Riley, V. (1975) Mouse mammary tumors: alteration of incidence as apparent function of stress. *Science* 189:465–467.

Sass, B. & Dunn, T.B. (1979) Classification of mouse mammary tumors in Dunn's miscellaneous group including recently reported types. *Journal of the National Cancer Institute* 62:1287–1293.

Pulmonary Neoplasia

Johnson, L., et al. (2001) Somatic activation of the K-ras oncogene causes early onset lung cancer in mice. *Nature (London)* 410:1111–1116.

Nitkin, A.Y., Alcaraz, A., Anver, M.R., Bronson, R.T., Cardiff, R.D., Dixon, D., Fraire, A.E., Gabrielson, E.W., Gunning, W.T., Haines, D.C., Kaufman, M.H., Linnoila, R.I., Maronpot, R.R., Rabson, A.S., Reddick, R.L., Rehm, S., Rozengurt, N., Schuller, H.M., Shmidt, E.N., Travis, W.D., Ward, J.M., & Jacks, T. (2004) Classification of proliferative pulmonary lesions of the mouse: Recommendations of the Mouse Models of Human Cancer Consortium. *Cancer Research* 64:2307–2316.

Pilling, A.M., Mifsud, N.A., Jones, S.A., Endersby-Wood, H.J., & Turton, J.A. (1999) Expression of surfactant protein mRNA in normal and neoplastic lung of B6C3F$_1$ mice as demonstrated by in situ hybridization. *Veterinary Pathology* 36:57–63.

Shmidt, E.N. & Nitkin, A.Y. (2004) Pathology of mouse models of human lung cancer. *Comparative Medicine* 54:23–26.

Hepatocellular Neoplasia

Becker, F.F. (1982) Morphological classification of mouse liver tumors based on biological characteristics. *Cancer Research* 42:3918–3923.

Frith, C.H. & Ward, J.M. (1980) A morphologic classification of proliferative and neoplastic hepatic lesions in mice. *Journal of Environmental Pathology and Toxicology* 3:329–351.

Frith, C.H. & Wiley, L. (1982) Spontaneous hepatocellular neoplasms and hepatic hemangiosarcomas in several strains of mice. *Laboratory Animal Science* 32:157–162.

Harderian Gland Neoplasia

Ihara, M., Tajima, M., Yamate, J., & Shibuya, K. (1994) Morphology of spontaneous Harderian gland tumors in aged B6C3F$_1$ mice. *Journal of Veterinary Medical Science* 56:775–778.

Myoepitheliomas

Sundberg, J.P., Hanson, C.A., Roop, D.R., Brown, K.S., & Bedigian, H.G. (1991) Myoepitheliomas in inbred laboratory mice. *Veterinary Pathology* 28:313–323.

Neoplasms of Mesenchymal Tissues

Booth, C.J. & Sundberg, J.P. (1995) Hemangiomas and hemangiosarcomas in inbred laboratory mice. *Laboratory Animal Science* 45:497–502.

Harvey, M., McArthur, M.J., Montgomery, C.A., Jr., Butel, J.S., Bradley, A., & Donehower, L.A. (1993) Spontaneous and carcinogen-induced carcinogenesis in p53-deficient mice. *Nature Genetics* 5:225–229.

Kavirayani, A.M. & Foreman, O. (2010) Retrospective study of spontaneous osteosarcomas in the nonobese diabetic and nonobese diabetic-derived substrains of mice. *Veterinary Pathology* 47:482–487.

Kavirayani, A.M., Sundberg, J.P., & Foreman, O. (2012) Primary neoplasms of bones in mice: retrospective study and review of the literature. *Veterinary Pathology* 49:182–205.

Mitchel, R.E.J., Jackson, J.S., Morrison, D.P., & Carlisle, S.M. (2003) Low doses of radiation increase the latency of spontaneous lymphomas and spinal osteosarcomas in cancer-prone, radiation-sensitive Trp53 heterozygous mice. *Radiation Research* 159:320–327.

Sher, R.B., Cox, G.A., Mills, K.D., & Sundberg, J.P. (2011) Rhabdomyosarcomas in aging A/J mice. *PLoS One* 6:e23498.

Sundberg, J.P., Adkison, D.L., & Bedigian, H.G. (1991) Skeletal muscle rhabdomyosarcomas in inbred laboratory mice. *Veterinary Pathology* 28:200–206.

Wilson, J.T., Hauser, R.E., & Ryffel, B. (1985) Osteomas in OF-1 mice: no alteration in biologic behavior during long-term treatment with cyclosporine. *Journal of the National Cancer Institute* 75:897–903.

Teratomas

Blackshear, P., Mahler, J., Bennett, L.M., McAllister, K.A., Forsythe, D., & Davis, B.J. (1999) Extragonadal teratocarcinoma in chimeric mice. *Veterinary Pathology* 36:457–460.

Hardy, K.P., Carthew, P., Handyside, A.H., & Hooper, M.L. (1990) Extragonadal teratocarcinoma derived from embryonal stem cells in chimaeric mice. *Journal of Pathology* 160:71–76.

Jiang, L.I. & Nadeau, J.H. (2001) 129/Sv mice: a model system for studying germ cell biology and testicular cancer. *Mammalian Genome* 12:89–94.

Stevens, L.C. (1973) A new inbred subline of mice (129-terSV) with a high incidence of spontaneous congenital teratomas. *Journal of the National Cancer Institute* 50:235–242.

2 Rat

INTRODUCTION

There are well over 100 species categorized in the genus *Rattus*. However, rats used in research laboratories today evolved from the Brown Norway (BN) rat, *Rattus norvegicus*. This species originated in central Asia, and disseminated worldwide relatively recently within the last 200 years. Early in the 19th century, "rat baiting" was a popular spectator sport in Western Europe. Albino rats were occasionally trapped during the acquisition of live rats for this "sport" and selectively bred as pets or show animals. They are considered to be a primary source of the laboratory rat stocks for use in research laboratories today. The Brown Norway rat appears to be the first mammalian species to be domesticated primarily for scientific purposes. Fancy rats coevolved during this time. Laboratory rats are represented by fewer numbers of outbred stocks and inbred strains than laboratory mice. Small numbers of transgenic rats now exist, and it is likely that transgenic rats will become more prevalent, but never to the degree of mice. The genetic background of rats is as important a consideration as in mice for expression of disease. Rats are subject to infection with fewer viruses than mice but seem to make up for this with more clinically significant bacterial infections.

Wild rats tend to live in association with human environments. They live in social hierarchies consisting of a dominant male with a number of females and younger or submissive males. Intraspecies communication is complex, utilizing olfaction, pheromones, ultrasonic vocalizations, and tactile cues. Wild rats inhabit complex burrow systems, usually near water, with chambers for nesting and food storage. Domesticated rats are remarkably more docile than their wild counterparts, but aggressiveness varies among stocks and strains of laboratory rats. Brown Norway and F344 rats tend to be more aggressive than outbred stocks.

ANATOMIC FEATURES

Hematology

The predominant peripheral blood leukocyte in rats is the lymphocyte, which makes up approximately 80% of the cell population. Nuclear ring forms are common among granulocytes in tissues, as in the mouse. Eosinophils tend to possess annular, ring-shaped nuclei without lobation. Basophils are rare. Mature male rats have higher total leukocyte counts than do females, in both lymphocytes and granulocytes. Splenic hematopoiesis occurs in the adult rat, but not to the extent seen in mice. Prominent hematopoietic activity usually denotes an underlying disease state. In pathogen-free rats, splenic hematopoiesis is minimal, with only a few megakaryocytes present.

Lymphoreticular System

The rat thymus remains prominent into young adulthood and involutes thereafter. Occasionally, the thymus has involuted to the point where it is no longer identifiable by as early as 1 year of age, particularly in males. Hemosiderin progressively accumulates in splenic macrophages throughout life, particularly in breeding females. Splenic white pulp has a prominent marginal zone, compared to mice (Fig. 2.1). Rats lack tonsillar lymphoid tissue.

Respiratory System

The rat is anatomically similar to the mouse. Rats possess serous cells in respiratory epithelium, which are unique to this species.

Gastrointestinal System

The rat is anatomically similar to the mouse. As in mice, salivary gland sexual dimorphism also occurs in rats. Intestinal Paneth cells have smaller granules than in

Pathology of Laboratory Rodents and Rabbits, Fourth Edition. Stephen W. Barthold, Stephen M. Griffey, and Dean H. Percy.
© 2016 John Wiley & Sons, Inc. Published 2016 by John Wiley & Sons, Inc.

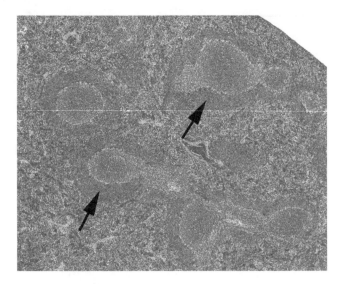

FIG. 2.1. *Splenic white pulp of a rat, depicting the prominent marginal zone in normal rats (arrows).*

mice. Unlike mice, the rat liver is consistently lobated into 4 major lobes and lacks a gall bladder. Hepatocytes in the rat are more uniform in size than in the mouse. However, polyploidy is a common morphological feature in adult animals, and the number of binucleate cells increases with age. Bile is not concentrated. Foci of "altered hepatocytes" are well documented in this species. They are generally of more concern to pathologists working in the pharmaceutical industry than to pathologists in the diagnostic laboratory. Focal hepatitis with mononuclear cell infiltration in the absence of an identifiable infectious agent occasionally occurs as an incidental finding in laboratory rats. The liver may also reflect general disease states. Atrophy of hepatic cords is a common manifestation of reduced (or absence of) food intake (Fig. 2.2). Atrophy of hepatic cords has been

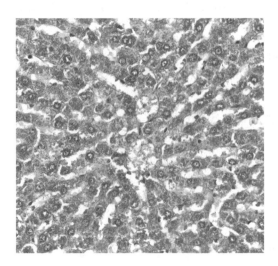

FIG. 2.2. *Liver from an adult rat with atrophy of hepatic cords. The reduction in hepatocellular cytoplasmic volume is consistent with reduced food intake and is often seen in disease states.*

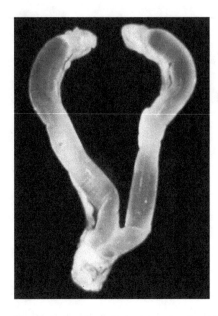

FIG. 2.3. *Uterus of a female rat during proestrus, in which the uterine horns are filled with clear fluid.*

observed in adult male and female rats following fasting periods as short as 18 hours. The rat pancreas is diffuse.

Urogenital System

The male and female rat reproductive organs are basically similar to those of the mouse. Adult female rats develop cyclic uterine infiltrates of eosinophils in response to estrogen, which can be misconstrued as abnormal. During proestrus, the uterus is filled with clear fluid (Fig. 2.3), which is normal. Rats have 3 pairs of pectoral and 3 pairs of inguinal mammary glands. As in the mouse, mammary tissue extends throughout much of the subcutis of the sides and necks of rats. Proteinuria is normal in rats, due to tubular production of alpha globulins. Proteinuria due to loss of serum proteins is not normal (see "Chronic Progressive Nephropathy").

Skeletal System

As in mice and hamsters, bones lack Haversian systems. Adult rats, particularly males of some strains, continue to grow, and physeal ossification is not complete until after 1 year of age. Hematopoiesis remains active in long bones throughout life.

Other Anatomic Features

Adrenals of wild rats are remarkably larger than that of their domesticated cousins. Adrenals of females are larger than those of males. Rats are endowed with prominent brown fat, as in mice. The exorbital lacrimal glands of rats display striking epithelial megalokarya and polykarya, particularly in older males (Fig. 2.4). This increases with age and should not be confused

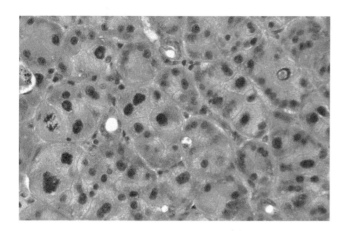

FIG. 2.4. *Exorbital gland from a mature male rat. Note the megalokarya and polykarya of acinar epithelial cells, a normal finding, particularly in old males.*

with a disease state. The fur of male albino rats tends to yellow with age.

BIBLIOGRAPHY FOR BEHAVIORAL AND ANATOMIC FEATURES

Car, B.D., Eng, V.M., Everds, N., & Bounous, D.I. (2005) Clinical pathology of the rat. In: *The Laboratory Rat*, 2nd edn (eds. M.A. Suckow, S.H. Weisbroth, & C.L. Franklin), pp. 127–146. Academic Press, New York.

Casteleyn, C., Breugelmans, S., Simoens, P., & Van den Broeck, W. (2011) The tonsils revisited: review of the anatomical localization and histological characteristics of the tonsils of domestic and laboratory animals. *Clinical and Developmental Immunology* ePub 2011:472460.

Cesta, M.F. (2006) Normal structure, function, and histology of the spleen. *Toxicologic Pathology* 34:455–465.

Gaertner, D.J., Lindsey, J.R., & Stevens, J.O. (1988) Cytomegalic changes and "inclusions" in lacrimal glands of laboratory rats. *Laboratory Animal Science* 38:79–82.

Greene, E.C. (1970) *Anatomy of the Rat.* Hafner Publishing Company, New York.

Kuper, C.F., Beems, R.B., & Hollanders, V.M. (1986) Spontaneous pathology of the thymus in aging Wistar (Cpb:WU) rats. *Veterinary Pathology* 23:270–277.

Richter, C.P. (1954) The effects of domestication and selection on the behavior of the Norway rat. *Journal of the National Cancer Institute* 15:727–728.

Sanderson, J.H. & Phillips, C.E. (1981) *An Atlas of Laboratory Animal Haematology.* Clarendon, Oxford.

Turner, P.V., Albassam, M.A., & Walker, R.M. (2001) The effects of overnight fasting, feeding, or sucrose supplementation prior to necropsy in rats. *Contemporary Topics in Laboratory Animal Science* 40:36–40.

GENERAL REFERENCES ON DISEASES OF RATS

The following references have been extensively used throughout this chapter as sources of information. Many of these citations have multiple contributors, but for the sake of space, individual contributors within review books are not cited. Various sections of this chapter refer back to these basic general references, rather than repeat them for each section.

Boorman, G.A., Eustis, S.L., Elwell, M.R., Montgomery, C.A., Jr., & MacKenzie, W.F. (1990) *Pathology of the Fischer Rat.* Academic Press, New York.

Burek, J.D. (1978) *Pathology of Aging Rats.* CRC Press, Boca Raton, FL.

Hard, G.C., Alden, C.L., Bruner, R.H., Frith, C.H., Owen, R.A., Krieg, K., & Durchfield-Meyer, B. (1999) Non-proliferative lesions of the kidney and lower urinary tract in rats. *Guides for Toxicologic Pathology.* STP/ARP/AFIP, Washington, DC.

Jones, T.C., Capen, C.C., & Mohr, U. (1996) *Respiratory System,* Monographs on Pathology of Laboratory Animals, 2nd edn. Springer, New York.

Jones, T.C., Capen, C.C., & Mohr, U. (1996) *Endocrine System,* Monographs on Pathology of Laboratory Animals, 2nd edn. Springer, New York.

Jones, T.C., Hard, G.C., & Mohr, U. (1998) *Urinary System,* Monographs on Pathology of Laboratory Animals, 2nd edn. Springer, New York.

Jones, T.C., Mohr, U., & Hunt, R.E. (1988) *Nervous System,* Monographs on Pathology of Laboratory Animals, 2nd edn. Springer, New York.

Jones, T.C., Mohr, U., & Popp, J.A. (1997) *Hemopoietic System,* Monographs on Pathology of Laboratory Animals, 2nd edn. Springer, New York.

Jones, T.C., Popp, J.A., & Mohr, U. (1997) *Digestive System,* Monographs on Pathology of Laboratory Animals, 2nd edn. Springer, New York.

Kohn, D.F. & Clifford, C.B. (2007) Biology and diseases of rats. In: *Laboratory Animal Medicine,* 2nd edn (eds. J.G. Fox, L.C. Anderson, F.M. Loew, & F.W. Quimby), pp. 121–165. Academic Press, New York.

Krinke, G.J. (2000) *The Laboratory Rat,* Handbook of Experimental Animals. Academic Press, New York.

Mohr, U. (2001) *International Classification of Rodent Tumors: The Mouse.* Springer, Berlin.

Mohr, U., Dungworth, D.L., & Capen, C.C. (1992) *Pathobiology of the Aging Rat,* Vols. 1 and 2. International Life Sciences Institute Press, Washington, DC.

Renne, R., Brix, A., Harkema, J., Herbert, R., Kittel, B., Lewis, D., March, T., Nagano, K., Pino, M., Rittinghausen, S., Rosenbruch, M., Tellier, P., & Wohrmann, T. (2009) Proliferative and nonproliferative lesions of the rat and mouse respiratory tract. *Toxicologic Pathology* 37:5S–73S.

Suckow, M.A., Weisbroth, S.H., & Franklin, C.L. (2005) *The Laboratory Rat,* 2nd edn. Academic Press, New York.

Suttie, A.W., Leininger, J.R., & Bradley, A.E. (2014) *Boorman's Pathology of the Laboratory Rat,* 2nd edn. Academic Press, New York.

Thoolen, B., Maronpot, R.R., Harada, T., Nyska, A., Rousseaux, C., Nolte, T., Malarkey, D.E., Kaufman, W., Kuttler, K., Deschl, U., Nakae, D., Gregson, R., Vinlove, M.P., Brix, A.E., Singh, B., Belpoggi, F., & Ward, J.W. (2010) Proliferative and nonproliferative lesions of the rat and mouse hepatobiliary system. *Toxicolic Pathology* 38:5S–81S.

DNA VIRAL INFECTIONS

Rat Adenovirus Infection

Disease due to adenovirus in rats is absent, but lesions, consisting of intranuclear inclusions within small intestinal enterocytes, represent incidental findings (Fig. 2.5). Intranuclear inclusions have been induced by treatment of rats with chemotherapeutic agents, presumably activating subliminal infection. Attempts to isolate the rat adenovirus have failed.

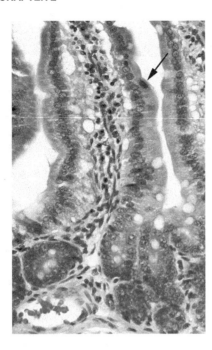

FIG. 2.5. *Small intestine from a rat, illustrating an adenoviral intranuclear inclusion body (arrow) in villus epithelium. Enteric adenoviral inclusions are typically located in nuclei of enterocytes that have lost their basal polarity.*

Serological surveys indicate that rats commonly seroconvert to mouse adenovirus MAdV-2. Rats could not be infected with mouse adenoviruses MAdV-1 or MAdV-2, suggesting that rats are naturally infected with serologically related but rat-specific adenovirus(es).

Rat Cytomegalovirus Infection

Rats are host to their own rat-specific cytomegalovirus (RCMV). Based upon presence of lesions in salivary glands, RCMV is common among wild rats, but appears to be nonexistent in laboratory rats. RCMV infects the salivary and lacrimal glands, causing cytomegaly with both intracytoplasmic and intranuclear inclusions in ductal epithelium, with nonsuppurative interstitial inflammation. Intracerebral inoculation of suckling rats with RCMV will produce nonsuppurative encephalitis with karyomegaly, intranuclear and intracytoplasmic inclusion bodies in neural tissue, and polykaryocyte formation. Serological tests are available but not generally applied because of their rarity in laboratory rat populations.

Rat Papillomavirus Infection

Papilloma viruses have not been associated with lesions in rats, but 2 papillomaviruses, rat papilloma virus-1 (RnPV1) and rat papillomavirus-2 (RnPV-2) have been amplified and sequenced from the oral cavity, rectal mucosa, and facial hairs of wild Norway rats in Europe. RnPV-1 belongs to the *Pipa-papillomavirus* genus, and RnPv-2 belongs to the *Iota-papillomavirus* genus. The existence of these 2 distantly related papillomaviruses in subclinically infected wild rats suggests that such infections may be widespread among rats, and it remains to be determined if laboratory rats carry papillomaviruses. The recent observation of an outbreak of viral papillomas among laboratory athymic nude mice due to an unrelated mouse papillomavirus (see Mouse Chapter 1, "Papillomavirus infections") underscores the concept that not all viral infections of laboratory rodents have been discovered and the growing use of immunodeficient rodents may contribute to future discoveries.

Rat Polyomavirus Infection

Rat polyomavirus (Rat-PyV), serologically distinct from polyoma and K viruses of mice, can infect rats, but its prevalence is unknown. Rat-PyV initially became apparent in a colony of Rowett (athymic) nude (*rnu*) rats, in which 10–15% developed a wasting disease, dyspnea with pneumonia and parotid sialadenitis. Intranuclear inclusions were present in duct epithelium and, to a lesser extent, acini of parotid glands, and lungs. Euthymic rats did not develop the disease. Viral antigen was found in salivary glands, larynx, and, less often, bronchiolar epithelium and kidney. Since the virus has not been isolated, serological screens of laboratory rat populations for this agent are not performed. Conspicuous intranuclear inclusions can be seen in salivary gland epithelium (Fig. 2.6), bronchiolar epithelium, and alveolar lining cells, resulting in interstitial pneumonia and weight loss. Other organs appear to be histologically normal. This infection has periodically arisen on multiple occasions among *rnu* rats.

Parvovirus Infections

Laboratory rats are naturally susceptible to 4 serotypes of parvovirus: rat virus (RV, or Kilham's rat virus), H-1 virus (or Toolan's H-1 virus), rat parvovirus (RPV), and rat minute virus (RMV). RV, H-1, and RMV are antigenically and genetically closely related, whereas RPV is more disparate. Each group contains a number of isolates.

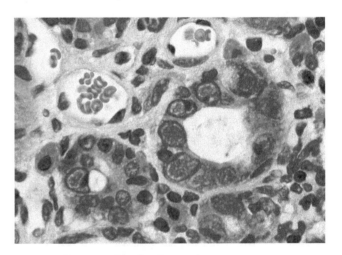

FIG. 2.6. *Submandibular salivary gland of a nude rat naturally infected with rat polyomavirus. Note the multiple prominent intranuclear inclusions with margination of nuclear chromatin.*

Epizootiology and Pathogenesis

Serological surveys indicate that subclinical infections with various rat parvoviruses are common among laboratory rats. Transmission appears to occur primarily by oronasal contact with infected animals, or by contaminated fomites. Virus shedding has been documented in urine, feces, and oropharynx. RV is recognized to be the most pathogenic of rat parvoviruses under both field and experimental conditions and may be the only strain that produces clinical disease under natural conditions. Transplacental transmission of RV has been demonstrated in pregnant rats inoculated orally with high doses of RV, resulting in infertility and fetal resorption. RV may persist in colonies for long periods of time. Rats born to seropositive dams receive maternal antibodies during the neonatal period and usually acquire RV at 2–7 months of age. Virus may also be shed in the milk during lactation. In seronegative 2-day-old suckling rats inoculated oronasally with RV, inoculated animals were able to transmit virus for up to 10 weeks, and for at least 7 weeks after seroconversion had occurred. Rats inoculated as juveniles shed RV for at least 3 weeks postinoculation. Virus may be reactivated by immunosuppression, resulting in acute systemic disease. Although persistence can theoretically occur in individual rats, persistence of parvovirus infections in colonies of rats is dependent on the continuous availability of new susceptible animals to permit propagation of the virus. The widespread distribution of parvoviruses and their requirements for dividing cells for replication results in the frequent contamination of tumor cell lines and tumor virus stocks that have been passaged in laboratory rats.

In experimentally induced infections in newborn rats, target tissues for RV replication include primordial cells of the cerebellar cortex, periventricular region, hepatocytes, endothelial cells, and bone marrow. Other target organs include kidney, lung, and genital tract. The multiple hemorrhages seen in the experimental and naturally occurring disease are attributed to the endothelial cell and megakaryocyte damage associated with viral replication in these tissues. Intestinal mucosal lesions, which are so prominent in feline and canine parvoviral infections, do not occur in rats, which may be due to a lack of viral receptors on enterocytes. Documented descriptions of spontaneous outbreaks of parvovirus disease in rats are rare. In 1 report, juvenile rats were clinically affected. Clinical signs included dyspnea, ruffled hair coat, muscular weakness, and cyanotic scrotums. In this outbreak, rats seroconverted to RV, and later to H-1, suggesting that H-1 may have potentiated the development of the disease. Naturally occurring disease has not been attributed to H-1 viruses or RPVs. Experimental studies indicate that both of these types of parvovirus are also prone to persistence, and RPV has a strong tropism for lymphoid tissue, which may cause immunomodulation in experimental studies.

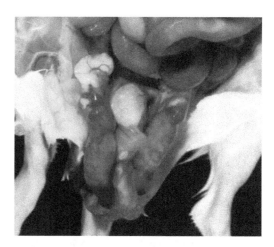

FIG. 2.7. *Rat virus (RV) infection in a young rat. Note the acute hemorrhage and fibrinous exudation in the peritesticular region. (Source: Coleman, et al. 1983. Reproduced with permission from SAGE Publications.)*

Pathology

In the adult form of RV disease, there is congestion of lymph nodes, loss of body fat, and scrotal hemorrhage, with peri-testicular fibrinous exudation (Fig. 2.7). Splenomegaly, icterus, and ascites are variable findings. Microscopic changes may be present in the brain, liver, and testes. Disseminated foci of hemorrhage occur in the cerebrum and cerebellum in a random distribution involving gray and white matter with malacia and obliteration of the normal architecture (Fig. 2.8). In the testes and epididymis, there may be multifocal coagulation necrosis and hemorrhage consistent with infarction, with thrombosis of regional vessels. Focal hepatocellular necrosis may occur, and amphophilic, intranuclear inclusions may be present in hepatocytes (Fig. 2.9), endothelial cells, and bile duct

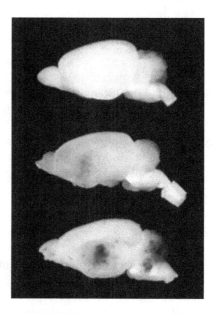

FIG. 2.8. *Brains of juvenile rats experimentally infected with RV, depicting hemorrhagic encephalopathy. (Source: R.O. Jacoby. Yale University, New Haven, CT. Reproduced with permission from R.O. Jacoby.)*

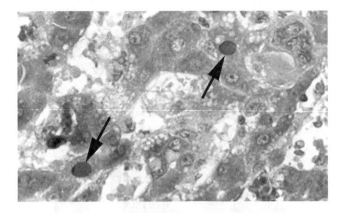

FIG. 2.9. *Liver from a juvenile rat with RV infection, illustrating intranuclear inclusions (arrows) in hepatocytes. (Source: R.O. Jacoby. Yale University, New Haven, CT. Reproduced with permission from R.O. Jacoby.)*

epithelium. Neonatal or infant rats can develop granulo-prival cerebellar hypoplasia, hepatitis, and jaundice. Lesions present in recovered rats may include focal angiectasis (peliosis hepatis), and nodular hyperplasia with portal scarring. Infertility, fetal resorption, and abortion may occur in pregnant females.

Diagnosis

The provisional diagnosis, based on the presence of typical lesions and inclusions, can be confirmed by the demonstration of viral antigen by immunohistochemistry or detection of DNA by PCR. Seroconversion may be detected by various procedures, but contemporary methods now utilize recombinant VP2 and NS1 antigens. VP antigens reflect virus strain specificity, whereas NS antigens are highly conserved and cross-reactive among all of the rat (and mouse) parvoviruses. RPV does not share homologous cross-reacting structural VP antigens with RV, H-1, or MVR, but possesses conserved cross-reacting NS nonstructural antigens. Likewise, PCR assays may target either NS1 or VP2 gene sequences. PCR has been used to detect rodent parvoviruses in contaminated biomaterials, mesenteric lymph node, spleen, feces, and environmental surfaces. Differential diagnoses include bacterial septicemias, chronic wasting due to agents such as *Mycoplasma pulmonis*, and trauma. Infertility and fetal resorption must be differentiated from conditions such as nutritional disorders, disruption of normal light cycles, and mycoplasmal infections.

Cowpox Virus Infection

Cowpox virus (CPXV), despite its name, is enzootic among wild rodents in Europe and Eurasia, but is infectious for humans, cattle, felids, and other hosts, including rats. Human exposure is most often contracted through infected cats, but recently, a number of human cases have arisen through contact with pet rats in Europe. Natural infection of laboratory rats with CPXV, which at the time was termed Turkmenia rodent poxvirus, was reported in the former Soviet Union in the

late 1970s. Clinical signs in rats were similar to ectromelia virus in mice, and ranged from inapparent infections, dermal pox, and tail amputation to an acute pulmonary form with high mortality. There have been multiple documented reports of transmission of CPXV from rats to human and nonhuman primates. CPXV is an *Orthopoxvirus* that is genetically related to variola, vaccinia, and monkeypox viruses.

Pathology

Experimental infection of laboratory rats demonstrated that intradermal or contact inoculation with CPXV generally resulted in mild dermal manifestations, characterized as vesiculopustular dermatitis. Intranasal inoculation resulted in severe dyspnea with peracute mortality. Histopathology revealed focal necrotizing lesions in respiratory mucosa with large eosinophilic intracytoplasmic inclusion bodies (Guarnieri bodies), bronchointerstitial pneumonia, pulmonary congestion and edema, and lymphoid necrosis. Intradermally inoculated rats also developed necrotizing rhinitis, laryngitis, and bronchointerstitial pneumonia. Dermal lesions were typically proliferative and necrotizing, involving limbs (Fig. 2.10), nose, lips, tongue, and inguinal skin with intracytoplasmic inclusions within epithelium (Fig. 2.11).

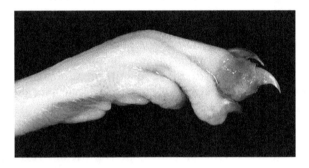

FIG. 2.10. *Digit of a rat with cowpox virus lesion. (Source: Briethaupt et al. 2012. Reproduced with permission from SAGE Publications.)*

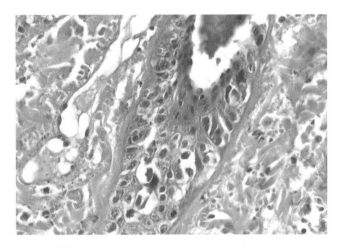

FIG. 2.11. *Skin from a rat infected with cowpox virus. Note the many intracytoplasmic inclusions in the follicular epithelium. (Source: Briethaupt et al. 2012. Reproduced with permission from SAGE Publications.)*

Diagnosis

Definitive diagnosis can be achieved by identification of typical pox viral inclusion bodies within lesions, immunohistochemistry, or PCR. Human exposure to infected rats is most often associated with skin lesions on the patient's neck. Severe flu-like illness may also be present. Serology, using ectromelia virus as antigen, may be used for surveillance in laboratory rat populations.

RNA VIRAL INFECTIONS

Rat Coronavirus Infection: Sialodacryoadenitis

Based upon past serological surveys, antibodies to rat coronaviruses were relatively common in both laboratory and wild rats, and outbreaks continue to occur sporadically in laboratory and pet rats. The 2 naturally occurring prototype coronaviruses isolated from this species are Parker's rat coronavirus (PRC) and sialodacryoadenitis virus (SDAV). SDAV is a morphological term, and represents any and all subsequent coronavirus isolates that produce necrotizing inflammation of salivary and lacrimal glands (sialodacryoadenitis). PRC was first isolated from the lungs of rats. Intranasal inoculation of newborn and weanling rats with PRC produced rhinitis, tracheitis, and interstitial pneumonia, with focal atelectasis and high mortality in infants. PRC also induces salivary and lacrimal gland lesions, but these were overlooked in the original descriptions. SDAV isolates produce lacrimal and salivary gland lesions, but also produce pulmonary disease in young rats. These viruses should be considered part of a single biological grouping (rat coronaviruses). Nevertheless, this dichotomy and terminology continues because of historical precedent. Like mouse hepatitis virus (MHV), the rat coronavirus group is likely to contain numerous, constantly changing strains that vary in virulence.

SDA is a disease of high morbidity and negligible mortality. Permanent ocular damage may occur in a small percentage of rats. Transient respiratory tract damage and hypersecretion may result in unexpected deaths in rats anesthetized during the acute stages of SDA. There is evidence that the virus has a significant additive effect in rats previously infected with *M. pulmonis*, and possibly the cilia-associated respiratory (CAR) bacillus. Behavioral changes and reproductive disorders including aberrations of the estrous cycle and neonatal mortality have also been associated with epizootics of the disease. Active infection has also been found to precipitate graft-versus-host disease in the salivary and lacrimal glands of rats with allogenic bone marrow grafts.

Epizootiology and Pathogenesis

Transmission is primarily through nasal secretions or saliva, and the virus spreads rapidly following introduction into a susceptible population of rats. In epizootics, there can be subclinical to high morbidity with virtually no mortality. Typical clinical signs associated with SDAV infection during the acute stages of the disease include sniffling, epiphora, blepharospasm, and cervical swelling. Dark red encrustations may be present around the eyes and external nares. These porphyrin-containing substances are released from damaged Harderian glands and emit a characteristic pink fluorescence under an ultraviolet light source. Other complications sometimes seen during the convalescent period include unilateral or bilateral ocular lesions. Reproductive disorders, including neonatal mortality and aberrations in the estrous cycle, have also been associated with SDAV. Prior exposure to the SDAV provides protection against the development of the disease upon reinfection for up to 15 months.

Pathology

Acutely infected rats may display excessive lacrimation or have red encrustations around the external nares and eyelids. Reflection of the skin of the ventral neck may reveal subcutaneous, periglandular, and interlobular edema of the parotid and/or the submandibular (submaxillary) salivary glands. In contrast to normal glands, affected glands are enlarged and blanched, with periglandular edema (Fig. 2.12). Similar changes are frequently evident in the Harderian, exorbital, and infraorbital lacrimal glands. Harderian glands often have blotchy brown pigmentation. During the acute stage of the disease, affected parotid and submandibular salivary glands and lacrimal glands have coagulation necrosis of the ductal epithelium, variable involvement of adjacent acini, with effacement of the normal architecture. Interstitial edema, with mononuclear and polymorphonuclear cell infiltration, frequently occurs (Figs. 2.13 and 2.14). During the reparative stages of the disease, beginning at 7–10 d postexposure, there is nonkeratinizing squamous metaplasia of ductal and acinar structures of salivary (Fig. 2.15) and lacrimal glands, with reactive hyperplasia of cervical lymph nodes. Cellular infiltrates in affected glands at this stage are primarily lymphocytes, plasma cells, mast cells, and

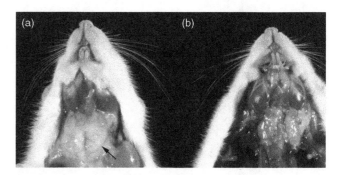

FIG. 2.12. *Sialodacryoadenitis virus (SDAV) infection of a rat during the acute stage of the disease. The submandibular salivary glands of the affected rat (a) are blanched and swollen (arrow), with periglandular edema, compared to an unaffected rat (b).*

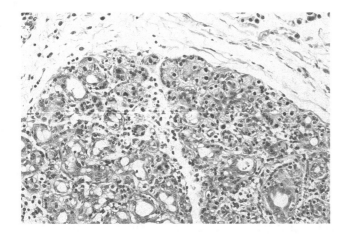

FIG. 2.13. *Submandibular salivary gland from a rat during acute SDAV infection. Note the epithelial necrosis, leukocytic infiltration, and interlobular and periglandular edema.*

macrophages. Squamous metaplasia is evident in salivary and lacrimal glands, and may be particularly marked in the Harderian glands (Fig. 2.16). In salivary glands, regeneration of acinar and ductal epithelial cells is usually complete by 3–4 weeks postexposure. There may be isolated ducts or acini lined by poorly differentiated epithelial cells, with scattered aggregations of mononuclear cells, including mast cells, but usually the salivary glands are essentially normal histologically at this stage. Focal residual inflammatory lesions associated with interstitial deposition of pigmented material may persist in the Harderian glands for several weeks. Ocular changes are secondary to impaired lacrimal gland function, resulting in keratitis sicca, impaired intraocular drainage, hyphema, and megaloglobus (Fig. 2.17), with subsequent permanent damage to the eye.

Necrotizing rhinitis, with mononuclear and polymorphonuclear cell infiltration, occurs during the acute stages of the disease. Both respiratory and olfactory

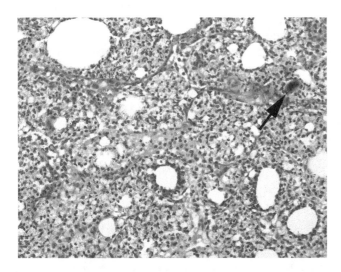

FIG. 2.14. *Harderian gland from a rat during acute SDAV infection. There is necrosis of glandular epithelium. Note the inspissated brown porphyrin pigment (arrow).*

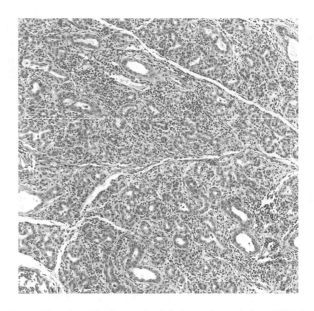

FIG. 2.15. *Parotid salivary gland during early resolution of SDAV infection. Ducts and acini are lined by undifferentiated hyperplastic epithelium and the interstitium is infiltrated with mononuclear leukocytes.*

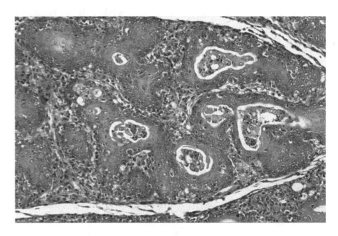

FIG. 2.16. *Harderian gland from a rat during recovery from SDAV infection. There is marked squamous metaplasia of ducts and acini.*

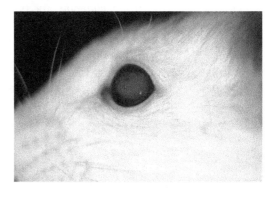

FIG. 2.17. *Megaloglobus with hyphema as a sequel of SDAV infection.*

epithelia are affected. The majority of the repair is complete by 14 days postexposure, although residual lesions may persist longer in specialized areas such as the vomeronasal organ. In the lower respiratory tract, there is transient tracheitis, and focal bronchitis and bronchiolitis, with leukocytic infiltration, hyperplasia of respiratory epithelial cells, and flattening and loss of ciliated cells. Focal alveolitis, when present, is characterized by hypercellularity of alveolar walls and mobilization of alveolar macrophages. Lesions in the lower respiratory tract are transient and usually have disappeared by 8–10 days postexposure.

Athymic nude rats are particularly susceptible to SDAV and develop chronic persistent infections and wasting disease. Chronic suppurative rhinitis, bronchopneumonia, and chronic inflammatory lesions in the salivary and lacrimal glands have been described. Viral antigen was evident in affected tissues, including epithelium of the urinary tract.

Diagnosis

The presence of the typical lesions of the salivary and lacrimal glands confirmed on microscopic examination is sufficient to make the diagnosis. Viral antigen may be present in the respiratory tract and affected salivary and lacrimal glands at 4–6 days postexposure, and PCR has been used for definitive diagnosis. Virus isolation is not a practical procedure in most circumstances. Serological testing is the recommended method to confirm prior exposure to SDAV. Differential diagnoses include nasal and ocular discharge associated with mycoplasma, Sendai virus, or pneumonia virus of mice (PVM) infections; subcutaneous edema of the head associated with *Pseudomonas aeruginosa*; ocular and nasal irritation associated with high environmental ammonia levels; and stress-associated chromodacryorrhea. The presence of porphyrin-containing red encrustations around the eyes and nose (chromodacryorrhea) are often present, but not diagnostic for SDA. Chronic disease states (e.g., chronic respiratory disease (CRD)) and stress-associated events may also result in the release of porphyrins from the Harderian glands.

Hantavirus Infection

Hantaviruses are significant zoonotic pathogens of laboratory rodents with potentially serious consequences for humans. Rats are susceptible to infection with hantaviruses, and thereby pose a zoonotic hazard to human contacts. The genus *Hantavirus* belongs to the family Bunyaviridae and contains at least 14 rodent-borne viruses. Members of this genus are spread by aerosol and contact, in contrast to other bunyaviruses, which are arthropod-borne. Phylogenetic trees comparing nucleotide sequences show 2 major lineages of hantaviruses. One represents viruses associated with hemorrhagic fever and renal syndrome (HFRS) in humans, and the other represents widespread viruses of the New World that are associated with hantavirus pulmonary syndrome (HPS) in humans. It is now apparent that hantaviruses originally evolved in the Old World; they then spread through rodents to the New World across the Bering land bridge. Humans are incidental hosts.

Hantaviruses have caused several laboratory rat-associated outbreaks of HFRS in Asia and Europe, and these have been traced to infected rats from breeders, wild rodents, and experimentally infected rodents, as well as immunocytomas grown in laboratory rats. The ubiquity of these viruses in wild rodents of North America, including *R. norvegicus*, dictates constant awareness of the hazard.

Epizootiology and Pathogenesis

Rats (*R. norvegicus* and *Rattus rattus*), several *Peromyscus* spp., and other rodents and insectivores are natural hosts for a variety of hantaviruses. In the rat, Hantaan virus and Seoul virus (members of the HFRS group) produce no clinical evidence of disease. In experimentally inoculated animals, viremia and virus shedding may occur in the saliva and urine, and intracage transmission may occur up to 2 months postinoculation. Bite wounds have also been proposed as a major means of intraspecies transmission. There is no evidence of transplacental transmission. Experimental infection of laboratory rats with Seoul virus has demonstrated subclinical, multisystemic persistent infection, with viral RNA within skin (vessels, panniculus carnosis, and epidermis), liver, lung, salivary gland, pancreas, kidney, and brain. Virus has a strong tropism for vascular smooth muscle and endothelium. The source of the virus in human infections is considered to be through contact with infected rodents and their urine. In human cases of HFRS, clinical symptoms include fever, thrombocytopenia, and capillary leakage resulting in myalgia, headache, and petechiation, with prominent retroperitoneal and renal hemorrhage. Humans infected with HPS develop fever and capillary leakage that is localized to the lungs. Death occurs from shock and cardiac complications.

Diagnosis

Serologic assays are available and should be used as part of routine safety precautions in laboratory animal programs using wild rodents or laboratory rats. Because of the high degree of genetic diversity among hantavirus isolates, PCR is not a practical approach to diagnosis.

Paramyxovirus Infections

Members of the family Paramyxoviridae, which infect rats, include members of the subfamily Paramyxovirinae: murine parainfluenza virus-1 (Sendai virus) and human parainfluenza virus-3 (PIV-3); and 1 member of the subfamily Pneumovirinae: PVM.

Sendai virus and PIV-3 are antigenically cross-reactive.

Sendai Virus Infection

Sendai virus (murine parainfluenza virus-1) is recognized to cause respiratory diseases in the laboratory mouse, rat, and hamster, and seroconversion also occurs in guinea pigs. Decades ago, Sendai virus was a common and significant pathogen in laboratory animal facilities. Although Sendai virus appears to have disappeared, it continues to be on the exclusion list for serologic surveillance for laboratory rodent colonies. Sendai virus in the laboratory rat is recognized to have an additive effect on respiratory infections with *M. pulmonis*. Sendai virus infection may also impair the normal immune response and has been associated with impaired fetal development and neonatal mortality by indirect means. In enzootically infected colonies, there is a danger of transmission to other susceptible species, including mice, hamsters, and guinea pigs. Humans may be susceptible to infection, and may play a role in introduction of this virus into rodent colonies.

Epizootiology and Pathogenesis

Although clinical disease and lesions of the respiratory tract are rarely attributed to Sendai virus infection in the rat, serological surveys from the past indicate that the virus was once relatively widespread in colonies of rats. Transmission occurs by direct contact or by aerosols. Following exposure, the virus replicates in the upper respiratory tract, and then extends down the trachea and smaller airways in a stepwise manner. Viral antigen is detectable from approximately 1–7 days. Virus has been recovered from the lung for up to 7 days postinoculation and for up to 12 days when inoculated in young rats. Serum antibody levels may be present for 7 or more months, dropping to low or undetectable levels by 9 months. The pathogenesis of Sendai virus infection in the rat is analogous to Sendai in genetically resistant strains of mice.

Pathology

In rats, necropsied during the acute stages of the disease, there is rhinitis, with focal to diffuse necrosis of respiratory epithelial cells. Leukocytic infiltrates consist of neutrophils, lymphocytes, and plasma cells. Residual lesions may persist in the nasal mucosa for 3 or more weeks. In the lower respiratory tract, there is a multifocal hyperplastic to suppurative bronchitis and bronchiolitis, and frequently, focal alveolitis. Alveolar septa are hypercellular, and infiltrating cells consist of alveolar macrophages, neutrophils, and lymphocytes. In the subacute and resolving stages, there is prominent perivascular and peribronchial cuffing with lymphocytes and plasma cells. Mononuclear cell infiltrates may persist for up to several weeks in alveolar septa, and there may be some evidence of residual interstitial fibrosis in alveolar walls (see Mouse Chapter 1, "Sendai Virus Infection").

Diagnosis

Rats are usually subclinically infected, thus the detection of pulmonary lesions on microscopic examination is frequently the first indication of a possible infectious disease. Acute bronchitis and bronchiolitis, when present, are diagnostic features of the disease. Other changes are not specific for Sendai virus, and confirmation requires demonstration of a rise in antibody. In suspected epizootics of Sendai virus infection, differential diagnoses must include PVM, PIV-3, and rat coronavirus infections. Seroconversion to Sendai virus antigen may occur with natural PIV-3 infection in rats due to cross-reactive antigens.

Parainfluenza Virus 3 Infection

Seroconversion to Sendai virus antigen was detected in rats in a pathogen-free laboratory rat colony without clinical signs, prompting further investigation. Using virus-specific hemagglutination inhibition serology, the agent was identified as PIV-3, possibly of human origin. The virus was isolated and sequenced, confirming it to be PIV-3 with >93% similarity to human PIV-3 isolates. Intranasal inoculation of rats resulted in transient respiratory epithelial necrosis and peribronchiolar mononuclear infiltrations. This event underscored the importance of differentiating natural infections of laboratory rats with PIV-3 from Sendai virus.

Pneumonia Virus of Mice Infection

Pneumonia virus of mice, despite its species-centric name, naturally infects mice, rats, hamsters, and possibly guinea pigs and gerbils. Infection is usually detected by seroconversion. Intranasal inoculation of F344 rats with PVM resulted in development of gross and microscopic lesions by 6 days postinoculation, without clinical evidence of disease. Histopathology includes multifocal, nonsuppurative perivasculitis and interstitial pneumonitis with hyperplasia of bronchus-associated lymphoid tissue. These lesions tend to persist for several weeks in the rat. The presence of interstitial pneumonia and perivasculitis attributed to PVM requires confirmation by seroconversion. Differential diagnoses include interstitial pneumonia due to Sendai virus, PIV-3, rat coronavirus, and *Pneumocystis* spp. PVM may be a copathogen in other respiratory diseases, such as mycoplasmal infections. The possibility of interspecies transmission to other laboratory animals, such as mice, hamsters, and gerbils, is another consideration.

Rat Theilovirus Infection

Rat theilovirus (RTV) is a Picornavirus within the *Cardiovirus* genus that is closely related to Theiler's murine encephalomyelitis virus (TMEV). Serosurveys have revealed that it is one of the most common infections in laboratory rat colonies. RTV was initially discovered in Sprague-Dawley rats, which exhibited central nervous system signs, with histopathologic lesions resembling TMEV in mice. The original isolate, known as MHG, induced posterior paresis in suckling rats and mice following intracerebral inoculation. Infection is typically subclinical and detected by seroconversion. Antibody is cross-reactive with TMEV antigen. Other strains that have been isolated include NSG910 and RTV1, which are genetically distinct from TMEV. Oral inoculation of rats with RTV has shown productive enteric infection and seroconversion. Viral antigen was detected within duodenal enterocytes, similar to TMEV in mice. Various inbred strains of rats had detectable virus for several weeks, and immunodeficient rats persistently carried high titers of virus. Lesions, including microscopic findings, were absent in the infected rats. Diagnosis is generally performed through serology, but immunohistochemistry and PCR may be used for confirmation.

Rotavirus Infection: Infectious Diarrhea of Infant Rats

An epizootic of diarrhea in infant rats known as infectious diarrhea of infant rats (IDIR) has been attributed to a group B rotavirus that is morphologically identical but antigenically distinct from most previously characterized (group A) rotaviruses. The agent is probably of human origin. Following oral inoculation of suckling rats, recipients developed diarrhea within 24–36 hours. Transient growth retardation, cracking and bleeding in the perianal region, and drying and flaking of skin were typical clinical signs. Rats were susceptible to experimental infection at all ages and to disease up to 12 days of age. They were resistant to clinical disease after 2 weeks of age. The stomach usually contained milk curd, with watery contents in the proximal small intestine. The distal small intestine and large intestine contained yellow-brown to green fluid and gas. Microscopic changes included intestinal villus attenuation, necrosis of enterocytes, and pathognomonic epithelial syncytia (Fig. 2.18). Changes were most evident in the ileal region. Eosinophilic intracytoplasmic inclusions were variably present in syncytia. Viral antigen could be demonstrated in small intestinal enterocytes and rarely in colonic epithelium, but only for 1–2 days. Viral precursor material and rotaviral particles were visualized in cells by electron microscopy. The IDIR agent is probably of human origin, and inoculation of suckling rats with human isolates of group B rotavirus resulted in diarrheal disease identical to IDIR. IDIR has not been reported since the initial observation, but the potential for re-emergence remains, since the agent was likely of human origin.

Reovirus Infection

Rats, in addition to a wide variety of other mammals, frequently seroconvert to reovirus, but natural or experimental disease does not occur in this species. Mice are the only laboratory animals that are susceptible to reovirus-induced disease.

Endogenous Viral Integrations

Rats, like mice, hamsters, guinea pigs, and other species, are infected with endogenous retroviruses, which are

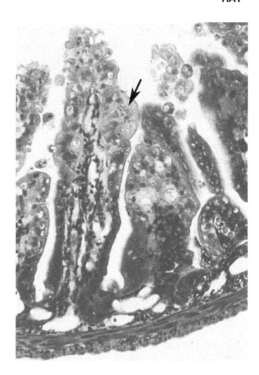

FIG. 2.18. *Distal small intestine from a suckling rat following inoculation with rotavirus (IDIR virus). Note pathognomonic syncytia (arrow). (Source: S. Vonderfecht.)*

transmitted vertically as provirus sequences in the genome. These viruses are of minimal practical significance but have been manipulated experimentally by combining with murine leukemia viruses and other rat leukemia viruses to form defective rat sarcoma viruses. Common laboratory sarcoma viruses of rat origin include the Harvey and Kirsten sarcoma agents. In addition, multiple Borna virus and parvovirus integrations have also been found within the genome of rats. The significance of endogenous viral integrations is minimal, but may influence PCR analysis for detection of parvovirus infection.

Viruses of Emerging Potential
Astrovirus Infection

Astroviruses have recently been found to be common among laboratory mice without clinical signs. Although not yet described among laboratory rats, astroviruses have been found in wild urban rats in Asia. Astroviruses are a major cause of gastroenteritis in humans, and the rat agent that was described appeared to be closely related to human isolates, based upon genetic sequencing.

Hepatitis E Virus

Recently, hepatitis E virus has been detected serologically and by PCR in wild rats in Europe, Asia, and the United States. The genotypes appear to be unique and distantly related to other known hepatitis E strains. Their significance as human pathogens has not been ascertained, but infectivity to rhesus macaques was not shown. Laboratory rats inoculated with a Los Angeles isolate developed mild focal necrotizing hepatitis and portal inflammation. The significance of hepatitis E virus in rats, its zoonotic potential, and prevalence in pet or laboratory rats remain to be determined.

BIBLIOGRAPHY FOR VIRAL INFECTIONS

General Bibliography for Virus Infections

Gaillard, E.T. & Clifford, C.B. (2000) Common diseases. In: *The Laboratory Rat*, Handbook of Experimental Animals (ed. G.J. Krinke), pp. 99–132. Academic Press, New York.

Jacoby, R.O. & Gaertner, D.J. (2005) Viral disease. In: *The Laboratory Rat*, 2nd edn (eds. M.A. Suckow, S.H. Weisbroth, & C.L. Franklin), pp. 423–451. Elsevier.

DNA Virus Infections

Rat Adenovirus Infection

Smith, A.L. & Barthold, S.W. (1987) Factors influencing susceptibility of laboratory rodents to infection with mouse adenovirus strains K87 and FL. *Archives of Virology* 95:143–148.

Smith, A.L., Winograd, D.F., & Burage, T.G. (1986) Comparative biological characterization of mouse adenovirus strains FL and K87 and seroprevalence in laboratory rodents. *Archives of Virology* 91:233–246.

Ward, J.M. & Young, D.M. (1976) Latent adenoviral infection of rats: intranuclear inclusions induced by treatment with a cancer chemotherapeutic agent. *Journal of the American Veterinary Medical Association* 169:952–953.

Rat Cytomegalovirus Infection

Bruggeman, C.A., Debie, W.M., Grauls, G., Majoor, G., & van Boven, C.P. (1983) Infection of laboratory rats with a new cytomegalo-like virus. *Archives of Virology* 76:189–199.

Kilham, L. & Margolis, G. (1975) Encephalitis in suckling rats induced with rat cytomegalovirus. *Laboratory Investigation* 33:200–206.

Lyon, H.W., Christian, J.J., & Mitler, C.W. (1959) Cytomegalic inclusion disease of lacrimal glands in male laboratory rats. *Proceedings of the Society for Experimental Biology and Medicine* 101:164–166.

Priscott, P.K. & Tyrell, D.A.J. (1982) The isolation and partial characterization of a cytomegalovirus from the brown rat, *Rattus norvegicus*. *Archives of Virology* 73:145–160.

Rat Papillomavirus Infection

Schulz, E., Gottschling, M., Ulrich, R.G., Richter, D., Stockfleth, E., & Nindl, I. (2012) Isolation of three novel rat and mouse papillomaviruses and their genomic characterization. *PLoS One* 7:e47164.

Schulz, E., Gottschling, M., Wibbelt, G., Stockfleth, E., & Nindl, I. (2009) Isolation and genomic characterization of the first Norway rat (*Rattus norvegicus*) papillomavirus and its phylogenetic position within *Pipapapillomavirus*, primarily infecting rodents. *Journal of General Virology* 90:2609–2614.

Rat Polyomavirus Infection

Ward, J.M., Lock, A., Collins, M.J., Gonda, M.A., & Reynolds, C.W. (1984) Papovaviral sialoadenitis in athymic nude rats. *Laboratory Animals* 18:84–89.

Parvovirus Infections

Ball-Goodrich, L.J., Leland, S.E., Johnson, E.A., Paturzo, F.X., & Jacoby, R.O. (1998) Rat parvovirus type 1: the prototype for a new rodent parvovirus serogroup. *Journal of Virology* 72:3289–3299.

Besselsen, D.G., Franklin, C.L., Livingston, R.S., & Riley, L.I. (2008) Lurking in the shadows: emerging rodent infectious diseases. *ILAR Journal* 49:277–290.

Coleman, G.L., Jacoby, R.O., Bhatt, P.N., Smith, A.L., & Jonas, A.M. (1983) Naturally occurring lethal parvovirus infection of juvenile and young-adult rats. *Veterinary Pathology* 20:49–56.

Dhawan, R.K., Wunderlich, M.L., Crowley, J.P., Ibriami, T., Dodge, M., Berg, E., & Shek, W.R. (2004) Virus-like particles as antigen for serologic detection of rat parvovirus antibodies. *Contemporary Topics in Laboratory Animal Science* 43:43–44.

Gaertner, D.J., Jacoby, R.O., Johnson, E.A., Paturzo, F.X., & Smith, A.L. (1995) Persistent rat virus infection in juvenile athymic rats and its modulation by immune serum. *Laboratory Animal Science* 45:249–253.

Henderson, K.S., Perkins, C.L., Banu, L.A., Jennings, S.M., Dhawan, R.K., & Niksa, P.L. (2006) Isolation of rat minute virus. *Journal of the American Association of Laboratory Animal Science* 45:86–87.

Jacoby, R.O., Ball-Goodrich, L.J., Besselsen, D.G., McKisic, M.D., Riley, L.K., & Smith, A.L. (1996) Rodent parvovirus infections. *Laboratory Animal Science* 46:370–380.

Jacoby, R.O., Bhatt, P.N., Gaertner, D.J., Smith, A.L., & Johnson, E.A. (1987) The pathogenesis of rat virus infection in infant and juvenile rats after oronasal inoculation. *Archives of Virology* 95:251–270.

Kajiwara, N., Ueno, Y., Takahashi, A., Sugiyama, F., Sugiyama, Y., & Yagami, K. (1996) Vertical transmission to embryo and fetus in maternal infection with rat virus (RV). *Experimental Animals* 45:239–244.

Kilham, L. & Margolis, G. (1966) Spontaneous hepatitis and cerebellar "hypoplasia" in suckling rats due to congenital infection with rat virus. *American Journal of Pathology* 49:457–475.

Kilham, L. & Margolis, G. (1969) Transplacental infection of rats and hamsters induced by oral and parenteral inoculations of H-1 and rat viruses (RV). *Teratology* 2:111–124.

Margolis, G. & Kilham, L. (1972) Rat virus infection of megakaryocytes: a factor in hemorrhagic encephalopathy? *Experimental and Molecular Pathology* 16:326–340.

Redig, A.J. & Besselsen, D.G. (2001) Detection of rodent parvoviruses by fluorogenic nuclease polymerase chain reaction. *Comparative Medicine* 51:326–331.

Riley, L.K., Knowles, R., Purdy, G., Salome, N., Pintel, D., Hook, R.R., Jr, Franklin, C.L., & Besch-Williford, C.L. (1996) Expression of recombinant parvovirus NS1 protein by a baculovirus and application to serologic testing of rodents. *Journal of Clinical Microbiology* 34:440–444.

Ueno, Y., Sugiyama, F., & Yagami, K. (1996) Detection and in vivo transmission of rat orphan parvovirus (ROPV). *Laboratory Animals* 30:114–119.

Wan, C.-H., Soderlund-Venermo, M., Pintel, D., & Riley, L.K. (2002) Molecular characterization of three newly recognized rat parvoviruses. *Journal of General Virology*. 83:2075–2083.

Wan, C.-H., Soderlund-Venermo, M., Pintel, D., & Riley, L.K. (2006) Detection of rat parvovirus type 1 and rat minute virus type 1 by polymerase chain reaction. *Laboratory Animals* 40:63–69.

Cowpox Virus Infection

Breithaupt, A., Kalthoff, D., Deutskens, F., Konig, P., Hoffman, B., Beer, M., Meyer, H., & Teifke, J.P. (2012) Clinical course and pathology in rats (*Rattus norvegicus*) after experimental cowpox virus infection by percutaneous and intranasal application. *Veterinary Pathology* 49:941–949.

Iftimovici, R., Iacobescu, V., Mutui, A., & Puca, D. (1976) Enzootic with ectromelia symptomatology in Sprague-Dawley rats. *Virologie* 27:65–66.

Kraft, L.M., D'Amelio, E.D., & D'Amelio, F.E. (1982) Morphological evidence for natural poxvirus infection in rats. *Laboratory Animal Science* 32:648–654.

Krikun, V.A. (1977) Pox in rats: isolation and identification of pox virus. *Voprosy Virusologii* 22:371–373.

Marennikova, S.S. & Shelukhina, E.M. (1976) White rats as a source of pox infection in carnivora of the family Felidae. *Acta Virologica* 20:422.

Marennikova, S.S., Shelukhina, E.M., & Fimina, V.A. (1978) Pox infection in white rats. *Laboratory Animals* 12:33–36.

Vogel, S., Sardy, M., Glos, K., Korting, H.C., Ruzicka, T., & Wollenberg, A. (2012) The Munich outbreak of cutaneous cowpox infection: transmission by infected pet rats. *Acta Dermato-Venereologica* 92:126–131.

Wolfs, T.F., Wagenaar, J.A., Niesters, H.G., & Osterhaus, A.D. (2002) Rat to human transmission of cowpox infection. *Emerging Infectious Diseases* 8:1495–1496.

RNA Virus Infections

Rat Coronavirus Infection

Bhatt, P.N. & Jacoby, R.O. (1977) Experimental infection of axenic rats with Parker's rat coronavirus. *Archives of Virology* 54:345–352.

Bihun, C.G. & Percy, D.H. (1995) Morphologic changes in the nasal cavity associated with sialodacryoadenitis virus infection in the Wistar rat. *Veterinary Pathology* 32:1–10.

Compton, S.R., Smith, A.L., & Gaertner, D.J. (1999) Comparison of the pathogenicity in rats of rat coronaviruses of different neutralization groups. *Laboratory Animal Science* 49:514–518.

Compton, S.R., Vivas-Gonzales, B.E., & Macy, J.D. (1999) Reverse transcriptase chain reaction-based diagnosis and molecular characterization of a new rat coronavirus strain. *Laboratory Animal Science* 49:506–513.

Hajjar, A.M., DiGiacomo, R.F., Carpenter, J.K., Bingel, S.A., & Moazed, T.C. (1991) Chronic sialodacryoadenitis virus (SDAV) infection in athymic rats. *Laboratory Animal Science* 41:22–25.

Harkness, J.E. & Ridgeway, M.D. (1980) Chromodacryorrhea in laboratory rats (*Rattus norvegicus*): etiologic considerations. *Laboratory Animal Science* 30:841–844.

Jacoby, R.O., Bhatt, P.N., & Jonas, A.M. (1975) Pathogenesis of sialodacryoadenitis virus in gnotobiotic rats. *Veterinary Pathology* 12:196–209.

Macy, J.D., Weir, E.C., & Barthold, S.W. (1996) Reproductive abnormalities associated with coronavirus infection in rats. *Laboratory Animal Science* 46:129–132.

Maru, M. & Sato, K. (1982) Characterization of a coronavirus isolated from rats with sialoadenitis. *Archives of Virology* 73:33–43.

Parker, J.C., Cross, S.S., & Rowe, W.P. (1970) Rat coronavirus (RCV): a prevalent naturally occurring pneumotropic virus of rats. *Archiv fur die gesamte Virusforschung* 31:293–302.

Percy, D.H., Bond, S.J., Paturzo, F.X., & Bhatt, P.N. (1990) Duration of protection following reinfection with sialodacryoadenitis virus. *Laboratory Animal Science* 40:144–149.

Percy, D.H. & Williams, K.L. (1990) Experimental Parker's rat coronavirus infection in Wistar rats. *Laboratory Animal Science* 40:603–607.

Percy, D.H., Wojcinski, Z.W., & Schunk, M.K. (1989) Sequential changes in the Harderian and exorbital lacrimal glands in Wistar rats infected with sialodacryoadenitis virus. *Veterinary Pathology* 26:238–245.

Rossie, K.M., Sheridan, J.F., Barthold, S.W., & Tutschka, P.J. (1988) Graft-versus-host disease and sialodacryoadenitis viral infection in bone marrow transplanted rats. *Transplantation* 45:1012–1016.

Schoeb, T.R. & Lindsey, J.R. (1987) Exacerbation of murine respiratory mycoplasmosis by sialodacryoadenitis virus infection in gnotobiotic F344 rats. *Veterinary Pathology* 24:392–399.

Schunk, M.K., Percy, D.H., & Rosendal, S. (1995) Effect of time of exposure to rat coronavirus and *Mycoplasma pulmonis* on respiratory tract lesions in the Wistar rat. *Canadian Journal of Veterinary Research* 59:60–66.

Utsumi, K., Ishikawa, T., Maeda, T., Shimizu, S., Tatsumi, H., & Fujiwara, K. (1980) Infectious sialoadenitis and rat breeding. *Laboratory Animals* 14:303–307.

Weir, E.C., Jacoby, R.O., Paturzo, F.X., & Johnson, E.A. (1990) Infection of SDAV-immune rats with SDAV and rat coronavirus. *Laboratory Animal Science* 40:363–366.

Weir, E.C., Jacoby, R.O., Paturzo, F.X., Johnson, E.A., & Ardito, R.B. (1990) Persistence of sialodacryoadenitis virus in athymic rats. *Laboratory Animal Science* 40:138–143.

Wojcinski, Z.W. & Percy, D.H. (1986) Sialodacryoadenitis virus-associated lesions in the lower respiratory tract of rats. *Veterinary Pathology* 23:278–286.

Hantavirus Infection

Childs, J.E., Glass, G.E., Korch, G.W., Arthur, R.R., Shah, K.V., Glasser, D., Rossi, C., & Leduc, J.W. (1987) Epizootiology of *Hantavirus* infections of Baltimore: isolation of a virus from Norway rats and characteristics of infected rat populations. *American Journal of Epidemiology* 126:55–68.

Compton, S.R., Jacoby, R.O., Paturzo, F.X., & Smith, A.L. (2004) Persistent Seoul virus infection in Lewis rats. *Archives of Virology* 149:1325–1339.

Dohmae, K., Okabe, M., & Nishimune, Y. (1994) Experimental transmission of *Hantavirus* infection in laboratory rats. *Journal of Infectious Disease* 170:1589–1592.

Glass, G.E., Childs, J.E., Korch, G.W., & LeDuc, J.W. (1998) Association of intraspecific wounding with hantaviral infection in wild rats (*Rattus norvegicus*). *Epidemiology and Infection* 101:459–472.

Kariwa, H., Fujiki, M., Yoshimatsu, K., Arikawa, J., Takashima, I., & Hashimoto, N. (1998) Urine-associated horizontal transmission of Seoul virus among rats. *Archives of Virology* 143:365–374.

Kariwa, H., Kimura, M., Yoshizumi, S., Arikawa, J., Yoshimatsu, K,. Takashima, I., & Hashimoto, N. (1996) Modes of Seoul virus infections: persistency in newborn rats and transiency in adult rats. *Archives of Virology* 141:2327–2338.

Leduc, J.W., Smith, J.A., & Johnson, K.M. (1984) Hantaan-like viruses from domestic rats captured in the United States. *American Journal of Tropical Medicine and Hygiene* 33:992–998.

Lee, P.W., Yanagihara, R., Gibbs, C.J., Jr, & Gajdusek, D.C. (1986) Pathogenesis of experimental Hantaan virus infection in laboratory rats. *Archives of Virology* 88:57–66.

Lloyd, G. & Jones, N. (1986) Infection of laboratory workers with hantavirus acquired from immunocytomas propogated in laboratory rats. *Journal of Infection* 12:117–125.

Schmaljohn, C. & Hjelle, B. (1997) Hantaviruses: a global disease problem. *Emerging Infectious Diseases* 3:95–104.

Tanishita, O., Takahashi, Y., Okuno, Y., Tamura, M., Asada, H., Dantas, J.R., Jr., Yamanouchi, T., Domae, K., Kurata, T., & Tamanishi, K. (1986) Persistent infection of rats with haemorrhagic fever with renal syndrome virus and their antibody response. *Journal of General Virology* 67:2819–2824.

Sendai Virus Infection

Burek, J.D., Zurcher, C., Van Nunen, M.C., & Hollander, C.F. (1977) A naturally occurring epizootic caused by Sendai virus in breeding and aging rodent colonies. II. Infection in the rat. *Laboratory Animal Science* 27:963–971.

Carthew, P. & Aldred, P. (1988) Embryonic death in pregnant rats owing to intercurrent infection with Sendai virus and *Pasteurella pneumotropica*. *Laboratory Animals* 22:92–97.

Castleman, W.L. (1983) Respiratory tract lesions in weanling outbred rats infected with Sendai virus. *American Journal of Veterinary Research* 44:1024–1031.

Castleman, W.L., Brudnage-Anguish, L.J., Kreitzer, L., & Neuenschwander, S.B. (1987) Pathogenesis of bronchiolitis and pneumonia induced in neonatal and weaning rats by parainfluenza (Sendai) virus. *American Journal of Pathology* 129:277–296.

Coid, R. & Wardman, G. (1971) The effect of parainfluenza type 1 (Sendai) virus infection on early pregnancy in the rat. *Journal of Reproduction and Fertility* 24:39–43.

Garlinghouse, L.E. & Van Hoosier, G.L., Jr. (1978) Studies on adjuvant-induced arthritis, tumor transplantability, and serologic response to bovine serum albumin in Sendai virus-infected rats. *American Journal of Veterinary Research* 39:297–300.

Garlinghouse, L.E., Jr., Van Hoosier, G.L., Jr., & Giddens, W.E., Jr. (1987) Experimental Sendai virus infection in laboratory rats. I. Virus replication and immune response. *Laboratory Animal Science* 37:437–441.

Giddens, W.E., Jr., Van Hoosier, G.L., Jr., & Garlinghouse, L.E., Jr. (1987) Experimental Sendai virus infection in laboratory rats. II. Pathology and immunohistochemistry. *Laboratory Animal Science* 37:442–448.

Jakob, G.J. & Dick, E.C. (1973) Synergistic effect in viral-bacterial infection: combined infection of the murine respiratory tract with Sendai virus and *Pasteurella pneumotropica*. *Infection and Immunity* 8:762–768.

Schoeb, T.R., Kervin, K.C., & Lindsey, J.R. (1985) Exacerbation of murine respiratory mycoplasmosis in gnotobiotic F344/N rats by Sendai virus infection. *Veterinary Pathology* 22:272–282.

Parainfluenza Virus 3 Infection

Miyata, H., Kanazawa, T., Shibuya, K., & Hino, S. (2005) Contamination of a specific-pathogen-free rat breeding colony with *Human parainfluenzavirus type 3*. *Journal of General Virology* 86:733–741.

Pneumonia Virus of Mice Infection

Brownstein, D.G. (1985) Pneumonia virus of mice infection, lung, mouse and rat. In: *Respiratory System* Monographs on Pathology of Laboratory Animals (eds. T.C. Jones, U. Mohr, & R.D. Hunt), pp. 206–210. Springer, New York.

Vogtsberger, L.M., Stromberg, P.C., & Rice, J.M. (1982) Histological and serological response of B6C3F1 mice and F344 rats to experimental pneumonia virus of mice infection. *Laboratory Animal Science* 32:419.

Rat Theilovirus Infection

Drake, M.T., Besch-Williford, C., Myles, M.H., Davis, J.W., & Livingston, R.S. (2011) In vivo tropisms and kinetics of rat theilovirus infection in immunocompetent and immunodeficient rats. *Virus Research* 160:374–380.

Drake, M.T., Riley, L.K., & Livingston, R.S. (2008) Differential susceptibility of SD and CD rats to a novel rat theilovirus. *Comparative Medicine* 58:458–464.

Hemelt, I.E., Huxsoll, D.L., & Warner, A.R., Jr. (1974) Comparison of MHG virus with mouse encephalomyelitis viruses. *Laboratory Animal Science* 24:523–529.

McConnell, S.J., Huxsoll, D.L., Garner, F.M., Spertzel, R.O., Warner, A.R., Jr., & Yager, R.H. (1964) Isolation and characterization of a neurotropic agent (MHG virus) from adult rats. *Proceedings of the Society for Experimental Biology and Medicine* 115:362–367.

Ohsawa, K., Watanabe, Y., Miyata, H., & Sato, H. (2003) Genetic analysis of a theiler-like virus isolated from rats. *Comparative Medicine* 53:191–196.

Rodrigues, D.M., Martins, S.S., Gilioli, R., Guaraldo, A.M., & Gatti, M.S. (2005) Theiler's murine encephalomyelitis virus in non-barrier rat colonies. *Comparative Medicine* 55:459–464.

Rotavirus Infection

Huber, A.C., Yolken, R.H., Mader, L.C., Strandberg, J.D., & Vonderfecht, S.L. (1989) Pathology of infectious diarrhea of infant rats (IDIR) induced by an antigenically distant rotavirus. *Veterinary Pathology* 26:376–385.

Salim, A.F., Phillips, A.D., Walker-Smith, J.A., & Farthing, M.J. (1995) Sequential changes in small intestinal structure and function during rotavirus infection in neonatal rats. *Gut* 36:231–238.

Vonderfecht, S.L., Huber, A.C., Eiden, J., Mader, L.C., & Yolken, R.H. (1984) Infectious diarrhea of infant rats produced by a rotavirus-like agent. *Journal of Virology* 52:94–98.

Endogenous Viral Integrations

Belyi, V.A., Levine, A.J., & Skalka, A.M. (2010) Unexpected inheritance: multiple integrations of ancient Borna virus and Ebolavirus/Marbugvirus sequences in vertebrate genomes. *PLoS Pathogens* 6:e1001030.

Horie, M. & Tomonaga, K. (2011) Non-retroviral fossils in vertebrate genomes. *Viruses* 3:1836–1848.

Kapoor, A., Simmonds, P., & Lipkin, I. (2010) Discovery and characterization of mammalian endogenous parvoviruses. *Journal of Virology* 84:12628–12635.

Viruses of Emerging Potential

Chu, D.K.W., Chin, A.W.H., Smith, G.J., Chan, K.-H., Guan, Y., Peiris, S.M., & Poon, L.L.M. (2010) Detection of novel astroviruses in urban brown rats and previously known astroviruses in humans. *Journal of General Virology* 91:2457–2462.

Johne, R., Dremsek, P., Kindler, E., Schielke, A., Plenge-Bonig, A., Gregersen, H., Wessels, U., Schmidt, K., Rietschel, W., Groschup, M.H., Guenther, S., Heckel, G., & Ulrich, R.G. (2012) Rat hepatitis E virus: geographical clustering within Germany and serological detection in wild Norway rats (*Rattus norvegicus*). *Journal of Molecular Epidemiology and Evolutionary Genetics of Infectious Diseases* 12:947–956.

Johne, R., Heckel, G., Plenge-Bonig, A., Kindler, E., Maresch, C., Reetz, J., Schielke, A., & Ulrich, R.G. (2010) Novel hepatitis E virus genotype in Norway rats, Germany. *Emerging Infectious Diseases* 16:1452–1455.

Lack, J., Volk, K., & Van Den Bussche, R.A. (2012) Hepatitis E virus genotype 3 in wild rats, United States. *Emerging Infectious Diseases* 18:1268–1281.

Li, T.-C., Ami, Y., Suzaki, Y., Yasuda, S.P., Yoshimatsu, K., Arikawa, J., Takeda, N., & Takaji, W. (2013) Characterization of full genome of rat hepatitis E virus strain from Vietnam. *Emerging Infectious Diseases* 19:115–118.

Purcell, R.H., Engle, R.E., Rood, M.P., Kabrane-Lazizi, Y., Nguyen, H.T., Govindarajan, S., St. Claire, M., & Emerson, S.U. (2011) Hepatitis E virus in rats, Los Angeles, California, USA. *Emerging Infectious Diseases* 17:2216–2222.

BACTERIAL INFECTIONS

Rats are susceptible to a number of important bacterial pathogens. Recognizing that any scheme is imperfect and overlapping, the following text has been organized into 3 sections: pathogens that are (i) primary enteric infections, (ii) primary respiratory infections, and (iii) other bacterial infections. Alphabetical listing is used within each category. This approach can best assist the pathologist with differential diagnoses.

Primary Respiratory Infections
Bordetella bronchiseptica *Infection*

Bordetella bronchiseptica is an uncommon, typically opportunistic pathogen that has been associated with respiratory disease in laboratory rats. The organism is a more common inhabitant of the upper respiratory tract of species such as the guinea pig and domestic rabbit. The organism tends to colonize the apices of respiratory epithelial cells, resulting in impaired clearance by ciliated epithelial cells.

Pathology

Aerosol exposure to *B. bronchiseptica* in laboratory rats has resulted in lesions characterized by suppurative rhinitis, multifocal bronchopneumonia with polymorphonuclear cell and lymphocytic infiltration, and peribronchial lymphoid hyperplasia. In animals examined at 2 or more weeks postinoculation, there was fibroblast proliferation and mononuclear cell infiltration. Spontaneous cases of bronchopneumonia associated with *B. bronchiseptica* infection in rats feature a suppurative bronchopneumonia with consolidation of affected anteroventral areas of the lung. Frequently, there is an identifiable concurrent infection, such as rat coronavirus or *Mycoplasma* infection. Experimental infection of SPF rats resulted in transient infection without spread to contact rats, lending credence to coinfection as a critical element for natural disease.

Diagnosis

Isolation of the organism in large numbers from affected tissues is required for definitive diagnosis. Identification of copathogens should also be considered.

Cilia-Associated Respiratory (CAR) Bacillus Infection

Naturally occurring respiratory disease in rats has been associated with Cilia-associated respiratory (CAR) bacillus, a filamentous, argyrophilic bacterium with gliding motility that colonizes the ciliated epithelium of airways. CAR bacillus has not been definitively classified, but it is closely related to members of the Flavobacter/Flexibacter group based upon 16S rRNA gene sequence analysis. The organism is Gram-negative and is difficult to grow on conventional cell-free media. It has also been demonstrated on respiratory epithelium in other species including mice, rabbits, cattle, goats, and pigs. Sequence analysis of 16S rRNA genes, antigenic comparisons, and experimental infectivity studies suggest that the rat CAR bacillus is closely related to isolates from other rodents, but distinct from the CAR bacillus of rabbits, cattle, and goats. CAR bacillus is associated with chronic respiratory disease (CRD) in the rat, frequently as a coinfection with *M. pulmonis*. Both CAR bacillus and M. *pulmonis* infect ciliated respiratory epithelium, resulting in perturbation of mucociliary clearance and development of CRD. Although CRD is often the result of coinfection with CAR bacillus and M. *pulmonis*, each of these agents can be found as single infections resulting in similar disease. CRD is often multifactorial, including environmental factors (ammonia) and viruses (Sendai virus). Although CAR bacillus was first described in 1980, there is evidence that the organism has been associated with respiratory disease in rats for decades, based upon retrospective staining of tissue sections. CAR bacillus is transmitted by direct

contact, usually during the neonatal period. Experimental inoculation of various strains and stocks of rats (F344, LEW, and SD) has shown that rats are uniformly susceptible to CAR bacillus-induced disease, but CAR bacillus isolates differ in pathogenicity.

Pathology

Infection may be subclinical with minimal or no microscopic lesions. Chronic suppurative bronchitis and bronchiolitis, with peribronchiolar cuffing with lymphocytes and plasma cells, are typical microscopic findings when disease is present. There is marked leukocytic infiltration in the lamina propria of affected airways. Bronchiolectasis, with mucin and leukocyte accumulation, may result in bulging of the serosal surfaces of the lung, which is often asymmetrical in distribution (see "*M. pulmonis* infection"). Although organisms are discernable in H&E sections, they are particularly evident when stained with the Warthin–Starry method, revealing slender, argyrophilic bacilli inserted along the apices of the ciliated respiratory epithelium (Fig. 2.19).

Diagnosis

The typical slender CAR bacteria are best demonstrated in tissue sections by silver stains, such as the Warthin–Starry stain. The organisms are also readily seen as electron-dense bacilli oriented between the cilia of respiratory epithelial cells by electron microscopy (Fig. 2.20). Serology can be used to detect seropositive animals. However, the use of CAR bacillus whole cell lysates as antigen for serology is problematic, in that this bacterium has a number of cross-reacting antigens among other bacteria. Other diagnostic techniques include the demonstration of the CAR bacillus in silver-stained tracheal scrapings using Steiner's silver stain, or in nasal swabs using PCR. The organism has been grown in embryonated chick eggs, cell culture, and, more recently, in cell-free media. Differential diagnoses include *M. pulmonis* infection and pneumonia due to conventional bacteria, with possible complications due to concurrent infections with other

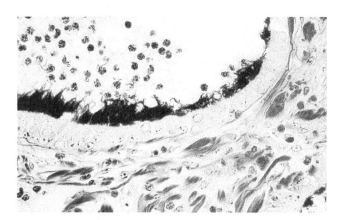

FIG. 2.19. *Bronchiole from a rat infected with CAR bacillus. The cilia have been completely effaced by overgrowth of CAR bacilli (Warthin–Starry stain).*

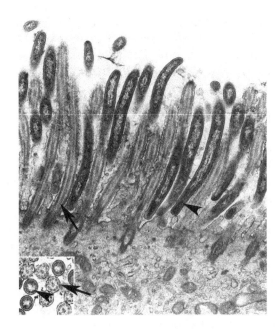

FIG. 2.20. *Electron micrograph of bronchiolar epithelium colonized by CAR bacilli. Note the end-on attachment of the bacilli (arrowheads) among the cilia (arrows). The inset represents a cross section of bacilli among the cilia. (Source: Ganaway et al. 1985. Reproduced with permission from American Society for Microbiology.)*

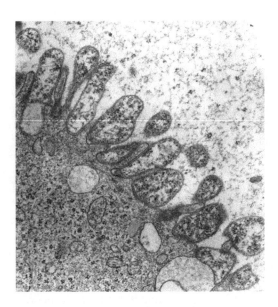

FIG. 2.21. *Electron micrograph of bronchiolar epithelium heavily colonized with* Mycoplasma pulmonis, *resulting in complete loss of cilia.*

respiratory tract pathogens (Sendai virus, PVM, rat coronavirus, or *Pneumocystis*).

Mycoplasma pulmonis *Infection: Murine Respiratory Mycoplasmosis*

Chronic respiratory disease in rats has undergone an interesting historical evolution. Initially believed to be multifactorial, it later became apparent that *M. pulmonis* could be the primary pathogen in this disease. This gave rise to the term murine respiratory mycoplasmosis (MRM) as the preferred terminology over CRD. However, other pathogens of the respiratory tract were shown to play a role in CRD, including CAR bacillus, respiratory viruses, and environmental factors, thereby returning the term CRD as the most appropriate and inclusive moniker for this disease. Nevertheless, *M. pulmonis* remains the major pathogen in cases of CRD. *Mycoplasma pulmonis* is a member of the order Mycoplasmatales, small pleomorphic bacteria devoid of cell walls that have specialized tip structures that play a key role in attachment to host cells. Respiratory disease results from loss of cilia following colonization of respiratory epithelium (Fig. 2.21). Some antigenic heterogeneity occurs among strains of *M. pulmonis*. There are demonstrable common cross-reactive antigens among 2 other naturally occurring murine mycoplasmas, *M. neurolyticum* (mice) and *M. arthritidis*, but *M. pulmonis* is the only clinically significant *Mycoplasma* sp. in rodents.

Epizootiology and Pathogenesis

Quality control programs in laboratory animal medicine have resulted in a marked reduction in the incidence of myocoplasmosis in rats. However, based on serological surveys, seropositive colonies continue to be identified, and infection in wild and pet rats is common. Transmission of *M. pulmonis* among cage-mates and to adjacent cages occurs inefficiently by aerosols. It may require up to several months to establish an infection in contact animals, and clinical disease may not occur until up to 6 months after infection. Intrauterine transmission may also occur, although newborn pups appear to be frequently infected by exposure to the infected dam during the postnatal period. Placentitis and fetal bronchopneumonia have been produced in pregnant rats inoculated intravaginally with *M. pulmonis* prior to breeding. The incidence and intensity of the disease are influenced by a variety of factors, such as strain of rat, concurrent infections, and environmental conditions. For example, LEW rats develop a more severe disease than do F344 rats. Concurrent infections with organisms, such as Sendai virus, rat coronavirus, or CAR bacillus, have an additive effect on CRD. Similarly, other opportunistic secondary bacterial invaders frequently play a role in the progression of the disease. Ammonia concentrations at the cage level of greater than 25 ppm may enhance the progression of CRD.

Mycoplasma pulmonis has an affinity for respiratory epithelium, middle ear, endometrium, and less commonly, synovium. Invasion of the middle ear probably occurs via the Eustachian tube. This usually results in a chronic otitis media, since the Eustachian tube opens into the tympanic bulla on the dorsal aspect, affording poor drainage to the nasopharynx. Colonization of respiratory epithelium results in ciliostasis, with resulting impaired airway clearance and accumulation of lysozyme-rich inflammatory exudate. Since intrapulmonary airways lack cartilage, bronchioles are subject to bronchiolar expansion and bronchiolectasis. Host cell damage may occur by a variety of means including uptake of essential cell metabolites and release of cytotoxic substances such as H_2O_2. Both the intact organisms and the cell membranes are nonspecific B-cell mitogens, resulting in marked peribronchiolar lymphocytic infiltration, which is a hallmark of CRD in the rat.

Pathology

Clinical signs vary, including subclinical infections, but can include minimal to florid respiratory distress, sniffling, torticollis, infertility, and arthritis. In severely affected animals, dyspnea, ruffled hair coat, and weight loss may occur. Porphyrin-containing dark red encrustations may be present around the eyes and external nares. At necropsy, serous to catarrhal exudate may be present in the nasal passages, trachea, and major airways. In animals with profuse viscid exudate in the airways, there may be patchy vesicular to bullous emphysema in the lungs. Early pulmonary lesions are usually manifested as pinpoint gray lesions. As peripheral bronchiolectasis becomes apparent, varying sized foci are present with clear mucous- or pus-filled lumina. Affected lobes and areas are usually cranioventral in distribution, unilateral or bilateral, often asymmetric in severity, and dark plumcolored to light tan (Fig. 2.22). One or both tympanic bullae may contain serous to inspissated purulent material, with thickening of the tympanic membrane. The uterine horns, ovarian bursae, and oviducts may contain purulent exudate, but involvement of these sites may only be confirmed microscopically. Disseminated

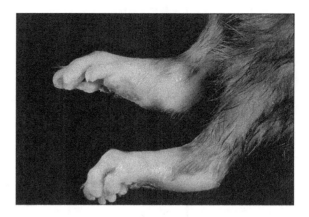

FIG. 2.23. *Bilateral swelling of tibiotarsal joints in a young rat with naturally acquired systemic* Mycoplasma pulmonis *infection. Arthritis is a rare component of mycoplasmosis in the rat.*

infection may occasionally result in arthritis, with swelling of the tibiotarsus (Fig. 2.23).

Microscopic changes in the affected tympanic bullae, turbinates, and major airways are characterized by a leukocytic infiltrate in the submucosa consisting of neutrophils, lymphocytes, and plasma cells. Epithelial cells in affected areas are often cuboidal to squamous, with loss of cilia, and hyperplasia of goblet cells. Leukocytes, mucus, and cell debris are frequently present on the surface in affected areas. Peribronchial, peribronchiolar, and perivascular infiltration with lymphocytes and plasma cells is a prominent feature at all stages of CRD (Fig. 2.24). Chronic bronchitis and bronchiolitis frequently progress to bronchiolectasis, characterized by dilation of airways, rupture of airways, and abscessation (Fig. 2.25). Collections of mucus, leukocytes, and cellular debris are present in the lumen (Fig. 2.26). There may be rupture of the bronchiolar walls, with release of inflammatory cells, mucus, and debris into the adjacent parenchyma and abscessation. Alveolar changes are often

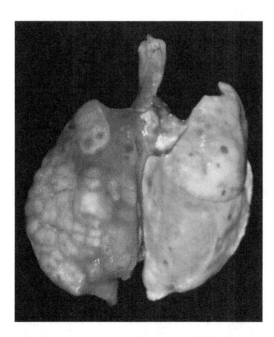

FIG. 2.22. *Chronic respiratory disease in a rat associated with* Mycoplasma pulmonis *infection. Note the asymmetric involvement of lung lobes and the irregular surface of affected areas due to bronchiolectasis and peribronchiolar lymphocytic infiltration.*

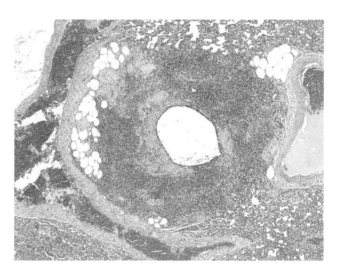

FIG. 2.24. *Peribronchiolar cuffing with lymphocytes and plasma cells, a characteristic feature of* Mycoplasma pulmonis *infection in rats.*

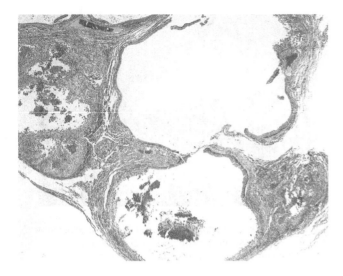

FIG. 2.25.   *Pulmonary lesions associated with an advanced case of mycoplasmosis. There is marked bronchiolectasis, rupture of airways, and abscessation.*

focal to segmental in distribution. Macrophages, neutrophils, and mucus may be present in alveolar spaces, with lymphocytic infiltration in the alveolar septa. There may be variable degrees of alveolar emphysema, with focal to patchy rupture of alveolar septa. Genital tract lesions, when present, consist of perioophoritis and endometritis, with mononuclear and polymorphonuclear cell infiltration in the stratum compactum and endometrium. In some cases, the lumen may be packed with leukocytes. Inflammatory lesions may also arise in the male genital tract.

Diagnosis

CRD caused by *M. pulmonis*, CAR bacillus, or both has similar macroscopic and microscopic features. The role of CAR bacillus can be confirmed as already described.

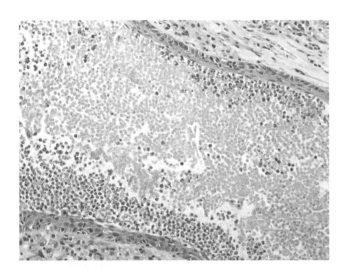

FIG. 2.26.   *Chronic bronchiolitis associated with murine respiratory mycoplasmosis. Note the squamous metaplasia of respiratory epithelium, loss of cilia, and necrotic cellular debris filling the lumen.*

Mycoplasma organisms are not readily visible microscopically, but their presence may be inferred by lack of cilia on respiratory epithelium. *Mycoplasma pulmonis* can usually be cultured from nasopharyngeal washes or affected sites such as the upper and lower respiratory tract and uterus using appropriate media, and can also be detected by PCR or immunohistochemistry. Cultures may fail to detect the organism in some infected animals. Serology is commonly used for surveillance within a population. However, animals may be falsely seropositive due to exposure to *M. arthritidis*. In addition, rats naturally exposed to *M. pulmonis* may be seronegative for up to 4 months postexposure. Thus, there are limitations to relying solely on serology to confirm the diagnosis. The collection of tissues and sera from retired breeders is recommended as a useful means of screening for mycoplasmal infections. Serological testing for antibodies against coinfecting respiratory viruses such as Sendai virus, PVM, and rat coronavirus are recommended, particularly when lower respiratory disease is severe. These agents can have an additive effect on the progression of CRD. Cultures for conventional bacteria are critical, since there may be concurrent infections with other bacteria, such as *Pasteurella pneumotropica* or *Streptococcus pneumoniae*. Infection should be considered chronic, with no merit in antibiotic treatment other than palliating clinical signs. Differential diagnoses include pulmonary abscessation due to *Corynebacterium kutscheri* infection, chronic respiratory infections due to the CAR bacillus, otitis media due to conventional bacteria, and suppurative metritis due to *P. pneumotropica* infection.

Primary Enteric Infections
Campylobacter jejuni *Infection*

Campylobacter jejuni infects a wide range of animals, including laboratory rats. Because of its wide host range, this bacterium can be introduced to laboratory animal units through a number of means and can spread between species within a facility. Infection in rats is usually subclinical, but young rats may manifest mild diarrhea or soft feces. Experimental oral inoculation of outbred rats induced mild acute lesions in the small intestine, including enterocyte swelling, basal subnuclear vacuolation, villus tip disruption, villus widening, and mild crypt hyperplasia. Infection was also transient, with no detectable infection by 32 days after inoculation. Humans are susceptible to gastroenteritis when infected with *C. jejuni*.

Clostridium difficile *Infection*

Unlike other species covered in this text, *C. difficile* enterotoxemia is rare in rats. Nevertheless, germ-free rats that were experimentally monoassociated with toxigenic *C. difficile* developed pseudomembranous colitis. Thus, laboratory rats may, under certain circumstances, develop enterotoxemia.

Clostridium piliforme *Infection: Tyzzer's Disease*

The Tyzzer's bacillus, *C. piliforme*, was previously named *Bacillus piliformis*, which gave rise to the sometimes used, but inappropriate name of *Clostridium piliformis*. It has a wide host range, but *C. piliforme* isolates tend to be host-specific, with minimal antigenic cross-reactivity among isolates. Infection involves the vegetative form, and spores are shed in the feces, which may remain infectious in contaminated bedding for up to 1 year (for additional information on epizootiology and pathogenesis, see Rabbit Chapter 6, "*Clostridium Piliforme Infection*"). Outbreaks in laboratory rats usually occur in young rats during the postweaning period. Transmission is achieved through oral ingestion of spores. Transplacental transmission has been demonstrated in seropositive rats treated with prednisolone during the last week of pregnancy. Subclinically infected rats can transmit the organism to naïve rats via contaminated bedding, but the organism can be eliminated from immunocompetent rats by cesarean section and appropriate disinfection techniques. Tyzzer's disease is typically an enterohepatic disease, with variable involvement of the heart. In naturally occurring outbreaks, clinical signs may include depression, ruffled hair coat, abdominal distension, low morbidity, and high mortality in clinically affected animals. Clinical disease with low mortality has also been reported. Clinically normal seropositive rats have been identified in colonies, indicating that inapparent infections may occur.

Pathology

Rats with Tyzzer's disease may develop necrohemorrhagic ileitis, with pronounced dilation of the terminal small intestine (megaloileitis) (Fig. 2.27). The flaccid ileum may be distended up to 3–4 times the normal diameter, with variable involvement of the jejunum and cecum. Megaloileitis does not always occur in rats with Tyzzer's disease. Enteritis may be evident only at the microscopic level. The mesenteric lymph nodes are swollen and edematous. Disseminated pale foci of necrosis up to several millimeters in diameter are scattered throughout the parenchyma of the liver. They may also be circumscribed to linear pale foci present on the heart (Fig. 2.28). Microscopic changes are confined primarily to the ileum, liver, and myocardium. In the intestine, there is frequently a necrotizing transmural ileitis, with segmental involvement of affected areas. There is necrosis and sloughing of enterocytes and edema of the lamina propria and submucosa, often with fragmentation and hypercellularity of the muscular layers. Infiltrating inflammatory cells are primarily mononuclear cells, with a sprinkling of neutrophils. In the liver, the histological characteristics vary from foci of acute coagulation necrosis to focal hepatitis, with polymorphonuclear and mononuclear leukocyte infiltration (Fig. 2.29). Hepatic lesions of some duration are characterized by fibrosis, with

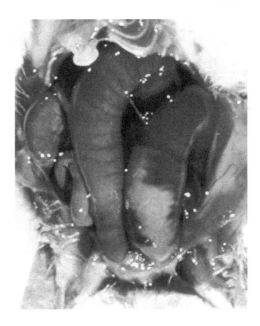

FIG. 2.27. *Tyzzer's disease, manifesting as necrotizing and hemorrhagic ileitis with adynamic ileus (megaloileitis) in a young rat infected with* Clostridium piliforme.

multinucleated giant cells and mineralized debris in reparative foci. In the heart, lesions may vary from necrosis of isolated myofibers to destruction of relatively large segments of myocardium. There is vacuolation to fragmentation of the sarcoplasm, with interstitial edema and mononuclear and polymorphonuclear leukocyte infiltration. Giemsa, Warthin–Starry, or PAS stains may used to demonstrate bundles of slender bacilli in the cytoplasm of enterocytes in ileal lesions, in hepatocytes surrounding

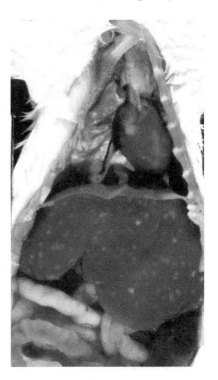

FIG. 2.28. *Tyzzer's disease in a young rat. Note the multifocal hepatitis and the multifocal to coalescing myocardial lesions.*

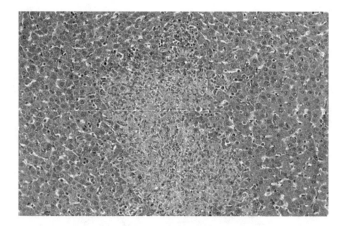

FIG. 2.29. *Tyzzer's disease in a juvenile rat. There is acute focal necrosis of hepatocytes with polymorphonuclear cell infiltration.*

necrotic foci, and scattered in the sarcoplasm in myocardial lesions (Fig. 2.30).

Diagnosis

Diagnosis is achieved by the demonstration of the organisms in tissue sections. Visualization of diagnostically typical fascicles of intracytoplasmic bacilli, particularly in liver, may require arduous searching. The triad of organs usually affected in Tyzzer's disease (intestine, liver, and heart) are also useful diagnostic features, if present. Serologic tests are now widely used, but use of a single isolate as antigen may not detect seroconversion among different host species (including between mice and rats) due to significant antigenic heterogeneity. PCR has also been developed for detection of the organism in feces. Differential diagnoses include salmonellosis and ileus following the intraperitoneal administration of chloral hydrate for general anesthesia.

Enterococcus *spp. Infection: Enterococcal Enteropathy*

Epizootics of enteric disease with high morbidity and mortality have been observed in suckling rats. In a

number of outbreaks, the etiologies have been identified as *Enterococcus* spp., including *E. durans*, *E. hirae*, and other isolates that have not been speciated. The disease has been reproduced in suckling rats inoculated with pure cultures of the *Enterococcus* isolated from affected rats. *Enterococci* are no longer considered to be members of the *Streptococcus* genus, but this disease has been referred to as "streptococcal enteropathy."

Pathology

Animals are stunted, with distended abdomens and fecal soiling in the perineal region. The stomachs are usually distended with milk, and there is dilation of the small and large intestine with fluid and gas. On microscopic examination, large numbers of coccoid bacteria are present on the brush border of histologically normal villi of the small intestine, with minimal or no inflammatory response (Fig. 2.31). Organisms can be readily visualized with Gram stains (Fig. 2.32). Ultrastructurally, the organisms possess a prominent glycocalyx and superficially populate the brush border of enterocytes (Fig. 2.33).

Diagnosis

Diagnosis is achieved by demonstration of typical lesions in affected rats. Isolation of *Enterococcus* spp. from the intestine of rats is not diagnostic, since *Enterococci* are part of the normal microbiome of conventional rats. This fact poses the question of an underlying contributing factor in this disease, which has not been explored.

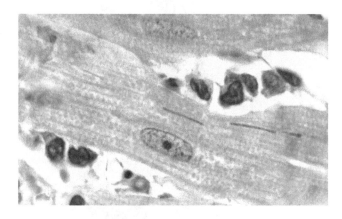

FIG. 2.30. *Myocardium from a rat with Tyzzer's disease. Tyzzer's bacilli are present within myofibers. Giemsa stain. (Source: R. Feinstein, The National Veterinary Institute, Sweden. Reproduced with permisison from R. Feinstein.)*

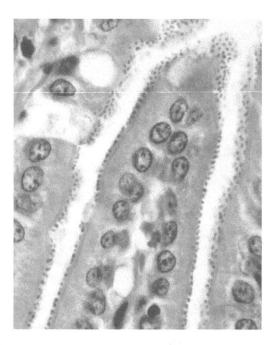

FIG. 2.31. *Small intestine from a suckling rat with streptococcal (enterococcal) enteropathy. The morphology of the villi and enterocytes are essentially normal, with numerous coccoid organisms adherent to the brush border.*

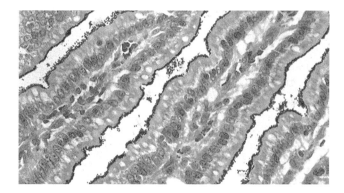

FIG. 2.32. *Small intestine from the case of streptococcal (enterococcal) enteropathy depicted in the previous figure. Note the aggregations of Gram-positive cocci on the surface of the villi (Brown and Brenn stain).*

Helicobacter *spp. Infections*

Although infections with *Helicobacter* spp. occur in laboratory rats, they have not assumed the importance of counterpart infections in the mouse. Species identified to date in the rat include *Helicobacter bilis*, *Helicobacter trogontum*, *Helicobacter muridarum*, and *Helicobacter pullorum*. There is no evidence that any of the *Helicobacter* isolates currently identified produce disease in immunocompetent rats. In contrast, proliferative and ulcerative typhlitis, colitis, and proctitis have been observed in athymic nude rats naturally infected with *H. bilis* (Figs. 2.34 and 2.35). Intraperitoneal inoculation of this isolate into athymic rats produced similar lesions in the intestinal tract. Laboratory Brown Norway rats have been shown to be infected with *H. pullorum*. Experimental studies demonstrated that Brown Norway, but not Sprague-Dawley, rats were susceptible to experimental infection with *H. pullorum*. Based on data from diagnostic laboratories, the prevalence of *Helicobacter*-positive colonies of laboratory rats may approach 20%. Fecal PCR is generally used as a screening method to detect *Helicobacter* infections in rodents.

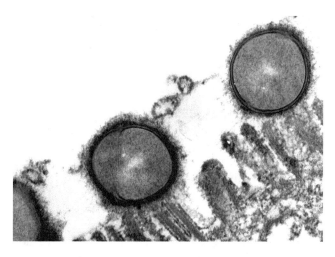

FIG. 2.33. *Electron micrograph of small intestinal mucosa from a case of streptococcal (enterococcal) enteropathy. Note the prominent glycocalyx surrounding the bacteria and their relationship to the brush border.*

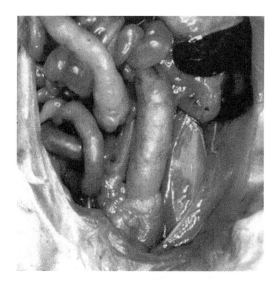

FIG. 2.34. *Helicobacter-associated colitis in an athymic rat with thickening of the colon due to mucosal hyperplasia. (Source: J.M. Ward, Montgomery Village, MD. Reproduced with permission from J.M. Ward.)*

Lawsonia intracellularis *Infection*

Along with other species (particularly hamsters and rabbits), rats are susceptible to infection with *L. intracellularis*. Natural infection of laboratory Wistar rats has been reported, in which multiple rats were described that developed adenocarcinomas of the ascending colon. With Warthin–Starry staining and electron microscopy, lesions contained typical intracytoplasmic bacteria within the apical cytoplasm of hyperplastic enterocytes. At the time, the bacteria were considered to be *Campylobacter*-like organisms, and *C. jejuni*-like bacteria were isolated from affected rats, contributing to the assumption of etiology. In retrospect, the intracytoplasmic bacteria had pathognomonic features of *L. intracellularis*. Lesions resembled the invasive hyperplastic crypt epithelium and histiocytic inflammation in hamsters infected with *L. intracellularis*, with formation of multiple cystic granulomatous subserosal nodules and occasional extension into mesenteric lymph nodes. In all

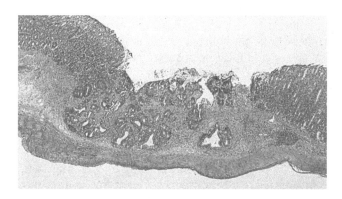

FIG. 2.35. *Helicobacter-associated colitis in an athymic rat. The colonic mucosa is hyperplastic, with focal crypt atypia and crypt herniation. (Source: J.M. Ward, Montgomery Village, MD. Reproduced with permission from J.M. Ward.)*

probability, the lesions were not neoplastic, but the epithelial invasiveness typical of this disease has led to that conclusion in hamsters as well.

Salmonella enterica *Infection*

Salmonella enterica infects and produces disease in a wide variety of animals, including humans. For this reason, it can be introduced to laboratory animal populations in a number of ways. During the early years of the 20th century, *Salmonella* infections represented an important infectious disease in laboratory rodents. However, with improved sanitation, health-monitoring methods, and feeding practices, the disease now rarely occurs in laboratory animal colonies. During 1895–1910, serotype Enteritidis was used as a rodenticide to control populations of wild rats in Europe and the United States. Enthusiasm waned when the public health implications became apparent. Of the multitude of serotypes of *S. enterica* capable of causing disease in the laboratory rat, serotypes Enteritidis and Typhimurium have been most frequently implicated.

Pathology

Clinical signs include depression, ruffled hair coat, porphyrin crusting around the eyes, hunched posture, weight loss, and variations in the nature of the feces from softer, lighter, formed feces to fluid feces. Subclinical infections without discernible lesions are frequent. In clinically affected rats, the ileum and cecum are often distended with liquid contents and flecks of blood, and there may be thickening of the gut wall in affected areas. Focal ulcerations may be present in the mucosa of the cecum and ileum. Splenomegaly frequently occurs. On microscopic examination, lesions in the ileum and cecum are characterized by hyperplasia of crypt epithelial cells, edema of the lamina propria, and leukocytic infiltration with focal ulceration. There is hyperplasia of the mesenteric lymph nodes, spleen, and Peyer's patches, with focal necrosis and leukocytic infiltration. In acute cases, lesions in other viscera are consistent with a Gram-negative septicemia, with focal embolization within spleen, liver, and lymph nodes. Emboli consist of bacteria, fibrinous exudate, and cellular debris. In the spleen, focal granulomas, fibrinous exudation, and focal necrosis are typical lesions present in the red pulp. Sinusoidal congestion and focal coagulation necrosis are frequent findings in the liver.

Diagnosis

Isolation and identification of the organism from animals with lesions or from inapparent carriers are necessary to confirm the diagnosis of *S. enterica* infection. Salmonellae are intermittently present in the intestine, especially in carrier animals. Repeated fecal samplings may be required in order to detect inapparent carrier animals. At necropsy, mesenteric lymph nodes are a tissue of choice, as they tend to yield *Salmonella* in

rats with negative fecal culture. Differential diagnoses include Tyzzer's disease, pseudomoniasis, *C. jejuni* infection, Enterococcus enteritis, rotaviral enteritis, cryptosporidiosis, and management-related problems due to failure to provide feed or water.

Other Bacterial Infections
Corynebacterium kutscheri *Infection: Pseudotuberculosis; Corynebacteriosis*

Corynebacterium kutscheri is a Gram-positive bacillus that can infect mice, rats, and guinea pigs.

The organism is frequently harbored as an inapparent infection. The organism may be carried for several weeks in the oropharynx and adjacent lymph nodes in the absence of inflammatory lesions. In clinical cases, hematogenous spread occurs from these sites, with resultant dissemination to the thoracic and abdominal viscera. Visceral abscesses will eventually heal by scarring and become culture-negative. Clinically, all age groups may be infected.

Disease and mortality are usually associated with concomitant disease states, such as immunosuppression or nutritional deficiencies. Infections with viral pathogens such as rat coronavirus, Sendai virus, or parvovirus do not appear to alter the course of the disease experimentally.

Pathology

Weight loss, respiratory distress, and ruffled hair coat are typical clinical signs, when present. At necropsy, dark red encrustations may be present around the eyes and external nares, or there may be a mucopurulent exudate around the nose. In the lung, there are frequently raised pale foci of suppuration of variable size with a characteristic hyperemic peripheral zone (Fig. 2.36). Affected areas frequently coalesce with adjacent lesions. Raised foci may be present in other organs, particularly the liver and kidney (Fig. 2.37). Fibrinous exudate may be present on the pleura and/or pericardium.

Lesions most frequently occur in the lung. There are foci of coagulation to caseation necrosis, with leukocytic infiltration. Neutrophils are the predominant cellular infiltrates in the early stages. Subsequently, there are mononuclear cells composed of macrophages, lymphocytes, and plasma cells. Lesions arise hematogenously, and early lesions can be found in association with blood vessels (Fig. 2.38). Adjacent pulmonary parenchyma may have interstitial pneumonia, with hypercellularity of alveolar septa, perivascular cuffing, and pulmonary edema. Some airways adjacent to affected areas may contain purulent exudate. Lesions of several days duration are suppurative in nature, with peripheral mononuclear cell infiltration and fibrosis. Large bacterial colonies are pathognomonic in lesions that have not resolved (Fig. 2.39), and appear as amorphous basophilic material in H&E stained tissue sections. Lymphoid hyperplasia is a frequent finding in chronic cases of

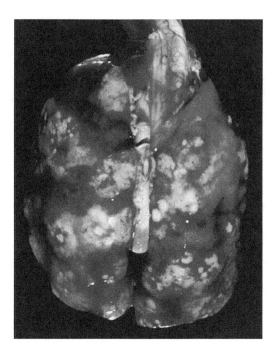

FIG. 2.36. Corynebacterium kutscheri *infection (pseudotuberculosis) in an adult rat. Note the multiple foci of abscessation with peripheral reddening and consolidation in the lung.*

corynebacteriosis, and residual scars may be present in target tissues in recovered animals.

Diagnosis

The distribution and nature of the lesions require confirmation by bacterial culture of affected organs or oropharyngeal washings. Gram, Warthin–Starry, or Giemsa stains will reveal the diphtheroid appearance of the bacilli, with "Chinese letter" configurations. Detection

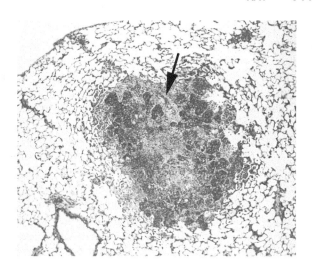

FIG. 2.38. *Lung from a case of early* Corynebacterium kutscheri *dissemination. Note inflammation arising at the terminus of a small artery (arrow), indicative of hematogenous dissemination.*

of carrier animals is best accomplished by culture or PCR of oropharyngeal washes or cervical lymph nodes. Serology is available for detecting seropositive rats. Differential diagnoses include pulmonary abscessation associated with advanced cases of chronic respiratory disease, acute to chronic pseudomoniasis, or diplococcal infections.

Erysipelas rhusiopathiae *Infection*

Erysipelas rhusiopathiae infections were observed in an outbreak that occurred in laboratory rats in Scandinavia. Lesions included chronic fibrinopurulent polyarthritis, myocarditis, and endocarditis. *Erysipelas* was isolated from affected joints.

Haemophilus *spp. and V-Factor-Dependent* Pasteurellaceae *Infection*

Haemophilus spp. and V-factor-dependent Pasteurellaceae belong to the family Pasteurellaceae. Specific pathogen-free rats are often colonized with *Haemophilus* spp.

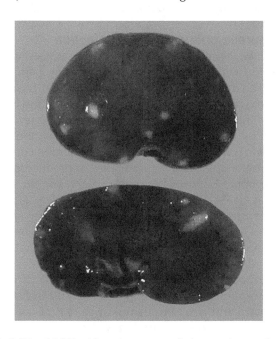

FIG. 2.37. *Multifocal hematogenous renal abscesses in a rat due to* Corynebacterium kutscheri *infection.*

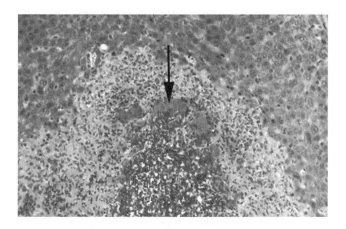

FIG. 2.39. Corynebacterium kutscheri *abscess in the liver of a rat. Note the prominent colonies of bacteria (arrow) adjacent to the necrotic center of the lesion.*

and V-factor-dependent Pasteurellaceae, which are generally commensal in nature, but can be opportunistic pathogens under some circumstances. An undefined species of *Haemophilus* has been isolated from the nasal cavity, trachea, lungs, and female genital tract of rats. In rats sampled from one vendor, the organism was recovered from a significant percentage of animals, and antibodies to the *Haemophilus* sp. were detected in close to 50% of animals tested. On microscopic examination, mild inflammatory cell infiltrates were present in the lower respiratory tract. Coinfection with other respiratory pathogens was not fully investigated. Experimental intranasal inoculation of athymic F344-*rnu* rats with V-factor-dependent Pasteurellaceae isolates resulted in colonization of the respiratory tract, but without discernable clinical signs or lesions. There is a very blurred distinction between commensal and pathogen within this family, so that the Federation for European Laboratory Animal Science Associations (FELASA) recommends screening for all members of Pasteurellaceae by serology, culture, and/or PCR.

Klebsiella pneumoniae *Infection*

Klebsiella pneumoniae is an opportunistic pathogen in the rat, since it can be isolated from feces of normal animals. However, this organism has been associated with abscesses of cervical, inguinal, and mesenteric lymph nodes and of kidney. This organism has also been associated with mild suppurative rhinitis in otherwise pathogen-free rats.

Leptospira *spp. Infection*

Leptospirosis in humans is the most widespread zoonotic disease throughout the world, and wild rats and mice play an important role as maintenance hosts for pathogenic *Leptospira*. Among the 13 recognized species of pathogenic *Leptospira*, there are numerous serogroups and serovars, but neither serogroup nor serovar is predictive of species (see Mouse Chapter 1, "*Leptospira* spp. infection" for a discussion of nomenclature). Rats are clinically silent chronic carriers of *Leptospira*, and both pet rats and laboratory rats have also been found to carry pathogenic *Leptospira* and be sources of human infection. Pathology in rats is minimal, consisting of mild nonsuppurative interstitial nephritis. Leptospires populate the proximal tubules (Fig. 2.40) in large numbers, and are shed through urine. They can be visualized in tissue sections with Warthin–Starry or other silver stains, and cultured from kidney tissue. Speciation is accomplished through DNA hybridization analysis.

Mycoplasma haemomuris *Infection*

Formerly known as *Hemobartonella muris*, *Mycoplasma haemomuris* is now classified as a member of the genus *Mycoplasma*. It is a hemotropic *Mycoplasma* that infects wild rats and other rodents and at one time was common in laboratory rats. It is transmitted primarily by *Polyplax*

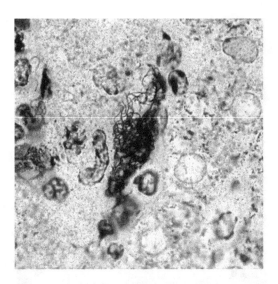

FIG. 2.40. *Colonization of a renal tubular lumen with* Leptospira *sp. in an infected rat (Warthin–Starry stain). (Source: Tucunduva de Faria et al. 2007. Reproduced with permission from Elsevier.)*

spinulosa and can also be transmitted in utero, but apparently inefficiently, since cesarean section is usually successful at eliminating the organism. *Mycoplasma haemomuris* can contaminate biological products derived from infected rodents and is infectious in both rats and mice. Natural infections are invariably inapparent, with mild transient bacteremia, splenomegaly, and erythrocytic reticulocytosis. The reticuloendothelial system, especially the spleen, is critical for clearing the bacteremia. Splenectomy of carrier rats may result in hemolytic anemia with hemoglobinuria and death. Immunosuppression with corticosteroids is ineffective in activating a subclinical infection. Diagnosis can now be achieved by PCR of blood from infected rodents.

Pasteurella pneumotropica *Infection*

Pasteurella pneumotropica commonly colonizes rodent intestine, where it may be carried for long periods of time. The organism can also be isolated from the nasopharynx, conjunctiva, lower respiratory tract, and uterus as an inapparent infection. Transmission probably occurs by direct contact or fecal contamination. The organism is frequently isolated in the absence of disease, and intranasal inoculation has failed to produce lesions in the upper or lower respiratory tract. On the other hand, it may represent an important secondary bacterial invader and opportunistic infection in primary *M. pulmonis* or Sendai virus infections. Interstitial pneumonia with polymorphonuclear cell infiltration has been observed in pregnant rats with primary Sendai virus and secondary *P. pneumotropica* infection. Fetal death and resorption occurred in approximately 30% of fetuses in infected animals. Abundant growth of *P. pneumotropica* was recovered from the lungs of affected dams. An outbreak of chronic necrotizing mastitis in Fischer 344 rats has also been attributed to the organism. Intranasal inoculation of athymic F344-rnu rats with a number of *P. pneumontropica* isolates resulted in colonization of the respiratory tract, but variable disease. When present, clinical signs included sneezing, and lesions consisted of mild nasal mucosal necrosis and inflammation. These studies underscored the concept that pathogenicity of *P. pneumotropica* is generally mild and bacterial strain dependent.

Pathology

Although infection is often subclinical in the absence of lesions, lesions may include rhinitis, sinusitis, conjunctivitis, otitis media, suppurative bronchopneumonia, subcutaneous abscessation, suppurative or chronic necrotizing mastitis, and pyometra.

Diagnosis

Recovery of the organism from lesions in pure culture is an important step in confirming the diagnosis. *Pasteurella pneumotropica* has bipolar staining properties and grows on conventional media under aerobic conditions. PCR can also be used to screen for *P. pneumotropica* as well as other *Pasteurellaceae*. Differential diagnosis includes other pyogenic organisms such as *Staphylococcus*, *Corynebacterium*, or *Pseudomonas*.

Pseudomonas aeruginosa *Infection: Pseudomoniasis*

Pseudomonas aeruginosa is an opportunistic Gram-negative bacillus that contaminates a variety of environments, including food, bedding, water bottles, bottle stoppers, and sipper tubes. *Pseudomonas* has also been recovered from human carriers, including feces. Ungloved hands are considered to be a source of the organism in animal facilities. Upon exposure, the organism transiently localizes in the oropharynx, upper respiratory tract, and the large intestine. Maintenance of infection requires continuous exposure, which is most expeditiously maintained through sipper tubes. Following exposure to *P. aeruginosa*, the incidence of inapparent healthy carriers is usually around 5–20%. Antibiotic treatment facilitates colonization with *P. aeruginosa*, presumably by reducing the inhibitory effect of normal microflora. Disease is typically precipitated by predisposing factors that result in neutropenia, including irradiation and treatment with steroids or other immunosuppressants. In addition, surgical procedures such as the implantation of indwelling jugular catheters may result in acute to chronic pseudomoniasis. Among populations at risk, detection of carriers by culturing sipper tubes, improved sanitation, and chlorination or acidification of the drinking water are recommended.

Pathology

In acute cases, there may be pulmonary edema, splenomegaly, and visceral ecchymoses, consistent with a Gram-negative bacterial septicemia. In rats that succumb during the subacute to chronic stages of the disease, multifocal necrosis with abscessation may be present in organs such as lung, spleen, and kidney. In animals with indwelling jugular catheters, vegetative lesions may be present on the tricuspid valves. On microscopic examination, lesions in acute cases are those of an acute bacterial septicemia, with vasculitis, thrombosis, hemorrhage, and polymorphonuclear leukocyte infiltration. In affected foci, changes vary from acute coagulative necrosis to suppuration, with obliteration of the normal architecture. Lesions are usually most extensive in the lung. In addition to thromboembolic changes with hemorrhage, bacterial colonies and proteinaceous fluid are frequently present in alveoli.

Diagnosis

The history of procedures that induce neutropenia or certain surgical manipulations, coupled with typical gross and microscopic changes, should be sufficient to provide a provisional diagnosis. The Gram-negative organisms are usually identifiable in sections stained with tissue Gram stains. The organism can usually be recovered from heart blood or spleen in septicemic animals. In subacute to chronic cases, *P. aeruginosa* may be isolated from visceral lesions. Differential diagnoses include visceral abscessation due to *C. kutscheri* or *P. pneumotropica* infections, salmonellosis, and pulmonary abscessation associated with chronic respiratory disease.

Staphylococcus aureus *Infection: Ulcerative Dermatitis*

Staphylococcus aureus is a ubiquitous commensal bacterium that inhabits the skin and mucous membranes of laboratory rodents. Infection is usually subclinical, but *S. aureus* may be associated with ulcerative skin lesions among adult rats and occasionally vesicular dermatitis in infant rats. The incidence of ulcerative dermatitis may vary from 1–2% to over 20% in certain populations of rats. The syndrome is particularly common in NK-deficient beige (Chediak–Higashi syndrome) rats. Lesions are most common in males. Trauma with persistent irritation appears to be an important contributing factor. Toenail clipping or amputation of the toes of the hind feet has resulted in remission of skin lesions, emphasizing the role of self-trauma in the disease. Changes ranging from alopecia to superficial ulceration have been associated with linoleic acid deficiency in Dahl rats. Linoleic acid plays a role in the cornification process and the maintenance of healthy skin. A marked increase in the numbers of *S. aureus* has been observed on the skin of mice deficient in linoleic acid. The significance, if any, of these findings in naturally occurring cases of ulcerative dermatitis in rats is unknown.

Pathology

Irregular, circumscribed red ulcerative skin lesions occur over the shoulder and rib cage, submandibular regions,

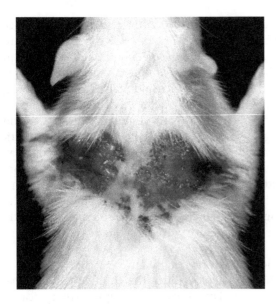

FIG. 2.41. *Ulcerative dermatitis of the dorsal neck and interscapular regions in a Sprague-Dawley rat. This syndrome is associated with* Staphylococcus aureus *infection.*

neck, ears, and head (Fig. 2.41). In acute cases, microscopic examination of lesions reveals an ulcerative dermatitis, with underlying coagulation necrosis of the underlying dermis. In adjacent areas, there is hyperplasia of the epidermis, with leukocytic infiltration into the underlying dermis (Fig. 2.42). Colonies of Gram-positive coccoid bacteria may be present within the proteinaceous material on the surface of lesions. There may be variable degeneration and leukocytic infiltration of the adnexae in affected areas. In lesions of some duration, dermal sclerosis and mononuclear cell infiltration are prominent features. Healed lesions frequently have dense collagenous tissue in the dermis, with loss of hair follicles and other adnexae. Histopathology suggests a role of epidermolytic toxin, as early stages are reminiscent of burn lesions. Lesions in deeper tissues may manifest botryomycotic features of the Splendore–Hoeppli response, with colonies of Gram-positive cocci

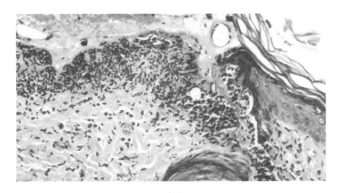

FIG. 2.42. *Skin of a rat with ulcerative dermatitis. There is a sharply demarcated area of epidermal coagulation necrosis with underlying leukocytic infiltration. Discrete colonies of darkly staining coccoid bacteria are present within the surface exudate. (Source: T.W. Forest.)*

surrounded by radiate eosinophilic material. Mastitis, subcutaneous abscesses, and infection of prepucial glands may also be associated with *S. aureus* infection.

Diagnosis

The presence of the typical ulcerative lesion with colonization by Gram-positive cocci is diagnostic. Bacterial cultures yield coagulase-positive *S. aureus*. Differential diagnoses include mycotic infections, fighting injuries, and, rarely, skin lesions associated with epitheliotropic lymphoid tumors (mycosis fungoides).

Streptobacillus moniliformis *Infection: Rat Bite Fever*

Streptobacillus moniliformis is a Gram-negative, pleomorphic rod or filamentous commensal organism that inhabits the nasopharynx of rats. It may also be present in the blood and urine of infected animals. Infection is common in wild rats and is rarely found in some populations of laboratory rats. Infection of pet rats has also been documented. It can be associated with opportunistic respiratory infections and can cause wound infections and abscesses. It has been found in bronchiolectatic abscesses of rats with chronic respiratory disease, in concert with *M. pulmonis* and CAR bacillus. Of particular concern is its pathogenicity in humans and mice. In humans, it is the cause of rat bite fever. There have been documented cases of systemic infections with mortality in children and in previously healthy adults. In human patients, clinical signs include maculopapular and pustular rash, fever, headache, and polyarthritis. Transmission may occur by bites, close contact with infected rats, or the inadvertent ingestion of rat excreta. A similar syndrome, called Haverill fever, has been associated with ingestion of rat-contaminated foodstuffs, particularly milk. Another commensal bacterium, *Spirillum muris*, has also been associated with rat bite fever (particularly in Asian countries). Laboratory rats should be monitored for infection by culture of blood or nasopharygeal swabs in appropriate media, serology, and/or PCR. Infected colonies should be depopulated because of zoonotic risk.

Streptococcus pneumoniae *Infection: Pneumococcal or Diplococcal Infection*

In the past, diplococcal (pneumococcal) infections due to *S. pneumoniae* were recognized to be a common problem in laboratory rats. Today, outbreaks of clinical disease are rarely recognized in well-managed, barrier-maintained facilities. The organism is carried primarily in the nasoturbinates and tympanic bullae in clinically normal rats. Some of the serotypes isolated from rats are identical to those isolated from human cases, and human carriers have been implicated as a possible source of the organism. Conversely, *S. pneumonia*-infected rats represent a potential zoonotic hazard. *Streptococcus pneumoniae* may cause acute primary disease with mortality, but frequently it represents an important secondary invader, particularly in respiratory infections. An abundant polysaccharide capsule enables the organism to resist phagocytosis by the host cells. Pneumococci are not known to produce soluble toxins. However, several of the recognized serotypes produce tissue damage by activation of the alternate complement pathway. In clinically normal animals infected with the organism, predisposing factors such as concurrent infections or environmental changes may precipitate disease.

Pathology

Clinical signs may include serosanguinous nasal discharge, rhinitis, sinusitis, conjunctivitis, and vestibular signs consistent with middle ear infection. At necropsy, there may be serous to mucopurulent exudate present in the nasal passages, with variable involvement of the tympanic bullae. In the acute systemic form of the disease, there are variable patterns of characteristic fibrinopurulent polyserositis, including pleuritis, pericarditis (Fig. 2.43), peritonitis, periorchitis, and meningitis. Fibrinopurulent lesions may be confined to the leptomeninges in some fatal cases. There may be consolidation of one or more lung lobes. Affected areas are dark red to dull tan and relatively firm and nonresilient. On microscopic examination, in the acute form of the disease, fibrinopurulent pleuritis and pericarditis are typical findings. Pulmonary changes vary from localized suppurative bronchopneumonia to acute fibrinopurulent bronchopneumonia, with obliteration of the normal architecture in affected lobes. Fibrinopurulent peritonitis, perihepatitis, and/or leptomeningitis are frequent findings. Suppurative rhinitis and otitis media may also occur. Embolic suppurative lesions have been observed in organs such as liver, spleen, and kidney. In more chronic, localized disease states, pneumococcal

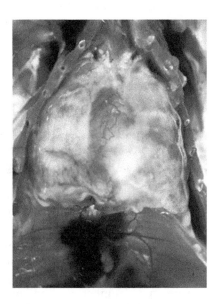

FIG. 2.43. *Fibrinous pericarditis and pleuritis in a young rat with acute diplococcal* (Streptococcus pneumoniae) *infection.*

infections have been associated with suppurative bronchopneumonia in chronic respiratory disease, as well as otitis media.

Diagnosis

The presence of fibrinopurulent serositis is characteristic when present, and demonstration of the typical encapsulated diplococci in Gram-stained smears from lesions will provide a provisional diagnosis. Confirmation of streptococcosis requires the collection and culture of material from lesions and identification of the alpha-hemolytic organism. Nasal lavage at necropsy is a recommended procedure to recover the organism for bacterial culture. Differential diagnoses include corynebacteriosis, salmonellosis, pseudomoniasis, and pasteurellosis.

Bacterial Pyelonephritis/Nephritis

Suppurative pyelonephritis is more commonly encountered in male rats, and may be associated with a concurrent disease process, such as cystitis or prostatitis. A variety of bacteria have been recovered from affected kidneys, including *Escherichia coli*, *Klebsiella* sp., *P. aeruginosa*, *Corynebacterium* sp., *Streptococcus* sp., *Enterococcus* spp., and *Proteus* sp. The lower urinary tract is considered to be the most likely portal of entry in pyelonephritis. Excavation of the renal papilla, dilation of the renal pelves, and the accumulation of suppurative inflammatory exudates are typical findings. In cases of suppurative nephritis involving the renal interstitium, descending infections with bacterial emboli are the usual source of the infection. *Streptococci* are the most common isolates. Lesions are similar to those seen in other species with suppurative disease processes of this system.

FUNGAL INFECTIONS

Aspergillus spp. Infection

There have been isolated reports of outbreaks and sporadic cases of upper respiratory tract infections in laboratory rats due to *Aspergillus fumigatus* or *Aspergillus niger*. On microscopic examination, the changes are consistent with a chronic rhinitis with epithelial changes varying from hyperplasia to squamous metaplasia. Pulmonary aspergillosis has also been reported in laboratory rats. Fungal hyphae are readily demonstrated on epithelial surfaces of affected nasal passages or lung lesions with PAS or silver stains. Possible predisposing factors include contaminated bedding, air quality, the presence of concurrent infections, and immune status of the host.

Blastomyces dermatitidis Infection

Pulmonary lesions, consisting of multifocal to coalescing gray-white nodules, due to *Blastomyces* spp. infection have been documented in a laboratory rat. Microscopic findings included bronchopneumonia with multifocal pyogranulomas containing thick-walled yeast forms.

Speciation of the causative agent was achieved by PCR and DNA sequencing. The source of infection was not found.

Dermatophyte Infection: Dermatophytosis, Ringworm

Recognized infections with dermatophytes are relatively rare in contemporary laboratory rats, although infection appears to occur more frequently in wild and pet rats. Dermatophyte infections in rats are most commonly caused by *Trichophyton mentagrophytes*, which poses a zoonotic risk to human handlers. In confirmed outbreaks of the disease, patterns vary from subclinical carriers to rats with florid skin lesions. Lesions, when present, are most frequently observed on the neck, back, and at the base of the tail. There is patchy hair loss, and affected areas of skin are usually raised, erythematous, dry to moist, and pustular in appearance. On microscopic examination, hyperkeratosis, epidermal hyperplasia, and leukocytic infiltration in the underlying dermis with folliculitis are typical findings. Arthrospores investing hair shafts may be seen on H & E-stained tissue sections, but the fungi are better demonstrated with PAS or methenamine silver stains (Fig. 2.44). The skin scrapings with wet mount preparations in 10% KOH and fungal culture are recommended procedures.

Encephalitozoon cuniculi Infection

Encephalitozoon cuniculi infection of laboratory rats is not common, but has been associated with nonsuppurative focal lesions in the brain, kidneys, and occasionally liver. See Rabbit Chapter 6, "*Encephalitozoon cuniculi* infection" for a more complete description of this disease.

Phycomycotic Infection

Immature rats have been found to rarely develop phycomycotic meningoencephalitis, with necropurulent

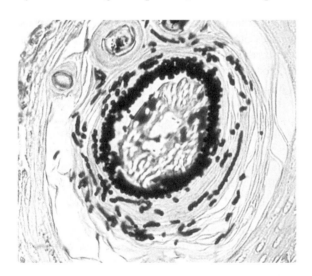

FIG. 2.44. *Skin from a rat with* Trichophyton mentagrophytes *dermatophytosis. Numerous arthrospores are present within the hair follicle (methenamine silver stain).*

inflammation containing nonseptate hyphae that are demonstrable with various fungal stains. Older rats within the same populations were unaffected.

Pneumocystis carinii *and* Pneumocystis wakefieldiae *Infections: Pneumocystosis*

Laboratory rats have been central to understanding the biology of *Pneumocystis*. Rats were recognized to develop pneumonias caused by a new organism that had features similar to human disease. Although not the first host species to be shown to be infected with *Pneumocystis* (guinea pigs get that honor), rats were definitively shown to be infected with a similar agent that was the first *Pneumocystis* to be named: *Pneumocystis carinii*. Because the organism cannot be cultured or propagated in vitro, the rat became an important model and source of infectious organisms, which has given way to immunodeficient mice in recent years. For many years, *Pneumocystis* was thought to be a protozoan, giving way to terminology that continues in use today, including trophozoites, cysts, and sporozoites. It became apparent in early studies that there was a high degree of host species specificity among *Pneumocystis* organisms. The advent of molecular sequencing revealed the true complexity of this genus, finally recognizing *Pneumocystis* to be a fungus, and giving rise to a multitude of new names and species. Human pneumocystosis is now recognized to be caused by human-specific *Pneumocystis jiroveci*, but physicians continue to use "PCP" (*P. carinii* pneumonia) as a common term for the human condition. Since *P. carinii* was initially assigned to the rat, rats have been awarded this species as their own. It is now recognized that rats can serve as hosts to at least 5 species of *Pneumocystis*, and laboratory rats have been shown to be host to 2 of those species, including *P. carinii* and *P. wakefieldiae*. The former is the most common among laboratory rats, but dual infections occur. The mouse agent is genetically distinct, and named *Pneumocystis murina*.

Pulmonary lesions associated with *Pneumocystis* infection and propagation of organisms have been produced in young laboratory rats from infected colonies that were treated for several weeks with immunosuppressants such as cortisone and fed a protein-deficient diet. Steroid-treated female rats develop the disease at a faster rate than male rats. Spontaneous pneumocystosis has been recognized in athymic rats. During the late 1990s, inflammatory lesions were noted in young immunocompetent rats, which were attributed to a putative viral agent called "rat respiratory virus (RRV)." Recent studies have revealed that RRV is *Pneumocystis*, rather than a virus. *Pneumocystis* is transmitted by aerosol exposure during the neonatal period. Six- to twelve-week-old rats are optimal shedders of *Pneumocystis*, after which time *Pneumocystis* numbers decline until they are completely cleared from the immunocompetent host. Infection within an enzootically infected population is

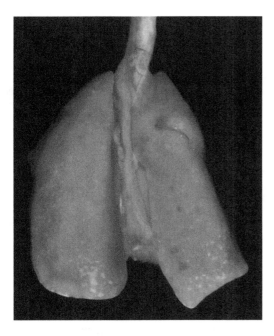

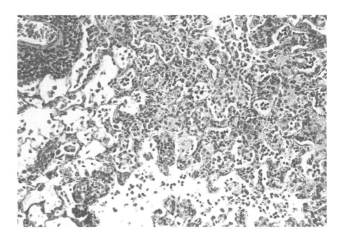

FIG. 2.47. *Lung from a young rat with pulmonary lesions that were once attributed to "rat respiratory virus" infection, but have been found to be due to* Pneumocystis *sp. infection. Note the perivascular lymphocytic infiltrates, interstitial pneumonia, and the marked alveolar histiocytosis.*

FIG. 2.45. *Lungs from an immunocompromised rat with pneumocystosis. Note the failure to collapse and the raised foci in the subpleural regions consistent with focal cellular infiltrates.*

maintained by spore-shedding young rats that transmit infection to 3–4-week-old weanling rats with declining maternal antibody.

Pathology

In severely affected animals, clinical signs include dyspnea, cyanosis, and weight loss. There is diffuse to focal consolidation, lungs collapse poorly, and frequently, they have an opaque pale pink color (Fig. 2.45). On microscopic examination, there is alveolar flooding with foamy, eosinophilic material, presenting a honeycomb appearance (Fig. 2.46). In athymic rats, pulmonary lesions vary from mild interstitial pneumonia with

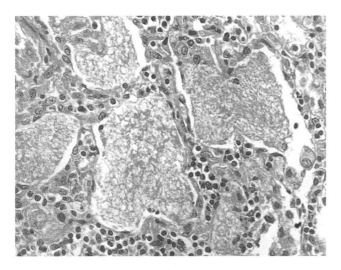

FIG. 2.46. *Lung from a rat with pneumocytosis. Alveoli are flooded with foamy material containing* Pneumocystis *organisms and the interstitium is infiltrated with mononuclear leukocytes.*

scattered alveolar macrophages to severe interstitial pneumonia with the alveoli distended with typical foamy material. In more advanced cases, in addition to the infiltrating inflammatory cells and the foamy alveolar exudate, there is marked proliferation of type II pneumocytes and interstitial fibrosis. In sections stained using procedures such as the Grocott modification of Gomori's methenamine silver technique, numerous black trophozoites and yeast-like cysts 3–5 μm in diameter are present singly or in groups within alveoli. Ultrastructural examination reveals trophozoites with filapodia in close association with type I pneumocytes.

Conventionally housed, young immunocompetent rats may develop transient multifocal nonsuppurative perivasculitis and interstitial pneumonia (Fig. 2.47), which may persist for several weeks. A scattering of neutrophils and focal hyperplasia of type II pneumocytes have also been observed during the course of the infection. Airways are usually spared, although there may be lymphocytic infiltrates around some bronchioles. These lesions were once considered to be due to RRV, but are now known to be associated with *Pneumocystis* infection. In the absence of an immunodeficient state (e.g., athymic rats), these lesions are far more likely to be encountered than the classic lesions of pulmonary pneumocystosis.

Diagnosis

The distinctive pulmonary lesions and the demonstration of the cyst forms (see Mouse Chapter 1, "*Pneumocystis murina* Infection") during active infection, using silver-staining procedures on impression smears of lung or in paraffin-embedded specimens, is generally used to confirm the diagnosis. PCR can be used to detect the organism in specimens collected from lung tissue, by bronchioalveolar lavage, or with oral swabs.

BIBLIOGRAPHY FOR BACTERIAL AND FUNGAL INFECTIONS

See "General References on Diseases of Rats"

Primary Respiratory Infections

Bordetella bronchiseptica Infection

Bemis, D.A., Shek, W.R., & Clifford, C.B. (2003) *Bordetella bronchiseptica* infection of mice and rats. *Comparative Medicine* 53:11–20.

Bemis, D.A. & Wilson, S.A. (1985) Influence of potential virulence determinants on *Bordetella bronchiseptica*-induced ciliostasis. *Infection and Immunity* 50:35–42.

Burek, J.D., Jersey, G.C., Whitehair, C.K., & Carter, G.R. (1972) The pathology and pathogenesis of *Bordetella bronchiseptica* and *Pasteurella pneumotropica* infection in conventional and germ-free rats. *Laboratory Animal Science* 22:844–849.

Cilia-Associated Respiratory (CAR) Bacillus Infection

Franklin, C.L., Pletz, J.D., Riley, L.K., Livingston, B.A., Hook, R.R., Jr., & Besch-Williford, C.L. (1999) Detection of cilia-associated respiratory (CAR) bacillus in nasal-swab specimens from infected rats by use of polymerase chain reaction. *Laboratory Animal Science* 49:114–117.

Ganaway, J.R., Spencer, T.R., Moore, T.D., & Allen, A.M. (1985) Isolation, propagation, and characterization of a newly recognized pathogen, cilia-associated respiratory bacillus of rats, an etiological agent of chronic respiratory disease. *Infection and Immunity* 47:472–479.

Hook, R.R., Franklin, C.L., Riley, L.K., Livingston, B.A., & Besch-Williford, C.L. (1998) Antigenic analyses of cilia-associated respiratory (CAR) bacillus isolates by use of monoclonal antibodies. *Laboratory Animal Science* 48:234–239.

Kawano, A., Nenoi, M., Matsushita, S., Matsumoto, T., & Mita, K. (2000) Sequence of 16S rRNA gene of rat-origin cilia-associated respiratory (CAR) bacillus SMR strain. *Journal of Veterinary Medical Science* 62:797–800.

MacKenzie, W.F., Magill, L.S., & Hulse, M. (1981) A filamentous bacterium associated with respiratory disease in wild rats. *Veterinary Pathology* 18:836–839.

Matsushita, S. (1986) Spontaneous respiratory disease associated with cilia-associated respiratory (CAR) bacillus in a rat. *Japanese Journal of Veterinary Science* 48:437–440.

Matsushita, S. & Joshima, H. (1989) Pathology of rats intranasally inoculated with cilia-associated respiratory bacillus. *Laboratory Animals* 23:89–95.

Medina, L.V., Chladnym, J., Fortman, J.D., Artwohol, J.E., Bunte, R.M., & Bennett, B.T. (1996) Rapid way to identify the cilia-associated respiratory bacillus: tracheal mucosal scraping with a modified microwave Steiner silver impregnation. *Laboratory Animal Science* 46:113–115.

Medina, L.V., Fortman, J.D., Bunte, R.M., & Bennett, B.T. (1994) Respiratory disease in a rat colony: identification of CAR bacillus without other respiratory pathogens by standard diagnostic screening methods. *Laboratory Animal Science* 44:521–525.

Schoeb, T.R., Davidson, M.K., & Davis, J.K. (1997) Pathogenicity of cilia-associated respiratory (CAR) bacillus isolates for F344, LEW, and SD rats. *Veterinary Pathology* 34:263–270.

Schoeb, T.R., Dybvig, K., Davidson, M.K., & Davis, J.K. (1993) Cultivation of cilia-associated respiratory bacillus in artificial medium and determination of the 16S rRNA gene sequence. *Journal of Clinical Microbiology* 31:2751–2757.

Van Zwieten, M.J., Sulleveld, H.A., Lindsey, J.R. de Groot, F.G., Zurcher, C., & Hollander, C.F. (1980) Respiratory disease in rats associated with a filamentous bacterium: a preliminary report. *Laboratory Animal Science* 30:215–221.

Mycoplasma pulmonis Infection

Aguila, H.N., Wayne, C.L., Lu, Y.S., & Pakes, S.P. (1988) Experimental *Mycoplasma pulmonis* infection of rats suppresses humoral but not cellular immune response. *Laboratory Animal Science* 38:138–142.

Brennan, P.C., Fritz, T.E., & Flynn, R.J. (1969) The role of *Pasteurella pneumotropica* and *Mycoplasma pulmonis* in murine pneumonia. *Journal of Bacteriology* 97:337–349.

Broderson, J.R., Lindsey, J.R., & Crawford, J.E. (1976) Role of environmental ammonia in respiratory mycoplasmosis of the rat. *American Journal of Pathology* 85:115–130.

Brunnert, S.R., Dai, Y., & Kohn, D. (1994) Comparison of polymerase chain reaction and immunohistochemistry for the detection of *Mycoplasma pulmonis* in paraffin-embedded tissue. *Laboratory Animal Science* 44:257–260.

Cassell, G.H. (1982) The pathogenic potential of mycoplasmas: *Mycoplasma pulmonis* as a model. *Reviews of Infectious Diseases* 4:S18–S34.

Cassell, G.H., Davis, J.K., Simecka, J.W., Lindsey, J.R., Cox, N.R., Ross, S., & Fallon, M. (1986) Mycoplasmal infections: disease pathogenesis, implications for biomedical research, and control. In: *Viral and Mycoplasmal Infections of Laboratory Rodents: Effects on Biomedical Research* (eds. P.N. Bhatt, R.O. Jacoby, H.C. Morse, III, & A.E. New), pp. 87–136. Academic Press, New York.

Davis, J.K. & Cassell, G.H. (1982) Murine respiratory mycoplasmosis in LEW and F344 rats: strain differences in lesion severity. *Veterinary Pathology* 19:280–293.

Schoeb, T.R., Kervin, K.C., & Lindsey, J.R. (1985) Exacerbation of murine respiratory mycoplasmosis in gnotobiotic F344/N rats by Sendai virus infection. *Veterinary Pathology* 22:272–282.

Schoeb, T.R. & Lindsey, J.R. (1987) Exacerbation of murine respiratory mycoplasmosis by sialodacryoadenitis virus infection in gnotobiotic F344 rats. *Veterinary Pathology* 24:392–399.

Steiner, D.A., Uhl, E.W., & Brown, M.D. (1993) In utero transmission of *Mycoplasma pulmonis* in experimentally infected Sprague-Dawley rats. *Infection and Immunity* 61:2985–2990.

Tully, J.G. (1986) Biology of rodent mycoplasmas. In: *Viral and Mycoplasmal Infections of Laboratory Rodents: Effects on Biomedical Research* (eds. P.N. Bhatt, R.O. Jacoby, H.C. Morse, III, & A.E. New) pp. 64–85. Academic Press, New York.

Primary Enteric Infections

Campylobacter jejuni Infection

Epoke, J. & Coker, A.O. (1991) Intestinal colonization of rats following experimental infection with *Campylobacter jejuni*. *East African Medical Journal* 68:348–351.

Meanger, J.D. & Marshall, R.B. (1989) *Campylobacter jejuni* infection within a laboratory animal production unit. *Laboratory Animals* 23:126–132.

Morales, W., Pimentel, M., Hwang, L., Kunkel, D., Pokkunuri, V., Basseri, B., Low, K., Wang, H., Conklin, J.L., & Chang, C. (2011) Acute and chronic histological changes of the small bowel secondary to *C. jejuni* infection in a rat model for post-infectious IBS. *Digestive Disease Science* 56:2575–2584.

Clostridium difficile Infection

Czuprynski, C.J., Johnson, W.J., Balish, E., & Wilkins, T. (1983) Pseudomembranous colitis in *Clostridium difficile*-monoassociated rats. *Infection and Immunity* 39:1368–1376.

Clostridium piliforme Infection

Fries, A.S. (1979) Studies on Tyzzer's disease: transplacental transmission of *Bacillus piliformis* in rats. *Laboratory Animals* 13:43–46.

Franklin, C.L., Motzel, S.L., Besch-Williford, C.L., Hook, R.R., Jr., & Riley, L.K. (1994) Tyzzer's infection: host specificity of *Clostridium piliforme* isolates. *Laboratory Animal Science* 44:568–572.

Fries, A.S. & Svendsen, O. (1978) Studies on Tyzzer's disease in rats. *Laboratory Animals* 12:1–4.

Fujiwara, K., Nakayama, M., & Takahashi, K. (1981) Serologic detection of inapparent Tyzzer's disease in rats. *Japanese Journal of Experimental Medicine* 51:197–200.

Furukawa, T., Furumoto, K., Fujieda, M., & Okada, E. (2002) Detection by PCR of the Tyzzer's disease organism (*Clostridium piliforme*). *Experimental Animals* 51:513–516.

Hansen, A.K., Skovgaard-Jensen, H.J., Thomsen, P., Svendsen, O., Dagnaes-Hansen, F., & Mollegaard-Hansen, K.E. (1992) Rederivation of rat colonies seropositive for *Bacillus piliformis* and subsequent screening for antibodies. *Laboratory Animal Science* 42:444–448.

Jonas, A.M., Percy, D., & Craft, J. (1970) Tyzzer's disease in the rat: its possible relationship with megaloileitis. *Archives of Pathology* 90:516–528.

Motzel, S.L. & Riley, L.K. (1992) Subclinical infection and transmission of Tyzzer's disease in rats. *Laboratory Animal Science* 42:439–443.

Riley, L.K., Besch-Williford, C., & Waggie, K.S. (1990) Protein and antigenic heterogeneity among isolates of *Bacillus piliformis*. *Infection and Immunity* 58:1010–1016.

Enterococcus spp. Infection

Etheridge, M.E. & Vonderfecht, S.L. (1992) Diarrhea caused by a slow-growing *Enterococcus*-like agent in neonatal rats. *Laboratory Animal Science* 42:548–550.

Etheridge, M.E., Yolken, R.H., & Vonderfecht, S.L. (1988) *Enterococcus hirae* implicated as a cause of diarrhea in suckling rats. *Journal of Clinical Microbiology* 26:1741–1744.

Gades, N.M., Mandrell, T.D., & Rogers, W.P. (1999) Diarrhea in neonatal rats. *Contemporary Topics in Laboratory Animal Science* 38:44–46.

Hoover, D., Bendele, S.A., Wightman, S.R., Thompson, C.Z., & Hoyt, J.A. (1985) Streptococcal enteropathy in infant rats. *Laboratory Animal Science* 35:653–641.

Helicobacter spp. Infections

Beckwith, C.S., Franklin, C.L., Hook, R.R., Jr., Besch-Williford, C.L., & Riley, L.K. (1997) Fecal PCR assay for diagnosis of *Helicobacter* infection in laboratory rodents. *Journal of Clinical Microbiology* 35:1620–1623.

Cacioppo, L.D., Shen, Z., Parry, J.M., & Fox, J.G. (2012) Resistance of Sprague-Dawley rats to infection with *Helicobacter pullorum*. *Journal of the American Association for Laboratory Animal Science* 51:803–807.

Cacioppo, L.D., Turk, M.L., Shen, Z., Ge, Z., Parry, N., Whary, M.T., Boutin, S.R., Klein, H.J., & Fox, J.G. (2012) Natural and experimental *Helicobacter pullorum* infection in Brown Norway rats. *Journal of Medical Microbiology* 61:1319–1323.

Haines, D.C., Goerlick, P.L., Battles, J.K., Pike, K.M., Anderson, R.J., Fox, J.G., Taylor, N.S., Shen, Z., Dewhirst, F.E., Anver, M.R., & Ward, J.M. (1998) Inflammatory large bowel disease in immunodeficient rats naturally and experimentally infected with *Helicobacter bilis*. *Veterinary Pathology* 35:202–208.

Lee, A.M.W. 1992. *Helicobacter muridarum* sp. nov., a microaerophilic helical bacterium with novel ultrastructure isolated from the intestinal mucosa of rodents. *International Journal of Systematic Bacteriology* 42:27–36.

Mendes, E.N., Quieroz, D.M.M., Dewhirst, F.E., Paster, B.J., Moura, S.B., & Fox, J.G. (1996) *Helicobacter trogontum* sp. nov. isolated from the rat intestine. *International Journal of Systematic Bacteriology* 46:916–921.

Phillips, M.W. & Lee, A. (1983) Isolation and characterization of a spiral bacterium from the crypts of rodent gastrointestinal tracts. *Applied Environmental Microbiology* 45:675–683.

Vandenberghe, J., Verheyen, A., Lauwers, S., & Geboes, K. (1985) Spontaneous adenocarcinoma of the ascending colon in Wistar rats: the intracytoplasmic presence of a *Campylobacter*-like bacterium. *Journal of Comparative Pathology* 95:45–55.

Whary, M.T. & Fox, J.G. (2004) Natural and experimental *Helicobacter* infections. *Comparative Medicine* 54:128–158.

Whary, M.T. & Fox, J.G. (2006) Detection, eradication, and research implications of *Helicobacter* infections in laboratory rodents. *Laboratory Animals (NY)*. 35:25–27, 30–36.

Lawsonia intracellularis Infection

Salmonella enterica Infection

Maenza, R.M., Powell, D.W., Plotkin, G.R., Focmal, S.B., Jervis, H.R., & Sprinz, H. (1970) Experimental diarrhea: *Salmonella* enterocolitis in the rat. *Journal of Infectious Diseases* 121:475–485.

Pappenheimer, A.M. & Von Wedel, H. (1914) Observations on a spontaneous typhoid-like epidemic of white rats. *Journal of Infectious Diseases* 14:180–185.

Thygesen, P., Martinsen, C., Hongen, H.P., Hattori, R., Stenvang, J.P., & Ryngaard, J. (2000) Histologic, cytologic, and bacteriologic examinations of experimentally induced *Salmonella typhimurium* infection in Lewis rats. *Comparative Medicine* 50:124–132.

Other Bacterial Infections

Corynebacterium kutscheri Infection

Ackerman, J.I., Fox, J.G., & Murphy, J.C. (1984) An enzyme linked immunoabsorbent assay for detection of antibodies to *Corynebacterium kutscheri* in experimentally infected rats. *Laboratory Animal Science* 34:38–43.

Amao, H., Komukai, Y., Akimoto, T., Sugiyama, M., Takahashi, K.W., Sawada, T., & Saito, M. (1995) Natural and subclinical *Corynebacterium kutscheri* infection in rats. *Laboratory Animal Science* 45:11–14.

Barthold, S.W. & Brownstein, D.G. (1988) The effect of selected viruses on *Corynebacterium kutscheri* infection in rats. *Laboratory Animal Science* 38:580–583.

Boot, R., Thuis, H., Bakker, R., & Veenema, J.L. (1995) Serological studies of *Corynebacterium kutscheri* and coryneform bacteria using an enzyme-linked immunosorbent assay. *Laboratory Animals* 29:294–299.

Brownstein, D.G., Barthold, S.W., Adams, R.L., Terwilliger, G.A., & Aftosmis, J.G. (1985) Experimental *Corynebacterium kutscheri* infection in rats: bacteriology and serology. *Laboratory Animal Science* 35:135–138.

Fox, J.G., Niemi, S.M., Ackerman, J., & Murphy, J.C. (1987) Comparison of methods to diagnose an epizootic of *Corynebacterium kutscheri* pneumonia in rats. *Laboratory Animal Science* 37:72–75.

Giddens, W.E., Keahey, K.K., Carter, G.R., & Whitehair, C.K. (1969) Pneumonia in rats due to infection with *Corynebacterium kutscheri*. *Pathologia Veterinaria* 5:227–237.

McEwen, S.A. & Percy, D.H. (1985) Diagnostic exercise: pneumonia in a rat. *Laboratory Animal Science* 35:485–487.

Erysipelas rhusiopathiae Infection

Feinstein, R.E. & Eld, K. (1989) Naturally occurring erysipelas in rats. *Laboratory Animals* 23:256–260.

Haemophilus spp. Infection

Boot, R., van den Berg, L., Van Lith, H.A., & Veenema, J.L. (2005) Rat strains differ in antibody response to natural *Haemophilus* species infection. *Laboratory Animals* 39:413–420.

Boot, R., Vlemminx, M.J., & Reubsaet, F.A. (2009) Comparison of polymerase chain reaction primer sets for amplification of rodent Pasteurellaceae. *Laboratory Animals* 43:371–375.

Bootz, F., Kirschnek, S., Nicklas, W., Wyss, S.K., & Homberger, F.R. (1998) Detection of Pasteurellaceae in rodents by polymerase chain reaction analysis. *Laboratory Animal Science* 48:542–546.

Hayashimoto, N., Yasuda, M., Ueno, M., Goto, K., & Takakura, A. (2008) Experimental infection studies of *Pasteurella pneumotropica* and V-factor dependent *Pasteurellaceae* for F344-*rnu* rats. *Experimental Animals* 57:57–63.

Nicklas, W. (1989) *Haemophilus* infection in a colony of laboratory rats. *Journal of Clinical Microbiology* 27:1636–1639.

Nicklas, W., Staut, M., & Benner, A. (1993) Prevalence and biochemical properties of V factor-dependent *Pasteurellaceae* from rodents. *Zentralblatt fur Bakteriologie* 279:114–124.

Klebsiella pneumoniae Infection

Jackson, N.N., Wall, H.G., Miller, C.A., & Rogul, M. (1980) Naturally acquired infections of *Klebsiella pneumonia* in Wistar rats. *Laboratory Animals* 14:357–361.

Leptospira spp. Infection

Athanazio, D.A., Silva, E.F., Santos, C., Rocha, G.M., Vannier-Santos, M.A., McBride, A.J.A., Ko, A.I., & Reis, M.G. (2008) *Rattus norvegicus* as a model for persistent renal colonization by pathogenic *Leptospira interrogans*. *Acta Tropica* 105:176–180.

Evangelista, K.V. & Coburn, J. (2010) *Leptospira* as an emerging pathogen: a review of its biology, pathogenesis and host immune responses. *Future Microbiology* 5:1413–1425.

Fuzi, M. & Csoka, R. (1961) Leptospirosis in white laboratory rats. *Nature* 191:1123.

Jansen, A. & Schneider, T. (2011) Weil's disease in a rat owner. *Lancet Infectious Diseases* 11:152.

Tucunduva de Faria, M.T., Athanazio, D.A., Goncalves Ramos, E.A., Silva, E.F., Reis, M.G. & Ko, A.I. (2007) Morphological alterations in the kidney of rats with natural and experimental *Leptospira* infection. *Journal of Comparative Pathology* 137:231–238.

Mycoplasma haemomuris Infection

Neimark, H., Johansson, K.E., Rikihisa, Y., & Tully, J.G. (2002) Revision of haemotropic *Mycoplasma* species names. *International Journal of Systematic and Evolutionary Microbiology* 52:683.

Zhang, C. & Rikihisa, Y. (2002) Evaluation of sensitivity and specificity of a *Mycoplasma haemomuris*-specific polymerase chain reaction test. *Comparative Medicine* 52:313–315.

Pasteurella pneumotropica Infection

Boot, R., Vlemminx, M.J., & Reubsaet, F.A. (2009) Comparison of polymerase chain reaction primer sets for amplification of rodent Pasteurellaceae. *Laboratory Animals* 43:371–375.

Brennan, P.C., Fritz, T.E., & Flynn, R.J. (1969) The role of *Pasteurella pneumotropica* and *Mycoplasma pulmonis* in murine pneumonia. *Journal of Bacteriology* 97:337–349.

Burek, J.D., Jersey, G.C., Whitehair, C.K., & Carter, G.R. (1972) The pathology and pathogenesis of *Bordetella bronchiseptica* and *Pasteurella pneumotropica* infection in conventional and germfree rats. *Laboratory Animal Science* 22:844–849.

Carthew, P. & Aldred, P. (1988) Embryonic death in pregnant rats owing to intercurrent infection with Sendai virus and *Pasteurella pneumotropica*. *Laboratory Animals* 22:92–97.

Hayashimoto, N., Yasuda, M., Ueno, M., Goto, K., & Takakura, A. (2008) Experimental infection studies of *Pasteurella pneumotropica* and V-factor dependent *Pasteurellaceae* for F344-*rnu* rats. *Experimental Animals* 57:57–63.

Hong, C.C. & Ediger, R.D. (1978) Chronic necrotizing mastitis in rats caused by *Pasteurella pneumotropica*. *Laboratory Animal Science* 28:317–320.

Moore, T.D., Allen, A.M., & Ganaway, J.R. (1973) Latent *Pasteurella pneumotropica* infection in the intestine of gnotobiotic and barrier-held rats. *Laboratory Animal Science* 23:657–661.

Pseudomonas aeruginosa Infection

Flynn, R.J. (1963) Introduction: *Pseudomonas aeruginosa* infection and its effects on biological and medical research. *Laboratory Animal Science* 13:1–6.

Wyand, D.S. & Jonas, A.M. (1967) *Pseudomonas aeruginosa* infection in rats following implantation of an indwelling jugular catheter. *Laboratory Animal Care* 17:261–266.

Staphylococcus aureus Infection

Ash, G.W. (1971) An epidemic of chronic skin ulceration in rats. *Laboratory Animals* 5:115–122.

Fox, J.G., Niemi, S.M., Murphy, J.C., & Quimby, F.W. (1977) Ulcerative dermatitis in the rat. *Laboratory Animal Science* 27:671–678.

Godfrey, D.M., Gaumond, G.A., Delano, M.L., & Silverman, J. (2005) Clinical linoleic acid deficiency in Dahl salt-sensitive (SS/Jr) rats. *Comparative Medicine* 55:470–475.

Kunstyr, I., Ernst, H., & Lenz, W. (1995) Granulomatous dermatitis and mastitis in two SPF rats associated with a slowly growing *Staphylococcus aureus*: a case report. *Laboratory Animals* 29:177–179.

Ozaki, K., Nishikawa, T., Nishimura, M., & Narama, I. (1997) Spontaneous skin lesions in beige rats (Chediak–Higashi syndrome of rats). *Journal of Veterinary Medical Science* 59:651–655.

Wagner, J.E., Owens, D.R., LaRegina, M.C., & Vogler, G.A. (1977) Self-trauma and *Staphylococcus aureus* in ulcerative dermatitis of rats. *Journal of the American Veterinary Medical Association* 171:839–841.

Streptobacillus moniliformis Infection

Anderson, L.C., Leary, S.L., & Manning, P.J. (1983) Rat-bite fever in animal research laboratory personnel. *Laboratory Animal Science* 33:292–294.

Boot, R., Oosterhuis, A., & Thuis, H.C. (2002) PCR for the detection of *Streptobacillus moniliformis*. *Laboratory Animals* 36:200–208.

Graves, M.H. & Janda, M.J. (2001) Rat-bite fever (*Streptobacillus moniliformis*): a potential emerging disease. *International Journal of Infectious Diseases* 5:151–154.

Wullenweber, M. (1994) *Streptobacillus moniliformis*: a zoonotic pathogen. Taxonomic considerations, host species, diagnosis, therapy, geographical distribution. *Laboratory Animals* 29:1–15.

Streptococcus pneumoniae Infection

Borkowski, G.L. & Griffith, J.W. (1990) Diagnostic exercise: pneumonia and pleuritis in a rat. *Laboratory Animal Science* 40:323–325.

Fallon, M.T., Reinhard, M.K., Gray, B.M., Davis, T.W., & Lindsey, J.R. (1988) Inapparent *Streptococcus pneumoniae* type 35 infections in commercial rats and mice. *Laboratory Animal Science* 38:129–132.

Weisbroth, S.H. & Freimer, E.H. (1969) Laboratory rats from commercial breeders as carriers of pathogenic pneumococci. *Laboratory Animal Care* 19:473–478.

Yoneda, K. & Coonrod, J.D. (1980) Experimental type 25 pneumococcal pneumonia in rats. *American Journal of Pathology* 99:231–242.

Fungal Infections

Aspergillus spp. Infection

Gupta, B.N. (1978) Pulmonary aspergilloma in a rat. *Journal of the American Veterinary Medical Association* 173:1196–1197.

Hubbs, A.F., Hahn, F.F., & Lundgren, D.C. (1991) Invasive tracheobronchial aspergillosis in an F344/N rat. *Laboratory Animal Science* 41:521–524.

Rehm, S., Waalkes, M.P., & Ward, J.M. (1988) *Aspergillus rhinitis* in Wistar (Crl(WI)BR) rats. *Laboratory Animal Science* 38:162–166.

Rozengurt, N. & Sanchez, S. (1993) *Aspergillus niger* isolated from an outbreak of rhinitis in rats. *Veterinary Record* 132:656–657.

Singh, B. & Chawla, R.S. (1974) A note on an outbreak of pulmonary aspergillosis in albino rat colony. *Indian Journal of Animal Science* 44:804–807.

Blastomyces dermatitidis Infection

Chang, S.C., Hsuan, S.L., Lin, C.C., Lee, W.C., Chien, M.S., Chen, L.C., Wu, J.H., Cheng, S.J., Chen, C.L., & Liao, J.W. (2012) Probably *Blastomyces dermatitidis* infection in a young rat. *Veterinary Pathology* 50:343–346.

Dermatophyte Infection

Balsardi, A., Bianchi, C., Cocilovo, A., Dragoni, I., Poli, G., & Ponti, W. (1981) Dermatophytes in clinically healthy laboratory animals. *Laboratory Animals* 15:75–77.

Phycomycotic Infection

Moody, K.D., Griffith, J.W., & Lang, C.M. (1986) Fungal meningo-encephalitis in a laboratory rat. *Journal of the American Veterinary Medical Association* 189:1152–1153.

Rapp, J.P. & McGrath, J.T. (1975) Mycotic encephalitis in weanling rats. *Laboratory Animal Science* 25:477–480.

Pneumocystis spp. Infection

Albers, T. & Clifford, C. (2003) Transmission of rat respiratory virus in a rat colony: gross and histopathological progression of lesions. *Contemporary Topics in Laboratory Animal Science* 42:73–74.

Albers, T.M., Simon, M.A., & Clifford, C.B. (2009) Histopathology of naturally transmitted "rat respiratory virus": progression of lesions and proposed diagnostic criteria. *Veterinary Pathology* 46:992–999.

An, C.L., Cigliotti, F., & Harmsen, A.G. (2003) Exposure of immunocompetent adult mice to *Pneumocystis carinii* f. sp. *muris* by cohousing: growth of *P. carinii* f. sp. *muris* and host immune response. *Infection and Immunity* 71:2065–2070.

Armstrong, M.Y., Smith, A.L., & Richards, F.F. (1991) *Pneumocystis carinii* pneumonia in the rat model. *Journal of Protozoology* 38:136S–138S.

Barton, E.G. & Campbell, W.G. (1969) *Pneumocystis carinii* in lungs of rats treated with cortisone acetate: ultrastructural observations relating to the life cycle. *American Journal of Pathology* 54:209–236.

Cushion, M.T. (2004) Molecular and phenotypic description of *Pneumocystis wakefieldiae* sp. nov., a new species in rats. *Mycologicia* 96:429–438.

Cushion, M.T. (2004) *Pneumocystis*: unraveling the cloak of obscurity. *Trends in Microbiology* 12:243–249.

Deerberg, F., Pohlmeyer, G., Wullenweber, M., & Hedrich, H.J. (1993) History and pathology of an enzootic *Pneumocystis carinii* pneumonia in athymic Han:RNU and Han:NZNU rats. *Journal of Experimental Animal Science* 36-1-11.

Ellwell, M.R., Mahler, J.F., & Rao, G.N. (1997) Have you seen this? Inflammatory lesions in the lungs of rats. *Toxicologic Pathology* 25:529–531.

Feldman, S.H., Weisbroth, S.P., & Weisbroth, S.H. (1996) Detection of *Pneumocystis carinii* in rats by polymerase chain reaction: comparison of lung tissue and bronchoalveolar lavage specimens. *Laboratory Animal Science* 46:628–634.

Furuta, T., Fujita, M., Machii, R., Kobayashi, K., Kojima, S., & Veda, K. (1993) Fatal spontaneous pneumocystosis in nude rats. *Laboratory Animal Science* 43:551–556.

Henderson, K.S., Dole, V., Parker, N.J., Momtsios, P., Banu, L., Brouillette, R., Simon, M.A., Albers, T.M., Pritchett-Corning, K.R., Clifford, C.B., & Shek, W.R. (2012) *Pneumocystis carinii* causes a distinctive interstitial pneumonia in immunocompetent laboratory rats that had been attributed to "rat respiratory virus." *Veterinary Pathology* 49:440–452.

Icenhour, C.R., Rebholz, S.L., Collins, M.S., & Cushion, M.T. (2001) Widespread occurrence of *Pneumocystis carinii* in commercial rat colonies detected using targeted PCR and oral swabs. *Journal of Clinical Microbiology* 39:3437–3441.

Icenhour, C.R., Rebholz, S.L., Collins, M.S., & Cushion, M.T. (2002) Early acquisition of *Pneumocystis carinii* in neonatal rats as evidence by PCR and oral swabs. *Eukaryotic Cell* 1:414–419.

Livingston, R.S., Besch-Williford, C.L., Myles, M.H., Franklin, C.L., Crim, M.J., & Riley, L.K. (2011) *Pneumocystis carinii* infection causes lung lesions historically attributed to rat respiratory virus. *Comparative Medicine* 61:45–59.

Nahimana, A., Cushion, M.T., Blanc, D.S., & Hauser, P.M. (2001) Rapid PCR-single-strand conformation polymorphism method to differentiate and estimate relative abundance of *Pneumocystis carinii* special forms infecting rats. *Journal of Clinical Microbiology* 39:4563–4565.

Oz, H.S. & Hughes, W.T. (1996) Effect of sex and dexamethazone dose on the experimental host for *Pneumocystis carinii*. *Laboratory Animal Science* 46:109–110.

Pohlmeyer, G., & Deerberg, F. (1993) Nude rats as a model of *Pneumocystis carinii* pneumonia: sequential morphologic study of lung lesions. *Journal of Comparative Pathology* 109:217–230.

Slaoui, M., Dreef, H.C., & van Esch, E. (1998) Inflammatory lesions in the lungs of Wistar rats. *Toxicologic Pathology* 26:712–713.

Encephalitozoon cuniculi Infection

Attwood, H.D. & Sutton, R.D. (1965) Encephalitozoon granuloma in rats. *Journal of Pathology and Bacteriology* 89:735–738.

PARASITIC DISEASES

In addition to the parasites outlined in this section, there are other parasites that are rarely seen in rats maintained in well-managed facilities. Various sources and reviews on rat parasites include many agents that are rarely, if ever, pathogenic and questionably parasitic. Although interesting in many respects, significance of many of these agents is basically up to the beholder. For additional information on the biology and identification of parasites in rats, refer to Baker (2006, 2007).

Protozoal Infections

Molecular methodology has unveiled the complexity of unicellular organisms to the point that the term protozoa is no longer strictly valid. Nevertheless, we use the term loosely in its historical context to collectively cover eukaryotic parasitic unicellular organisms. As in other rodents covered in this text, rats are host to numerous commensal protozoa in their alimentary tract. Wild, pet, and laboratory rats are variably colonized by *Giardia muris*, *Spironucleus muris*, *Hexamastix muris*, *Chilomastix bettencourti*, *Tritrichomonas muris*, *Tritrichomonas minuta*, *Tetratrichomonas microtii*, *Pentatrichomonas hominis*, *Entamoeba muris*, *Balantidium coli*, and others. All of these agents are essentially nonpathogenic commensals. Sporozoa are eukaryotic parasites that belong within the phylum Apicomplexa, members of which are defined by the presence of an apical complex that is utilized for penetration and infection of host cells. Rat sporozoa include *Hepatozoon muris*, *Toxoplasma gondii*, *Hammondia hammondi*, *Sarcocystis* spp., *Frenkelia* spp., and several species of *Eimeria*. Although some of these agents have been recognized in laboratory rats, particularly decades ago, none are overtly pathogenic in rats under natural conditions.

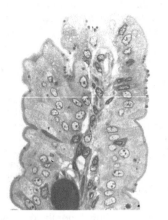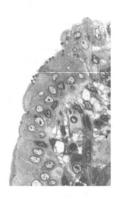

FIG. 2.48. *Epon-embedded section of villus from a young rat infected with* Cryptosporidium *sp. Note the trophozoites embedded within the brush border.*

Cryptosporidium *spp. Infection: Cryptosporidiosis*

An outbreak of diarrhea and high mortality among infant rats of the Rapp hypertensive strain has been described. Surviving pups were runted and their fur was stained with feces. Lesions in convalescing 21-day-old rats were restricted to the mucosa of the small intestine, primarily jejunum. The mucosa was hyperplastic and villi were shortened and fused, with cryptosporidia attached to the brush borders of enterocytes toward the villus tips (Fig. 2.48). Cryptosporidiosis can be induced experimentally in rats, but is transient and mild unless rats are immunosuppressed or athymic.

Trypanosoma lewisi: *Trypanosomiasis*

Naturally occurring infections with *Trypanosoma lewisi* are now a rarity in laboratory rats. However, there have been isolated reports of infections with *T. lewisi* in laboratory and wild rats in developing countries. This flagellate is a species-specific nonpathogenic blood parasite. Infected rats are normally subclinical, and procedures such as irradiation are used to induce parasitemia in subclinically infected animals. Rats are infected principally by the ingestion of infected fleas or flea feces from *T. lewisi*-infected rats. The diagnosis of trypanosomiasis is usually made by identification of the organism in Giemsa-stained blood films. A PCR technique has also been developed to identify infected animals.

Helminth Infestations
Syphacia muris, Syphacia obvelata *and* Aspiculuris tetraptera: *Pinworms*

Rats may serve as hosts to 3 species of pinworms: *S. muris*, *S. obvelata*, and *A. tetraptera*, which are generally found in the cecum and colon in infested animals. *Syphacia muris* commonly occurs in laboratory and wild rats and is transmissible to the laboratory mouse. In contrast, *S. obvelata* is primarily a pinworm of mice that may

infest rats. These parasites have a direct life cycle. Eggs are deposited in the colon or on the perianal area. The eggs embryonate and become infectious within a few hours. Rats may become infested by direct ingestion of embryonated eggs from the perianal region, ingestion of eggs in contaminated food and water or from fomites, or direct migration of larvae via the anus to the large intestine. Infestation is frequently subclinical, but younger animals with heavy infestations may exhibit various signs, including diarrhea, poor weight gains, impactions, rectal prolapse, and intussusceptions. *Aspiculuris tetraptera* frequently occurs in conventional rats and mice. The life cycle is also direct. Eggs are passed in the feces and, therefore, are not found in the perianal region.

Diagnosis

The microscopic demonstration of the characteristic eggs on touch preparations of the anal region (using transparent adhesive tape) is a useful method for detection of *Syphacia*, but has little value for detection of *Aspiculuris*. Eggs of all 3 species can be demonstrated in fecal samples, and adults are visible as small, thread-like worms in the cecum and colon. Adults are also readily seen in tissue sections of large intestine, identifiable as nematodes with typical oxyurid lateral alae (Fig. 2.49). Occasionally, focal submucosal granulomas may be evident in sections of the large intestine on microscopic examination. *Syphacia* and *Aspiculuris* can be differentiated by morphologic features of the adults and eggs.

Trichosomoides crassicauda *Infestation*

Trichosomoides crassicauda nematodes occur in the urinary tract of wild rats and, rarely, in laboratory rats. infested animals are usually clinically normal. The thread-like adult worms are found in the lumen and mucosa of the urinary bladder and renal pelvis at necropsy. In tissue sections examined microscopically, migratory-stage larvae and immature worms may be present in multiple tissues, particularly in the lungs.

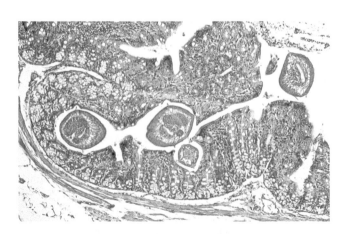

FIG. 2.49. *Cecum from a rat with pinworm infestation. Note cross sections of nematodes with characteristic lateral alae.*

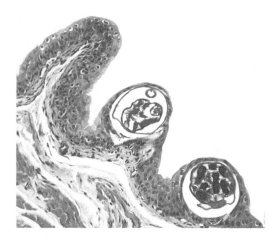

FIG. 2.50. *Urinary bladder mucosa of a rat infested with* Trichosomoides crassicauda *(bladder threadworm). Female worms burrow into the urothelium.*

Adult females reside in the epithelium of the renal pelvis and the urinary bladder (Fig. 2.50), which may elicit a chronic inflammatory response. Males are much smaller than females and live within the urinary tract lumen or within the uterus of the larger females. Typical double-operculated eggs are passed in the urine, and intracage transmission readily occurs. Urinary calculi and bladder tumors have been associated with this parasitic infestation.

Other Nematode Infestations

Wild rats are host to many nematodes that rarely infest laboratory rats, but there is ample evidence of wild rats serving as sources of laboratory rat infestations, generally through contamination of feed and bedding and occasionally through arthropod intermediate hosts, such as cockroaches. One survey of wild rats in urban Baltimore revealed a remarkably high prevalence of *Nippostrongylus braziliensis*, *Rodenolepis nana*, *Hymenolepis diminuta*, *Heterakis spumosa*, and *Trichuris muris*. In addition, a survey of wild rats in New Haven, CT by one of the authors (SWB) also found a high prevalence of *Gonglyonema neoplasticum*, *Calodium (Capillaria) hepaticum*, and *T. crassicauda*.

Rodentolepis *and* Hymenolepis *Infestations*

Several species of animals, including mice, rats, hamsters, humans, and nonhuman primates, may acquire tapeworms including *Rodentolepis nana* (formerly *Hymenolepis nana*), *Rodentolepis microstoma*, and *H. diminuta*. All 3 species infest the small intestine. With *Rodentolepis* spp., the life cycle may be either direct or indirect. In the direct cycle, intermediate stages can develop directly in the wall of the intestine without an intermediate host. Scoleces, or cysticercoids, may be identified in smears or in tissue sections of small intestine infested with *Rodentolepis*. In the indirect life cycle, embryonated eggs are ingested by an arthropod host, such as grain beetles or fleas. Ingestion of these arthropods by a susceptible host will then serve as the source of the parasite eggs. In

H. diminuta infestations, an intermediate host, such as beetles or fleas, is essential for the completion of the life cycle. Eggs can be shown in the feces to confirm the diagnosis. In heavy infestations, there may be poor weight gain and sometimes, catarrhal enteritis. See Chapter 3 Hamster, "Fig. 3.23 and 3.24" for figures of these tapeworms in tissue sections.

Taenia taeniaformis *Infestation*

The larval stage of *T. taeniaformis*, the cat tapeworm, is termed *Cysticercus fasciolaris*. When eggs of this tapeworm are ingested, they migrate through the bowel and often encyst in the liver of rats, mice, and other rodents. Laboratory rats and mice become infested by contamination of food or bedding with cat feces. Usually, only 1 or 2 cysts will be found in an affected animal. Parasitism in rats has been associated with the development of fibrosarcomas in the reactive tissue around the cyst.

Arthropod Infestations

Arthropod ectoparasites are not an important consideration in laboratory rats, although they are relatively common in wild and pet rats. Rats are host to 2 species of lice, *Polyplax spinulosa* (spined rat louse) and *Hoplopleura pacifica* (tropical rat louse), of which only the former has been described in laboratory rats. *Polyplax* was once an important vector for *M. haemomuris* among rats. It can be associated with pruritis, irritability, and anemia, caused directly by feeding and indirectly by *M. haemomuris*. Fleas of several genera, including *Xenopsylla*, *Leptopsylla*, and *Nosopsyllus*, infest wild rats and, rarely, laboratory rats. Several different types of mites can infest rats, but all are rare in laboratory rats, except *Radfordia ensifera* (*Myobia ratti*), the fur mite, which can be common in some populations. Pruritis, hair loss, and loss of condition are associated with heavy infestations. The mite can be demonstrated in the pellage and may also be evident in tissue sections of affected skin (Fig. 2.51). Mesostigmatid mites, including *Ornithonyssus bacoti* (tropical rat mite),

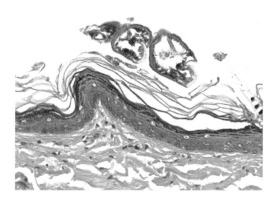

FIG. 2.51. *Skin from rat with* Radfordia ensifora *infestation. These fur mites are present on the stratum corneum, with minimal reaction in the underlying skin.*

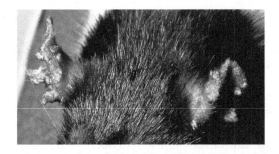

FIG. 2.52.   *Ear mange in a rat due to infestation with* Notoedres muris. *Note the disfigurement of the ears associated with proliferative dermatitis. (Source: N.J. Schoemaker, University of Utrecht, Netherlands. Reproduced with permission from N.J. Schoemaker.)*

Laelaps echidnina (spiny rat mite), and *Liponyssoides* sp. (house mouse mite), are blood-sucking mites that are common in wild rodents, and are known to periodically infest laboratory rats. These mites are associated with rats only while feeding. They seek refuge in the surrounding environment. Their bites are pruritic, as animal handlers can attest. Both *O. bacoti* and *L. echidnina* readily feed on humans, and *O. bacoti* in particular has been associated with dermatitis in humans exposed to rat-infested environments. These mites can cause anemia, debility, and infertility in rats. Rats may also be accidental hosts for a number of other mites. Other mites that reside permanently in or on the skin or fur of rats include *Demodex* spp., which have been found in follicles as an incidental finding in several populations of laboratory rats. *Rattus norvegicus* has been found to host 4 species of *Demodex*: *D. nanus*, *D. ratti*, *D. ratticola*, and *D. norvegicus*. The single report of *Demodex* infestation of laboratory rats suggested that the species was *D. nanus*. The prevalence of *Demodex* mites among laboratory rats is unknown, as these mites are generally only detected incidentally when skin sections are examined. *Notoedres muris*, a mange mite that burrows in the cornified epithelium of the ear and other hairless skin sites, is common among pet rats in Europe and often results in extensive proliferative lesions involving the ears and ear canal (Fig. 2.52). It has also appeared in laboratory rats following incursion of wild rats into an animal facility.

BIBLIOGRAPHY FOR PARASITIC DISEASES

General References for Parasitic Diseases
Baker, D.G. (2006) Parasitic diseases. In: *The Laboratory Rat*, 2nd edn (eds. M.A. Suckow, S.H. Weisbroth, & C.L. Franklin), pp. 453–478. Academic Press, New York.
Baker, D.G. (2007) *Flynn's Parasites of Laboratory Animals*, 2nd edn. Wiley-Blackwell.

Protozoal Infections
Desquesnes, M., Ravel, S., & Cuny, G. (2002) PCR identification of *Trypanosoma lewisi*, a common parasite of laboratory rats. *Kinetoplastid Biology and Disease* 1:1475–1483.
Gardner, A.L., Roche, J.K., Weikel, C.S., & Guerrant, R. (1991) Intestinal cryptosporidiosis: pathophysiologic alterations and specific cellular and humoral immune responses in RNU/+ and RNU/RNU (athymic) rats. *American Journal of Tropical Medicine and Hygiene* 44:49–62.
Moody, K.D., Brownstein, D.G., & Johnson, E.A. (1991) Cryptosporidiosis in suckling laboratory rats. *Laboratory Animal Science* 41:625–627.

Helminth Infestations
Easterbrook, J.D., Kaplan, J.B., Glass, G.E., Watson, J., & Klein, S.L. (2008) A survey of rodent-borne pathogens carried by wild-caught Norway rats: a potential threat to laboratory rodent colonies. *Laboratory Animals* 42:92–98.
Hanes, M.A. (1995) Fibrosarcomas in two rats arising from hepatic cysts of *Cysticercus fasciolaris*. *Veterinary Pathology* 32:441–444.
Schwabe, C.W. (1955) Helminth parasites and neoplasia. *American Journal of Veterinary Research* 16:455–458.
Zubaidy, A.J. & Majeed, S.K. (1981) Pathology of the nematode *Trichosomoides crassicauda* in the urinary bladder of laboratory rats. *Laboratory Animals* 15:381–384.

Arthropod Infestations
Izdebska, J.N. & Rolbiecki, L. (2012) Demodectic mites of the brown rat *Rattus norvegicus* (Berkenhout, 1769) (Rodentia, Muridae) with a new finding of *Demodex ratticola* Bukva, 1995 (Acari, Demodecidae). *Annals of Parasitology* 58:71–74.
Peper, R.L. (1994) Diagnostic exercise: mite infestation in a laboratory rat colony. *Laboratory Animal Science* 44:172–174.
Walberg, J.A., Stark, D.M., Desch, C., & McBride, D.F. (1981) Demodicidosis in laboratory rats (*Rattus norvegicus*). *Laboratory Animmal Science* 31:60–62.
Watson, J. (2008) New building, old parasite: mesostigmatid mites—an ever-present threat to barrier rodent facilities. *ILAR Journal* 49:303–309.

AGE-RELATED DISORDERS

Rats develop a myriad of age-related lesions. Several reviews provide encyclopedic coverage of noninfectious and neoplastic lesions of rats (see "General References on Diseases of Rats").

Degenerative Changes in the Nervous System

Age-related abnormalities seen in aged rats include Wallerian degeneration in focal areas of the spinal cord and segmental demyelination of the peripheral nervous system, particularly in the sciatic nerves. Wallerian degeneration in the spinal cord is characterized by the presence of enlarged axons containing eosinophilic material (spheroids). In the brain and spinal cord, there may be degeneration of scattered neurons, with astrogliosis. Lipochrome pigment may be present in some neurons in the brain and spinal cord.

Radiculoneuropathy

Radiculoneuropathy is a degenerative disease of the spinal cord and spinal roots, with concurrent atrophy of skeletal muscle in the lumbar region and hind limbs. Lesions occur in the spinal cord and spinal nerve roots (Fig. 2.53). Lesions consist of demyelination, swollen axon sheaths, and axonal loss. These changes are restricted to white matter, and are most severe in the

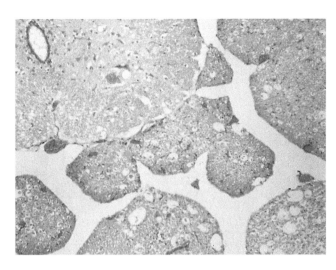

FIG. 2.53. *Lumbar spinal cord from an aged rat with radiculoneuropathy. Note the axon sheath swelling in nerve bundles of the cauda equina.*

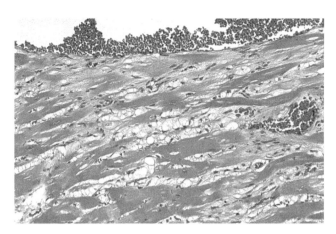

Fig. 2.55. *Myocardial degeneration and interstitial fibrosis in an aged rat.*

lateral and ventral funiculi and cauda equina. This syndrome is common in aged laboratory and pet rats, and is manifest clinically as posterior weakness or paresis.

Alveolar Histiocytosis

Aggregates of macrophages within the subpleural alveolar spaces are seen occasionally in the lungs of older laboratory rats. On gross examination, they usually appear as dull pale yellow foci (Fig. 2.54), and become accentuated when lungs are fixed in formalin. On histopathology, there are intra-alveolar collections macrophages with abundant foamy cytoplasm. This lesion is common in many species of animals.

Myocardial Degeneration/Fibrosis

Focal to diffuse areas of myocardial degeneration and fibrosis are frequently seen microscopically in conventional and specific pathogen-free rats, particularly after 1 year of age. Lesions are more common in male rats. The prevalence may be over 80% in some rat strains. At necropsy, there may be moderate to marked ventricular hypertrophy, and pale streaks may be evident on the epicardium. On microscopic examination, degenerative changes are usually most evident in the papillary muscles of the left ventricle, although the interventricular septum may also be involved. Atrophy of myofibers, vacuolation and fragmentation of sarcoplasm, loss of cross-striations, mononuclear cell infiltration, and fibrosis are typical changes (Fig. 2.55). Large reactive nuclei are occasionally observed. Interstitial fibrosis is an important feature of the disease, which is particularly evident in Trichrome-stained tissue sections (Fig. 2.56). Although this condition is frequently present in older rats, there may be little or no evidence of cardiac insufficiency.

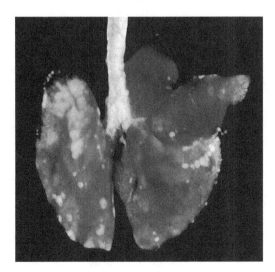

FIG. 2.54. *Alveolar histiocytosis in an aged rat. Note the raised pale foci in the subpleural regions consistent with intra-alveolar aggregations of macrophages.*

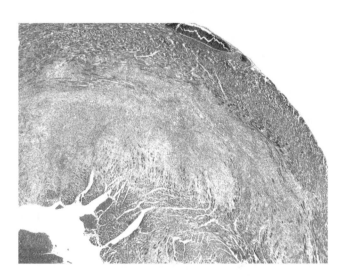

FIG. 2.56. *Left ventricle of an aged rat with marked myocardial fibrosis. Note the abundant blue-stained collagen. (Masson's trichrome stain).*

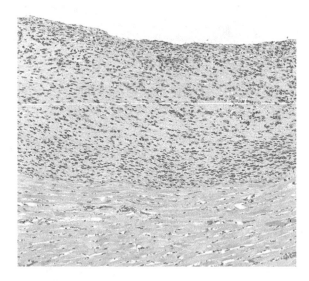

FIG. 2.57. *Endocardial spindle cell proliferation lining the ventricular lumen (top). This spontaneous lesion may arise in various strains and stocks of rats.*

Cardiac Valvular Angiectasis

A relatively high incidence of single and multifocal vascular anomalies were reported to arise on the atrioventricular valves of Sprague-Dawley rats from different commercial sources. The blood-filled structures were lined with normal-appearing endothelium and were often connected to one another by vascular channels. They arose most frequently on the septal cusp of the right atrioventricular valve near the atrioventricular ostium, although others were on other cusps and the left atrioventricular valve.

Endocardial Spindle Cell Proliferation

Proliferation of spindle-shaped cells resembling fibroblasts arise in the endocardium and subendocardial tissue (Fig. 2.57) as a frequent lesion in various stocks and strains of rats. These lesions may become expansive and invade the myocardium. They have been characterized as fibroproliferative, giving rise to terms including endocardial fibromatosis, fibroelastosis, endocardiosis, and endocardial fibromatous proliferation. It has also been suggested that these changes are precursors to schwannomas.

Polyarteritis Nodosa

Polyarteritis is frequently seen in aging rats. The prevalence is higher in males. Arterial lesions most frequently occur in medium-size arteries of the mesentery, pancreas, kidney, pancreaticoduodenal artery, testis, and most other organs, except the lung. The disease most frequently occurs in the Sprague-Dawley and spontaneous hypertensive rat (SHR) strains, and in rats with late-stage chronic nephropathy. At necropsy, affected vessels are enlarged and thickened in a segmental pattern, with marked tortuosity, particularly in the mesenteric vessels

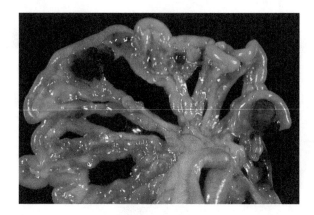

FIG. 2.58. *Mesentery and intestines of an aged rat with polyarteritis. Note the nodular dilation and tortuosity of the mesenteric vessels. (Source: D. Imai, University of California, Davis, CA. Reproduced with permission from D. Imai.)*

(Fig. 2.58). On microscopic examination, there is intimal fibrinoid degeneration and thickening of the media of affected arteries, with smudging of the normal architecture. Infiltrating leukocytes consist of mononuclear cells, with a few neutrophils (Fig. 2.59). There are marked variations in the size and contours in the lumen of affected vessels, and thromboses, occasionally with recanalization, may occur.

Aging Lesions of the Liver

Rats develop polyploidy, megalokarya, binuclear hepatocytes, intranuclear cytoplasmic invagination, and intracytoplasmic inclusions of hepatocytes that are similar to but not as striking as in the aging mouse. Although not remarkable in younger animals, the shift to increased ploidy occurs relatively early in life. There is strain-related variation in the incidence of polyploidy in rats. Foci of sinusoidal dilatation and peliosis, either spontaneous or drug-induced, do occur, especially in older animals. Foci of cytoplasmic alteration vary phenotypically from areas of clearing to acidophilic to

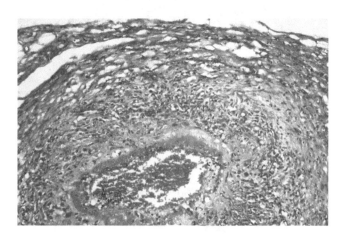

FIG. 2.59. *Mesenteric artery from a rat with polyarteritis. There is fibrinoid change in the intima, with inflammation of the media and adventitia.*

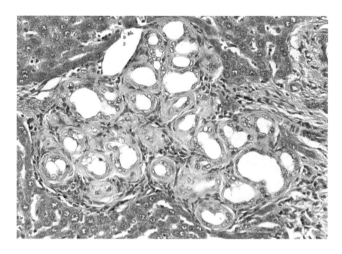

FIG. 2.60. *Hepatic portal region from an aged rat, illustrating bile ductular proliferation and fibrosis.*

basophilic staining. These changes are of particular interest to the toxicologic pathologist. A striking lesion that is frequently observed in aging rats is bile ductular proliferation. Initially, there are increased numbers of bile ductules in portal tracts, which become progressively dilated, lined by atrophic epithelium, and surrounded by collagenous connective tissue (Fig. 2.60). Extramedullary hematopoiesis may occur in older rats with conditions such as severe chronic renal disease.

Pancreatic Islet Hypertrophy and Fibrosis
Aging rats develop pancreatic islet hypertrophy, which progresses to increasingly severe dissecting fibrosis of pancreatic islets (Fig. 2.61). This lesion has been reported in aging Sprague-Dawley rats, but it occurs in other strains as well.

Chronic Progressive Nephropathy
This disease has been referred to by a variety of other terms, including "glomerulosclerosis," "progressive glomerulonephrosis," and "old rat nephropathy," among others. Chronic progressive nephropathy (CPN), the

preferred term used herein, is an extremely common life-limiting disease of aged rats. The prevalence of CPN in older rats varies but may exceed 75% in susceptible strains. A variety of predisposing factors play a role in the development of CPN. (i) *Age*: lesions are usually most extensive in animals at least 12 months of age. (ii) *Sex*: CPN is more common and more severe in males. (iii) *Strain*: the prevalence is usually significantly higher and more severe in Sprague-Dawley and Fischer 344 rats compared to other rat strains. (iv) *Diet*: high-protein diets are an important contributing factor, although total dietary restriction, rather than protein content, may be more important in reducing the progression of CPN. (v) *Immunological factors*: mesangial deposition of IgM has been observed in affected glomeruli, consistent with noncomplement-fixing immune complexes, but CPN does not appear to be primarily an immunologically mediated disease. (vi) *Endocrine*: prolactin levels have been implicated as a contributing factor. (vii) *Microbial status*: axenic rats tend not to develop CPN, living much longer than microbe-associated rats.

Pathology
Clinical signs associated with CPN include proteinuria, weight loss, and in advanced cases elevated plasma creatinine levels consistent with renal insufficiency. The renal cortices are usually pitted and sometimes irregular, with variable degrees of enlargement and pallor in some affected animals. On cut surface, there may be irregularities and linear streaks in the cortex and medulla, with varying degrees of brown pigmentation (Fig. 2.62). Microscopic changes are consistent with a chronic glomerulopathy. Glomerular changes vary from minimal thickening of the basement membranes to marked thickening of glomerular tufts, with segmental sclerosis and adhesions to Bowman's capsule (Fig. 2.63). Proteinaceous casts are often present in dilated tubules in the cortex and medulla (Fig. 2.64). Eosinophilic, PAS-positive and iron-positive resorption droplets are

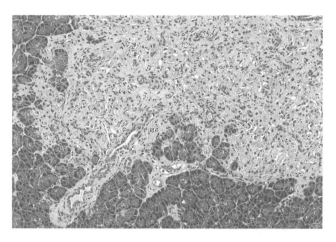

FIG. 2.61. *Pancreatic islet fibrosis in an aged rat.*

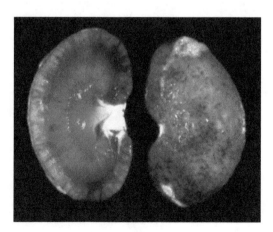

FIG. 2.62. *Chronic progressive nephropathy in an aged rat. Note the granular appearance to cortical surface, linear streaks on cut surface, and irregular pigmentation.*

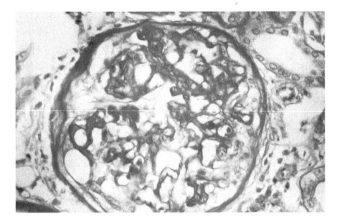

FIG. 2.63.   *Chronic progressive nephropathy in an aged rat. Note the thickening and splitting of Bowman's capsular basement membrane, thickening of glomerular capillary basement membranes, and glomerular synechiae (PAS stain).*

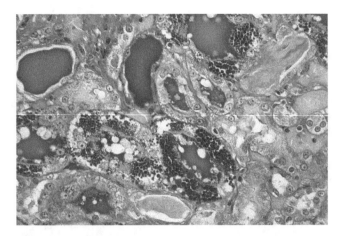

FIG. 2.65.   *Chronic progressive nephropathy. Note the proteinaceous casts in dilated tubules and the variable-sized granules (resorption droplets) in the cytoplasm of tubular epithelial cells (PTAH stain).*

frequently present in epithelial cells lining affected nephrons (Fig. 2.65). Tubules are frequently dilated and lined by flattened epithelial cells, contracted and lined by poorly differentiated, cuboidal, basophilic epithelial cells, or sclerotic. There may be varying degrees of thickening and splitting of Bowman's capsular and proximal tubular basement membranes, interstitial fibrosis, and interstitial mononuclear cell infiltration. Macrophages and myofibroblasts appear to play an important role in the development of the interstitial fibrosis. In advanced cases, there may be secondary hyperparathyroidism, with mineralized deposits in tissues such as kidney, gastric mucosa, lungs, and the media of larger arteries. CPN contributes to hypertension, and is often associated with polyarteritis. Hypercholesterolemia, hypoproteinemia, and elevated blood urea nitrogen consistent with renal insufficiency/failure may be evident in advanced cases. Elevated serum cholesterol and marked

proteinuria (>300 mg/dl of urine) are useful diagnostic parameters. In advanced CPN, urine proteins electrophoretically mimic serum protein profiles. Animals with severe disease appear to cope well, but may rapidly decompensate and die.

Nephrocalcinosis

Renal mineralization has been observed on occasion in laboratory rats, including animals on standard commercial diets. The disease has been produced by a variety of dietary manipulations, including those with a low-magnesium content, high-calcium content, high concentrations of phosphorus, and preparations with a low calcium-phosphorus ratio. Lesions are characterized by the deposition of lamellar calcium phosphates in the interstitium of the corticomedullary junction, with intratubular aggregations in the same region. In advanced cases, there may be detectable manifestations of renal dysfunction, including albuminuria.

Urolithiasis

Urolithiasis in laboratory rats is normally rare and usually sporadic. When present in the urinary bladder (Fig. 2.66),

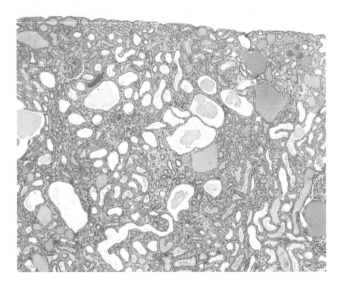

Fig. 2.64.   *Chronic progressive nephropathy in an aged rat. The cortex has severe tubular dilation with eosinophilic protein casts and interstitial fibrosis with mononuclear leukocyte infiltration.*

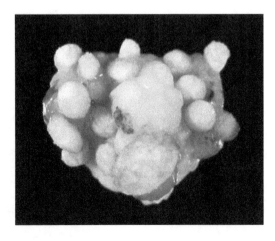

FIG. 2.66.   *Multiple calculi in the urinary bladder of a rat.*

calculi may be associated with hemorrhagic cystitis, hematuria, and urinary obstruction. Calculi may also be located at other sites (e.g., renal pelvis, ureter, and urethra). The composition of calculi is variable. Analyses have revealed combinations such as ammonium magnesium phosphate, mixed carbonate and oxalate, and mixed carbonate and phosphate with magnesium and calcium. In male rats there are also erroneous reports of a high incidence of mucoid calculi, which are agonally excreted copulatory plugs into the urethra and bladder.

Hydronephrosis

Hydronephrosis is a relatively common incidental finding at necropsy and occurs in a variety of strains and stocks of rats. In some strains, there is a hereditary basis for the disorder. For example, in the Brown Norway rat, hydronephrosis appears to be an autosomal polygenetic disorder, with incomplete penetrance. In the Gunn rat, it is apparently inherited as a dominant gene and may be lethal when present in the homozygous state. In studies of hydronephrosis in outbred Sprague-Dawley rats, it was concluded that the condition is a highly heritable trait, probably involving more than 1 gene. Spontaneous hydronephrosis, particularly of the right kidney, is a well-recognized abnormality, especially in male rats. It has been proposed that the lesion in males may be due to the passage of the internal spermatic vessels across the ureter, resulting in mechanical obstruction to outflow and subsequent hydronephrosis of the affected kidney. However, sectioning of the right spermatic vessels in young male Wistar-derived rats failed to reduce the incidence of hydronephrosis, compared with control animals.

At necropsy, there may be varying degrees of involvement. In severely affected animals, the kidney consists of a fluid-filled sac containing clear serous fluid. On microscopic examination, there is marked dilation of the renal pelvis, with excavation of the renal medulla, reduction in the length of the collecting tubules, and absence of an inflammatory response. Differential diagnoses include pyelonephritis, polycystic kidneys, and renal papillary necrosis. In most strains, unilateral or bilateral hydronephrosis is often an incidental finding at necropsy. The defect may be fatal when bilateral. There may be an increased susceptibility to superimposed renal infections due to urine stasis.

Renal Papillary Hyperplasia

Intermittent hematuria has been reported in hybrid Lewis × Brown Norway rats. The syndrome occurred predominantly in males, but it also occurs in females. Some, but not all, of the rats had concommitant unilateral or bilateral hydronephrosis. Lesions were confined to the renal papillae and consisted of focal urothelial proliferative change, with hemorrhage and necrosis of the stroma (Fig. 2.67). Epithelial papillary proliferation has also been described in Brown Norway rats.

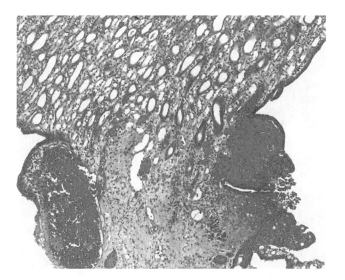

FIG. 2.67. *Renal papilla from adult rat with a history of hematuria. Note the proliferative vascular malformations with eroded surfaces and hemorrhage.*

Degenerative Osteoarthritis

Erosion of the articular cartilage occurs in sites such as the sternum and femur in aged rats, with degeneration of cartilaginous matrix, clefting, and cyst formation.

MISCELLANEOUS DISORDERS

Auricular Chondropathy

Inflammatory lesions of the auricular pinnae arise spontaneously in multiple strains of rats and mice, often, but not always, in association with metal ear tags. Lesions are characterized by chronic granulomatous inflammation with destruction of cartilage, nodular proliferation of new cartilage (Figs. 2.68 and 2.69), and foci of osseous metaplasia. When arising in association with ear tags, the contralateral ear is often involved. Lesions closely resemble those induced by immunization with type II

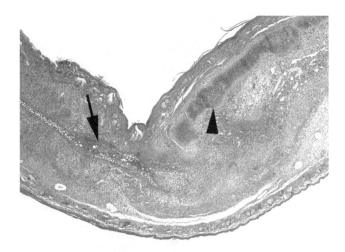

FIG. 2.68. *Auricular chondropathy in a rat, depicting irregular areas of cartilage destruction and inflammation (arrow) adjacent to reactive chondroid hyperplasia (arrowhead).*

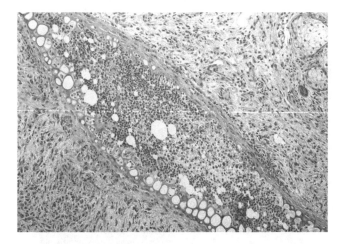

FIG. 2.69. *Higher magnification of the lesion depicted in the previous figure, showing cartilage destruction and inflammation.*

collagen, and are, therefore, believed to be immunologically mediated.

Malocclusion

Overgrowth of the incisor teeth occurs sporadically in rats. The condition occurs secondary to poor alignment of the upper and lower incisor teeth, with resultant failure to wear in the normal manner. The condition may be secondary to a broken upper or lower incisor tooth but is more often a spontaneous event and in many cases is considered to be due to genetic factors. Depending on the duration and severity of the problem, affected animals are frequently thin due to their inability to prehend and masticate food normally, and in advanced cases, severely affected lower or upper incisors may penetrate into the soft tissues of the palate or jaw (Fig. 2.70).

Hydrocephalus

Hydrocephalus arises sporadically among various strains of rats, but may have a genetic basis in some populations, such as WAG/Rig rats. Affected rats have a domed calvarium, with dilation of lateral ventricles and thin cerebral cortices. Rats with congenital hydrocephalus typically present with dehydration at weaning age, when they are no longer under the care of their mothers. Hydrocephalus, resulting from stenosis of the cerebral aqueduct, can be readily induced in newborn rats from dams that are deficient in vitamin B12.

Eosinophilic Granulomatous Pneumonia in Brown Norway Rats

The BN rat has been used to study the pathogenesis of asthma, since they readily develop increased bronchiolar responsiveness and elevated IgE following exposure to allergens. However, BN rats may develop a spontaneous eosinophil-rich granulomatous pneumonia in the absence of any experimental procedure. The changes have been attributed to inadvertent exposure to an allergen or environmental particulates. Lesions have been observed in BN rats of various ages, but particularly in young adults. Both sexes are susceptible. Typically, on gross examination, there are multifocal pale tan to gray to red 1–3 mm foci scattered throughout the parenchyma of the lung. In affected animals, there is a multifocal to diffuse granulomatous pneumonia with a cellular infiltrate consisting of epithelioid cells and, in some cases, a prominent multinucleated giant cell component. Frequently, there may be marked perivascular and peribronchiolar edema with an inflammatory cell infiltrate that is rich in eosinophils (Fig. 2.71). Attempts to demonstrate an infectious agent by serology, bacterial culture, and with special stains on affected lungs have been uniformly negative.

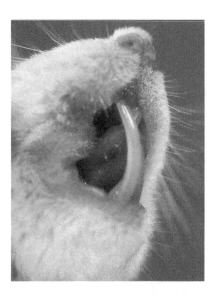

FIG. 2.70. *Incisor malocclusion in a laboratory rat. Note overgrowth of a lower incisor into the anterior palate.*

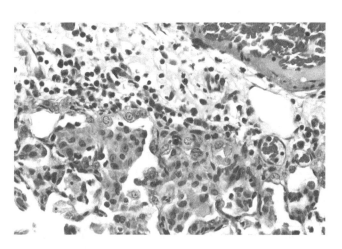

FIG. 2.71. *Perivascular edema with mixed leukocytic infiltrates, including eosinophils, and granulomatous inflammatory response in adjacent alveoli in a Brown Norway rat with eosinophilic granulomatous pneumonia. (Source: J. Kwiecien.)*

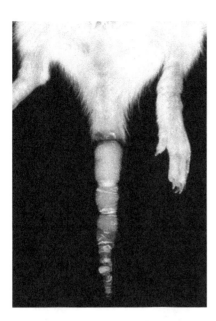

FIG. 2.72. *"Ringtail" in a suckling rat. There is prominent annular ridging and contraction with dry gangrene of the distal tail.*

Persistent Vaginal Septum

Sprague-Dawley and Wistar rats have been reported to have persistent transverse occlusive membranes, known as vaginal septa. The septa may be partially or completely occlusive, and are associated with retention of mucus, ascending bacterial infections, metritis, fetal death, and dystocia. The septa are lined on both sides by vaginal epithelium. The report in Sprague-Dawley rats documented an incidence of 6% among female rats.

ENVIRONMENTAL DISORDERS

Ringtail

Annular constrictions of the skin of the tail lead to dry gangrene of the distal tail (Fig. 2.72). This syndrome is most apt to occur in preweaning rats. Ringtail has been attributed to low environmental humidity (e.g., less than 25%). However, other factors, such as genetic susceptibility, low environmental temperatures, degree of hydration, and nutrition may be involved. In a study of specimens from a naturally occurring outbreak of ringtail in suckling rats, epidermal changes were observed to precede changes in the underlying tissues. Epidermal hyperplasia with orthokeratotic and parakeratotic hyperkeratosis were prominent features. Dilated and thrombosed vessels were observed in severe cases, accompanied by necrosis hemorrhage and coagulative necrosis of the overlying epidermis. Topical application of lanolin was found to be beneficial in the treatment of this disease.

Dehydration

Rats become dehydrated easily, usually from malfunction of water bottle sipper tubes. Dehydration is often accompanied by porphyrin staining around the eyes, a sign of general stress. Rats with hydrocephalus generally present with dehydration at weaning age.

High Environmental Temperature

High environmental temperature can cause infertility, particularly in male rats.

Light Cycle Aberrations

The female estrous cycle is sensitive to light cycles. For example, exposure to constant light for as little as 3 days may induce persistent estrus, hyperestrogenism, polycystic ovaries, and endometrial hypertrophy.

Phototoxic Retinopathy and Cataracts

Marked retinal degeneration can occur in albino rats subjected to light intensities that would be relatively harmless to animals with pigmented uveal tracts. Retinal changes may occur in rats exposed to cyclic light with an intensity of 130 lux or higher at the cage level. Typically, the changes are most severe in rats housed on the top shelves of racks nearest the ceiling light fixtures. There is a progressive reduction of the photoreceptor cell nuclei in the outer nuclear layer of the central retina. Advanced disease has marked depletion and alteration of the retinal layers, with concomitant cataract formation (Fig. 2.73). This must be differentiated from peripheral retinal degeneration, which occurs in some strains of rats as a genetically inherited disorder. Degenerative changes may also occur in the Harderian glands of rats exposed to high-intensity light.

Conjunctivitis, Keratitis, and Other Corneal Lesions

The underlying causes of spontaneous conjunctivitis vary from infectious agents (e.g., *Pasteurella* sp., rat coronavirus infections) to environmental factors. Spontaneous cases of conjunctivitis/blepharitis that occurred in a colony of nude rats were attributed to irritation and abrasions from a type of hardwood bedding. Their lack of eyelashes was considered to be an important predisposing factor. The problem was resolved when the original

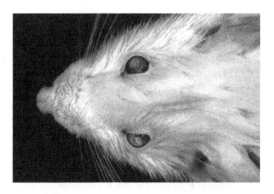

FIG. 2.73. *Bilateral cataracts in an albino rat exposed to excessive ambient light. This typically occurs in concert with light-induced retinal degeneration.*

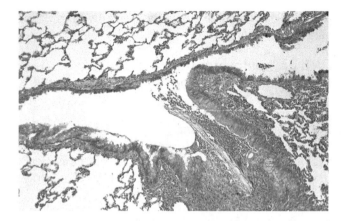

FIG. 2.74.   *Lung from a rat that aspirated plant material. Note the presence of the aspirated material in the lumen of the airway and an associated inflammatory response.*

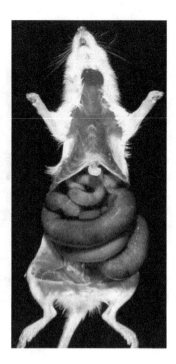

FIG. 2.75.   *Adynamic ileus in a juvenile rat following intraperitoneal administration of chloral hydrate as an anesthetic agent. There is marked dilation of the small intestine.*

bedding was replaced with a paper-based product. Keratitis sicca may be associated with lacrimal gland dysfunction following rat coronavirus infections (see "Rat Coronavirus Infection").

Quality of Bedding

Dusty bedding material can result in aspiration pneumonia (Fig. 2.74). This is often the aftermath of rough handling of shipping boxes. Blepharitis has been seen in nude rats housed on hardwood type bedding. High mortality has been observed in Sprague-Dawley rats housed on aromatic cedar wood shavings. Reduced weight gains were also observed. The mechanism(s) of the disease was not determined.

DRUG-RELATED DISORDERS

Ketamine–Xylazine Corneal Lesions

Corneal lesions have been observed in rats anesthetized with injectable ketamine–xylazine. Changes were attributed to drug-induced vasoconstriction of the ciliary and iridial vessels, and subsequent corneal hypoxia, corneal opacity, mineralization of the anterior limiting membrane of the cornea, and corneal ulceration.

Chloral Hydrate Ileus

Intraperitoneal injection of chloral hydrate or related compounds causes peritonitis and ileus. The ileus may not be apparent until up to 5 weeks after administration of the drug. Rats develop distended abdomens due to segmental atony and distension of the jejunum, ileum, and cecum (Fig. 2.75). Focal serosal hyperemia can also occur. This must be differentiated from megaloileitis that may arise in rats with Tyzzer's disease.

NSAIDS Renal Papillary and Tubular Necrosis

Rats are susceptible to renal proximal tubular and papillary necrosis in response to administration of salicylates and acetaminophen. Susceptibility is age-related, with older rats being most susceptible.

BIBLIOGRAPHY FOR AGE-, MISCELLANEOUS-, ENVIRONMENTAL- AND DRUG-RELATED DISORDERS

See "General References on Diseases of Rats"

General References on Age-Related Disorders

Anver, M.R., Cohen, B.J., Lattuada, C.P., & Foster, S.J. (1982) Age-associated lesions in barrier-reared male Sprague-Dawley rats: a comparison between Hap(SD) and Crl:COBS[R]CD[R](SD) stocks. *Experimental Aging Research* 8:3–24.

Coleman, G.L., Barthold, S.W., Osbaldiston, G.W., Foster, S.J., & Jonas, A.M. (1977) Pathological changes during aging in barrier-reared Fischer 344 male rats. *Journal of Gerontology* 32:258–278.

Dixon, D., Heider, K., & Elwell, M.R. (1995) Incidence of nonneoplastic lesions in historical control male and female Fischer 344 rats from 90-day toxicity studies. *Toxicologic Pathology* 23:338–348.

Goodman, D.G., Ward, J.M. Squire, R.A., Chu, K.C., & Linhart, M.S. (1979) Neoplastic and non-neoplastic lesions in aging F344 rats. *Toxicology and Applied Pharmacology* 48:237–248.

Goodman, D.G., Ward, J.M., Squire, R.A., Paxton, M.B., Reichardt, W.D., Chu, K.C., & Linhart, M.S. (1980) Neoplastic and non-neoplastic lesions in aging Osborne-Mendel rats. *Toxicologic Pathology* 55:433–447.

Age-Related Disorders

Alveolar Histiocytosis

Hook, G.E. (1991) Alveolar proteinosis and phospholipidosis of the lungs. *Toxicologic Pathology* 19:49–53.

Yang, Y.H., Yang, C.Y., & Grice, H.C. (1966) Multifocal histiocytosis in the lungs of rats. *Journal of Pathology and Bacteriology* 92:559–561.

Degenerative Changes in the Nervous System

Berg, B.N., Wolf, A., & Simms, H.S. (1962) Degenerative lesions of spinal roots and peripheral nerves of aging rats. *Gerontologia, Basel* 6:72–80.

Van Steenis, G. & Kroes, R. (1971) Changes in the nervous system and musculature of old rats. *Veterinary Pathology* 8:320–332.

Radiculoneuropathy

Burek, J.D., Van der Kogel, A.J., & Hollander, C.F. (1976) Degenerative myelopathy in three strains of aging rats. *Veterinary Pathology* 13:321–331.

Kazui, H. & Fujisawa, K. (1988) Radiculoneuropathy of aging rats: a quantitative study. *Neuropathology and Applied Neurobiology* 14:137–156.

Krinke, G. (1983) Spinal radiculoneuropathy in aging rats: demyelination secondary to neuronal dwindling? *Acta Neuropathologica* 59:63–69.

Mitsumori, K., Maita, K., & Shirasu, Y. (1981) An ultrastructural study of spinal nerve roots and dorsal root ganglia in aging rats with spontaneous radiculoneuropathy. *Veterinary Pathology* 18:714–726.

Van Steenis, G. & Kroes, R. (1971) Changes in the nervous system and musculature of old rats. *Veterinary Pathology* 8:320–332.

Cardiac Valvular Angiectasis

Fang, H., Howroyd, P.C., Fletcher, A.M., Diters, R.W., Woicke, J., Sasseville, V.G., Bregman, C.L., Freebern, W.J., Durham, S.K., & Mense, M.G. (2007) Atrioventricular valvular angiectasis in Sprague-Dawley rats. *Veterinary Pathology* 44:407–410.

Endocardial Fibromatous Proliferation

Alison, R.H., Elwell, M.R., Jokinen, M.P., Dittrich, K.L., & Boorman, G.A. (1987) Morphology and classification of 96 primary cardiac neoplasms in Fischer 344 rats. *Veterinary Pathology* 24:488–494.

Boorman, G.A., Zurcher, C., Hollander, C.F., & Feron, V.J. (1973) Naturally occurring endocardial disease in the rat. *Archives of Pathology* 96:39–45.

Frith, C.H., Farris, H.E., & Highman, B. (1977) Endocardial fibromatous proliferation in a rat. *Laboratory Animal Science* 27:114–117.

Novilla, M.N., Sandusky, G.E., Hoover, D.M., Ray, S.E., & Wightman, K.S. (1991) A retrospective survey of endocardial proliferative lesions in rats. *Veterinary Pathology* 28:156–165.

Zaidi, I., Sullivan, D.J., & Seiden, D. (1982) Endocardial thickening in the Sprague-Dawley rat. *Toxicologic Pathology* 10:27–32.

Polyarteritis Nodosa

Bishop, S.P. (1989) Animal models of vasculitis. *Toxicologic Pathology* 17:109–117.

Skold, B.H. (1961) Chronic arteritis in the laboratory rat. *Journal of the American Veterinary Medical Association* 138:204–207.

Yang, Y.H. (1965) Polyarteritis nodosa in laboratory rats. *Laboratory Investigation* 14:81–88.

Chronic Progressive Nephropathy

Barthold, S.W. (1979) Chronic progressive nephropathy in aging rats. *Toxicologic Pathology* 7:1–6.

Gray, J.E., van Zwieten, M.J., & Hollander, C.F. (1982) Early light microscopic changes in chronic progressive nephrosis in several strains of aging laboratory rats. *Journal of Gerontology* 37:142–150.

Gray, J.E., Weaver, R.N., & Purmalis, A. (1974) Ultrastructural observations of chronic progressive nephrosis in the Sprague-Dawley rat. *Veterinary Pathology* 11:153–164.

Natatsuji, S., Yamate, J., & Sakuma, S. (1998) Macrophages, fibroblasts, and extracellular matrix accumulation in interstitial fibrosis of chronic progressive nephropathy in aged rats. *Veterinary Pathology* 35:352–360.

Owen, R.A. & Heywood, R. (1986) Age-related variations in renal structure and function in Sprague-Dawley rats. *Toxicologic Pathology* 14:158–167.

Weaver, R.N., Gray, J.E., & Schultz, J.R. (1975) Urinary proteins in Sprague-Dawley rats with chronic progressive nephrosis. *Laboratory Animal Science* 25:705–710.

Nephrocalcinosis and Urolithiasis

Magnusson, G. & Ramsay, C.H. (1971) Urolithiasis in the rat. *Laboratory Animals* 5:153–162.

Paterson, M. (1979) Urolithiasis in the Sprague-Dawley rat. *Laboratory Animals* 13:17–20.

Ristskes-Hoitinga, J., Lemmons, A.G., & Beynen, A.C. (1989) Nutrition and kidney calcification in rats. *Laboratory Animals* 23:313–318.

Hydronephrosis

Van Winkle, T.J., Womack, J.E., Barbo, W.D., & Davis, T.W. (1988) Incidence of hydronephrosis among several production colonies of outbred Sprague-Dawley rats. *Laboratory Animal Science* 38:402–406.

Renal Papillary Hyperplasia

Stubb, C., Thon, R., Ritskes-Hoitinga, M., & Hansen, A.K. (2003) Renal epithelial proliferation and its clinical expression in Brown Norway (BN) rats. *Laboratory Animals* 38:85–91.

Treloar, A.F. & Armstrong, A. (1993) Intermittent hematuria in a colony of Lewis × Brown Norway hybrid rats. *Laboratory Animal Science* 43:640–641.

Osteoarthritis

Yamasaki, K. & Inui, S. (1985) Lesions of articular, sternal and growth plate cartilage in rats. *Veterinary Pathology* 22:46–50.

Miscellaneous Disorders

Auricular Chondropathy

Chiu, T. & Lee, K.P. (1984) Auricular chondropathy in aging rats. *Veterinary Pathology* 21:500–504.

Kitagaki, M., Suwa, T., Yanagi, M., & Shiratori, K. (2003) Auricular chondritis in young ear-tagged Crj:CD(SD)IGS rats. *Laboratory Animal Science* 37:249–253.

McEwen, B.J. & Barsoum, N.J. (1990) Auricular chondritis in Wistar rats. *Laboratory Animals* 24:280–283.

Meingassner, J.G. (1991) Sympathetic auricular chondritis in rats: a model of autoimmune disease? *Laboratory Animal Science* 25:68–78.

Prieur, D., Young, D.M., & Counts, D.F. (1984) Auricular chondritis in Fawn-Hooded rats: a spontaneous disorder resembling that induced by immunization with type II collagen. *American Journal of Pathology* 116:69–76.

Hydrocephalus

Woodward, J.C. & Newberne, P.M. (1967) The pathogenesis of hydrocephalus in newborn rats deficient in vitamin B12. *Journal of Embryology and Experimental Morphology* 17:177–187.

Eosinophilic Granulomatous Pneumonia in Brown Norway Rats

Albers, T.M. & Clifford, C.B. (2000) Eosinophilic granulomatous pneumonia: a strain-related lesion of high prevalence in the Brown Norway rat. *Contemporary Topics in Laboratory Animal Science* 39:61–62.

Germann, P.G., Hafner, D., Hanauer, G., & Drommer, W. (1998) Incidence and severity of granulomatous pneumonia in Brown Norway (BN) rats: breeder related variations. *Journal of Experimental Animal Science* 39:22–33.

Noritake, S., Ogawa, K., Suzuki, G., Ozawa, K., & Ikeda, T. (2007) Pulmonary inflammation in brown Norway rats: possible

association with environmental particles in the animal room environment. *Experimental Animals* 56:319–327.
Ohtsuka, R., Doi, K., & Itagaki, S. (1997) Histological characteristics of respiratory system in Brown Norway rat. *Experimental Animals* 46:127–133.

Persistent Vaginal Septum

De Schaepdrijver, L.M., Fransen, J.L., Van der Eycken, E.S., & Coussement, W.C. (1995) Transverse vaginal septum in the specific-pathogen-free Wistar rat. *Laboratory Animal Science* 45:181–183.
Lezmi, S., Duprey-Thibault, K., Bidaut, A., Hardy, P., Pino, M., Saint Macary, G., Barbellion, S., Brunel, P., Dorchies, O., Clifford, C., & Leconte, I. (2011) Spontaneous metritis related to the presence of vaginal septum in pregnant Sprague-Dawley Crl:CD (SD) rats: impact on reproductive toxicity studies. *Veterinary Pathology* 48:964–969.

Environmental Disorders

Bellhorn, R.W., Korte, G.E., & Abrutyn, D. (1988) Spontaneous corneal degeneration in the rat. *Laboratory Animal Science* 38:46–50.
Burkhart, C.A. & Robinson, J.L. (1978) High rat pup mortality attributed to the use of cedar-wood shavings as bedding. *Laboratory Animals* 12:221–222.
Cripps, L., Gobbi, A., Ceruti, R.M., Clifford, C.B., Remuzzi, A., & Scanziani, E. (2000) Ringtail in suckling Munich Wistar Frömter rats: a histopathologic study. *Comparative Medicine* 50:536–539.
Fleischman, R.W., McCracken, D., & Forbes, W. (1977) Adynamic ileus in the rat induced by chloral hydrate. *Laboratory Animal Science* 27:238–243.
Kurisu, K. Sawamoto, O., Watanabe, H., & Ito, A. (1996) Sequential changes in the Harderian gland of rats exposed to high intensity light. *Laboratory Animal Science* 46:71–76.
Losco, P.E. & Troup, C.M. (1988) Corneal dystrophy in Fischer 344 rats. *Laboratory Animal Science* 38:702–710.
Noell, W.K., Walker, V.S., Kang, B.S., & Berman, S. (1966) Retinal damage by light in rats. *Investigative Ophthalmology* 5:450–473.
Rao, G.N. (1991) Light intensity-associated eye lesions of Fischer 344 rats in long term studies. *Toxicologic Pathology* 19:148–155.
Semple-Rowland, S.L. & Dawson, W.W. (1987) Retinal cyclic light damage threshold for albino rats. *Laboratory Animal Science* 37:389–398.
Taylor, D.K., Rogers, M.M., & Hankenson, F.C. (2006) Lanolin as a treatment option for ringtail in transgenic rats. *Journal of the American Association for Laboratory Animal Science* 45:83–87.

Drug-Related Disorders

Alden, C.L. & Frith, C.H. (1991) Urinary system. In: *Handbook of Toxicologic Pathology* (eds. W.M. Haschek& Rousseaux), pp. 315–387. Academic Press, San Diego, CA.
Beierschmitt, W.P., Keenan, K.P., & Weiner, M. (1986) Age-related susceptibility of male Fischer-344 rats to acetaminophen nephrotoxicity. *Life Sciences* 39:2335–2342.
Fleischman, R.W., McCracken, D., & Forces, W. (1977) Adynamic ileus in the rat induced by chloral hydrate. *Laboratory Animal Science* 27:238–243.
Kufoy, E.A., Pakalnis, V.A., Parks, C.D., Wells, A., Yang, C.H., & Fox, A. (1989) Keratoconjunctivitis sicca and associated secondary uveitis elicited in rats after systemic ketamine/xylazine anesthesia. *Experimental Eye Research* 49:861–871.
Kyle, M.E. & Koscis, J.J. (1985) Effect of age on salicylate-induced nephrotoxicity in male rats. *Toxicology and Applied Pharmacology* 81:337–347.
Turner, P.V. & Albassam, M.A. (2005) Susceptibility of rats to corneal lesions after injectable anesthesia. *Comparative Medicine* 55:175–182.

NEOPLASMS

Neoplasia is very common in rats, and aged rats are often simultaneously afflicted with multiple types of neoplasia. It is beyond the scope of this chapter to give a detailed description of every neoplasm that might occur in this species. For additional information, refer to "General References on Diseases of Rats," in addition to "General References on Rat Neoplasms."

Zymbal's Gland and Preputial Gland Tumors

Tumors may arise from the Zymbal's holocrine glands within the subcutis at the base of the external ear. On gross examination, masses are circumscribed and lobulated (Fig. 2.76), and may become ulcerated. On microscopic examination, tumors consist of epithelial cells with abundant, vacuolated cytoplasm with squamous differentiation and keratinization (Fig. 2.77). Depending on their histologic pattern, they are classified as adenomas or adenocarcinomas. The malignant tumors are locally invasive, but are not metastatic. Similar tumors arise from the preputial glands of males (Figs. 2.78 and 2.79).

Mammary Fibroadenoma

Mammary fibroadenomas are a common occurrence in older female rats, particularly SD rats, although these tumors may also occur occasionally in male rats. Sex, age, genetic, dietary, and endocrine factors may all play a role in the incidence of spontaneous mammary tumors. There are significant variations in the incidence, depending on the source of rats of this strain. Ranges of 7–40% have been recorded in SD rats from different sources. The incidence of spontaneous mammary fibroadenomas is markedly reduced in ovarectomized rats. Restriction of food intake by 20% reduced the incidence of mammary tumors in female SD rats by fivefold, compared with controls. Prolactin levels have also been identified as a key factor. Serum prolactin values in females with mammary

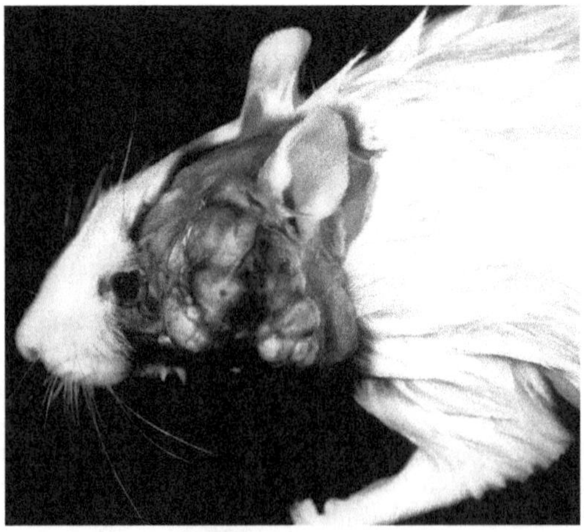

FIG. 2.76. *Lobulated tumor arising from the Zymbal's gland. The Zymbal's gland is located within the subcutis adjacent to the ear, with ductal drainage into the external ear canal.*

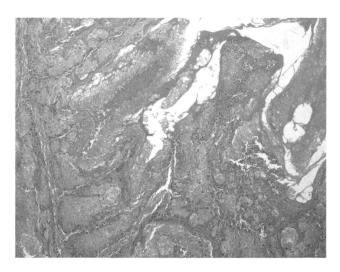

FIG. 2.77. *Zymbal's gland tumor composed of polyhedral cells with central keratinization and cellular debris.*

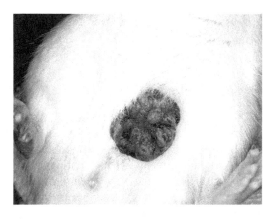

FIG. 2.78. *Preputial gland adenoma in a mature male rat. Note the distinct lobulated appearance to the tumor. (Source: T.R. Schoeb, University of Alabama, Tuscaloosa, Alabama. Reproduced with permission from T.R. Schoeb.)*

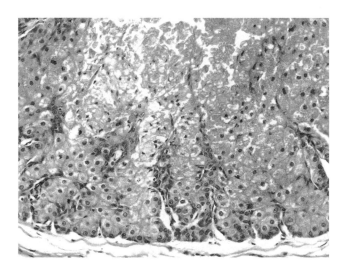

FIG. 2.79. *Preputial gland tumor shown in the previous figure. The mass consists of well-differentiated glandular epithelial cells. (Source: T.R. Schoeb, University of Alabama, Tuscaloosa, Alabama. Reproduced with permission from T.R. Schoeb.)*

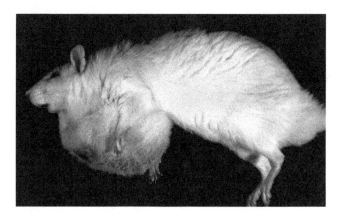

FIG. 2.80. *Mammary fibroadenoma in an aged rat. These tumors will often grow to very large size without malignant transformation or metastasis.*

tumors were over 25 times higher than in 6-month-old virgin females. There have been attempts to equate mammary tumors with the incidence of pituitary adenomas, but unequivocal correlations have not been made.

Mammary fibroadenomas may reach very large size (Fig. 2.80), and are typically circumscribed, movable, firm, and lobulated. They may be located within any of the 12 mammary glands along the mammary chain, and occasionally at other sites on the body. In larger tumors, there may be ulceration of the overlying skin. On cut section, tumors are lobulated (Fig. 2.81), with regions of highly fibrous to glandular tissue. The lobulated appearance is readily evident on cut surface. On microscopic examination, there is distinct interlobular and intralobular connective tissue surrounding relatively well-differentiated acinar structures (Figs. 2.82 and 2.83). There are markedly variable proportions of acinar and collagenous tissue, depending upon region of the tumor examined. Acini are lined by cuboidal epithelial cells, frequently with prominent vacuoles in the cytoplasm.

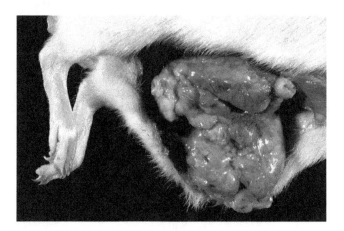

FIG. 2.81. *Mammary fibroadenoma in an adult female Sprague-Dawley rat. The prominent lobulations and interlobular fibrous tissue are characteristic gross findings seen with this neoplasm.*

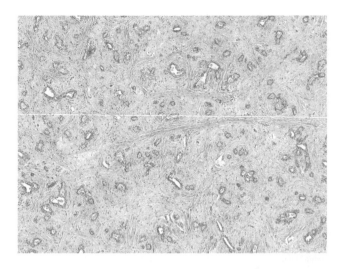

FIG. 2.82. *Mammary fibroadenoma, illustrating the acinar structures and prominent connective tissue components.*

Mammary Adenocarcinoma

Malignant mammary tumors represent a relatively small percentage of mammary tumors in the laboratory rat. However, diagnostic pathologists in some laboratories have reported an increase in malignant mammary tumors in this species. Mammary adenocarcinomas have also been produced experimentally by estrogen administration. A variety of patterns may be evident histologically. They have been classified by various terms, including "anaplastic adenocarcinoma" (Fig. 2.84), "cribriform," "tubular," "papillary," and "comedocarcinoma."

Lymphoreticular Tumors
Large Granular Lymphocytic (LGL) Leukemia

This signature neoplasm occurs in Fischer 344, Wistar, and Wistar-Furth rats. It is a major cause of death in aging F344 rats. Neoplastic cells arise in the spleen and then spread to other organs. Although once considered

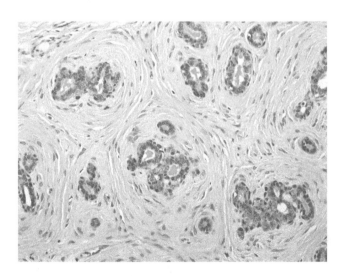

FIG. 2.83. *Mammary fibroadenoma, demonstrating the relatively well-differentiated epithelial cells lining acini and the prominent periacinar collagenous tissue.*

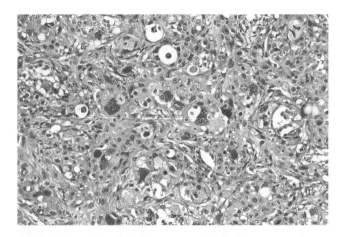

FIG. 2.84. *Anaplastic mammary adenocarcinoma in an adult female rat. The neoplasm features anaplastic epithelial cells.*

to be of natural killer (NK) cell origin, studies of cytotoxic activity and surface antigens suggest that these leukemias are of a heterogeneous lymphocytic cell origin. Clinical signs are characterized by weight loss, anemia, jaundice, and depression. LGL leukemia may be associated with elevated blood leukocyte counts of up to 400,000/ml^3. Morphologically, leukemic cells resemble large granular lymphocytes. The spleen is typically enlarged, and there may be moderate to marked enlargement of the liver (Fig. 2.85) and lymphadenopathy. Petechial hemorrhages are frequently present on the lung and lymph nodes. Stained impression smears of tissues such as spleen reveal LGL cells that are 10–15 μm in diameter, with irregular-shaped, frequently indented nuclei, pale cytoplasm, and azurophilic cytoplasmic granules (Fig. 2.86). On histological examination of tissue sections, there is diffuse infiltration with LGL cells in spleen, lymph nodes, liver, and lung. There is

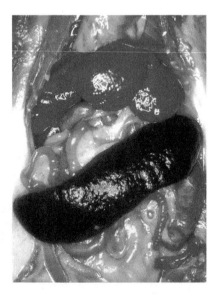

FIG. 2.85. *Abdominal viscera from a Fischer 344 rat with large granular lymphocyte (LGL) leukemia. There is marked splenomegaly and hepatomegaly. (Source: T.R. Schoeb, University of Alabama, Tuscaloosa, Alabama. Reproduced with permission from T.R. Schoeb.)*

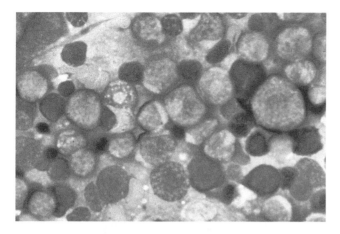

FIG. 2.86. *Impression smear of spleen from a case of LGL leukemia. There are large numbers of neoplastic lymphocytes intermixed with hematopoietic elements.*

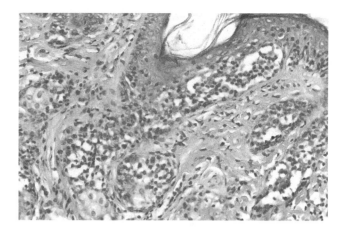

FIG. 2.88. *Skin from an adult rat with epitheliotropic lymphoma. Note the infiltrate of relatively well-differentiated lymphocytes at the dermoepidermal junction.*

frequently marked depletion of lymphoid follicles in the spleen and diffuse infiltration of leukemic cells in the sinusoids. Hepatocellular degeneration commonly occurs, probably a result of the concurrent anemia and neoplastic infiltrates. Erythrophagocytosis may be evident in the liver and spleen. There is usually a concurrent, immune-mediated hemolytic anemia, with thrombocytopenia and clotting abnormalities suggestive of disseminated intravascular coagulation.

Lymphoma and Lymphocytic Leukemia

Lymphoma and lymphocytic leukemia are relatively uncommon in most strains of rats. At necropsy, splenomegaly, enlarged lymph nodes (Fig. 2.87), and hepatomegaly are characteristic findings. On microscopic examination, there is frequently diffuse infiltration of neoplastic lymphocytes into organs such as spleen and liver, with obliteration of the normal architecture. Primary thymic lymphomas have also been described.

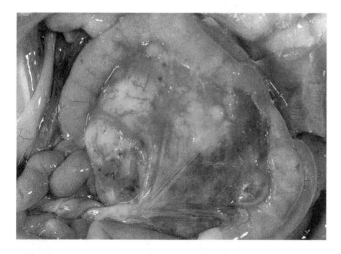

FIG. 2.87. *Lymphoma in a rat arising from mesenteric lymphoid tissue. Other than LGL leukemia, lymphoid tumors are rare in rats. (Source: D. Imai, University of California, Davis, CA. Reproduced with permission from D. Imai.)*

Cutaneous Lymphoma: Mycosis Fungoides

Epidermotropic lymphomas are relatively rare in rats. Clinically, the disease is characterized by the presence of circumscribed erythematous plaques on the skin that may progress to ulceration. Microscopically, there is epidermal hyperplasia with variable ulceration and marked infiltration with neoplastic lymphocytes in the dermis and epidermis. In the epidermis, the infiltrating cells occur singly or in clusters surrounded by a clear halo (Fig. 2.88). Similar changes are present in hair follicles in the region. The infiltrating lymphocytes are medium to large size and react with anti-CD3 antibody, providing confirmation that they are of T-cell origin. In cases documented to date, the neoplastic infiltrates have been confined to the skin.

Histiocytic Sarcoma

Histiocytic sarcomas occur most often in SD rats, but they also have been observed in other strains. The tumors are present primarily in animals over 12 months of age, and there is no obvious sex predisposition. At necropsy, sarcomas of this type may be present in the liver, lymph nodes, lung, spleen, mediastinum, retroperitoneum, or subcutaneous tissue. Neoplasms are pale and moderately firm, and they tend to infiltrate and displace normal tissue. Necrotic areas may be scattered in the mass. On microscopic examination, tumors consist of diffuse sheets of neoplastic cells, varying from elongated, pallisading fusiform cells to plump, pleomorphic histiocytic cells. The histiocytic cells have vesicular nuclei, prominent nucleoli, and abundant cytoplasm. Multinucleated giant cells are usually present in tumors with a prominent histiocytic component (Figs. 2.89 and 2.90). Based on electron microscopic and immunohistochemical studies, the histiocytic forms are derived from monocytes or histiocytes, while the origin of the fibrous types remains uncertain. Differential diagnoses include fibrosarcoma, lymphosarcoma, osteosarcoma, and granulomatous inflammatory tissue.

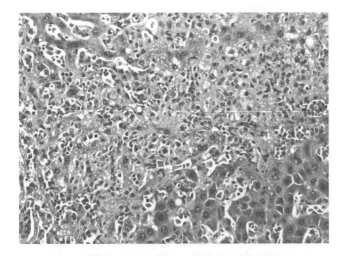

FIG. 2.89. *Histiocytic sarcoma infiltrating the liver of an aged rat. Note the indistinct cytoplasmic outlines, anisokaryosis, and pleomorphic appearance of the histiocytic cells that are dissecting through hepatic cords.*

Pituitary Gland Adenoma

Pituitary adenomas are very common tumors that arise in older animals, particularly in Sprague-Dawley and Wistar rats. In addition to age, genetic factors, diet, and breeding history may play a role. Reduction in food intake reduces the incidence of spontaneous pituitary tumors, and mated females have been shown to have a lower incidence of pituitary tumors than did virgin females. In some studies, there is a slightly higher incidence in females, but this is not a consistent finding. Clinical signs vary, from animals that are subclinical to animals with severe depression, frequently with incoordination. The majority of pituitary tumors are interpreted to be chromophobe adenomas. Acidophil and basophil tumors have also been described. Immunohistochemical techniques are required for positive

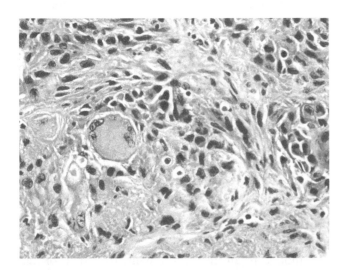

FIG. 2.90. *Histiocytic sarcoma in the liver of an aged rat, illustrating multinucleated giant cell formation, which is common in this type of neoplasm.*

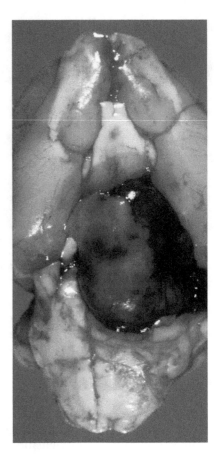

FIG. 2.91. *Pituitary gland adenoma in an aged female Wistar rat. Note the hemorrhagic appearance of the large fleshy mass.*

identification of cell type. In pituitary tumors studied by immunocytochemistry, prolactin-producing tumors are the most common type. Most tumors are interpreted to arise from the pars distalis, although tumors of the pars intermedia have also been described. Pituitary carcinomas are relatively uncommon.

Pathology

The pituitary is enlarged, frequently with prominent lobulations. Tumors are often dark red to brown and hemorrhagic in appearance (Fig. 2.91). In larger tumors, there may be minimal to marked compression of the overlying mesencephalon. On microscopic examination, the anterior pituitary consists of cords or nests of glandular cells bound by strands of connective tissue, with an abundant cavernous vascular capillary network. The cells typically have large nuclei and prominent nucleoli, with abundant, lightly basophilic to amphophilic cytoplasm consistent with a chromophobe adenoma (Fig. 2.92). Giant nuclei may be present in the mass. Mitotic figures are occasionally observed. A pseudocapsule composed of a fine band of connective tissue separates the tumor from the adjacent pituitary tissue. More than 1 tumor may be present in an affected gland. Nodules of hypertrophic or hyperplastic cells may be

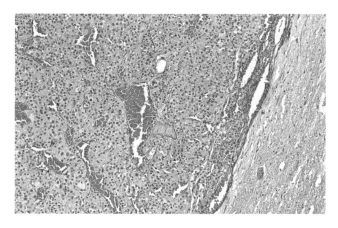

FIG. 2.92. *Pituitary adenoma, with prominent cords of epithelial cells interspersed within a vascular stroma.*

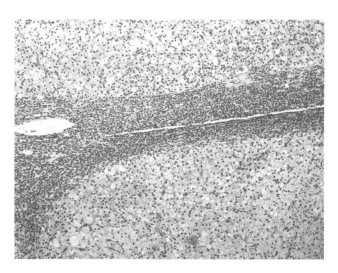

FIG. 2.94. *Interstitial cell tumor from an aged Fischer 344 rat. These tumors are typically composed of 2 morphologically distinct cell types, consisting of cells with minimal cytoplasm, which are usually at the periphery of nodules, and cells with abundant cytoplasm that are more centrally located. Both cell types are of Leydig cell origin.*

present in glands and must be differentiated from adenomas. They occur as islands of large cells, sometimes with mitoses, but there is no evidence of pseudo-encapsulation or compression of adjacent tissue.

Testicular Interstitial Cell Tumors

Interstitial cell tumors occur frequently in male F344 rats, reaching a prevalence of 100%. Tumors are often multicentric and involve one or both testes. On gross examination, they appear as circumscribed, lobulated, light yellow to hemorrhagic (Fig. 2.93). Microscopic changes are consistent with tumors of Leydig cell origin, with a spectrum of lesions ranging from small microscopic nodules to large tumors. Masses are composed of cells of 2 types: polyhedral to elongated cells with granular to vacuolated cytoplasm and smaller cells with hyperchromatic nuclei and scanty cytoplasm (Fig. 2.94). Interstitial cell tumors have been associated with concurrent hypercalcemia.

Mesothelioma

These neoplasms are occasionally encountered in laboratory rats, particularly the F344 strain. Affected rats frequently present with ascites, and at necropsy, there are multiple raised circumscribed yellow to brown nodules present in both the peritoneal and pleural cavities (Figs. 2.95 and 2.96). In most cases, the primary site is the tunica vaginalis of the testes, with subsequent implantation on the serosal surfaces of the peritoneal and pleural cavities. Microscopically, there are diffuse to nodular aggregations of cuboidal to polyhedral cells on serosal surfaces. It is

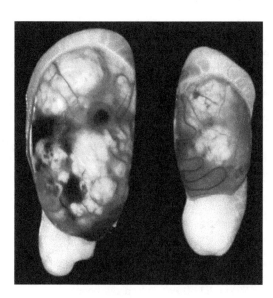

FIG. 2.93. *Testes from an aged Fischer 344 male rat, illustrating multiple interstitial (Leydig) cell tumors arising in both testes.*

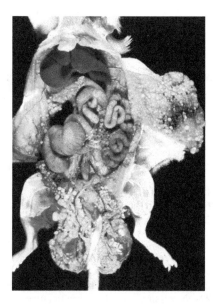

FIG. 2.95. *Fischer 344 rat with diffuse mesothelioma involving both the abdominal and thoracic cavities. Note the multiple raised circumscribed polypoid lesions on the serosal surfaces.*

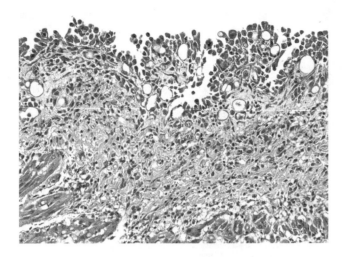

FIG. 2.96. *Mesothelioma on the pericardium of a Fischer 344 rat, depicting the papillary growth of neoplastic mesothelial cells on a fibrovascular stromal base.*

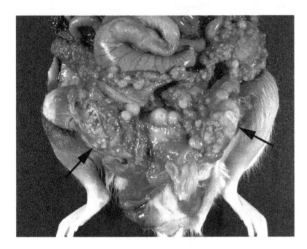

FIG. 2.97. *Mesothelioma and interstitial cell tumors (arrows) in an aged rat. Concommitant tumors are common in rats.*

fairly common to have simultaneous interstitial cell tumors in cases of mesothelioma (Fig 2.97).

BIBLIOGRAPHY FOR NEOPLASMS

General References on Rat Neoplasms

Dagle, G.E., Zwicker, G.M., & Renne, R.A. (1979) Morphology of spontaneous brain tumors in the rat. *Veterinary Pathology* 16:318–324.

Ikezaki, S., Takagi, M., & Tamura, K. (2011) Natural occurrence of neoplastic lesions in young Sprague-Dawley rats. *Journal of Toxicologic Pathology* 24:37–40.

MacKenzie, W.F. & Garner, F.M. (1973) Comparison of neoplasms from six sources of rats. *Journal of the National Cancer Institute* 50:1243–1257.

McMartin, D.N., Sahota, P.S., Gunson, D.E., Hsu, H.H., & Spaet, R.H. (1992) Neoplasms and related proliferative lesions in control Sprague-Dawley rats from carcinogenicity studies. Historical data and diagnostic considerations. *Toxicologic Pathology* 20:212–225.

Stinson, S.F., Schuller, H.M., & Reznik, G. (1990) *Atlas of Tumor Pathology of the Fischer Rat.* CRC Press, Boca Raton, FL.

Tucker, M.J. (1979) The effects of long-term food restriction on tumors in rodents. *International Journal of Cancer* 23:803–807.

Turusov, V.S. & Mohr, U. (1976) *Pathology of Tumours in Laboratory Animals: Tumours of the Rat*, Vol. 1. IARC Scientific Publications, Lyon, France.

Zwicker, G.M., Eyster, R.C., Sells, D.M., & Gass, J.H. (1992) Spontaneous renal neoplasms of aged Crl:CDBR rats. *Toxicologic Pathology* 20:125–130.

Zwicker, G.M., Eyster, R.C., Sells, D.M., & Gass, J.H. (1992) Naturally occurring intestinal epithelial neoplasms in aged CRL:CD BR rats. *Toxicologic Pathology* 20:253–259.

Zwicker, G.M., Eyster, R.C., Sells, D.M., & Gass, J.H. (1992) Spontaneous skin neoplasms in aged Sprague-Dawley rats. *Toxicologic Pathology* 20:327–340.

Zwicker, G.M., Eyster, R.C., Sells, D.M., & Gass, J.H. (1992) Spontaneous brain and spinal cord/nerve neoplasms in aged Sprague-Dawley rats. *Toxicologic Pathology* 20:576–584.

Zwicker, G.M., Eyster, R.C., Sells, D.M., & Gass, J.H. (1995) Spontaneous vascular neoplasms in aged Sprague-Dawley rats. *Toxicologic Pathology* 23:518–526.

Mammary Tumors

Barsoum, N.J., Gough, A.W., Sturgess, J.M., & de la Iglesia, F.A. (1984) Morphologic features and incidence of spontaneous hyperplastic and neoplastic mammary gland lesions in Wistar rats. *Toxicologic Pathology* 12:26–38.

Ito, A., Naito, M., Watanabe, H., & Yokoro, K. (1984) Prolactin and aging: X-irradiated and estrogen-induced rat mammary tumorigenesis. *Journal of the National Cancer Institute* 73:123–126.

Okada, M., Takeuchi, J., Sobue, M., Kataoka, K., Inagaki, Y., Shigemura, M., & Chiba, T. (1981) Characteristics of 106 spontaneous mammary tumours appearing in Sprague-Dawley female rats. *British Journal of Cancer* 43:689–695.

Lymphoreticular Tumors

Abbott, D.P., Prentice, D.E., & Cherry, C.P. (1983) Mononuclear cell leukemia in aged Sprague-Dawley rats. *Veterinary Pathology* 20:434–439.

Barsoum, N.J., Hanna, W., Gough, A.W., Smith, G.S., Sturgess, J.M., & de la Iglesia, F.A. (1984) Histiocytic sarcoma in Wistar rats: a light microscopic, immunohistochemical, and ultrastructural study. *Archives of Pathology and Laboratory Medicine* 108:802–807.

Frith, C.H., Ward, J.M., & Chandra, M. (1993) The morphology, immunohistochemistry, and incidence of hematopoietic neoplasms in mice and rats. *Veterinary Pathology* 21:206–218.

Greaves, P., Martin, J.M., & Masson, M.T. (1982) Spontaneous rat malignant tumors of fibrohistiocytic origin: an ultrastructural study. *Veterinary Pathology* 19:497–505.

Naylor, D.C., Krinke, G.J., & Ruefenacht, H.J. (1988) Primary tumors of the thymus in the rat. *Journal of Comparative Pathology* 99:187–203.

Prats, M., Fondevila, D., Rabanal, R.M., Marco, A., Domingo, M., & Ferrer, L. (1994) Epidermotropic cutaneous lymphoma (mycosis fungoides) in a SD rat. *Veterinary Pathology* 31:396–398.

Rosol, T.J. & Stromberg, P.C. (1990) Effects of large granular lymphocytic leukemia on bone in F344 rats. *Veterinary Pathology* 27:391–396.

Squire, R.A., Brinkous, K.M., Peiper, S.C., Firminger, H.I., Mann, R.B., & Standberg, J.D. (1981) Histiocytic sarcoma with a granuloma-like component occurring in a large colony of Sprague-Dawley rats. *American Journal of Pathology* 106:21–30.

Stromberg, P.C., Kociba, G.J., Grants, I.S., Krakowka, G.S., Rinehart, J.J., & Mezza, L.E. (1990) Spleen cell population changes and hemolytic anemia in F344 rats with large granular lymphocytic leukemia. *Veterinary Pathology* 27:397–403.

Stromberg, P.C. & Vogtsberger, L.M. (1983) Pathology of mononuclear cell leukemia of Fischer rats. I. Morphologic studies. *Veterinary Pathology* 20:698–708.

Ward, J.M. & Reynolds, C.W. (1983) Large granular lymphatic leukemia: a heterogeneous lymphocytic leukemia in F344 rats. *American Journal of Pathology* 111:1–10.

Pituitary Gland Tumors

McComb, D.J., Kovacs, K., Beri, J., & Zak, F. (1984) Pituitary adenomas in old Sprague-Dawley rats: a histologic, ultrastructural, and immunohistochemical study. *Journal of the National Cancer Institute* 73:1143–1166.

Nagatani, M., Miura, K., Tsuchitani, M., & Narama, I. (1987) Relationship between cellular morphology and immunocytological findings of spontaneous pituitary tumours in the aged rat. *Journal of Comparative Pathology* 97:11–20.

Pickering, C.E. & Pickering, R.G. (1984) The effect of diet on the incidence of pituitary tumours in female Wistar rats. *Laboratory Animals* 18:298–314.

Pickering, C.E. & Pickering, R.G. (1984) The effect of repeated reproduction on the incidence of pituitary tumours in Wistar rats. *Laboratory Animals* 18:371–378.

Sandusky, G.E., Van Pelt C.S., Todd, G.C., & Wightman, K. (1988) An immunocytochemical study of pituitary adenomas and focal hyperplasia in old Sprague-Dawley and Fischer rats. *Toxicologic Pathology* 16:376–380.

Testicular Tumors

Troyer, H., Sowers, J.R., & Babich, E. (1982) Leydig cell tumor induced hypercalcemia in the Fischer rat: morphometric and histochemical evidence for a humoral factor that activates osteoclasis. *American Journal of Pathology* 108:284–290.

3 Hamster

INTRODUCTION

The subfamily Cricetinae contains approximately 25 different hamster species worldwide. They are found primarily in southeastern Europe and Asia. A number of different genera and species of hamsters are used in the research laboratory: the Syrian or golden hamster (*Mesocricetus auratus*); Chinese or gray hamster (*Cricetulus griseus*); European or black-bellied hamster (*Cricetus cricetus*); Armenian or migratory hamster (*Cricetulus migratorius*); Dzungarian, Siberian, dwarf, winter-white, or striped hairy-footed hamster (*Phodopus sungorus*); South African hamster or white-tailed rat (*Mystromys albicaudatus*); and others. The majority of hamsters used in research are Syrian and Chinese hamsters. Syrian hamsters that are commonly used in research and kept as pets originated from a litter captured in Syria in 1930, and it is believed that subsequent progeny are descendants of a single sibling pairing. The original animals were bred in captivity at Hebrew University, and their offspring later served as the foundation stock for *M. auratus* in other countries. Although often referred to as outbred, Syrian hamsters are understandably genetically homozygous. It has been claimed that outbred Syrian hamsters are so inbred that they can accept tissue transplants among one another, evidence of which is provided in their unique susceptibility to a transmissible reticulum cell sarcoma. True inbred strains of Syrian hamsters have also been developed. *Cricetulus griseus* was first domesticated in Beijing, China, around 1920.

Syrian hamsters are susceptible to several serious enteric microbial infections, are remarkably susceptible to a number of xenogeneic viruses, and are prone to the induction of tumors with many such viruses. This is likely due to a limited major histocompatibility complex (MHC) repertoire resulting from their highly inbred nature. This chapter deals primarily with diseases of the Syrian hamster. Very little is known about diseases of other types of hamsters, and it must be kept in mind that generalizations cannot be made among hamster species, since hamsters represent different, distantly related genera.

In their natural habitat, Syrian hamsters live individually in burrows in close proximity to other hamsters and communicate using ultrasonic signals. Burrows are complex, with separate chambers devoted to food storage, nesting, and urination/defecation. Females tolerate adult males only when in estrus, and will reject and often kill males after mating. This solitary lifestyle is also evident when litters reach weaning age, at which time pups attempt to disseminate. If not separated at weaning, females will cannibalize their pups. Indeed, maternal cannibalization of pups is a major management challenge. Syrian hamsters may undergo true hibernation in response to variables such as low environmental temperature, decreased access to food, and exposure to diminishing hours of light. During hibernation, their metabolic rate may be reduced to 5% of normal. Hamsters may also undergo shorter periods of torpor. Hamsters are crepuscular, gathering food within their cheek pouches and hording food in their burrows. Using exercise wheel revolutions as a measurement of activity, female Syrian hamsters have been shown to travel distances equal to several kilometers during a 24-hour period while in estrus. Olfactory cues play an essential role in mating behavior. They are active chewers and adept at escape. Hamsters enjoy a well-constructed and comfortable nest and endeavor to cache impressive stores of food.

ANATOMIC FEATURES

The anatomy of the Syrian hamster has been reviewed by Bivin et al. (1987), Magalhaes (1968), and Murray (2012). Syrian hamsters have a characteristic compact body,

Pathology of Laboratory Rodents and Rabbits, Fourth Edition. Stephen W. Barthold, Stephen M. Griffey, and Dean H. Percy.

short legs, and very short glabrous tails. This is true for most other hamsters, with the exception of the Chinese hamster, which has a more elongated body and a longer tail. Hamsters possess 4 digits on the front feet and 5 on the rear feet. Syrian hamsters have remarkably abundant and loose skin. Adult female Syrian hamsters are larger than males. The female urethra has a separate opening from the vagina. Both sexes possess paired flank organs, which are most prominent in males. These organs consist of sebaceous glands, pigment cells, and terminal hair. They are darkly pigmented in mature males and appear to play a role in conversion of testosterone to dihydrotestosterone. The scent glands are located on the ventral midline in other species of hamsters. Hamsters have prominent depots of brown fat beneath and between the scapulae, in the axilla and neck, and around the adrenals and kidneys.

The gastrointestinal tract has a number of significant features. As in mice and rats, the incisors (but not the molars) grow continuously (elodont). Many, although not all, genera of hamsters possess buccal pouches, which extend dorsolaterally from the oral cavity on either side of the shoulder region. These structures have been utilized as immunologically privileged sites, which allow xenograft transplants to survive. The utility of hamster cheek pouches as an experimental tool has been largely supplanted by immunodeficient mice. The esophagus enters the stomach at the junction of the nonglandular and glandular stomachs, which are divided by a muscular sphincter (Fig. 3.1). The non-glandular stomach, or forestomach, features an elevated pH and a complex microbiome, which contribute to fermentative digestion. Paneth cells are a normal constituent of small intestinal crypts. The cecum is divided into apical and basal portions separated by a semilunar valve. In fact, there is a series of 4 valves in the ileoce-cocolic region of the hamster. As with other rodents and rabbits, hamsters rely on coprophagy for nutrition. The liver is divided into 4 lobes, with a gall bladder. As in the mouse and rat, intranuclear cytoplasmic invagination (inclusions) and eosinophilic cytoplasmic inclusions in hepatocytes can be found, particularly in diseased livers.

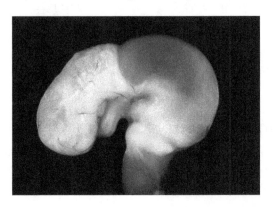

FIG. 3.1.   *Stomach from a hamster, depicting the nonglandular and glandular regions. Note the esophageal entry at the junction of each.*

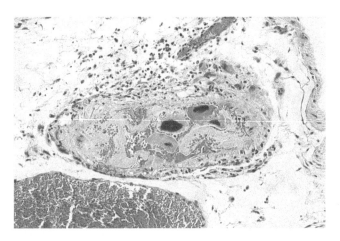

FIG. 3.2.   *Trophoblast cells within mesometrial vessel in a pregnant hamster.*

The respiratory tract is similar to that of other laboratory rodents, with no respiratory bronchioles. Lungs have a single left lobe and 5 lobes on the right side (cranial, middle, caudal, intermediate, and accessory). As desert animals, Syrian hamsters have water-conserving kidneys with elongated single papillae that extend into the ureters. The female reproductive tract consists of a duplex uterus with 2 cervical canals that merge into a single external cervical os. There are 7 pairs of mammary glands. The male testes and accessory glands, as with most rodents, are comparatively large and prominent. Adult males develop large adrenal glands, due to enlargement of the zona reticularis to 3 times the size of females. This enlargement is related to season and sexual maturity. The hamster placenta differs somewhat from the hemochorial placentation of other laboratory rodents and is termed "labyrinthine hemochorial." Trophoblastic giant cells of the fetal placenta are in direct contact with the maternal bloodstream and tend to migrate within the maternal vasculature. They have a tropism for arterial blood and can be found inside uterine vessels in the mesometrium (Fig. 3.2). They can persist for up to 3 weeks postpartum. On occasion, trophoblasts may be found in the pulmonary vessels of pregnant females.

Erythrocytic polychromasia is relatively common in hamsters, with moderate anisocytosis. Erythrocyte life spans vary from 50 to 78 days. Life spans are increased during hibernation. Leukocyte counts are 5,000–10,000/ml. Approximately 60–75% of the circulating leukocytes are lymphocytes. Neutrophils have densely staining eosinophilic granules and thus may be referred to as heterophils.

BIBLIOGRAPHY FOR INTRODUCTION AND ANATOMIC FEATURES

Bivin, W.S., Olsen, G.H., & Murray, K.A. (1987) Morphophysiology. In: *Laboratory Hamsters* (eds. G.L. Van Hoosier, Jr. & C.W. McPherson), pp. 9–41. Academic Press.

Burek, J.D., Goldberg, B., Hutchins, G., & Strandberg, J.D. (1979) The pregnant hamster as a model to study intravascular trophoblasts and associated maternal blood vessel changes. *Veterinary Pathology* 16:553–566.

Clark, J.D. (1987) Historical perspectives and taxonomy. In: *Laboratory Hamsters* (eds. G. L. Van Hoosier, Jr. & C. W. McPherson), pp. 3–7. Academic Press, New York.

Goshal, N.G. & Bal, H.S. (1990) Histomorphology of the hamster cheek pouch. *Laboratory Animals* 24:228–233.

Hankenson, F.C. & Van Hoosier, G.L. Jr. (2002) Biology and diseases of hamsters. In: *Laboratory Animal Medicine*, 2nd edn (eds. J.G. Fox, L.C. Anderson, F. M. Loew, & F. W. Quimby), pp. 167–202. Academic Press, New York.

Hoffman, R.A. (1968) Hibernation and effects of low temperature. In: *The Golden Hamster: Its Biology and Use in Medical Research* (ed. R.A. Hoffman), pp. 25–39. Iowa State University Press, Ames, IA.

Magalhaes, H. (1968) Gross anatomy. In: *The Golden Hamster: Its Biology and Use in Medical Research* (eds. R.A. Hoffman, P.F. Robinson, H. Magalhaes, K.M. Knigge, & S.A. Joseph), pp. 91–109. Iowa State University Press, Ames, IA.

Murray, K.A. (2012) Anatomy, physiology, and behavior. In: *The Laboratory Rabbit, Guinea Pig, Hamster, and Other Rodents* (eds. M.A. Suckow, K.A. Stevens, & R.P. Wilson), pp. 753–763. Academic Press, New York.

Richards, M.P.M. (1966) Activity measured by running wheels and observations during the oestrous cycle, pregnancy and pseudopregnancy in the golden hamster. *Animal Behavior* 14:450–458.

Smith, G.D. (2012) Taxonomy and history. In: *The Laboratory Rabbit, Guinea Pig, Hamster, and Other Rodents* (eds. M.A. Suckow, K.A. Stevens, & R.P. Wilson), pp. 747–752. Academic Press, New York.

Thomson, F.N. & Wardrop, K.J. (1987) Clinical chemistry and hematology. In: *Laboratory Hamsters* (eds. G.L. Van Hoosier, Jr. & C.W. McPherson), pp. 43–59. Academic Press, New York.

DNA VIRAL INFECTIONS

Adenovirus Infection

Adenoviral intranuclear inclusion bodies have been observed in ileal enterocytes in tissues collected from hamsters during the first few weeks of life. Typical adenoviral inclusions have been observed only in hamsters less than 4 weeks of age. In addition, antibodies to the MAdV-2 (K87) strain of mouse adenovirus are commonly present in hamsters from commercial suppliers, and antibodies to MAdV-1 have been occasionally detected. Large, amphophilic, intranuclear inclusions may be present in the enterocytes lining villi of the jejunum and ileum and rarely in the cryptal epithelial cells. Infection is subclinical, and there is no evidence of intestinal tract damage or inflammatory response. It is unclear if hamsters have their own indigenous adenovirus, or if it has been acquired from other species.

Cytomegalovirus Infection: Cricetid Herpesvirus, CrHV-1

Cytomegalovirus-like lesions have been observed in salivary glands of subclinically infected Chinese hamsters, but not other hamster species. Intranuclear and intracytoplasmic inclusions with cytomegaly were present in the acinar epithelium of the submaxillary salivary glands. Cytomegaloviruses are generally host-specific,

so it is unlikely that CrHV-1 infects other species of hamsters.

Papillomavirus Infections

Treatment of the lingual mucosa of Syrian hamsters with the carcinogen 9,10-dimethyl-1,2-benzanthracene (DMBA) and excisional wounding has been shown to result in development of dysplastic and neoplastic mucosal lesions in which papillomavirus antigen, viral particles, intranuclear and cytoplasmic inclusions, and koilocytosis were observed. Papillomavirus DNA was detected, fully sequenced, and named MsPV1. Using L1 gene sequence primers, specific DNA could be detected in normal, untreated mucosa. The source of the hamsters was not reported, and it is unknown how prevalent this virus is among Syrian hamsters in general. Another papillomavirus (PsPV1) has been amplified and fully sequenced from an anogenital lesion of a Siberian hamster. The nature of the lesion was not described and the prevalence of this virus among Siberian hamsters is unknown.

Parvovirus Infection

Fetal and neonatal Syrian hamsters are susceptible to experimental infection with a number of rodent parvoviruses, including minute virus of mice (MVM), mouse parvovirus (MPV), Kilham rat virus (RV), Toolan H-1 virus, and LuIII virus (unknown, but probably murine-origin virus isolated from cell culture). Tooth loss and discoloration, facial bone deformities, diarrhea, ataxia, and stunted growth have been observed. In addition, gross findings included intestinal hemorrhage, petechial hemorrhages, pale spleen or liver, testicular hypoplasia, and cerebellar hypoplasia. Virus localized to odontogenic stem cells, vascular endothelium, intestinal smooth muscle, hepatic Kupffer's cells, and granuloprival cells in the cerebellum. Although this book does not normally emphasize experimental disease, these studies are relevant to natural infections of hamsters. Serosurveillance for parvoviruses is not generally done for laboratory hamsters, but subclinical seroconversion of hamsters to H-1 virus has been documented, and natural disease due to infection with a parvovirus has also been reported, with parallels to experimentally induced parvoviral disease.

An outbreak of disease in a commercial breeding colony of Syrian hamsters was attributed to a newly recognized parvovirus, which was named hamster parvovirus (HaPV). The epizootic was confined to suckling and weanling hamsters. Affected animals presented with domed calvaria, potbellied appearance, marked discoloration, malformation and absence of the incisor teeth (Fig. 3.3), and high mortality. On microscopic examination, lesions associated with the infection included enamel hypoplasia of the incisor teeth, periodontitis, suppuration with mineralization, and hemorrhage in the dental pulp. Other lesions were observed,

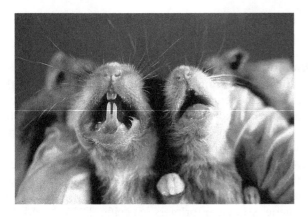

FIG. 3.3. *Weanling hamster with missing incisor teeth following infection with hamster parvovirus. Compare with normal weanling on the left. Source: Besselsen et al. 1999. Reproduced with permission from American Association for Laboratory Animal Science.*

including multifocal cerebral malacia, and testicular hypoplasia with multifocal necrosis and mineralization of cells lining seminiferous tubules. A similar pattern of disease with mortality was observed in suckling SPF hamsters inoculated with the HaPV isolate. Lesions included multifocal cerebellar and cerebral hemorrhage (Fig. 3.4), and thrombosis with transmural hemorrhage in the small intestine. HaPV DNA was detected in multiple tissues, and viral DNA was visualized in neuroglia and neurons of the cerebral cortex, hippocampus, and thalamus, as well as endothelium of brain and kidney. Intranuclear inclusions were observed in endothelium within the intestine. Based on PCR and gene sequencing, HaPV is closely related to the mouse parvovirus MPV-3. It was concluded that HaPV infections in hamsters may occur due to interspecies transmission of MPV-3 from mice, and that mice are the likely natural rodent host for this virus.

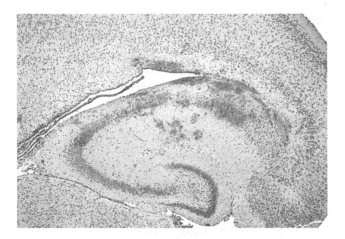

FIG. 3.4. *Brain from a 10-day-old hamster infected with hamster parvovirus. There are multiple hemorrhagic foci in the hippocampal region. Source: Besselsen et al. 1999. Reproduced with permission from American Association for Laboratory Animal Science.*

Hamster Polyoma Virus Infection: Transmissible Lymphoma

Hamster polyoma virus (HaPyV) is a polyomavirus that is structurally and biologically similar to polyoma virus of mice, but is a distinctly different virus (see Mouse Chapter 1, "Polyomavirus Infections"). HaPyV is the cause of transmissible lymphoma, which can occur in epizootics among young hamsters. HaPyV can cause devastating epizootics, which have caused the total loss of several inbred strains of Syrian hamsters. Once enzootic, the virus cannot be effectively eliminated without slaughter of the entire population and thorough decontamination of the premises. Even under these circumstances, repeated outbreaks have been known to occur, possibly because of the resistance of the virus to environmental decontamination.

Epizootiology and Pathogenesis

HaPyV is not common in laboratory hamsters, but may be found in some sources of pet hamsters. Infections of Syrian hamster colonies have been reported on several occasions in the United States and Europe. HaPyV is probably one of few truly hamster-origin viral agents, but its atypical virulence in Syrian hamsters is probably due to xenogeneic infection among distantly related hamster genera. It was probably introduced to laboratory Syrian hamsters in Eastern Europe through acquisition of wild European hamster (*C. cricetus*) stocks and mixing with laboratory Syrian hamsters. Natural latent infection, with isolation of virus from spleen and kidney tissue of subclinically infected European hamsters has been documented, suggesting that the European hamster is the natural host. HaPyV causes multisystemic persistent infection with shedding in the urine, which may be subclinical. HaPyV is also oncogenic, but tumor formation is a side effect of infection and not critical to the virus life cycle. HaPyV infection can result in the formation of lymphomas and hair follicle epitheliomas in hamsters. Other types of tumors have not been described. Typical of polyomaviruses, HaPyV can infect cells lytically with virus replication, or transform cells without virus replication. Thus, lymphomas do not have detectable infectious virus. On the other hand, HaPyV epitheliomas have HaPyV replication in keratinizing epithelium, similar to the behavior of papillomaviruses (and several polyomaviruses of other species). Hamsters are uniquely susceptible to the oncogenic effects of HaPyV beyond the neonatal period and following natural exposure.

With the above brief synopsis, the epizootiology of HaPyV can be understood. When first introduced to a naïve population of breeding hamsters, HaPyV may result in epizootics of lymphoma, with attack rates as high as 80% among young hamsters within 4–30 weeks postexposure. Infected hamsters may also have a variable incidence of trichoepitheliomas, usually around the face and feet, but they may arise anywhere on the body. Although the epitheliomas contain infectious virus, they are not necessary for virus transmission, which occurs primarily through the urine. Lymphomas do not contain infectious HaPyV, but HaPyV nucleic acid can be detected in their genome. Type C retrovirus particles (so-called hamster leukemia virus) also occur in these tumors, as they do in other tumors and normal tissues as an incidental finding. Once HaPV becomes enzootic, the incidence of lymphoma declines because young hamsters are presumably protected from infection by maternal antibody. In the enzootic context, the virus infects only older hamsters, which tend to resist the oncogenic effects. Infection of older hamsters often results in a clinically silent infection with persistent viruria. Enzootically infected hamsters, however, tend to develop a higher incidence of HaPyV skin tumors than do hamsters during the epizootic form, which develop lymphoma. These complex features have led to considerable confusion as to the etiology of transmissible lymphoma, including claims that it is caused by a DNA viroid-like agent. These claims have been refuted and the etiological role of HaPyV has been confirmed.

Pathology

Hamsters with HaPyV lymphoma appear thin, often with palpable masses in their abdomens. Lymphomas usually arise in the mesenteric lymph nodes (Fig. 3.5) and gut-associated lymphoid tissue without involvement of the spleen, but they can arise in axillary and cervical lymph nodes. Mesenteric masses typically involve the intestinal wall and lymph nodes, with

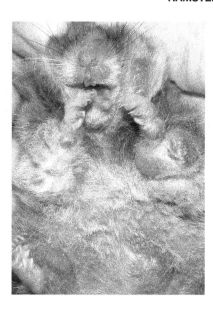

FIG. 3.6. *Multiple cutaneous nodules (trichoepitheliomas) in a hamster infected with hamster polyomavirus. Source: J. Simmons, Inside Diagnostic and Consulting, Pearland, TX. Reproduced with permission from J. Simmons.*

necrosis of the central region. This may result in intestinal ulceration and hemorrhage during the early stages of oncogenesis within the gut-associated lymphoid tissue. Infiltration of liver, kidney, thymus, and other organs can also occur. Tumors vary cytologically. They are usually lymphoid, but erythroblastic, reticulosarcomatous, and myeloid types have also been described. Lymphoid tumors are variably differentiated, usually immature, although sometimes they have plasmacytoid features. Lymphomas of the abdomen have been shown to possess B cell markers, and those of the thymus possess T cell markers. Affected hamsters may also present few to many nodular masses involving skin (Fig. 3.6). These lesions consist of keratinizing follicular structures reminiscent of trichoepitheliomas (Fig. 3.7).

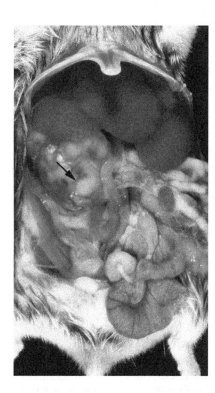

FIG. 3.5. *Hamster polyomavirus induced lymphoma in a hamster. Note the enlarged mesenteric lymph node (arrow) in the abdominal cavity. Source: Besselsen et al. 1999. Reproduced with permission from American Association for Laboratory Animal Science.*

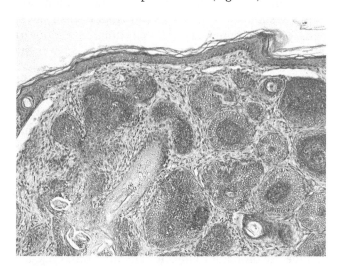

FIG. 3.7. *Trichoepithelioma in a hamster infected with hamster polyomavirus infection. These tumors allow virus replication in the keratinizing epithelium.*

Diagnosis

Epizootic HaPyV is unmistakable. Lymphoid tumors are otherwise rare in hamsters, and when they occur, it is usually in aged hamsters. As stated earlier, virus isolation or electron microscopy of lymphoid tumors in an effort to find HaPyV is a vacuous exercise. Trichoepitheliomas have not been described in hamsters unless associated with HaPyV. If present, they offer the opportunity to visualize HaPyV crystalloids in the nucleus of keratinizing epithelial cells, but only in that cell layer. A serological test for this virus is available, but it is generally not used routinely, and PCR amplification of HaPyV DNA is highly effective. Differential diagnoses must include transmissible ileal hyperplasia, which can cause palpable enlargement of the terminal ileum, spontaneous lymphoid tumors, and skin lesions such as Demodex folliculitis.

RNA VIRAL INFECTIONS

Lymphocytic Choriomeningitis Virus Infection

Lymphocytic choriomeningitis virus (LCMV) is an "Old World" arenavirus with a wide host range, including rodents and human and nonhuman primates. Its principal natural reservoir host is the wild house mouse (*Mus musculus*). Although originating in the Old World, LCMV occurs worldwide, largely due to colonization of *M. musculus*.

Epidemics of LCM have occurred among laboratory personnel exposed either to hamsters shedding virus or to infected cell lines. Pet hamsters are also the recognized source of virus in some human cases. In one outbreak in Europe, there were approximately 200 reported cases of LCM in humans after contact with subclinically infected pet hamsters. It was suggested that there may have been up to 4,000 additional cases of exposure in pet owners after hamsters were distributed to homes nationwide from the supplier of infected animals. In human cases, signs of infection may vary from subclinical infections to influenza-like symptoms. On rare occasions, viral meningitis or encephalomyelitis may occur. One report documented infection of 4 patients receiving solid-organ transplants from a single donor, of which 3 died due to LCMV infections. The source of the infection was traced to a pet store hamster recently purchased by the organ donor. These fatal cases serve to emphasize the increased risk to immunocompromised patients exposed to this virus.

Epizootiology and Pathogenesis

Infection with LCMV may occur by exposure to saliva or urine from animals shedding the virus. Portals of entry include the oronasal route and skin abrasions. Cage-to-cage transmission via aerosols (or transmission through soiled bedding) does not appear to play an important role in spread. Congenital infections also occur in hamsters. Cell cultures or transplantable tumors contaminated with the virus are an important source of the virus in the laboratory. The patterns of disease that occur in hamsters postexposure depend on the age of the animal, strain and dose of the virus, and route of administration. In 1 study, newborn hamsters were inoculated subcutaneously with LCMV. Approximately half of the recipients cleared the virus, with minimal to moderate lymphocytic infiltration in the viscera. In the remaining inoculated animals, viremia and viruria persisted for approximately 3 and 6 months, respectively. In addition, there was chronic wasting, and lymphocytic infiltration was observed in tissues such as liver, lung, spleen, meninges, and brain. Vasculitis and glomerulitis were present in hamsters examined histologically at 6 or more months postinoculation. Antigen–antibody complexes were demonstrated in arterioles and glomerular basement membranes.

Diagnosis

Pathology is varied, and seldom useful for definitive diagnosis. Serology is the recognized method for detecting infection among infected populations. Sera collected from hamsters infected early in life may have a high percentage of samples with anticomplementary activity, but the complement fixation test is generally not used any more. Antigen–antibody complexes may also obscure serologic detection. Hamsters that acquire LCMV infections as adults usually seroconvert early in the infection and remain seropositive for a long period of time. Immunohistochemistry can be used to demonstrate viral antigen during the acute stages of the disease, and PCR is now the method of choice for definitive diagnosis. The Mouse Antibody Production (MAP) test has been shown to be equally or more sensitive than PCR.

Pneumonia Virus of Mice (PVM) Infection

Laboratory hamsters, rats, and mice may be naturally infected with PVM. In an early report, interstitial pneumonia with consolidation was observed in hamsters inoculated with an infectious agent interpreted to be contaminated with PVM, but there are few details of the morphologic changes. Conventional colonies of hamsters may be seropositive, usually in the absence of clinical disease. It is evident that PVM infections in this species normally go unrecognized as a subclinical event.

Sendai Virus Infection

Sendai virus infections were once widespread among laboratory hamsters, but Sendai virus has largely disappeared from the laboratory animal scene. There are few reports of confirmed clinical disease due to Sendai virus infections in this species, although there are reports of mortality in newborn Syrian and Chinese hamsters. Young adult Syrian hamsters inoculated intranasally with Sendai virus remained subclinical, although there were changes in the upper and lower respiratory tract evident by light microscopy, and virus was recoverable from the lung during the acute stages of the infection. Hamsters seroconverted by day 7 postinoculation. Lesions included focal to segmental rhinitis progressing to necrotizing tracheitis and multifocal bronchoalveolitis. Immunohistochemistry may be used to demonstrate viral antigen in respiratory epithelial cells during the acute stages of the disease. In animals examined at 3–9 days postinoculation, lesions were very similar to those present in mice. In the reparative stages, features included hyperplasia of epithelial cells lining affected airways and peribronchial lymphocytic infiltration. In general, most lesions had resolved by 12 days postinfection.

Other Virus Infections of Minimal Significance

In addition to the viruses noted above, laboratory Syrian hamsters seroconvert to mouse encephalomyelitis virus, reovirus, and SV-5 (a paramyxovirus). Hamsters are also host to an endogenous retrovirus, which is expressed in tissues and cells as C-type particles without evidence of oncogenicity.

BIBLIOGRAPHY FOR VIRAL INFECTIONS

DNA Viral Infections

Adenovirus Infection
Gibson, S.V., Rottinghaus, A.A., Wagner, J.E., Srills, H.F., Jr., Stogsdil, P.L., & Kinden, D.A. (1990) Naturally acquired enteric adenovirus infection in Syrian hamsters (*Mesocricetus auratus*). *American Journal of Veterinary Research* 51:143–147.
Suzuki, E., Matsubara, J., Saito, M., Muto, T., Nakagawa, M., & Imaizumi, K. (1982) Serological survey of laboratory rodents for infection with Sendai virus, mouse hepatitis virus, reovirus 3 and mouse adenovirus. *Japanese Journal of Medical Science and Biology* 35:249–254.

Cytomegalovirus Infection
Kuttner, A.G. & Wang, S. (1934) The problem of the significance of the inclusion bodies in the salivary glands of infants, and the occurrence of inclusion bodies in the submaxillary glands of hamsters, white mice and wild rats (Peiping). *Journal of Experimental Medicine* 60:773–791.

Papillomavirus Infection
Iwasaki, T., Maeda, H., Kameyama, Y., Moriyama, M., Kanai, S., & Kurata, T. (1997) Presence of a novel hamster papillomavirus in dysplastic lesions of hamster lingual mucosa induced by application of dimethylbenzanthracene and excisional wounding: molecular cloning and complete nucleotide sequence. *Journal of General Virology* 78:1087–1093.
Kocjan, B.J., Kosnjak, L., Rocnik, J., Zadravec, M., & Poljak, M. (2014) Complete genome sequence of *Phodopus sungorus* papillomavirus type 1 (PsPV1), a novel member of the *Pipapapillomavirus* genus, isolated from a Siberian hamster. *Genome Announcements* 2:e00311–e00314.
Maeda, H., Kameyama, Y., Nakane, S., Takehana, S., & Sato, E. (1989) Epithelial dysplasia produced by carcinogen pretreatment and subsequent wounding. *Oral Surgery, Oral Medicine, Oral Pathology* 68:50–56.

Parvovirus Infection
Besselsen, D.G., Gibson, S.V., Besch-Williford, C.L., Purdy, G.A., Knowles, R.L., Wagner, J.E., Pintel, D.J., Franklin, C.L., Hook, R.R., Jr., & Riley, L.K. (1999) Natural and experimentally induced infection of Syrian hamsters with a newly recognized parvovirus. *Laboratory Animal Science* 49:308–312.
Christie, R.D., Marcus, E.C., Wagner, A.M., & Besselsen, D.G. (2010) Experimental infection of mice with hamster parvovirus: evidence for interspecies transmission of mouse parvovirus 3. *Comparative Medicine* 60:123–129.
Garant, P.R., Baer, P.N., & Kilham, L. (1980) Electron microscopic localization of virions in developing teeth of young hamsters infected with minute virus of mice. *Journal of Dental Research* 59:80–86.
Kilham, L. (1960) Mongolism associated with rat virus (RV) infection in hamsters. *Virology* 13:141–143.
Kilham, L. (1961) Rat virus (RV) infections in hamsters. *Proceedings of the Society for Experimental Biology and Medicine* 106:825–829.
Kilham, L. & Margolis, G. (1964) Cerebellar ataxia in hamsters inoculated with rat virus. *Science* 143:1047–1048.
Kilham, L. & Margolis, G. (1970) Pathogenicity of minute virus of mice (MVM) for rats, mice and hamsters. *Proceedings of the Society for Experimental Biology and Medicine* 133:1447–1452.
Lipton, H.L. & Johnson, R.T. (1972) The pathogenesis of rat virus infections in the newborn hamster. *Laboratory Investigation* 27:508–513.
Soike, K.R., Iatropoulis, M., & Siegl, G. (1976) Infection of newborn and fetal hamsters induced by inoculation of LuIII parvovirus. *Archives of Virology* 51:235–241.
Toolan, H.W. (1960) Experimental production of mongoloid hamsters. *Science* 131:1446–1448.

Hamster Polyomavirus Infection
Ambrose, K.R. & Coggin, J.H. (1975) An epizootic in hamsters of lymphomas of undetermined origin and mode of transmission. *Journal of the National Cancer Institute* 54:877–880.
Barthold, S.W., Bhatt, P.N., & Johnson, E.A. (1987) Further evidence for papovavirus as the probable etiology of transmissible lymphoma of Syrian hamsters. *Laboratory Animal Science* 37:283–288.
Coggin, J.H., Hyde, B.M., Heath, L.S., Leinbach, S.S., Fowler, E., & Stadtmore, L.S. (1985) Papovavirus in epitheliomas appearing on lymphoma-bearing hamsters: lack of association with horizontally transmitted lymphomas of Syrian hamsters. *Journal of the National Cancer Institute* 75:91–97.
Foster, A.P., Brown, P.J., Jandrig, B., Grosch, A., Voronkova, T., Scherneck, S., & Ulrich, R. (2002) Polyomavirus infection in hamsters and trichoepitheliomas/cutaneous adnexal tumours. *Veterinary Record* 151:13–17.
Graffi, A., Bender, E. Schramm, T., Kuhn, W., & Schneiders, F. (1969) Induction of transmissible lymphomas in Syrian hamsters by application of DNA from viral hamster papovavirus-induced tumors and by cell-free filtrates of human tumors. *Proceedings of the National Academy of Sciences of the United States of America* 64:1172–1175.
Graffi, A., Schramm, T., Graffi, I., Bierwolf, D., & Bender, E. (1968) Virus-associated skin tumors of the Syrian hamster: preliminary note. *Journal of the National Cancer Institute* 40:867–873.
Hannoun, C., Guillin, J.C., & Chatelain, J. (1974) Natural latent infection of the European hamster ("*Cricetus cricetus*", linne) with a papovavirus. I. Isolation of virus in golden hamster and new-born mice. *Annals of Microbiology (Paris)* 125A:215–226.
Manci, E.A., Heath, L.S., Leinbach, S.S., & Coggin, J.H., Jr. (1984) Lymphoma-associated ulcerative bowel disease in the hamster

(*Mesocricetus auratus*) induced by an unusual agent. *American Journal of Pathology* 116:1–8.

Simmons, J.H., Riley, L.K., Franklin, C.L., & Besch-Williford, C. (2001) Hamster polyomavirus infection in a pet Syrian hamster (*Mesocricetus auratus*). *Veterinary Pathology* 38:441–446.

RNA Viral Infections

Lymphocytic Choriomeningitis Virus Infection

Amman, B.R., Pavlin, B.I., Albarino, C.G., et al. (2007) Pet rodents and fatal lymphocytic choriomeningitis in transplant patients. *Emerging Infectious Diseases* 13:719–725.

Barthold, S.W. & Smith, A.L. (2007) Lymphocytic choriomeningitis virus. In: *The Mouse in Biomedical Research*, Vol. 2, 2nd edn. (eds. J.G. Fox, S.W. Barthold, M.T. Davisson, C.E. Newcomer, F.W. Quimby, & A.L. Smith), pp. 179–213. Academic Press, New York.

Besselsen, D., Wagner, A., & Loganbill, J. (2003) Detection of lymphocytic choriomeningitis virus by use of fluorogenic nuclease reverse transcriptase polymerase chain reaction analysis. *Comparative Medicine* 53:65–69.

Bhatt, P.N., Jacoby, R.O., & Barthold, S.W. (1986) Contamination of transplantable murine tumors with lymphocytic choriomeningitis virus. *Laboratory Animal Science* 36:136–139.

Biggar, R.J., Schmidt, T.J., & Woodall, J.P. (1977) Lymphocytic choriomeningitis in laboratory personnel exposed to hamsters inadvertently infected with LCM virus. *Journal of the American Veterinary Medical Association* 171:829–832.

Biggar, R.J., Woodall, J.P., Walter, P.D., & Haughie, G.E. (1975) Lymphocytic choriomeningitis outbreak associated with pet hamsters. Fifty-seven cases from New York State. *Journal of the American Medical Association* 232:494–500.

Bowen, G.S., Calisher, C.H., Winkler, W.G., Kraus, A.L., Fowler, E.H., Garman, R.H., Fraser, D.W., & Hinman, A.R. (1975) Laboratory studies of a lymphocytic choriomeningitis virus outbreak in man and laboratory animals. *American Journal of Epidemiology* 102:233–240.

Homberger, F.R., Romano, T.P., Seiler, P., Hansen, G.M., & Smith, A.L. (1995) Enzyme-linked immunosorbent assay for detection of antibody to lymphocytic choriomeningitis virus in mouse sera, with recombinant nucleoprotein as antigen. *Laboratory Animal Science* 45:493–496.

Parker, J.C., Igel, H.J., Reynolds, R.K., Lewis, A.M., Jr., & Rowe, W.P. (1976) Lymphocytic choriomeningitis virus infection in fetal, newborn, and young adult Syrian hamsters (*Mesocricetus auratus*). *Infection and Immunity* 13:967–981.

Sendai Virus Infection

Buthala, D.A. & Soret, M.G. (1964) Parainfluenza type 3 virus infection in hamsters: virologic, serologic, and pathologic studies. *Journal of Infectious Diseases* 114:226–234.

Pearson, H.E. & Eaton, M.D. (1940) A virus pneumonia of Syrian hamsters. *Proceedings of the Society of Experimental Biology and Medicine* 45:677–679.

Percy, D.H. & Palmer, D. (1997) Experimental Sendai virus infection in the Syrian hamster. *Laboratory Animal Science* 47:132–137.

Profeta, M.L., Leif, F.S., & Plotkin, S.A. (1969) Enzootic Sendai infection in laboratory hamsters. *American Journal of Epidemiology* 89:316–324.

BACTERIAL AND FUNGAL INFECTIONS

Bacterial Enteric Infections
Campylobacter jejuni Infection

Campylobacter jejuni has been isolated on numerous occasions from clinically normal hamsters, as well as hamsters with enteritis. Hamsters acquired from pet stores have been found to be commonly infected with *C. jejuni*. A few animals had watery diarrhea. Hamsters are relatively resistant to experimental disease. Manipulation may be required in order to produce clinical disease consistently in inoculated animals. Experimentally infected hamsters, which were preconditioned with magnesium sulfate as a purgative, were shown to develop edema, inflammation, and mild crypt hyperplasia of the ileal and cecal mucosa, with attachment of bacteria and disruption of the microvilli. Subclinically infected hamsters may shed the organism in the feces for up to several months. An outbreak of enterocecocolitis with mortality in a breeding colony of Syrian hamsters was attributed to concomitant infections with *Escherichia coli* and *Campylobacter*-like organisms. Adults were most frequently affected, and the cecum and colon were primarily involved. The organism can be a coinfecting pathogen during outbreaks of proliferative ileitis caused by *Lawsonia intracellularis*. *Campylobacter*-infected hamsters represent a zoonotic threat to both pet owners and laboratory animal personnel.

Clostridium difficile *Enterotoxemia*

Dysbiosis due to disruption of the intestinal microflora of hamsters results in *C. difficile* enterotoxemia. The most common precipitating cause is treatment of hamsters with antibiotics, including lincomycin, clindamycin, ampicillin, vancomycin, erythromycin, cephalosporins, gentamicin, and penicillin. Typhlocolitis has been documented in hamsters, following topical treatment with antibiotic ointment containing polymyxin B sulfate, neomycin sulfate, and bacitracin zinc. Spontaneous enterotoxemia may also occur in hamsters in the absence of antibiotic treatment. The exquisite susceptibility of hamsters to *C. difficile* enterotoxemia has made this species the primary animal model for study of this disease.

Epizootiology and Pathogenesis

The predominant bacterial flora in the hamster intestine are *Lactobacillus* and *Bacteroides*. Following therapy with certain narrow-spectrum antibiotics, overgrowth with *C. difficile* occurs, resulting in acute typhlocolitis, diarrhea, and death. In general, profuse diarrhea, with high mortality, occurs within 2–10 days following the oral or parenteral administration of certain narrow-spectrum antibiotics. The oral administration of cecal contents from normal animals has provided protection to the majority of recipients. Change may be precipitated by the loss of Gram-negative aerobic bacteria or other Clostridia following antibiotic treatment, but dietary manipulation has also been shown to precipitate *C. difficile* enterotoxemia. Alteration of the "inhibitory barrier" of the microbiome may then allow colonization of *C. difficile* with elaboration of toxins A and B. Fatal typhlitis attributed to *C. difficile* has been observed in hamsters housed in the same room as antibiotic-treated hamsters. There is also some evidence that *C. difficile*

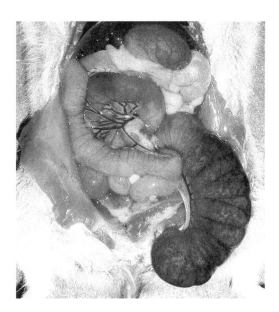

FIG. 3.8.   *Abdominal viscera of a hamster with* Clostridium difficile *enterotoxemia. Note the dilated bowel filled with fluid and the hyperemic and hemorrhagic cecum. Source: Keel and Songer. 2006. Reproduced with permission from SAGE Publications.*

may occur as an endogenous infection, and the organism has been isolated from the intestinal tract of normal hamsters.

Pathology

The intestine may be distended with gas and tan to red fluid. The cecal wall may be hyperemic with ecchymotic hemorrhages (Fig. 3.8). There may be distension and hyperemia of the terminal ileum and proximal colon. Histopathologic lesions vary from mild to acute pseudomembranous necrohemorrhagic typhlitis (Fig. 3.9). Microscopic changes in the cecum include effacement of the mucosal epithelium, edema of the lamina propria, leukocytic infiltration, and mucosal hyperplasia. There may be some involvement of the terminal ileum and colon.

Diagnosis

Clostridium difficile should be recoverable on anaerobic culture and its presence confirmed by PCR, but detection of toxin is essential to confirm cause. Due to the importance of this disease in humans, there are a number of commercially available assays for detection of *C. difficile* A and B cytotoxins, using fresh intestinal contents or feces. Differential diagnoses include Tyzzer's disease, salmonellosis, and enteropathogenic *E. coli* infections.

Cecal Mucosal Hyperplasia of Unknown Etiology

Spontaneous cases of cecal hyperplasia have been observed in suckling and weanling hamsters. Diarrhea, runting, and high mortality were associated with the disease. At necropsy, ceca are congested, contracted, and opaque due to mucosal thickening (Fig 3.10).

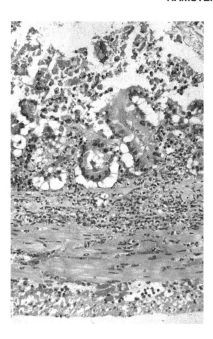

FIG. 3.9.   *Cecum from a hamster with spontaneous clostridial enteropathy not associated with prior antibiotic treatment. There is a necrotizing typhlitis with mucosal effacement and leukocytic infiltration.*

Microscopic changes included hyperplasia of enterocytes lining cecal crypts, as well as focal mucosal erosions. Bacterial cultures and ultrastructural studies failed to identify a specific causative agent. The syndrome probably represents the recovery phase of clostridial enteropathy.

Clostridium piliforme *Infection: Tyzzer's Disease*

Epizootics of Tyzzer's disease have been observed in Syrian hamsters in various parts of the world. The causative agent, *C. piliforme*, is a spore-forming bacillus that multiplies only within cells. The organism has a wide host range, including all of the species covered in this

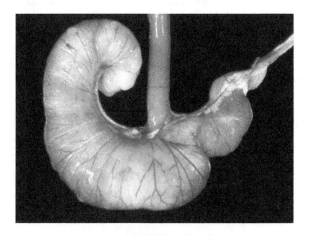

FIG. 3.10.   *Cecal mucosal hyperplasia in a hamster. This syndrome is probably the aftermath of clostridial enteropathy. Source: Barthold et al. 1987. Reproduced with permission from American Association for Laboratory Animal Science.*

book, but isolates from various host species have been found to have host specificity.

Epizootiology and Pathogenesis
Hamsters may become infected by contact with affected animals or by contaminated bedding, which remain infectious with environmentally resistant spores for many months. Predisposing factors, such as poor sanitation, intestinal parasitism, and inappropriate feeding practices, play a role in precipitating clinical outbreaks of the disease. Weanling hamsters are most often affected. In hamsters inoculated with infected liver homogenates, organisms, and lesions are detectable in the mucosa of the small and large intestine by 3 days postinoculation, and multiple lesions and bacilli may be present in the liver by day 6–8 postexposure.

Pathology
At necropsy, there is a variable distribution of lesions. In some epizootics, lesions may be confined to either the liver or the intestinal tract. Multifocal hepatic necrosis is evident in some cases. Intestinal lesions, when evident grossly, usually involve the lower ileum, cecum, and colon and are associated with diarrhea and soiling of the perineum. Affected areas are edematous and dilated, with fluid contents. Microscopically, there are foci of hepatocellular necrosis with leukocytic infiltration. Intracellular bundles of bacilli are usually best demonstrated at the periphery of hepatic lesions. When lesions are present in the intestinal tract, there is edema of the lamina propria, with polymorphonuclear leukocyte infiltration and effacement of the mucosal architecture. There may be extension of the inflammatory process into the underlying muscular layers. Typical bacilli are usually demonstrable within enterocytes in the region and in hepatocytes adjacent to necrotic foci (see Gerbil Chapter 4, "*Clostridium piliforme* Infection"). Focal granulomatous myocarditis, with conspicuous pale bulging nodules, has been associated with Tyzzer's disease in this species.

Diagnosis
Definitive diagnosis of acute Tyzzer's disease entails the demonstration of the typical intracellular bacilli in affected cells (enterocytes, hepatocytes, and myocytes), using Warthin–Starry or Giemsa stains. Differential diagnoses include clostridial enterotoxemia, salmonellosis, coliform enteritis, and Campylobacter enteritis. Both serologic and fecal PCR assays are commercially available, and are typically used for colony surveillance. PCR can be used to discriminate between rabbit and rodent *C. piliforme*, emphasizing the need to use the appropriate assay for the affected host species.

Escherichia coli *Infection*
Enteroinvasive *E. coli* strains 1056, 1126, and 4165 have been isolated from naturally occurring cases of hamster enteritis. When inoculated into ligated intestinal loops to test for enteropathogenicity, the pathogenic strains produced changes in most of the inoculated weanling hamsters and in some of the adult animals. One isolate of *E. coli*, strain 1056, has been recovered from ground ileal suspension prepared from a hamster with proliferative ileitis. Many of the weanling Syrian hamsters inoculated orally with this strain developed acute enteritis within 2 weeks postinoculation. Animals inoculated with a nonenteropathogenic *E. coli* strain remained unaffected throughout the study.

Pathology
The small intestine may contain yellow to dark red fluid material. On microscopic examination, blunting and fusion of villi are frequently observed. Degeneration and sloughing of enterocytes with polymorphonuclear leukocyte infiltration in the lamina propria commonly occurs. Changes in mesenteric lymph nodes may vary from lymphoid hyperplasia to diffuse polymorphonuclear leukocyte infiltration. Focal coagulation necrosis in the liver, with polymorphonuclear leukocyte infiltration, and gastric ulcers are other variable findings. Colitis and/or typhlitis may be present in some affected animals, sometimes with concomitant colonic intussusception. Ultrastructural studies of sections of ileum have revealed bacilli in the cytoplasm of enterocytes and blunting and irregularities in microvilli. Differential diagnoses include clostridial enterotoxemia, *Lawsonia*-associated proliferative ileitis, and salmonellosis.

Helicobacter *spp. Infection*
A variety of *Helicobacter* spp. colonize the gastrointestinal tracts of Syrian hamsters, including *Helicobacter aurati*, *Helicobacter cinaedi*, *Helicobacter cholecystitis*, *Helicobacter mesocricetorum*, and a *Helicobacter* sp. closely related to *Helicobacter bilis*. In many cases, infections are subclinical with no apparent microscopic lesions, but disease may arise in aged hamsters. Notably, *H. cinaedi* commonly infects immunocompromised humans, and thus poses a zoonotic risk to such individuals.

Pathology
Helicobacter aurati was isolated from the stomach and cecum of adult hamsters with gastritis, and chronic gastritis with intestinal metaplasia has been noted in hamsters naturally infected with *H. aurati* and 2 other microaerobic species. An invasive adenocarcinoma at the pyloric–duodenal junction was observed in a hamster at the site of *H. aurati*-associated inflammation. *Helicobacter cholecystus* has been isolated from the gall bladder of hamsters with cholangiofibrosis, bile ductular hyperplasia, portal hepatitis, and centrilobular pancreatitis. Spontaneous proliferative and dysplastic typhlocolitis associated with *Helicobacter* sp. infections has also been identified in aging hamsters. The agent genetically clustered closely with *H. bilis*. Lesions were most evident

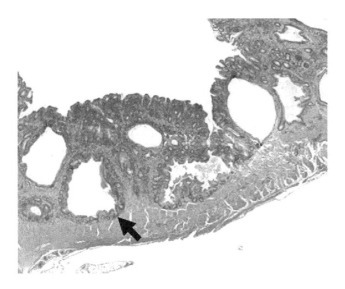

FIG. 3.11. *Cecum from a Syrian hamster with naturally occurring* Helicobacter *infection. There are multiple cystic areas (arrow) in the hyperplastic mucosa. Source: Nambiar et al. 2006. Reproduced with permission from SAGE Publications.*

at the ileocecocolic junction and terminal colon. Mucosal thickening and submucosal edema, hypertrophy of enterocytes, and hyperplasia of cells lining crypts were observed. Chronic inflammatory cell infiltrates in the lamina propria consisted primarily of lymphohistiocytic cells with a sprinkling of polymorphonuclear leukocytes (Figs. 3.11 and 3.12). Chronic hepatitis, portal fibrosis, biliary hyperplasia, and focal nodular dysplasia have also been found in aged hamsters infected with a *Helicobacter* spp. that clusters in the *H. bilis* clade. A round cell sarcoma and a histiocytic sarcoma were identified at the ileocecocolic junction in two of the affected animals. This *Helicobacter* sp. was also associated with hepatic

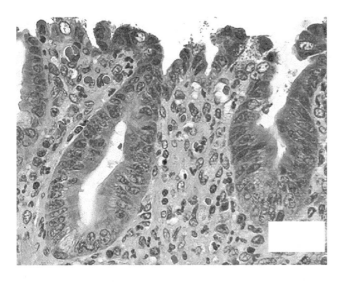

FIG. 3.12. *Colon from a hamster with chronic colitis associated with* Helicobacter *infection. Note the hyperplasia of enterocytes lining crypts and the cellular infiltrate in the lamina propria. Source: Nambiar et al. 2006. Reproduced with permission from SAGE Publications.*

portal fibrosis, which is a common sequel of enterohepatic *Helicobacter* infections.

Lawsonia intracellularis *Infection: Proliferative Ileitis, Transmissible Ileal Hyperplasia*

Proliferative ileitis is among the most commonly recognized diseases in the Syrian hamster. It usually results in high morbidity and mortality. This specific condition has been referred to by a variety of names, including regional ileitis, hamster enteritis, terminal enteritis, atypical ileal hyperplasia, enzootic intestinal adenocarcinoma, proliferative bowel disease, and wet tail. It seems that each individual or group that has become involved in the study of this syndrome has endowed it with a unique epithet. The term "wet tail" should not be used because it includes virtually all the numerous conditions that may cause diarrhea in hamsters.

After years of study by multiple investigators, the etiology of proliferative ileitis is now recognized to be *L. intracellularis*. The many past quests toward identifying the etiology of proliferative ileitis in hamsters have incriminated a number of apparently secondary and possibly contributory agents, including *E. coli*, *Campylobacter*, and *Cryptosporidium*. *Escherichia coli* isolates from cases of proliferative ileitis have been shown to be enteropathogenic in naïve hamsters, but did not induce proliferative disease. In another study, an organism was isolated and identified as a new species of Chlamydia. In subsequent studies, it was concluded that chlamydial infections do not play a primary role in the disease. The term "intracellular Disulfovibrio" (IDO) was proposed for a period of time. It is now widely recognized that *L. intracellularis* infects a wide variety of avian and mammalian species, producing similar proliferative bowel lesions. In 1994, proliferative ileitis was experimentally reproduced in hamsters infected with a porcine isolate grown in cell culture. Among laboratory animals covered in this text, mice, rats, hamsters, guinea pigs, and rabbits have all been found as hosts to this organism. The organism appears to be genetically homogeneous, regardless of host species origin, and can be readily transmitted among vastly unrelated host species with ease.

Epizootiology

Epizootics of the proliferative ileitis are usually confined to younger animals, particularly during the postweaning period. Hamsters are normally resistant to the experimental disease by 10–12 weeks of age. Overcrowding, transport, diet, and experimental manipulations have been identified as predisposing factors. In epizootics of the disease, there may be a morbidity rate of up to 60%, and mortality rates in affected animals may approach 90%.

Pathology

Clinical signs include runting, emaciation, lethargy, unkempt hair coat, anorexia, foul-smelling, watery

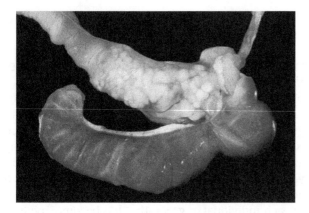

FIG. 3.13. *Proliferative ileitis in a young hamster due to* Lawsonia intracellularis *infection. The terminal ileum is thickened and the serosal surface is nodular due to granulomatous inflammation. Source: R.O. Jacoby. Yale University, New Haven, CT. Reproduced with permission from R.O. Jacoby.*

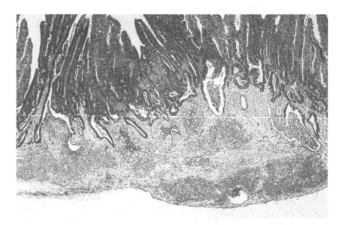

FIG. 3.15. *Chronic phase of proliferative ileitis in a hamster, illustrating mucosal hyperplasia with cryptal diverticula and transmural granulomatous inflammation. Source: R.O. Jacoby. Yale University, New Haven, CT. Reproduced with permission from R.O. Jacoby.*

diarrhea, soiling of the perineum, and dehydration. Rectal prolapse or intussusceptions frequently occur. At necropsy, the ileum is segmentally thickened, often with prominent serosal nodules (Fig. 3.13) and fibrinous peritoneal adhesions to adjacent structures. The opened bowel reveals an abrupt transition of the craniad, normal ileum, and the caudal cecum with the affected, hyperplastic mucosa. Microscopic lesions consist of marked crypt and villus epithelial hyperplasia, villus elongation, villus fusion, varying degrees of necrosis and hemorrhage, crypt invasion of underlying structures, destruction and inflammation of crypts, and granulomatous inflammation (Figs. 3.14 and 3.15). With silver or PAS stains, numerous and characteristic small bacteria can be seen in the apical cytoplasm of enterocytes (Fig. 3.16), and macrophages in the lamina propria and submucosa contain abundant granular PAS-positive material in their cytoplasm. The characteristic apical cytoplasmic niche of *L. intracellularis* can be observed ultrastructurally within infected enterocytes (Fig. 3.17).

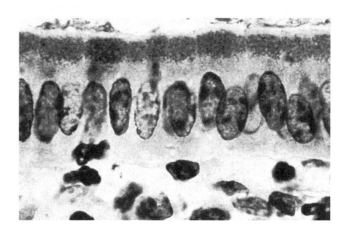

FIG. 3.16. *Ileal mucosa of hamster infected with* Lawsonia intracellularis. *Note clusters of argyrophilic organisms in the apical cytoplasm of enterocytes (Warthin–Starry stain). Source: R.O. Jacoby. Yale University, New Haven, CT. Reproduced with permission from R.O. Jacoby.*

Diagnosis
Demonstration of the typical ileal lesions should be sufficient to confirm the diagnosis. It is highly likely that coinfections are common and may even play an important role in the pathogenesis of ileal hyperplasia. *Lawsonia intracellularis* grows intracellularly in cell culture, but this is seldom done for diagnostic purposes.

Salmonella enterica *Infection*
Syrian hamsters are very susceptible to bacteremic *S. enterica* infections, but outbreaks in contemporary laboratory animal colonies are now rare. Unfortunately, *Salmonella* infections of pet rodents, including hamsters, have resulted in multiple zoonotic infections with multidrug-resistant isolates. *Salmonella enterica* serovars Typhimurium and Enteritidis are the most frequent isolates from hamsters. Transmission is probably by the ingestion of contaminated food or bedding, and interspecies transmission is likely to occur.

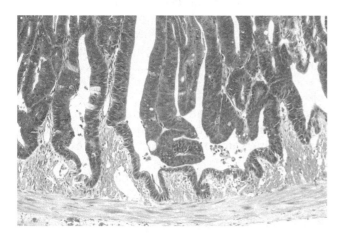

FIG. 3.14. *Proliferative ileitis in a young hamster. There is marked hyperplasia of enterocytes lining crypts and villi, with cryptal invasion into the muscularis externa. Source: R.O. Jacoby. Yale University, New Haven, CT. Reproduced with permission from R.O. Jacoby.*

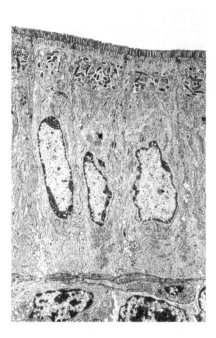

FIG. 3.17. *Ultrastructural section of ileal mucosa from a hamster infected with* Lawsonia intracellularis. *Note* Lawsonia *organisms within the apical cytoplasm of enterocytes.*

Pathology

Explosive outbreaks of salmonellosis are characterized by depression, ruffled hair coat, anorexia, dyspnea, and high mortality. At necropsy, there may be multifocal, pinpoint-size, pale areas in the liver, with patchy pulmonary hemorrhage and reddened hilar lymph nodes (Fig. 3.18). Microscopic changes in the lung are characterized by multifocal interstitial pneumonitis, with intraalveolar hemorrhage. There may be a septic thrombophlebitis in pulmonary veins and venules, with thrombi containing leukocytes, and erosion of venous walls (Fig. 3.19). Focal splenic necrosis and focal necrotizing hepatitis, with leukocytic infiltration and venous thrombosis, are typical lesions. Embolic glomerular lesions and focal splenitis may also occur.

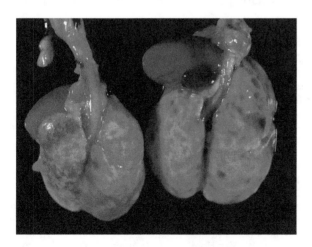

FIG. 3.18. *Multifocal pulmonary hemorrhages in hamsters with acute* Salmonella *septicemia. (Courtesy A. Wuenschmann.)*

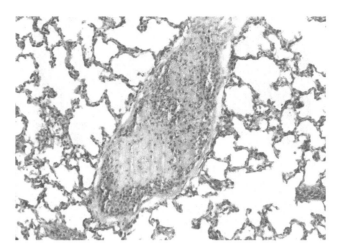

FIG. 3.19. *Pulmonary venous thrombosis in a hamster with acute salmonellosis.*

Diagnosis

In acute salmonellosis, the organism can usually be readily recovered from blood, lung, and other viscera. Differential diagnoses include Tyzzer's disease, pathogenic *E. coli* infections, and other acute bacteremic infections. Subclinical carriers may also be common among hamsters, requiring surveillance of feces by culture or PCR.

Other Bacterial Infections
Corynebacterium *spp. Infections*

Corynebacterium kutscheri has been isolated from the oral cavities of clinically normal adult Syrian hamsters. In addition, the organism has been recovered from sites such as esophagus, cecal contents, submaxillary lymph nodes, and upper respiratory tract. In 1 study, Syrian hamsters were inoculated subcutaneously or intramuscularly with *C. kutscheri*. Localized granulomatous and suppurative lesions were observed. Another species, *Corynebacterium paulometabulum*, was isolated from a hamster with respiratory signs, but its role as a primary pathogen is uncertain.

Francisella tularensis *Infection: Tularemia*

Tularemia, due to *F. tularensis* infection, is rare in laboratory hamsters, although it has been reported in a hamster breeding colony, resulting in 100% mortality. Hamsters were hunched, had ruffled fur, and died within 48 hours. Lungs were mottled with hemorrhage, livers were pale and swollen, and spleens were enlarged. Gut-associated lymphoid tissue was prominent and pale. Microscopic findings included lymphoid necrosis, focal hemorrhages, and bacteria. Others have noted the predominant gross lesion to be enlarged spleens with multiple pale foci in European hamsters, and similar findings have been noted in naturally infected Syrian hamsters (Fig. 3.20). Tularemia is endemic among many species, particularly the rabbit (see Rabbit Chapter 6, "Francisella tularensis Infection") and is regionally endemic among wild European hamsters (*C. cricetus*). Zoonotic infections have been documented among hunters of European

---

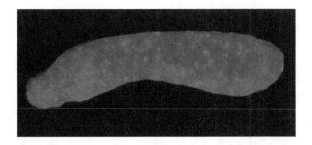

FIG. 3.20. *Enlarged spleen with multiple pale foci from a hamster with tularemia, caused by* Francisella tularensis *infection. Splenic involvement is a predominant feature of this disease in hamsters. Source: A. Wuenschmann, University of Minnesota, Minneapolis, Minnesota. Reproduced with permission from A Wuenschmann.*

hamsters. Zoonotic infection has been documented following exposure to infected pet hamsters in the United States (Centers for Disease Control) and Canada (Public Health Agency of Canada).

Leptospira ballum *Infection: Leptospirosis*

Hamsters have been inadvertently infected with *L. ballum* by inoculation with contaminated tissue from subclinically infected mice. The hamsters developed severe hemolytic disease, jaundice, hemoglobinuria, nephritis, and hepatitis within 4–6 days. Hamsters are highly susceptible to experimental inoculation with a number of *Leptospira* spp., and thus can be potentially susceptible to severe natural disease, although never reported.

Mycobacterium *spp. Infection*

Mycobacteriosis has been documented in both laboratory and pet hamsters, but it is apparently quite rare. Laboratory hamsters have been inadvertently infected with *Mycobacterium tuberculosis* following inoculation of human tissue, with one outbreak of disseminated tuberculosis occurring among multiple hamsters resulting from a contaminated inoculation needle. A pet hamster was reported to have severely enlarged feet and lymph nodes due to granulomatous inflammation associated with *Mycobacterium chelonai* infection.

Pasteurella pneumotropica *Infection*

The nasal cavity of hamsters may be colonized by *P. pneumotropica* without clinical effect, but there is a single report of hamsters developing prolapsed rectums, fecal discharge, and enteritis at day 7 after parturition. Prior to whelping, *P. pneumotropica* was isolated from the nasal cavity, but not from other organs, whereas during the epizootic, pure cultures of *P. pneumotropica* were isolated from the bowels of affected hamsters. Since *P. pneumotropica* is not known to be a primary enteric pathogen, the findings suggest an underlying dysbiosis, possibly related to *C. difficile*.

Yersinia pseudotuberculosis *Infection*

Hamsters have been known to incur infections of *Y. pseudotuberculosis* via contaminated food or bedding.

This organism produces chronic emaciation with intermittent diarrhea. Necropsy findings include necrotic caseous nodules in the intestine, mesenteric lymph nodes, liver, spleen, and lungs.

Miscellaneous Bacterial Infections

Upper respiratory disease, otitis, and bronchopneumonia in hamsters have been associated with a number of bacteria, including *P. pneumotropica*, *Pasteurella* spp., *Streptococcus pneumoniae*, *Streptococcus agalactiae*, and *Streptococcus* spp. The primary roles of these bacteria in respiratory disease in hamsters have not been definitively established. *Mycoplasma pulmonis* has been isolated from hamsters, but its pathogenic potential in hamsters is not known. Mastitis has been associated with beta-hemolytic *Streptococcus*, *P. pneumotropica*, and *E. coli*. Cutaneous and cervical abscesses have been found to be colonized with a variety of organisms, including *Actinomyces bovis*, *Staphylococcus aureus*, *Streptococcus* spp., and *P. pneumotropica*. *Pseudomonas aeruginosa* septicemia has also been observed in this species. Enteritis in postpartum dams has been attributed to *P. pneumotropica*, but a cause and effect relationship was not established.

Fungal Infections
Dermatomycosis

Spontaneous dermatophyte infections due to *Trichophyton* sp. and *Microsporum* sp. are rare in laboratory hamsters, and there are few reports of confirmed cases in the literature.

Encephalitozoon cuniculi

There is relatively little information on *E. cuniculi* infections in hamsters. One report describes *Encephalitozoon* infection of a transplantable ascites-plasmacytoma of hamsters, but details of pathologic findings were not included (for additional information, see Rabbit Chapter 6, "*Encephalitozoon cuniculi* Infection").

BIBLIOGRAPHY FOR BACTERIAL AND FUNGAL INFECTIONS

General Bibliography for Bacterial and Fungal Infections

Frisk, C.S. (1987) Bacterial and mycotic diseases. In: *Laboratory Hamsters* (eds. G.L. Van Hoosier, Jr.& C.W. McPherson), pp. 111–133. Academic Press, New York.

Frisk, C.S. (2012) Bacterial and fungal diseases. In: *The Laboratory Rabbit, Guinea Pig, Hamster, and Other Rodents* (eds. M.A. Suckow, K.A. Stevens, & R.P. Wilson), pp. 797–820. Academic Press, New York.

Hagen, C.A., Shefner, A.M., & Ehrlich, R. (1965) Intestinal microflora of normal hamsters. *Laboratory Animal Care* 15:185–193.

Renshaw, H.W., Van Hoosier, G.L., & Amend, N.D. (1975) A survey of naturally occurring diseases of the Syrian hamster. *Laboratory Animals* 9:179–191.

Bacterial Enteric Infections

Campylobacter jejuni Infection

Fox, J.G., Hering, A.M., Ackerman, J.I., & Taylor, N.S. (1983) The pet hamster as a potential reservoir of human campylobacteriosis. *Journal of Infectious Diseases* 147:784.

Fox, J.G., Zanotti, S., Jordan, H.V., & Murphy, J.C. (1986) Colonization of Syrian hamsters with streptomycin resistant *Campylobacter jejuni*. *Laboratory Animal Science* 36:28–31.

Humphrey, C.D., Montag, D.M., & Pittman, F.E. (1985) Experimental infection of hamsters with *Campylobacter jejuni*. *Journal of Infectious Diseases* 151:485–493.

Humphrey, C.D., Montag, D.M., & Pittman, F.E. (1986) Morphologic observations of experimental *Campylobacter jejuni* infection in the hamster intestinal tract. *American Journal of Pathology* 122:152–159.

Lentsch, R.H., McLaughlin, R.M., & Wagner, J.E. (1982) *Campylobacter fetus* ssp. *jejuni* isolated from Syrian hamsters with proliferative ileitis. *Laboratory Animal Science* 32:511–514.

Clostridium spp. Enterotoxemia

Alworth, L., Simmons, J., Franklin, C., & Fish, R. (2009) Clostridial typhlitis associated with topical antibiotic therapy in a Syrian hamster. *Laboratory Animals* 43:304–309.

Barthold, S.W. & Jacoby, R.O. (1978) An outbreak of cecal mucosal hyperplasia in hamsters. *Laboratory Animal Science* 28:723–727.

Bartlett, J.G., Chang, T.W., Moon, N., & Onderdonk, A.B. (1978) Antibiotic-induced lethal enterocolitis in hamsters: studies with eleven agents and evidence to support the pathogenic role of toxin-producing Clostridia. *American Journal of Veterinary Research* 39:1525–1530.

Blankenship-Paris, T.L., Chang, J., Dalldorf, F.G., & Gilligan, P.H. (1995) In vivo and in vitro studies of *Clostridium difficile*-induced disease in hamsters fed an atherogenic, high-fat diet. *Laboratory Animal Science* 45:47–53.

Eastwood, K., Else, P., Charlett, A., & Wilcox, M. (2009) Comparison of nine commercially available *Clostridium difficile* toxin detection assays, a real-time PCR assay for *Clostridium difficile* tcdB, and a glutamate dehydrogenase detection assay to cytotoxigenic culture methods. *Journal of Clinical Microbiology* 47:3211–3217.

Hawkins, C.C., Buggy, B.P., Fekety, R., & Schaberg, D.R. (1984) Epidemiology of colitis induced by *Clostridium difficile* in hamsters: application of bacteriophage and bacteriocin typing system. *Journal of Infectious Diseases* 149:775–780.

Iaconis, J.P. & Rolfe, R.D. (1986) *Clostridium difficile*-associated ileocecitis in clindamycin-treated infant hamsters. *Current Microbiology* 13:327–332.

Keel, M.K. & Songer, J.G. (2006) The comparative pathology of *Clostridium difficile*-associated disease. *Veterinary Pathology* 43:225–240.

Rehg, J.E. (1997) Clostridial enteropathies, hamster. In: *Monographs on Pathology of Laboratory Animals: Digestive System*, 2nd edn (eds. T.C. Jones, J.A. Popp, & U. Mohr), pp. 396–403. Springer, New York.

Rehg, J.E. & Lu, Y.-S. (1982) *Clostridium difficile* typhlitis in hamsters not associated with antibiotic therapy. *Journal of the American Veterinary Medical Association* 181:1422–1423.

Ryden, E.B., Lipman, N.S., Taylor, N.S., Ross, R., & Fox, J.G. (1990) Non-antibiotic-associated Clostridium *difficile* enterotoxemia in Syrian hamsters. *Laboratory Animal Science* 40:544.

Small, J.D. (1987) Drugs used in hamsters with a review of antibiotic-associated colitis. In: *Laboratory Hamsters* (eds. G.L. Van Hoosier, Jr. & C.W. McPherson), pp. 179–199. Academic Press, New York.

Wilson, K.H., Silva, J., & Fekety, F.R. (1981) Suppression of *Clostridium difficile* by hamster cecal flora and prevention of antibiotic-associated cecitis. *Infection and Immunity* 34:626–628.

Clostridium piliforme Infection

Feldman, S.H., Kiavand, A., Seidelin, M., & Reiske, H.R. (2006) Ribosomal RNA sequences of *Clostridium piliforme* isolated from rodent and rabbit: re-examining the phylogeny of the Tyzzer's disease agent and development of a diagnostic polymerase chain reaction assay. *Journal of the American Veterinary Medical Association* 45:65–73.

Franklin, C.L., Motzel, S.L., Besch-Williford, C.L., Hook, R.R., & Riley, L.K. (1994) Tyzzer's infection: host specificity of *Clostridium piliforme* isolates. *Laboratory Animal Science* 44:568–572.

Motzel, S.L. & Gibson, S.V. (1990) Tyzzer's disease in hamsters and gerbils from a pet store supplier. *Journal of the American Veterinary Medical Association* 197:1176–1178.

Nakayama, M., Machii, K., Goto, Y., & Fujiwara, K. (1976) Typhlohepatitis in hamsters infected perorally with Tyzzer's organism. *Japanese Journal of Experimental Medicine* 46:309–324.

Takasaki, Y., Oghiso, Y., Sato, K., & Fujiwara, K. (1974) Tyzzer's disease in hamsters. *Japanese Journal of Experimental Medicine* 44:267–270.

Waggie, K.S., Thornburg, L.P., Grove, K.J., & Wagner, J.E. (1987) Lesions of experimentally induced Tyzzer's disease in Syrian hamsters, guinea pigs, mice and rats. *Laboratory Animals* 21:155–160.

Zook, B.C., Huang, K., & Rhorer, R.G. (1977) Tyzzer's disease in Syrian hamsters. *Journal of the American Veterinary Medical Association* 171:833–836.

Escherichia coli Infection

Amend, N.K., Loeffler, D.G., Ward, B.C., & Van Hoosier, G.L., Jr. (1976) Transmission of enteritis in the Syrian hamster. *Laboratory Animal Science* 26:566–572.

Frisk, C.S. & Wagner, J.E. (1977) Experimental hamster enteritis: an electron microscopic study. *American Journal of Veterinary Research* 38:1861–1868.

Frisk, C.S., Wagner, J.E., & Owens, D.R. (1978) Enteropathogenicity of *Escherichia coli* isolated from hamsters (*Mesocricetus auratus*) with hamster ileitis. *Infection and Immunity* 20:319–320.

Frisk, C.S., Wagner, J.E., & Owens, D.R. (1981) Hamster (*Mesocricetus auratus*) enteritis caused by epithelial cell-invasive *Escherichia coli*. *Infection and Immunity* 31:1232–1238.

Helicobacter spp. Infection

Fox, J.G., Shen, Z., Muthupalani, S., Rogers, A.R., Kirchain, S.M., & Dewhirst, F.E. (2009) Chronic hepatitis, hepatic dysplasia, fibrosis, and biliary hyperplasia in hamsters naturally infected with a novel *Helicobacter* classified in the *H. bilis* cluster. *Journal of Clinical Microbiology* 47:3673–3681.

Franklin, C.L., Beckwith, C.S., Livingston, R.S., Riley, L.K., Gibson, S.V., Besch-Williford, C.L., & Hook, R.R., Jr. (1996) Isolation of a novel *Helicobacter* species, *Helicobacter cholecystus* sp. nov., from the gall bladders of Syrian hamsters with cholangiofibrosis and centrilobular pancreatitis. *Journal of Clinical Microbiology* 34:2952–2958.

Gebhart, C.J., Fennell, C.L., Murtaugh, M.P., & Stamm, W.E. (1989) *Campylobacter cinaedi* is normal intestinal flora in hamsters. *Journal of Clinical Microbiology* 27:1692–1694.

Nambiar, P.R., Kirchain, S.M., Courmier, K., Xu, S., Taylor, N.S., Theve, E.J., Patterson, M.M., & Fox, J.G. (2006) Progressive proliferative and dysplastic typhlocolitis in aging Syrian hamsters naturally infected with *Helicobacter* spp.: a spontaneous model of inflammatory bowel disease. *Veterinary Pathology* 43:2–14.

Nambiar, P.R., Kirchain, S., & Fox, J.G. (2005) Gastritis-associated adenocarcinoma and intestinal metaplasia in a Syrian hamster naturally infected with *Helicobacter* species. *Veterinary Pathology* 42:386–390.

Patterson, M.M., Schrenzel, M.D., Feng, Y., & Fox, J.G. (2000) Gastritis and intestinal metaplasia in Syrian hamsters infected with *Helicobacter aurati* and two other microaerobes. *Veterinary Pathology* 37:589–596.

Patterson, M.M., Schrenzel, M.D., Feng, Y., Xu, S., Dewhirst, F.E., Paster, B.J., Thibodeau, S.A., Versalovic, J., & Fox, J.G. (2000) *Helicobacter aurati* sp. nov., a urease-positive *Helicobacter* species cultured from the gastrointestinal tissues of Syrian hamsters. *Journal of Clinical Microbiology* 38:3722–3728.

Simmons, J.H., Riley, L.K., Besch-Williford, C.L., & Franklin, C.L. (2000) *Helicobacter mesocricetorum* sp. nov., a novel *Helicobacter* isolated from the feces of Syrian hamsters. *Journal of Clinical Microbiology* 38:1811–1817.

Whary, M.T. & Fox, J.G. (2004) Natural and experimental *Helicobacter* infections. *Comparative Medicine* 54:128–158.

Lawsonia intracellularis Infection

Boothe, A.D. & Cheville, N.F. (1967) The pathology of proliferative ileitis in the golden hamster. *Pathologia Veterinaria* 4:31–44.

Cooper, D.M. & Gebhart, C.J. (1998) Comparative aspects of proliferative enteritis. *Journal of the American Veterinary Medical Association* 212:1446–1451.

Davis, A.J. & Jenkins, S.J. (1986) Cryptosporidiosis and proliferative ileitis in a hamster. *Veterinary Pathology* 23:632–633.

Dillehay, D.L., Paul, K.S., Boosinger, T.R., & Fox, J.G. (1994) Enterocolitis associated with *Escherichia coli* and *Campylobacter*-like organisms in a hamster (*Mesocricetus auratus*) colony. *Laboratory Animal Science* 44:12–16.

Fox, J.G., Dewhirst, F.E., Fraser, J.G., Paster, B.J., Shames, B., & Murphy, J.C. (1994) The intracellular *Campylobacter*-like organism from ferrets and hamsters with proliferative bowel disease is a *Disulfovibrio* sp. *Journal of Clinical Microbiology* 32:1229–1237.

Fox, J.G., Stills, H.F., Paster, B.J., Dewhirst, F.E., Yan, L., Palley, L., & Prostak, K. (1993) Antigenic specificity and morphologic characterization of *Chlamydia trachomatis*, strain SFPD, isolated from hamsters with proliferative ileitis. *Laboratory Animal Science* 43:405–410.

Jacoby, R.O. (1978) Transmissible ileal hyperplasia of hamsters. I. Histogenesis and immunohistochemistry. *American Journal of Pathology* 91:433–450.

Jacoby, R.O. & Johnson, E.A. (1981) Transmissible ileal hyperplasia. *Advances in Experimental Medicine and Biology* 34:267–289.

Jasni, S., McOrist, S., & Lawson, G.H.K. (1994) Reproduction of proliferative enteritis in hamsters with a pure culture of porcine ileal symbiont intracellularis. *Veterinary Microbiology* 41:1–9.

Jasni, S., McOrist, S., & Lawson, G.H.K. (1994) Experimentally-induced proliferative enteritis in hamsters: an ultrastructural study. *Research in Veterinary Science* 56:186–192.

Stills, H.F., Jr. (1991) Isolation of an intracellular bacterium from hamsters (*Mesocricetus auratus*) with proliferative ileitis and reproduction of the disease with pure culture. *Infection and Immunity* 59:3227–3236.

Salmonella enterica Infection

Innes, J.R.M., Wilson, C., & Ross, M.A. (1956) Epizootic *Salmonella enteritidis* infection causing pulmonary phlebothrombosis in hamsters. *Journal of Infectious Diseases* 98:133–141.

Ray, J.P. & Mallick, B.B. (1970) Public health significance of *Salmonella* infections in laboratory animals. *Indian Veterinary Journal* 47:1033–1037.

Swanson, S.J., Snider, C., Braden, C.R., Boxrud, D., Wunschmann, A., Rudrofff, JA., Lockett, J., & Smith, K.E. (2007) Multidrug-resistant *Salmonella enterica* serotype Typhimurium associated with pet rodents. *New England Journal of Medicine* 356:21–28.

Other Bacterial Infections

Corynebacterium spp. Infections

Amao, H., Akimoto, T., Takahashi, K.W., Nakagawa, M., & Saito, M. (1991) Isolation of *Corynebacterium kutscheri* from aged Syrian hamsters (*Mesocricetus auratus*). *Laboratory Animal Science* 41:265–268.

Amao, H., Kanamoto, T., Komukai, Y., Takahashi, K.W., Sawada, T., Saito, M., & Sugiyama, M. (1995) Pathogenicity of *Corynebacterium kutscheri* in the Syrian hamster. *Journal of Veterinary Medical Science* 57:715–719.

Tansey, G., Roy, A.F., & Bivin, W.S. (1995) Acute pneumonia in a Syrian hamster: isolation of a *Corynebacterium* species. *Laboratory Animal Science* 45:366–367.

Francisella tularensis Infection

Centers for Disease Control (2005) Tularemia associated with a hamster bite: Colorado. *Morbidity and Mortality Weekly Report* 53:1202–1203.

Glyuranecz, M., Denes, B., Rigo, K., Foldvari, G., Szeredi, L., Fodor, L., Alexandra, S., Janosi, K., Erdelyi, K., Krisztalovics, K., & Makrai, L. (2010) Susceptibility of the common hamster (*Cricetus cricetus*) to *Francisella tularensis* and its effect on the epizootiology of tularemia in an area where both are endemic. *Journal of Wildlife Diseases* 46:1316–1320.

Perman, V. & Bergeland, M.E. (1967) A tularemia enzootic in a closed hamster breeding colony. *Laboratory Animal Care* 17:563–568.

Leptospira spp. Infection

Frenkel, J.K. (1972) Infection and immunity in hamsters. *Progress in Experimental Tumor Research* 16:326–367.

Mycobacterium spp. Infection

Chesterman, F.C. (1972) Background pathology in a colony of golden hamsters. *Progress in Experimental Tumor Research* 16:51–68.

Chute, R.N., Kenton, H.B., & Sommers, S.C. (1954) A laboratory epidemic of human-type tuberculosis in hamsters. *American Journal of Clinical Pathology* 24:223–226.

Karbe, E. (1987) Disseminated mycobacteriosis in the golden hamster. *Zentralblatt fur Veterinarmedizin B* 34:391–394.

Pasteurella pneumotropica Infection

Lesher, R.J., Jeszenka, E.V., & Swan, M.E. (1985) Enteritis caused by *Pasteurella pneumotropica* infection in hamsters. *Journal of Clinical Microbiology* 23:448.

Miscellaneous Bacterial Infections

Frisk, C.S., Wagner, J.E., & Owens, D.R. (1976) Streptococcal mastitis in golden hamsters. *Laboratory Animal Science* 26:97.

Huerkamp, M.J. & Dillehay, D.L. (1990) Coliform mastitis in a golden Syrian hamster. *Laboratory Animal Science* 40:325–327.

Lesher, R.J., Jeszenka, E.V., & Swan, M.E. (1985) Enteritis caused by *Pasteurella pneumotropica* infection in hamsters. *Journal of Clinical Microbiology* 22:448.

Fungal Infections

Meisser, J., Kinzel, V., & Jirovec, O. (1971) Nosematosis as an accompanying infection of plasmacytoma ascites in Syrian golden hamsters. *Pathologia et Microbiologia* 37:249–260.

Sebesteny, A. (1979) Syrian hamsters. In: *Handbook of Laboratory Animals* (eds. J.M. Hime & P.N. O'Donoghue), pp. 111–113. Heinemann Veterinary Books, London.

PARASITIC DISEASES

Protozoal Infections

Hamsters are host to numerous enteric protozoa, which are often listed and discussed in reviews of parasites, but very few protozoa have any pathogenic significance in the hamster.

Cryptosporidium *spp. Infections*

Hamsters are naturally and experimentally susceptible to infection with *Cryptosporidium muris* and *Cryptosporidium parvum*. Hamster isolates of *C. muris* have been shown to belong to a distinct genotype that differs from *C. muris* isolated from bovine and camel hosts. Experimental infections with *C. parvum* have revealed that aged hamsters (20–24 months) shed higher numbers of oocysts compared to younger hamsters (8–12 weeks). Microscopic findings in the aged hamsters included the presence of organisms attached to villus enterocytes, villus attenuation, and crypt hyperplasia within the small intestine, whereas lesions were absent in juvenile hamsters. In another study with *C. muris*, very young hamsters (1 week old) were more susceptible than adult hamsters (5 and 10 weeks of age). Collectively, these studies revealed that immune senescence in aged hamsters and immunodeficiency in infant hamsters contributed to higher susceptibility. Natural infections with unidentified *Cryptosporidium* spp. have been documented as incidental findings in hamsters with proliferative ileitis (*Lawsonia intracellularis* infection). Cryptosporidiosis may be common, but overlooked and inapparent, relative to the frequency and significance of other enteric infections in hamsters. Diagnosis is generally achieved by visualization of typical organisms embedded in the brush border of villus enterocytes.

Giardia muris *Infection*

Natural infections with *G. muris* are common in laboratory rodents, including hamsters. There appears to be some degree of host species specificity, as *G. muris* from mice and hamsters are reciprocally infectious, but not to rats. Natural infections are usually subclinical. However, chronic emaciation and diarrhea have been associated with *G. muris* infection of aged hamsters with concomitant advanced amyloidosis. These hamsters had the classic lesions of chronic giardiasis, with diffuse mural thickening of the small and large intestine (Figs. 3.21). In tissue sections of the small intestine, pear-shaped to ellipsoidal trophozoites are present along the brush borders of enterocytes and the lamina propria is infiltrated with lymphocytes and plasma cells (Fig. 3.22). Trophozoites normally congregate in the crypts of the duodenum, but in severe infections they may be present in the intervillus regions, extending to the tips of the villi as well as throughout the small and large intestine of aged hamsters. They may also be found in the stomach of hamsters with *Helicobacter aurati* gastritis in association with areas of intestinal metaplasia of the gastric mucosa. Wet mount preparations from the duodenal region should reveal the pear-shaped trophozoites that move with a characteristic rolling tumbling movement. The banded cyst forms can be visualized in wet mount preparations using phase contrast microscopy or with Giemsa-stained preparations. Typical thick-walled

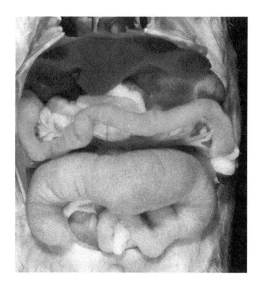

FIG. 3.21. *Aged hamster with chronic giardiasis. Note the diffuse thickening of small intestine, cecum, and colon.*

ellipsoidal cysts containing 4 nuclei can be visualized microscopically by fecal flotation or in fecal smears stained with Lugol's iodine.

Spironucleus muris *Infection*

Spironucleus muris is a common intestinal flagellate of many rodents, including hamsters. Clinical signs attributable to spironucleosis appear to be restricted to laboratory mice, usually in mice that have been recently weaned, coinfected with mouse hepatitis virus, or are immunocompromised. The organism has been identified frequently in hamster stocks from commercial

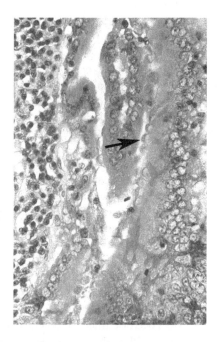

FIG. 3.22. *Duodenal mucosa of a hamster with chronic giardiasis. Note the* Giardia *organisms associated with the surface of the villi (arrow) and infiltration of the lamina propria with mononuclear leukocytes.*

suppliers. Concomitant infection with *Giardia* sp. has been reported, in which large numbers of *S. muris* organisms were present within hyperplastic crypts of the jejunum. The organisms normally feed on intestinal bacteria, and their presence is an incidental finding. These flagellates have been found in the peripheral blood of hamsters with enteritis. There appears to be a strong degree of host specificity for various *S. muris* isolates. Reciprocal interspecies transmission has been shown using clones of *S. muris* isolated from mice and Syrian hamsters, but not between these species and rats. Isolates from European hamsters were shown to be infectious for Syrian hamsters, but not rats or mice, including severe combined immunodeficient mice. Diagnosis of *S. muris* infection can be confirmed by demonstration of the flagellated organisms in tissue sections and mucosal wet mounts, examination of feces for banded cysts, or by fecal PCR.

Other Enteric Protozoa

The above-mentioned protozoa, under the best of circumstances, are marginally pathogenic. Other common hamster enteric microfauna include *Chilomastix* sp., *Monocercomonoides* sp., *Octomitus* sp., *Tritrichomonas* sp., and *Entamoeba muris*, among others. Other than the thrill of discovery by the enthusiastic observer, these protozoa have no significance.

Helminth Infestations
Pinworm Infestations

Syrian hamsters are remarkably susceptible to pinworm infestations originating from a number of other rodent host species. These include *Syphacia criceti*, *Syphacia peromysci*, *Syphacia stroma*; the mouse and rat pinworms *Syphacia obvelata*, *S. muris*, and *Aspiculuris tetraptera*; and the gerbil pinworm *Dentostomella translucida*. *Syphacia mesocriceti* may be the only pinworm species that is native to hamsters. Concomitant infections are common in pet hamsters. Notably, there is host species preference of various pinworms between those of mice and rats and those of mice and gerbils, but hamsters appear to be universally susceptible to them all. Parasitism with pinworms has not been reported to result in any clinical disease among hamsters. Differential speciation can be achieved by morphology of ova upon fecal floatation and perianal tape specimens, or morphology of adult nematodes in the intestine at necropsy (see Burr, et al. 2012).

Trichosomoides nasalis *Infestation*

A number of reports have documented infestation of the nasal cavity of hamsters with *T. nasalis*. Involvement of laboratory hamsters was documented several decades ago, but sporadic cases are likely to be observed in pet hamsters. The primary hosts for this nematode are other wild rodents. Double-operculated ova in feces are diagnostic, but must be differentiated from equally rare *Capillaria* spp.

Tapeworm Infestations

Hamsters, like other rodents, have been found with liver cysts of *Cysticercus fasciolaris*, the intermediate stage of *Taenia taeniaeformis*, a tapeworm of cats. Infestation is incurred by contamination of food with feces from the definitive hosts. Hamsters may be hosts to 3 tapeworms of the family Hymenolepidae, including *Hymenolepis diminuta*, *Rodentolepis microstoma*, and *Rodentolepis nana* (the dwarf tapeworm). In the past, infestations with *H. diminuta* and *R. nana* were relatively common in hamsters, and *R. nana* continues to be common in pet hamsters. *Rodentolepis microstoma* and *R. nana* adults are usually found in the lower small intestine, whereas *H. diminuta* adults tend to reside in the upper small intestine. Unless there is a heavy infestation, hamsters do not show clinical signs. All 3 of these tapeworms may utilize arthropod intermediate hosts (indirect life cycle), but *R. nana* may also complete a direct life cycle within its mammalian host, thereby posing a higher zoonotic risk of transmission to human contacts. *Rodentolepis nana* is the most common human tapeworm worldwide, but laboratory rodents (mice, rats, and hamsters) have been found to be resistant to infection with human isolates of *R. nana*. Diagnosis is made by identification of the eggs in fecal samples or in crush preparations, by demonstration of the adult worms at necropsy, or on histological examination. *Rodentolepis nana* adults are relatively small (Fig. 3.23), whereas *H. diminuta* and *R. microstoma* adults are considerably larger (Fig. 3.24).

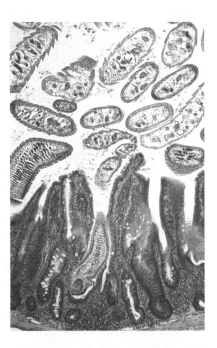

FIG. 3.23. *Small intestine from a hamster infested with* Rodentolepis nana. *Note the small size of the adult tapeworms relative to the size of villi.*

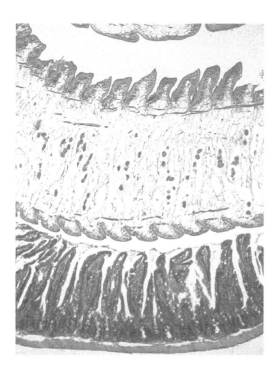

FIG. 3.24. *Small intestine from another animal infested with* Hymenolepis diminuta. *Note the large size of the adult parasite in relation to the intestinal villi (versus* R. nana*).*

Ectoparasitic Infestations
Demodex *spp. Infestation*

Two species of the *Demodex* genus, *Demodex aurati* and *D. criceti*, occur as natural infestations in Syrian hamsters. These mites are relatively common in animal facilities. In 1 survey, the majority of animals in colonies surveyed were infested with *D. aurati* and/or *D. criceti*, and all colonies examined were positive. Hamsters born to infested dams acquire the parasite during the suckling period. Demodex mites are normally of low pathogenicity, and clinical signs rarely occur in hamsters. Lesions have been observed occasionally, particularly in older animals and hamsters under experimental manipulation. Hair loss may occur over the back, neck, and hindquarters. Denuded areas are nonpruritic, dry, and scaling (Fig. 3.25). Microscopically, *D. criceti* are usually present in epidermal "pits," with sparing of the dermis, whereas *D. aurati* are found in hair follicles and canals of the sebaceous glands (Fig. 3.26). Hair follicles infested with the slender forms of *D. aurati* may be dilated with mites and debris, usually with minimal inflammatory response. When skin lesions do occur, there are usually other predisposing factors, such as experimental manipulations and/or advanced age. The mites are species-specific, and there is no evidence of interspecies spread.

Specimens should be collected from male hamsters, since males usually have a larger mite parasite load than females. Mites can be demonstrated in skin scrapings cleared in 10% KOH or NaOH. Differential diagnoses include bacterial dermatitis, bite wounds, and dermatophyte infections.

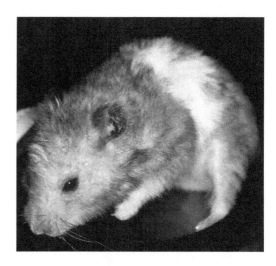

FIG. 3.25. *Aged hamster with diffuse scaling dermatitis due to chronic* Demodex *sp. infestation.*

Notoedres *spp. Infestation*

Hamsters have been found to be infested with *Notoedres notoedres*, a mange mite that burrows in the stratum corneum. Scabby lesions are typically found on the ears, nose, feet (Fig. 3.27), and perianal areas, including large scabious masses around the anus. Numerous mites are present in skin scrapings and sections. Notoedric mange is rare, but can be focally common in some hamster colonies. An outbreak of notoedric mange has also been described in which hamsters were infested with *Notoedres cati*.

Miscellaneous Mite Infestations

In Europe, nasal mite (*Speleorodens clethrionomys*) infestations were observed in 3 separate hamster breeding colonies. Hamsters can also be host to *Ornithonyssus bacoti*, the tropical rat mite, and *Ornithonyssus sylviarum*, the northern fowl mite.

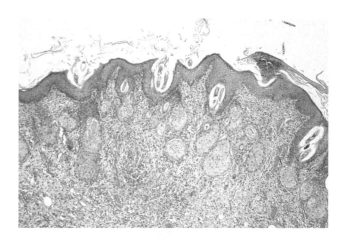

FIG. 3.26. *Section of skin from hamster with demodicosis. Mites and debris are present in dilated hair follicles, the epidermis is diffusely hyperplastic and the underlying dermis is infiltrated with leukocytes.*

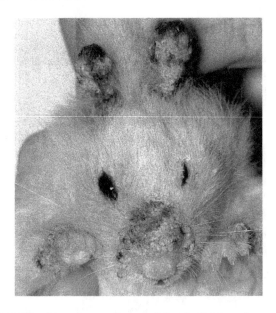

FIG. 3.27.   *Mange in a pet hamster infested with* Notoedres muris. *Note the proliferative crusts on nose, feet, and ears. Source: Beco et al. 2001. Reproduced with permission from BMJ Publishing Group Ltd.*

Myiasis

Rare cases of myiasis in hamsters can occur, due to *Wohlfahrtia vigil, Sarcophaga haemorrhoidalis,* and *Musca domestica.*

BIBLIOGRAPHY FOR PARASITIC DISEASES

General References for Parasitic Diseases

Baker, D.G. (2007) *Flynn's Parasites of Laboratory Animals*, 2nd edn. Blackwell Publishing.

Burr, H.N., Paluch, L.-R., Roble, G.S., & Lipman, N.S. (2012) Parasitic diseases. In: *The Laboratory Rabbit, Guinea Pig, Hamster, and Other Rodents* (eds. M.A. Suckow, K.A. Stevens, & R.P. Wilson), pp. 839–866. Academic Press, New York.

Hasegawa, H., Sato, H., Iwakiri, E., Ikeda, Y., & Une, Y. (2008) Helminths collected from imported pet murids, with special reference to concomitant infection of the golden hamsters with three pinworm species of the genus *Syphacia* (Nematoda: Oxyuridae). *Journal of Parasitology* 94:752–754.

Kunstyr, I. & Friedhoff, K.T. (1980) Parasitic and mycotic infections of laboratory animals. In: *Animal Quality and Models in Research* (ed. A. Spiegel), pp. 181–192. Gustav Fischer Verlag, Stuttgart.

Pinto, R.M., Goncalves, L., Gomes, D.C., & Noronha, D. (2001) Helminth fauna of the golden hamster *Mesocricetus auratus* in Brazil. *Contemporary Topics in Laboratory Animal Science* 40:21–26.

Wagner, J.E. (1987) Parasitic diseases. In: *Laboratory Hamsters* (eds. G.L. Van Hoosier, Jr. & C.W. McPherson), pp. 135–156. Academic Press, New York.

Protozoal Infections

Cryptosporidium spp. Infection

Davis, A.J. & Jenkins, S.J. (1986) Cryptosporidiosis and proliferative ileitis in a hamster. *Veterinary Pathology* 23:632–633.

Orr, J.P. (1988) *Cryptosporidium* infection associated with proliferative enteritis (wet tail) in Syrian hamsters. *Canadian Veterinary Journal* 29:843–844.

Rasmussen, K.R. & Healey, M.C. (1992) *Crytosporidium parvum*: experimental infections in aged Syrian golden hamsters. *Journal of Infectious Diseases* 165:769–772.

Rhee, J.K., So, W.S., & Kim, H.C. (1999) Age-dependent resistance to *Cryptosporidium muris* (strain MCR) infection in golden hamsters and mice. *Korean Journal of Parasitology* 37:33–37.

Giardia muris Infection

Kunstyr, I., Schoeneberg, U., & Friedhoff, K.T. (1992) Host specificity of *Giardia muris* isolates from mouse and golden hamster. *Parasitology Research* 78:621–622.

Patterson, M.M., Schrenzel, M.D., Feng, Y., & Fox, J.G. (2000) Gastritis and intestinal metaplasia in Syrian hamsters infected with *Helicobacter aurati* and two other microaerobes. *Veterinary Pathology* 37:589–596.

Spironucleus muris Infection

Barthold, S.W. (1997) *Spironucleus muris* infection, intestine, mouse, rat, and hamster. In: *Monographs on Pathology of Laboratory Animals: Digestive System* (eds. T.C. Jones, J.A. Popp, & U. Mohr), pp. 419–422. Springer, New York.

Jackson, G.A., Livingston, R.S., Riley, L.K., Livingston, B.A., & Franklin, C.L. (2013) Development of a PCR assay for the detection of *Spironucleus muris*. *Journal of the American Association of Laboratory Animal Science* 52:165–170.

Kunstyr, I., Poppinga, G., & Friedhoff, K.T. (1993) Host specificity of cloned *Spironucleus* sp. originating from the European hamster. *Laboratory Animals* 27:77–80.

Schagemann, G., Bohnet, W., Kunstyr, I., & Friedhoff, K.T. (1990) Host specificity of cloned *Spironucleus muris* in laboratory rodents. *Laboratory Animals* 24:234–239.

Sebesteny, A. (1979) Transmission of *Spironucleus* and *Giardia* spp. and some nonpathogenic intestinal protozoa from infested hamsters to mice. *Laboratory Animals* 13:189–191.

Sheppard, B.J., Walden, H.D.S., & Kondo, H. (2013) Syrian hamsters (*Mesocricetus auratus*) with simultaneous intestinal *Giardia* sp., *Spironucleus* sp., and trichomonad infections. *Journal of Veterinary Diagnostic Investigation* XX:1–6.

Wagner, J.E., Doyle, R.E., Ronald, N.C., Garrison, R.G., & Schmitz, J.A. (1974) Hexamitiasis in laboratory mice, hamsters, and rats. *Laboratory Animal Science* 24:349–354.

Helminth Infestations

Pinworm Infestations

Dick, T.A., Quentin, J.C., & Freeman, R.S. (1973) Redescription of *Syphacia mesocriceti* (Nematoda: Oxyuridae) parasite of the golden hamster. *Journal of Parasitology* 59:256–259.

Greve, J.H. (1985) *Dentostomella translucida*, a nematode of the golden hamster. *Laboratory Animal Science* 35:497–498.

Ross, C.R., Wagner, J.E., Wightman, S.R., & Dill, S.E. (1980) Experimental transmission of *Syphacia muris* among rats, mice, hamsters and gerbils. *Laboratory Animal Science* 30:35–37.

Trichosomoides nasalis Infestation

Chesterman, F.C. (1972) Background pathology in a colony of golden hamsters. *Progress in Experimental Tumor Research* 16:51–68.

Chesterman, F.C. & Buckley, J.J.C. (1965) *Trichosomoides* sp. (? *nasalis* Biocca and Aurizi 1961) from the nasal cavities of a hamster. *Transactions of the Royal Society of Tropical Medicine and Hygiene* 59:8.

Redha, F. & Horning, B. (1980) Nematode infection (*Trichosomoides nasalis*) in the nasal cavities of a golden hamster. *Schweizer Archiv für Tierheilkunde* 122:357–358.

Tapeworm Infestations

Macnish, M.G., Morgan, U.M., Behnke, J.M., & Thompson, R.C. (2002) Failure to infect laboratory rodent hosts with human isolates of *Rodentolepis* (= *Hymenolepis*) *nana*. *Journal of Helminthology* 76:37–43.

Macnish, M.G., Ryan, U.M., Behnke, J.M., & Thompson, R.C. (2003) Detection of the rodent tapeworm *Rodentolepis* (= *Hymenolepis*) *microstoma* in humans. A new zoonosis? *International Journal of Parasitology* 33:1079–1085.

Ectoparasite Infestations
Beco, L., Petite, A., & Olivry, T. (2001) Comparison of subcutaneous ivermectin and oral moxidectin for the treatment of notoedric acariasis in hamsters. *Veterinary Record* 149:324–327.

Bornstein, S. & Iwarsson, K. (1980) Nasal mites in a colony of Syrian hamsters. *Laboratory Animals* 14:31–33.

Estes, P.C., Richter, C.B., & Franklin, J.A. (1971) Demodectic mange in the golden hamster. *Laboratory Animal Science* 21:825–828.

Flatt, R.E. & Kerber, W.T. (1968) Demodectic mite infestation in golden hamsters. *Laboratory Animal Digest* 4:6–7.

Owen, D. & Young, C. (1973) The occurrence of *Demodex aurati* and *Demodex criceti* in the Syrian hamster (*Mesocricetus auratus*) in the United Kingdom. *Veterinary Record* 92:282–284.

NUTRITIONAL AND METABOLIC DISORDERS

Spontaneous Hemorrhagic Necrosis of the Central Nervous System of Fetal Hamsters

Spontaneous hemorrhagic necrosis (SHN) has been recognized in fetal hamsters examined during the last trimester of pregnancy and in newborn hamsters. In affected litters, animals are stillborn or weak at birth and are frequently cannibalized by the dam. Microscopic changes are usually most extensive in the prosencephalon. Symmetrical, subependymal vascular degeneration occurs, with edema and hemorrhage in the neuropil (Fig. 3.28). Intraventricular hemorrhage has been observed, and lesions may extend down the neuroaxis. There appear to be strain-related variations in susceptibility to the disease. SHN has been reproduced by feeding dams a diet deficient in available vitamin E and alleviated by vitamin E supplementation.

Diabetes Mellitus

Diabetes mellitus is a genetically recessive disorder of Chinese hamsters, which occurs in high incidence in some inbred lines. Hamsters display weight loss, glucose intolerance, mild to severe hyperglycemia, polyuria, polydipsia, glycosuria, hypoinsulinemia, ketonuria, and high levels of free fatty acids in the blood. Microscopic changes in the pancreas include islet involution with nuclear pyknosis; shrunken, eosinophilic cytoplasm; cytoplasmic vacuolation; and degranulation.

Hyperadrenocorticism: Cushing's-Like Syndrome

Cushings-like syndrome is apparently common among aging pet Syrian hamsters, but the underlying cause has seldom been determined. In limited studies, it has been associated with pituitary chromophobe adenoma or adrenocortical adenocarcinoma. Affected hamsters present with alopecia (Fig. 3.29) and cutaneous hyperpigmentation. Adrenal tumors are among the most common tumors of hamsters, and are likely to be the underlying cause of clinical hyperadrenocorticism.

Pregnancy Toxemia: Eclampsia

Late-term pregnant hamsters have been reported to develop a syndrome with high mortality that is similar to eclampsia in women. Affected hamsters have disseminated intravascular coagulation in which there are fibrin thrombi in capillaries, particularly involving renal

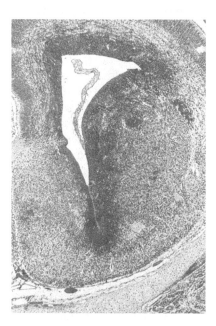

FIG. 3.28. *Brain from a newborn Syrian hamster with hemorrhagic encephalopathy associated with vitamin E deficiency. There is acute extravasation of erythrocytes with disruption of the neuropil.*

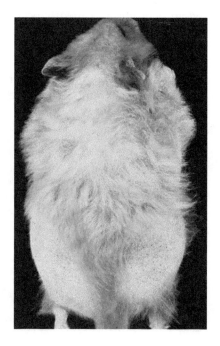

FIG. 3.29. *Adult hamster with Cushing's disease. Note the obesity and bilateral alopecia in the lumbosacral region.*

glomeruli. Severe cases may feature ischemic tubular degeneration and cortical necrosis.

DISEASES ASSOCIATED WITH AGING

Amyloidosis

Amyloidosis frequently occurs in older hamsters, and is a major life-limiting disease in this species. There is a marked variation in the prevalence, depending on the colony under study. There is an approximately threefold increase in the prevalence of amyloidosis in females compared to males. A "hamster female protein" with functional characteristics similar to amyloid P has been identified in the sera, particularly in female hamsters. Testosterone administration will inhibit the expression of this female protein and reduce the prevalence of amyloidosis in female hamsters. Amyloid deposition may be detected as early as 5 months, but it is much more common in hamsters examined at 15 or more months of age. There may be a drop in serum albumin and a rise in serum globulins. Amyloidosis may be produced experimentally in adult hamsters with regular injections of casein.

Pathology

The kidneys are pale with an irregular, granular capsular surface (Fig. 3.30), and affected livers are swollen, with a prominent lobular pattern. On microscopic examination, the liver, kidneys (Fig. 3.31), and adrenal glands are most frequently involved. Other tissues that can be affected include spleen, stomach, testes, and intestine. In the liver, deposition of eosinophilic, homogeneous material is evident around portal triads and within vessel walls, with variable involvement of the sinusoidal regions. Amyloid deposition frequently occurs initially in the glomerular tufts. The early changes may be characterized by the appearance of PAS-positive hyaline-like deposits along the glomerular basement membranes. The early deposits may have the typical amyloid fibrils evident by electron microscopy but may be negative for

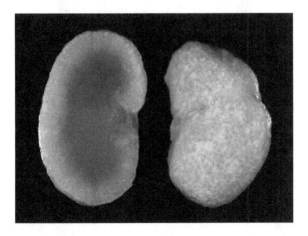

FIG. 3.30.   *Renal amyloidosis in an aged hamster. The kidneys are pale and swollen.*

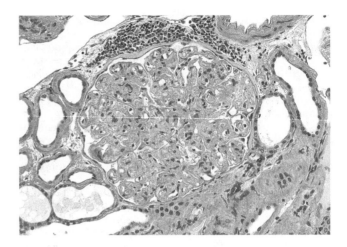

FIG. 3.31.   *Kidney from a hamster with advanced renal amyloidosis. There is complete obliteration of the glomerular architecture.*

amyloid (paramyloid), using the usual histochemical stains. In addition to deposition along glomerular basement membranes, the basement membranes of tubules are also frequently affected. In the adrenal glands, extensive cortical deposition may occur, with distortion of the normal architecture. Atrial thrombosis is relatively common in advanced renal amyloidosis. The loss of antithrombin III in the urine resulting in a hypercoagulable state is considered to be an important predisposing factor.

Diagnosis

The presence of amyloid can be verified using techniques such as Congo red or thioflavin T staining procedures. Deposits may be negative for amyloid using the Alcian blue–PAS staining method. The primary differential diagnosis is hamster glomerulonephropathy.

Atrial Thrombosis

Thrombosis, involving the cardiac auricles and atria, is a common occurrence in older hamsters. Either left- or right-sided atria may be involved, but left atrial thrombosis is most common. Females are usually affected earlier than males, and the syndrome is often associated with amyloidosis. Changes also occur in coagulation and fibrinolytic parameters consistent with consumptive coagulopathy. Atrial thrombosis may be in part due to local blood stasis secondary to cardiac insufficiency. Frequently, there may be concurrent myocardial degeneration and left- or right-sided congestive heart failure.

Pathology

Hamsters with this disorder often present with severe dyspnea due to left-sided congestive heart failure resulting from thrombosis of the left auricle and atrium (Fig. 3.32). A moderately firm to friable, pale thrombus may be adherent to the adjacent endocardium. Bilateral ventricular hypertrophy is a common finding. Lungs become congested and edematous. Microscopically,

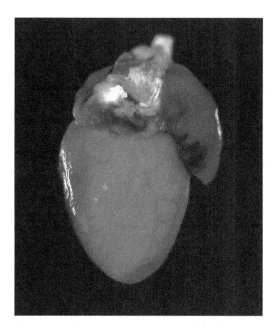

FIG. 3.32. *Thrombosis of the left cardiac auricle in an aged hamster. Left auricular thrombosis is associated with left-sided heart failure. The right auricle may also become thrombosed, resulting in right-sided heart failure.*

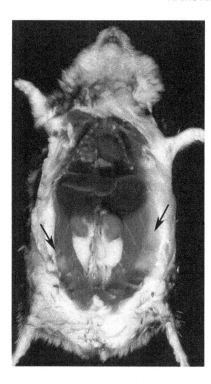

FIG. 3.33. *Subcutaneous edema (arrows) in a hamster with right-sided congestive heart failure due to auricular thrombosis.*

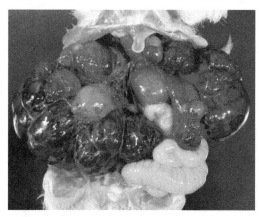

FIG. 3.34. *Severe polycystic disease in an aged hamster. There are multiple cystic areas in the liver with compression and disruption of the parenchyma. Source: A. Griffey, Winters, CA. Reproduced with permission from A. Griffey.*

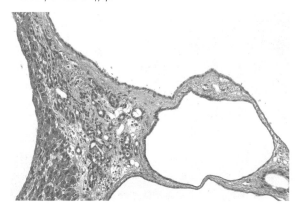

FIG. 3.35. *Liver with polycystic disease. The cystic areas are lined by squamous to cuboidal epithelium.*

there may be some degree of organization of the layered thrombus. Focal to diffuse myocardial degeneration, when present, is characterized by nuclear hypertrophy, vacuolation of sarcoplasm, fiber atrophy, and interstitial fibrosis. There may be concurrent focal medial degeneration and calcification of coronary arteries. In the valves, fibrosis and myxomatous change may occur. Thrombosis of the right auricle may also occur, resulting in right-sided heart failure. Affected hamsters have been referred to as "jelly hamsters" because of the marked subcutaneous edema (Fig. 3.33).

Polycystic Disease: Polycystic Liver Disease

Multiple hepatic cysts may occasionally be found as an incidental finding in older hamsters at necropsy. They are considered to be of congenital origin and due to either failure of fusion of the intralobular and interlobular ducts or failure of superfluous bile ducts to disappear. Raised, cystic areas of variable size, up to 2 cm in diameter, are present on the capsule and within the parenchyma of the liver (Fig. 3.34). True cysts may also be present in other tissues such as epididymis, seminal vesicles, pancreas, and endometrium. In 1 report, over 75% of hamsters studied had cystic lesions at necropsy and many had lesions at multiple sites. Cysts were most common in the liver and epididymis, followed by seminal vesicles and pancreas. The cysts are thin-walled and contain clear, straw-colored fluid. On microscopic examination, there are multiple unilocular and multilocular cystic areas composed of a band of collagenous tissue and lined by flattened to cuboidal epithelial cells (Fig. 3.35). In the adjacent parenchyma of the liver, changes may include pressure atrophy of hepatic cords, hemosiderin deposition, proliferation of bile ducts, and periportal lymphocytic infiltration.

Bile Ductular Hyperplasia: Hepatic Cirrhosis
This spontaneous disorder occurs sporadically among laboratory hamsters, reaching a prevalence of up to 20% in some colonies. It occurs in aged animals, particularly females. Grossly, there is uniform nodularity to the capsular surface, with microscopic evidence of periportal fibrosis and bile duct proliferation, analogous to the liver lesion encountered in aging rats. There may also be nodular hepatocellular proliferation with concurrent degeneration, necrosis, and mixed leukocyte infiltration. *Helicobacter* spp. have been associated with this lesion in hamsters and other laboratory rodents.

Glomerulonephropathy
Degenerative renal disease represents an important cause of morbidity and mortality in older hamsters. The disease occurs more frequently in females than in males. The etiology and pathogenesis of the disease is poorly understood. The disease in the hamster has been interpreted to be similar to chronic progressive nephropathy in aged rats. It has been suggested that there is a direct relationship between the concentration of dietary protein and the severity of the renal lesions. Proteinuria is present, but no IgG or amyloid has been found in the glomeruli. Renovascular hypertension has been suggested as a possible cause of the disease.

Pathology
Affected kidneys are pale and granular in appearance, with irregular cortical depressions (Fig. 3.36). There may be radiating cortical scarring evident on the cut surface. On microscopic examination, glomerular changes vary from segmental to diffuse thickening of basement membranes, with deposition of eosinophilic material. In severely affected animals, there may be complete obliteration of glomerular structures. In advanced cases, there is often concurrent amyloid deposition on glomerular basement membranes and dilation and atrophy of

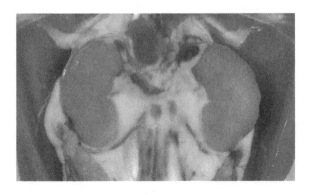

FIG. 3.36. *Adult hamster with advanced glomerulonephropathy. Note the pale, irregular cortical surfaces.*

degenerating tubules. Some tubules may be lined by poorly differentiated epithelial cells, and epithelial changes in other tubules vary from flattening to degeneration. There is a variable degree of interstitial fibrosis in a diffuse to segmental pattern, with thickening of basement membranes and minimal inflammatory cell response. Proteinaceous, eosinophilic casts may be present in many tubules. Fibrinoid change may be present in the media of intrarenal vessels, but this is not a consistent finding.

Diagnosis
Differential diagnoses include toxic nephropathy and uncomplicated amyloidosis. Amyloid deposition frequently occurs as a concurrent event, particularly in advanced cases of glomerulonephropathy.

Other Changes Associated with Aging
Alveolar histiocytosis, fibrinoid degeneration of arterioles, and cerebral mineralization are lesions that have been observed in older animals. Focal cerebral mineralization may be seen microscopically as an incidental finding at necropsy. There are foci of mineralization in the neuropil, with displacement of adjacent structures and minimal cellular response.

ENVIRONOMENTAL, GENETIC, AND OTHER DISORDERS
Bedding-Associated Dermatitis
Leg lesions have been associated with contact bedding in Chinese and Syrian hamsters. Lesions in animals housed on wood shavings are primarily on the footpads and are characterized by degeneration and atrophy of the digits, with granulomatous inflammatory response. Necrotic areas with ulceration may spread to the legs and shoulders. On histological examination, wood shavings and sawdust are frequently detectable in the dermis and subcutis, with leukocytic infiltration and multinucleate giant cell formation. The site of entry is likely the footpad, with subsequent subcutaneous migration to proximal areas. Rats and mice housed on the same bedding are not affected. Differential diagnoses include trauma and cannibalism.

Malocclusion
Like other rodents, hamsters can develop malocclusion or broken incisors, resulting in overgrowth of incisor teeth that are not in good opposition.

Periodontal Disease
Hamsters have served as experimental models of both periodontal disease and caries, which are induced by a combination of dietary and microbial factors. Spontaneous periodontal disease does occur, but is apparently rare. Hamster parvovirus (MPV-3) infection may cause abnormalities in tooth growth.

Congenital/Hereditary Hydrocephalus

Spontaneous cases of hydrocephalus have been identified in Syrian hamsters housed in a research facility in Switzerland. No obvious behavioral changes were detected in affected animals. There was no evidence of impairment of reproductive activity in affected animals, and viable offspring were produced. Examination of brains of hydrocephalic hamsters revealed various gradations of involvement, ranging from marked dilation of the lateral ventricles to barely perceptible hydrocephalus detectable only on microscopic examination. Doming of calvaria was absent, and the limitation of the dilation to the lateral ventricles was consistent with stenosis of the cerebral aqueduct. Additional studies failed to identify any infectious or toxic agent that could be the underlying cause. The entity appears to be widespread in hamster stocks in central Europe.

BIBLIOGRAPHY FOR NONINFECTIOUS DISEASES

General References for Noninfectious Diseases

Hubbard, G.B. & Schmidt, R.E. (1987) Noninfectious Diseases. In: *Laboratory Hamsters* (eds. G.L. Van Hoosier, Jr.& C.W. McPherson), pp. 169–178. Academic Press, New York.

Karolewski, B., Mayer, T.W., & Ruble, G. (2012) Non-infectious diseases. In: *The Laboratory Rabbit, Guinea Pig, Hamster, and Other Rodents* (eds. M.A. Suckow, K.A. Stevens, & R.P. Wilson), pp. 867–873. Academic Press, New York.

Pour, P., Althoff, J., Salmasi, S.Z., & Stepan, K. (1979) Spontaneous tumors and common diseases in three types of hamsters. *Journal of the National Cancer Institute* 63:797–811.

Pour, P., Knoch, N., Greiser, E., Mohr, U., Althoff, J., & Cardesa, A. (1976) Spontaneous tumors and common diseases in two colonies of Syrian hamsters. I. Incidence and sites. *Journal of the National Cancer Institute* 56:931–935.

Schmidt, R.E. (1983) *Pathology of Aging Syrian Hamsters.* CRC Press, Boca Raton, FL.

Nutritional and Metabolic Disorders

Bauck, L., Orr, J.P., & Lawrence, K.H. (1984) Hyperadrenocorticism in three teddy bear hamsters. *Canadian Veterinary Journal* 25:247–250.

Galton, M. & Slater, S.M. (1996) Naturally occurring fatal disease of the pregnant golden hamster. *Proceedings of the Society for Experimental Biology and Medicine* 120:873–876.

Keeler, R.F. & Young, S. (1979) Role of vitamin E in the etiology of spontaneous hemorrhagic necrosis of the central nervous system of fetal hamsters. *Teratology* 20:127–132.

Margolis, G. & Kilham, L. (1976) Hemorrhagic necrosis of the central nervous system: a spontaneous disease of fetal hamsters. *Veterinary Pathology* 13:484–490.

Richter, A.G., Lausen, N.C., & Lage, A.L. (1984) Pregnancy toxemia (eclampsia) in Syrian golden hamsters. *Journal of the American Veterinary Medical Association* 185:1357–1358.

Young, S. & Keeler, R.F. (1978) Hemorrhagic necrosis of the central nervous system of fetal hamsters: litter incidence and age-related pathological changes. *Teratology* 17:293–301.

Amyloidosis

Coe, J.E. & Ross, J.J. (1990) Amyloidosis and female protein in the Syrian hamster: concurrent regulation by sex hormones. *Journal of Experimental Medicine* 171:1257–1266.

Gleiser, C.A. (1971) Amyloidosis and renal paramyloid in a closed hamster colony. *Laboratory Animal Science* 21:197–202.

Gruys, E., Timmermans, H.J., & van Ederen, A.M. (1979) Deposition of amyloid in the liver of hamsters: an enzyme-histochemical and electron-microscopical study. *Laboratory Animals* 13:1–9.

Lewis, R.M. & Mezza, L.E. (1998) Spontaneous amyloidosis, Syrian hamster. In: *Monographs on Pathology of Laboratory Animals: Urinary System*, 2nd edn (eds. T.C. Jones, G.C. Hard, & U. Mohr), pp. 225–227. Springer, New York.

Atrial Thrombosis

Doi, K., Yamamoto, T., Isegawa, N., Doi, C., & Mitsouka, T. (1987) Age-related non-neoplastic lesions in the heart and kidneys of Syrian hamsters of the APA strain. *Laboratory Animals* 21:241–248.

McMartin, D.N. & Dodds, W.J. (1982) Atrial thrombosis in aging Syrian hamsters: an animal model of human disease. *American Journal of Pathology* 107:277–279.

Sichuk, G., Bettigole, R.E., Der, B.K., & Fortner, J.G. (1965) Influence of sex hormones on thrombosis of left atrium in Syrian (golden) hamsters. *American Journal of Physiology* 208:465–470.

Polycystic Disease

Gleiser, C.A., Van Hoosier, G.L., & Sheldon, W.G. (1970) A polycystic disease of hamsters in a closed colony. *Laboratory Animal Care* 20:923–929.

Kaup, F.J., Konstyr, I., & Drommer, W. (1990) Characteristic of spontaneous intraperitoneal cysts in golden hamsters and European hamsters. *Experimental Pathology* 40:205–212.

Somvanshi, R., Iyer, P.K., Biswas, J.C., & Koul, G.L. (1987) Polycystic liver disease in golden hamsters. *Journal of Comparative Pathology* 97:615–618.

Bile Ductular Hyperplasia: Hepatic Cirrhosis

Chesterman, F.C. & Pomerance, A. (1965) Cirrhosis and liver tumours in a closed colony of golden hamsters. *British Journal of Cancer* 19:802–811.

Glomerulonephropathy

Slausen, D.O., Hobbs, C.H., & Crain, C. (1978) Arteriolar nephrosclerosis in the Syrian hamster. *Veterinary Pathology* 15:1–11.

Van Marck, E.A., Jacob, W., Deelder, A.M., & Gigase, P.L. (1978) Spontaneous glomerular basement membrane changes in the golden hamster (*Mesocricetus auratus*): a light and electron microscopic study. *Laboratory Animals* 12:207–211.

Environmental, Genetic, and Other Disorders

Edwards, J.F., Gebhardt-Henrich, S., Fischer, K., Hauzenberger, A., Konar, M., & Steiger, A. (2006) Hereditary hydrocephalus in laboratory-reared golden hamsters (*Mesocricetus auratus*). *Veterinary Pathology* 43:523–529.

Griffin, H.E., Gbadamosi, S.G., & Perry, R.L. (1989) Hamster limb loss. *Laboratory Animals* 18:19–20.

Meshorer, A. (1976) Leg lesions in hamsters caused by wood shavings. *Laboratory Animal Science* 26:827–829.

Murphy, M.R. & Schneider, G.E. (1970) Olfactory bulb removal eliminates mating behavior in the male golden hamster. *Science* 167:302–303.

NEOPLASMS

Hamsters were once commonly used for the experimental induction of tumors by a number of xenogeneic viruses, including adenoviruses, papillomaviruses, and polyomaviruses. Spontaneous tumors are relatively rare among hamsters. There is a marked variation in the prevalence of neoplasms in different colonies. This

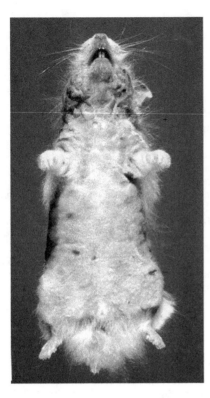

FIG. 3.37. *Aged hamster with multifocal raised ulcerated areas on the skin and erythroderma due to epidermotropic lymphoma.*

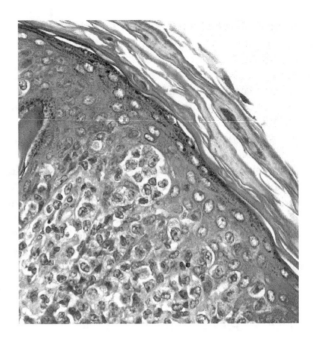

FIG. 3.38. *Skin from an aged hamster with epidermotropic lymphoma. Note the infiltrate of poorly differentiated mononuclear cells in the dermis and excavation of the adjacent epidermis.*

probably reflects the influence of genetic and environmental conditions. Lymphomas and epithelial tumors associated with hamster polyomavirus (HaPyV) have been discussed previously in the "Viral Infections" section. In addition, spontaneous lymphomas arise in aged hamsters that are not associated with HaPV. They are multicentric, often involving thymus, thoracic lymph nodes, mesenteric lymph nodes, superficial lymph nodes, spleen, liver, and other sites. Cell types are variable. Cutaneous lymphoma resembling mycosis fungoides has been observed in adult hamsters. Lethargy, anorexia, weight loss, patchy alopecia, and exfoliative erythroderma have been observed in affected animals (Fig. 3.37). Microscopic changes include infiltrates of neoplastic lymphocytes in the dermis, with extension into the epidermis (Fig. 3.38). During the 1960s and 1970s, a contagious reticulum cell sarcoma was known to occur within some laboratory hamster colonies. Tumor cells were transmissible by direct contact and by feeding. Although not reported in recent years, conditions may allow recurrence of this phenomenon.

Among other tumors that occur in this species, the majority are benign, and frequently arise from the endocrine system or alimentary tract. Adrenocortical adenomas are among the most frequently recorded tumors. For additional information on neoplasms, see Pour et al. (1976), Pour et al. (1979), Strandberg (1987), Turusov et al. (1996), Van Hoosier and Trentin (1979), and Barthold (1996).

BIBLIOGRAPHY FOR NEOPLASMS

Barthold, S.W. (1996) Tumours of the haematopoietic system. In: *Pathology of Tumours in Laboratory Animals. III. Tumors of the Hamster*, 2nd edn (eds. V.S. Turusov& U. Mohr), pp. 365–383. IARC Scientific Publications, Lyon, France.

Brindley, D.C. & Banfield, W.G. (1961) A contagious tumor of the hamster. *Journal of the National Cancer Institute* 26:549–557.

Copper, H.L., Mackay, C.M., & Banfield, W.G. (1964) Chromosome studies of a contagious reticulum cell sarcoma of the Syrian hamster. *Journal of the National Cancer Institute* 33:691–706.

Harvey, R.G., Whitbread, T.J., Ferrer, L., & Copper, J.E. (1992) Epidermotropic cutaneous T-cell lymphoma (mycosis fungoides) in Syrian hamsters (*Mesocricetus auratus*). A report of six cases and the demonstration of T-cell specificity. *Veterinary Dermatology* 3:13–19.

Pour, P., Althoff, J., Salmasi, S.Z. & Stepan, K. (1979) Spontaneous tumors and common diseases in three types of hamsters. *Journal of the National Cancer Institute* 63:797–811.

Pour, P., Knoch, N., Greiser, E., Mohr, U., Althoff, J., & Cardesa, A. (1976) Spontaneous tumors and common diseases in two colonies of Syrian hamsters. I. Incidence and sites. *Journal of the National Cancer Institute* 56:931–935.

Saunders, G.K. & Scott, D.W. (1988) Cutaneous lymphoma resembling mycosis fungoides in the Syrian hamster (*Mesocricetus auratus*). *Laboratory Animal Science* 38:616–617.

Strandberg, J.D. (1987) Neoplastic diseases. In: *Laboratory Hamsters* (eds. G.L. Van Hoosier, Jr.& C.W. McPherson), pp. 157–168. Academic Press, New York.

Turusov, V.S. & Mohr, U. (1996) *Pathology of Tumours in Laboratory Animals. III. Tumours of the Hamster*, 2nd edn. IARC Scientific Publications, Lyon, France.

Van Hoosier, G.L., Jr. & Trentin, J.J. (1979) Naturally occurring tumors of the Syrian hamster. *Progress in Experimental Tumor Research* 23:1–12.

4 Gerbil

INTRODUCTION

Gerbils belong to the family Muridae, subfamily Gerbillinae, which contains approximately 110 species native to Africa and Asia. The Mongolian gerbil (*Meriones unguiculatus*) is indigenous to Mongolia, southern Siberia, and northern China. It is the most common laboratory gerbil, and is commercially available as such. Like other laboratory rodents, the pet trade has adopted these animals as well. All laboratory Mongolian gerbils are derived from 20 pairs trapped in eastern Mongolia in 1935, which were taken to Japan's Kitasato Institute, from which a subcolony was established at the Central Laboratories for Experimental Animals in Tokyo. Eleven pairs from the Tokyo subcolony were imported into the United States in 1954, and subcolonies from that stock have been used to establish other breeding stocks in the United States and Europe. Gerbils are indigenous to desert climates, live in social groups based upon a bonded pair, and live in simple burrows. The Mongolian gerbil is also known as the Clawed Jird (the term jird is derived from an unrelated critter, the jerboa). Gerbils are used in research because they are highly susceptible to cerebral infarction following unilateral carotid ligation, their predisposition to epilepsy (with inbred seizure-sensitive and seizure-resistant lines), and other uses. Gerbils are susceptible to a wide variety of experimental infectious diseases and infestations with parasites of other species. A few other species of gerbils are used for research purposes, but most of the information available on pathology of gerbils relates to *M. unguiculatus*, as does this chapter. Most commercially available gerbils are outbred, although inbred strains exist.

Gerbils are relatively docile and easily handled. Their means of locomotion is saltatorial (hopping). Gerbils form monogamous pairs by 10–12 weeks of age and will stay together for life. In the absence of the opposite sex, isosexual pairs will bond. Females have a postpartum estrus, and if bred at this time, their pregnancy may be prolonged (from 25 up to 42 days) due to delayed implantation. Males contribute to rearing of pups. They tolerate each other very well if grouped before maturity, but mixing unfamiliar adult gerbils will usually provoke fighting, with death of the weaker animal. Separation of bonded animals for a period of time will also provoke fighting when reintroduced. It is important to breed gerbils as a single pair, as multiple females will fight over a male. Being desert animals, gerbils are highly efficient at conserving water (see "Anatomy"). As a result, they excrete very little urine and their feces are very dry. Given the opportunity, they will burrow and build nests, whether or not they are actively breeding. Gerbils adapt well to a wide range of temperatures, particularly if allowed to burrow and build nests, and do best with low humidity (less than 50%). An important behavioral characteristic is "sand bathing," which is essential for proper grooming and maintaining optimal health, particularly for prevention of "sore nose" (see "Nasal Dermatitis"). When humidity is high, their fur stands out and takes on a matted appearance. Gerbils are intermittently active day and night. Foot stomping is a common signal of startling, communication, and aggression.

ANATOMIC FEATURES

Hematology

The most conspicuous peculiarity of the gerbil is a high proportion of red cells with polychromasia, basophilic stippling, and reticulocytosis. This is particularly obvious in young gerbils up to 20 weeks of age, but occurs throughout life. This may be a reflection of the short half-life of erythrocytes (approximately 10 days), compared with other species. The predominant peripheral blood leukocyte is the lymphocyte, with a 3:1 to 4:1 ratio

Pathology of Laboratory Rodents and Rabbits, Fourth Edition. Stephen W. Barthold, Stephen M. Griffey, and Dean H. Percy.
© 2016 John Wiley & Sons, Inc. Published 2016 by John Wiley & Sons, Inc.

over granulocytes. Gerbils are normally lipemic (hyper-cholesterolemic) on standard diets, especially adult males.

Anatomy

The gross anatomy of the gerbil is similar to that of other rodents, except that they have well-developed hind limbs that facilitate their saltatorial gait. Unlike other laboratory rodents, their tails are nonglabrous. Females have 4 nipples (1 pair thoracic and 1 pair abdominal), and nipples are not apparent in males. Gerbils are utilized in stroke research because of their susceptibility to cerebral ischemia following common carotid artery ligation. This is because gerbils often have an incomplete circle of Willis, which is of minimal practical significance relative to spontaneous disease. Incisor teeth grow continuously (elodont), but molar teeth are rooted. Lung lobation is similar to that of mice and rats, and like mice and rats, they have no intrapulmonary bronchi. Mongolian gerbils have a prominent scent gland on the midline of the ventral abdomen composed of sebaceous glands and specialized hair structures. It is inconspicuous in females, but is prominent in sexually mature males. Gerbils do not have preputial glands. Auditory bullae are distinctively large, reflecting their highly adapted specialization for acute hearing. Microscopic adaptations in ear structure are also evident. The thymus persists into adulthood. The adrenal glands of the gerbil are quite large relative to other species of laboratory rodents. The uterus is bicornuate, and placentation is hemotrichorial. Intravascular dissemination of placental trophoblasts may be present in pregnant gerbils, as in hamsters. Renal function is adapted for urine concentration. The kidney has a very long papilla, and the ratio of papilla plus inner medulla to cortex is about twice that of a laboratory rat. This is a reflection of very long loops of Henle. Some Bowman's capsules in sexually mature male gerbils can be thickened due to the presence of cells that are morphologically intermediate between fibroblasts and smooth muscle cells (myofibroblasts). This lamina muscularis is unique to *Meriones* (Fig. 4.1).

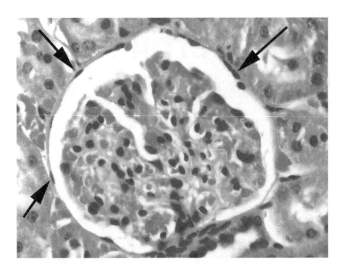

FIG. 4.1. *Lamina muscularis (arrows) lining Bowman's capsule of a renal glomerulus from a male Mongolian gerbil.*

Harkness, J.E. & Wagner, J.E. (1983) *Biology and Medicine of Rabbits and Rodents*, 2nd edn. Lea & Febiger, Philadelphia, PA.

Laber-Laird, K. (1996) Gerbils. In: *Handbook of Rodent and Rabbit Medicine* (eds. K. Laber-Laird, P. Flecknell, & M. Swindle), pp. 39–55. Elsevier, New York.

Lay, D.M. (1972) The anatomy, physiology, functional significance and evolution of specialized hearing organs of gerbilline rodents. *Journal of Morphology* 138:41–56.

Levine, S. & Sohn, D. (1969) Cerebral ischemia in infant and adult gerbils: relation to incomplete circle of Willis. *Archives of Pathology* 87:315–317.

Loew, F.M. (1971) The management and diseases of gerbils. In: *Current Veterinary Therapy IV* (ed. R.W. Kirk), pp. 450–452. W.B. Saunders Co., Toronto, ON.

Marston, J.H. & Chang, M.C. (1965) The breeding management and reproductive physiology of the Mongolian gerbil (*Meriones unguiculatus*). *Laboratory Animal Care* 15:34–48.

Mays, A., Jr. (1969) Baseline hematological and blood biochemical parameters of the Mongolian gerbil. *Laboratory Animal Care* 19:838–842.

Ruhren, R. (1965) Normal values for hemoglobin concentration and cellular elements in the blood of Mongolian gerbils. *Laboratory Animal Care* 15:313–320.

Sales, N. (1973) The ventral gland of the male gerbil (*Meriones unguiculatus*, Gerbillidae): I. Histochemical features of the mucopolysaccharides. *Annals of Histochemistry* 18:171–178.

Smith, R.A., Termer, E.A., & Glomski, C.A. (1976) Erythrocyte basophilic stippling in the Mongolian gerbil. *Laboratory Animals* 10:379–383.

BIBLIOGRAPHY FOR ANATOMIC FEATURES

Batchelder, M., Keller, L.S., Ball Sauer, M., & West, W.L. (2012) Gerbils. In: *The Laboratory Rabbit, Guinea Pig, Hamster, and Other Rodents* (eds. M.A. Suckow, K.A. Stevens, & R.P. Wilson), pp. 1131–1155. Academic Press, New York.

Buchanan, J.G. & Stewart, A.D. (1974) Neurohypophysial storage of vasopressin in the normal and dehydrated gerbil (*Meriones unguiculatus*) with a note on kidney structure. *Journal of Endocrinology* 60:381–382.

Bucher, O.M. & Kristic, R.V. (1979) Pericapsular smooth muscle cells in renal corpuscles of the Mongolian gerbil (*Meriones unguiculatus*). *Cell and Tissue Research* 199:75–82.

Dillon, W.G. & Glomski, C.A. (1975) The Mongolian gerbil: qualitative and quantitative aspects of the cellular blood picture. *Laboratory Animals* 9:283–287.

VIRAL INFECTIONS

There are no reported naturally occurring viral infections of gerbils, but this is probably a reflection of ignorance rather than reality. Certainly, clinically significant viral infections are not recognized to be a problem. Nevertheless, laboratory gerbil colonies are often screened for antibodies to a panel of rodent viruses with zoonotic significance or significance to other laboratory rodents, including lymphocytic choriomeningitis virus, pneumonia virus of mice (PVM), minute virus of mice (MVM), parainfluenza virus, hantavirus, mouse hepatitis virus (MHV), reovirus 3, Sendai virus, and Simian virus 5.

Data on the natural seroprevalence of these agents among laboratory gerbils have not been reported. A recent study examined the actual susceptibility of gerbils to oronasal inoculation with murine norovirus, MHV, PVM, mouse cytomegalovirus, Sendai virus, reovirus 3, and rotavirus (epizootic diarrhea of infant mice (EDIM) virus). Gerbils inoculated with Sendai virus, reovirus 3, and EDIM virus seroconverted, and PVM viral genomes were detected by PCR in tissues of inoculated gerbils, but none of the gerbils exhibited clinical signs. No serologic evidence of infection could be documented with the other agents, although laboratory mice were susceptible to all agents used in the study. Newborn gerbils experimentally inoculated with reovirus 3 have also been shown to develop degenerative lesions in the pancreas and focal necrotizing encephalitis, similar to lesions found in reovirus-infected mice.

BIBLIOGRAPHY FOR VIRAL INFECTIONS

Bleich, E.-M., Keubler, L.M., Smoczek, A., Mahler, M., & Bleich, A. (2012) Hygienic monitoring of Mongolian gerbils: which mouse viruses should be included? *Laboratory Animals* 46:173–175.

Rehbinder, C., Baneux, P., Forbes, D., van Herck, H., Nicklas, W., Rugaya, Z., & Winkler, G. (1996) FELASA recommendations for the health monitoring of mouse, rat, hamster, gerbil, guinea pig and rabbit experimental units. Report of the Federation of European Laboratory Animal Science Associations (FELASA) Working Group on Animal Health accepted by the FELASA Board of Management, November 1995. *Laboratory Animals* 30:193–208.

BACTERIAL INFECTIONS

Bordetella bronchiseptica Infection

This bacterium is a potential problem for gerbils, but has not been reported as a natural disease. Young gerbils inoculated intranasally with *B. bronchiseptica* developed severe disease with high mortality, while older gerbils appeared to be more resistant. Both *M. unguiculatus* and *Meriones shawi* were susceptible. Because of the frequency of *B. bronchiseptica* in laboratory guinea pigs and rabbits, contact of gerbils with these species should be avoided.

Cilia-Associated Respiratory (CAR) Bacillus Infection

Gerbils are susceptible to experimentally induced infections with the CAR bacillus. Young gerbils inoculated intranasally with a rat isolate were subclinically infected during the study. However, at necropsy, there was colonization of the apices of epithelial cells lining the trachea and airways, with marked peritracheal and peribronchial lymphocytic infiltration. The relevance of these findings under natural conditions remains unclear.

Citrobacter rodentium Infection

An outbreak of diarrhea in a Spanish laboratory animal facility was attributed to infection with *C. rodentium*. The presenting signs were bloody diarrhea, rough hair coat, wasting, high mortality, and, on gross and microscopic examination, thickening of the colonic and rectal walls, with goblet cell metaplasia. *Citrobacter rodentium* was isolated from the large intestines of animals sampled during the acute stages of the disease.

Clostridium difficile Enterocolitis: Antibiotic Toxicity

Typhlocolitis with mortality has occurred in gerbils that received a combination of amoxicillin and metronidazole in their food. Deaths occurred beginning on day 7 following treatment, and typhlitis and colitis were the lesions observed at necropsy. *Clostridium difficile* was recovered on anaerobic culture, and *C. difficile* exotoxins were demonstrated by ELISA. This is a complication following oral antibiotic treatment designed to eliminate naturally occurring *Helicobacter* spp. infections in gerbils.

Clostridium piliforme Infection: Tyzzer's Disease

Mongolian gerbils are exquisitely susceptible to fatal Tyzzer's disease, caused by *C. piliforme*. There have been numerous documented cases of Tyzzer's disease in this species. Typically, the experimental induction of the disease in rodents requires treatment with immunosuppressive drugs, such as cortisone. However, Tyzzer's disease can be produced readily in gerbils without benefit of immunosuppression. Young gerbils have developed the typical disease following the oral inoculation of isolates from other species. Gerbils appear to be more susceptible to clinical disease following exposure to *C. piliforme* than do immunosuppressed mice. Gerbils caged with nonautoclaved soiled bedding suspected to be contaminated with the organism have been used as sentinels for detection of subclinical infections or environmental contamination with *C. piliforme*. Typical clinical signs associated with Tyzzer's disease in gerbils include depression, ruffled hair coat, hunched posture, anorexia, and watery diarrhea. Following oral inoculation, severely affected animals usually die within 5–7 days postinoculation. In addition to focal hepatic necrosis, bacterial antigen has been observed in ileocecal enterocytes by 3 days. Extensive lesions and bacterial antigen have been demonstrated in the jejunum, ileum, and cecum by 5–6 days. In affected gerbils, bacterial antigen may also be present in the muscle layers of the intestine and in Peyer's patches. Ileal enterocytes and Peyer's patches may be the initial sites for bacterial growth.

Pathology

Pinpoint, pale foci up to 2 mm in diameter are usually present in the liver. Ecchymoses on the small intestine and cecum are variable findings. The walls of the small intestine and cecum are usually edematous. Intestinal contents are fluid and sometimes contain blood. The

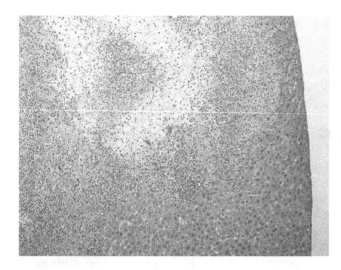

FIG. 4.2. *Focal necrotizing hepatitis in a young Mongolian gerbil with acute Tyzzer's disease.*

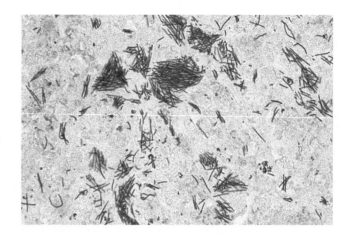

FIG. 4.4. *Hepatic lesion from a Mongolian gerbil with Tyzzer's disease, stained with the Warthin–Starry method. Note the bundles of intracytoplasmic* Clostridium piliforme *bacilli in hepatocytes.*

mesenteric lymph nodes may be enlarged and edematous. On microscopic examination, liver lesions are frequently concentrated in the periportal regions. In acute cases, there are foci of coagulation to caseation necrosis, with variable leukocytic infiltration, neutrophils predominating (Fig. 4.2). Intracytoplasmic bacilli are most numerous in hepatocytes adjacent to necrotic foci (Figs. 4.3 and 4.4). In hepatic lesions interpreted to be several days in duration, there may be focal fibrosis with mineralization. Intestinal lesions are usually most extensive in the ileum and cecum. Necrosis and sloughing of enterocytes, blunting of villi in affected areas, and transmural edema occur. Leukocytic infiltrates in the lamina propria consist of neutrophils and mononuclear cells. There may be necrosis of the adjacent intestinal smooth muscle, with leukocytic infiltration (Fig. 4.5).

Frequently focal necrosis of Peyer's patches and mesenteric lymph nodes occurs. Intracytoplasmic bacilli are usually evident in enterocytes and sometimes in smooth muscle cells. Myocardial lesions, when present, consist of focal coagulation necrosis, with collapse of myofibers, and leukocytic infiltration (Fig. 4.6). There may be mineralization of cell debris. Bundles of bacilli may be evident in cardiac myofibers bordering necrotic foci using Warthin–Starry or Giemsa stains. Diffuse suppurative encephalitis is another possible manifestation of Tyzzer's disease in this species.

Diagnosis

The presence of the typical gross and microscopic lesions and the histochemical demonstration of intracellular fascicles of bacilli are sufficient to confirm the diagnosis. Differential diagnoses include bacterial enterocolitis associated with *C. rodentium*, *C. difficile*, and *Salmonella* spp. infections.

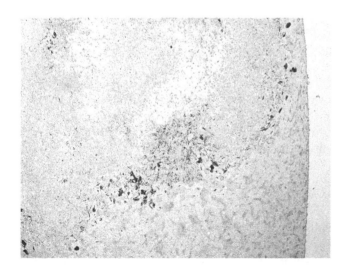

FIG. 4.3. *Same region as the previous figure, stained with Warthin–Starry method. Note the argyrophilic* Clostridium piliforme *bacteria at the periphery of the necrosis.*

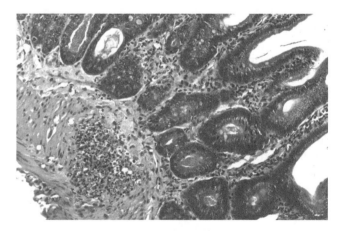

FIG. 4.5. *Ileum from a Mongolian gerbil with Tyzzer's disease. Note the leukocytic infiltrate in the lamina propria and the focus of leukocytic infiltration in the adjacent muscularis.*

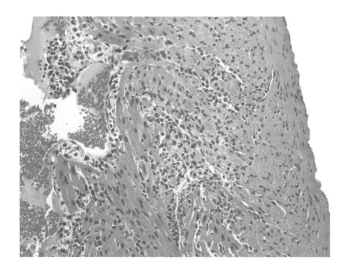

FIG. 4.6.   *Focal nonsuppurative myocarditis in a Mongolian gerbil with Tyzzer's disease.*

Helicobacter spp. Infections

Naturally occurring enteric *Helicobacter* spp. infections have been identified in gerbils. In a survey conducted in Japan, *Helicobacter hepaticus* was detected in the feces of gerbils collected from several premises, *Helicobacter bilis* was detected in the feces of gerbils acquired from a commercial supplier in the United States, and *Helicobacter rodentium* has also been detected in inbred gerbils from Japan. Lesions and clinical signs were absent in these animals. Diagnosis can be achieved by culture or PCR of feces or intestine. Following experimental inoculation with *Helicobacter pylori*, Mongolian gerbils develop chronic gastritis, gastric ulcers, intestinal metaplasia, and gastric adenocarcinomas. The Mongolian gerbil is an established animal model for the study of gastric carcinogenesis associated with chronic *H. pylori* infection.

Leptospira spp. Infection: Leptospirosis

Leptospirosis has not been reported as a natural infection in gerbils, but gerbils are quite susceptible to experimental infection with a number of *Leptospira* serovars, although different stocks of gerbils may vary in susceptibility. Acute disease is characterized by hemolytic icterus, with pale, mottled livers. Microscopically, there is degeneration of renal distal convoluted tubules and centrilobular hepatocytes with conspicuous erythrophagocytosis in the spleen. Spirochetes are present in kidney and liver in large numbers. Chronic infection occurs frequently, with chronic nonsuppurative inflammation, interstitial fibrosis, and development of progressively severe tubular degeneration and cyst formation. The infection may persist in the kidney for months to years. Thus, leptospirosis remains a yet to be reported natural infection in gerbils, but has high potential as a disease to be discovered in gerbils.

Listeria monocytogenes Infection: Listeriosis

Listeriosis occurs naturally in a number of rodents and lagomorphs. Natural infection of Mongolian gerbils with *L. monocytogenes* has not been reported, but a natural outbreak of listeriosis was observed in bushy-tailed jirds (*Sekeetamys calurus*). Affected animals died acutely with no prior clinical signs. Necrotizing lesions with large numbers of Gram-positive coccobacilli were present in liver, intestine, spleen, hepatic lymph nodes, and mesenteric lymph nodes. Most of the animals also had pneumonitis, with fewer numbers of visible bacteria. Diagnosis can be confirmed by culture, which is enhanced when tissues are preincubated at low temperatures prior to culture.

Salmonella enterica Infection: Salmonellosis

Disease and mortality have been observed in young gerbils 3–10 weeks of age that were naturally infected with *S. enterica* serovar Typhimurium. Clinical signs included moderate to severe diarrhea, dehydration, weight loss, and leukocytosis with neutrophilia. The mortality rate reached over 90%. In 1 report, animals also had a heavy infestation with *Rodentolepis nana*. An outbreak of salmonellosis in a gerbil colony due to a *S. enterica* serovar Enteritidis (O antigen Group D) has also been reported. Salmonella-infected cockroaches were implicated as a possible source of the infection.

The gastrointestinal tract is usually distended with gas and fluid ingesta. Fibrinopurulent exudate may be present in the peritoneal cavity in some animals. Microscopic hepatic lesions may vary from foci of leukocytic infiltration to larger foci consisting of central caseation necrosis with variable mineralization with epithelioid cells, lymphocytes, and neutrophils oriented around the periphery. Exudation of neutrophils into crypt lumina is occasionally present in the intestine. Focal hepatitis, splenic necrosis, suppurative orchitis, interstitial pneumonia, and purulent or pyogranulomatous leptomeningitis have been observed microscopically in gerbils. *Salmonella* may be cultured from sites such as the small intestine, liver, spleen, and heart blood. The primary differential diagnosis would be Tyzzer's disease.

Staphylococcus aureus Infection: Staphylococcal Dermatitis

Acute, diffuse dermatitis has been associated with beta-hemolytic *S. aureus* infection. The disease appears to affect primarily young gerbils, and there may be a relatively high morbidity and mortality. The disease was reproduced in gerbils inoculated in the nasal region with the staphylococcal isolate. On gross examination, there may be a diffuse moist dermatitis involving the face, nose, feet, legs, and ventral body surface. Alopecia, erythema, and moist brown exudate have been associated with the typical lesions. Microscopic changes are those of a suppurative dermatitis, with neutrophils infiltrating into the superficial and deep dermis and adnexae, with concurrent acanthosis and hyperkeratosis. Ulcerations may occur. Focal suppurative hepatitis may be present in some fatal cases of the disease. *Staphylococcus aureus* and *Staphylococcus xylosus* have been associated with the syndrome nasal dermatitis (sore nose), probably as opportunistic infections (see "Nasal Dermatitis").

BIBLIOGRAPHY FOR BACTERIAL INFECTIONS

Bordetella bronchiseptica Infection
Winsser, J. (1960) A study of *Bordetella bronchiseptica*. *Proceedings of the Animal Care Panel* 10:87–104.

Cilia-Associated Respiratory Bacillus Infection
St. Claire, M.B., Besch-Williford, C.L., Riley, L.K., Hook, R.R., & Franklin, C.L. (1999) Experimentally-induced infection of gerbils with cilia-associated respiratory bacillus. *Laboratory Animal Science* 49:421–423.

Citrobacter rodentium Infection
de la Puente-Rodondo, V.A., Gutierrez-Martin, C.B., Perez-Martinez, C., del Blanco, N.G., Garcia-Iglesias, M.J., Perez-Garcia, C.C., & Rodriguez-Ferri, E.F. (1999) Epidemic infection caused by *Citrobacter rodentium* in a gerbil colony. *Veterinary Record* 145:400–403.

Clostridium difficile Infection
Bergin, I.L., Taylor, N.S., Nambiar, P.R., & Fox, J.G. (2005) Eradication of enteric *Helicobacters* in Mongolian gerbils is complicated by the occurrence of *Clostridium difficile* enterotoxemia. *Comparative Medicine* 55:265–268.

Clostridium piliforme Infection
Carter, G.R., Whitenack, D.L., & Julius, L.A. (1969) Natural Tyzzer's disease in Mongolian gerbils (*Meriones unguiculatus*). *Laboratory Animal Care* 19:648–651.
Gibson, S.V., Waggie, K.S., Wagner, J.E., & Ganaway, J.R. (1987) Diagnosis of subclinical *Bacillus piliformis* infection in a barrier-maintained mouse production colony. *Laboratory Animal Science* 37:786–791.
Motzel, S.L. & Gibson, S.V. (1990) Tyzzer's disease in hamsters and gerbils from a pet store supplier. *Journal of the American Veterinary Medical Association* 197:1176–1178.
Port, C.D., Richter, W.R., & Moize, S.M. (1971) An ultrastructural study of Tyzzer's disease in the Mongolian gerbil (*Meriones unguiculatus*). *Laboratory Investigation* 25:81–87.
Veazey, R.S., 2nd., Paulsen, D.B., & Schaeffer, D.O. (1992) Encephalitis in gerbils due to naturally occurring infection with *Bacillus piliformis* (Tyzzer's disease). *Laboratory Animal Science* 42:516–518.
Waggie, K.S., Ganaway, J.R., Wagner, J.E., & Spencer, T.H. (1984) Experimentally induced Tyzzer's disease in Mongolian gerbils (*Meriones unguiculatus*). *Laboratory Animal Science* 34:53–57.
Yokomori, K., Okada, N., Murai, Y., Goto, N., & Fujiwara, K. (1989) Enterohepatitis in Mongolian gerbils (*Meriones unguiculatus*) inoculated perorally with Tyzzer's organism (*Bacillus piliformis*). *Laboratory Animal Science* 39:16–20.

Helicobacter spp. Infections
Bergin, I.L., Taylor, N.S., & Fox, J.G. (1999) *Helicobacter pylori*-induced gastritis in U.S.-bred Mongolian gerbils. *Contemporary Topics in Laboratory Animal Science* 38:27.

Bergin, I.L., Taylor, N.S., Nambiar, P.R., & Fox, J.G. (2005) Eradication of enteric *Helicobacters* in Mongolian gerbils is complicated by the occurrence of *Clostridium difficile* enterotoxemia. *Comparative Medicine* 55:265–268.
Fox, J.G. & Wang, T.C. (2014) Dietary factors modulate *Helicobacter*-associated gastric cancer in rodent models. *Toxicologic Pathology* 42:162–181.
Goto, K., Ohashi, H., Takakura, A., & Itoh, T. (2000) Current status of *Helicobacter* contamination of laboratory mice, rats, gerbils, and house musk shrews in Japan. *Current Microbiology* 41:161–166.
Kodama, M., Murakami, K., Sato, R., Okimoto, T., Nishizono, A., & Fujioka, T. (2005) *Helicobacter pylori*-infected animal models are extremely suitable for the investigation of gastric carcinogenesis. *World Journal of Gastroenterology* 45:7063–7071.
Watanabe, T., Tada, M., Nagai, H., Sasaki, S., & Nakao, M. (1998) *Helicobacter pylori* infection induces gastric cancer in Mongolian gerbils. *Gastroenterology* 115:642–648.
Whary, M.T. & Fox, J.G. (2004) Natural and experimental *Helicobacter* infections. *Comparative Medicine* 54:128–158.

Leptospira spp. Infection
Lewis, C. & Grey, J.E. (1961) Experimental *Leptospira pomona* infection in the Mongolian gerbil (*Meriones unguiculatus*). *Journal of Infectious Diseases* 109:194–204.
Tripathy, D.N. & Hanson, L.E. (1976) Some observations on chronic leptospiral carrier state in gerbils experimentally infected with *Leptospira grippotyphosa*. *Journal of Wildlife Diseases* 12:55–58.
Yamada, M. (1991) Differential susceptibility of two stocks of Mongolian gerbils (*Meriones unguiculatus*) to *Leptospira*. *Journal of Experimental Animal Science* 34:1–5.

Listeria monocytogenes Infection
Tappe, J.P., Chandler, F.W., Westrom, W.K., Liu, S.K., & Dolensek, E.P. (1984) Listeriosis in seven bushy-tailed jirds. *Journal of the American Veterinary Medical Association* 185:1367–1370.

Salmonella enterica Infection
Clark, J.D., Shotts, E.B., Jr., Hill, J.E., & McCall, J.W. (1992) Salmonellosis in gerbils induced by a nonrelated experimental procedure. *Laboratory Animal Science* 42:161–163.
Olson, G.A., Shields, R.P., & Gaskin, J.M. (1977) Salmonellosis in a gerbil colony. *Journal of the American Veterinary Medical Association* 171:970–972.

Staphylococcus aureus Infection
Peckham, J.C., Cole, J.R., Chapman, W.A., Jr., Malone, J.B. Jr., McCall, J.W., & Thompson, P.E. (1974) Staphylococcal dermatitis in Mongolian gerbils (*Meriones unguiculatus*). *Laboratory Animal Science* 24:43–47.

PARASITIC DISEASES

Gerbils are experimentally susceptible to a wide variety of protozoal, helminth, and arthropod parasites that are not naturally indigenous to gerbils. Those with potential for natural infection of gerbils, through exposure to other laboratory rodents or through management practices, are covered in this section.

Protozoal Infections
Although natural cryptosporidiosis has not been observed in gerbils, infant and adult gerbils are experimentally susceptible to infection with a number of *Cryptosporidium* species without immunosuppression,

including *Cryptosporidium parvum*, *Cryptosporidium muris*, and *Cryptosporidium andersoni*. *Cryptosporidium parvum* infects the small intestine and biliary epithelium, and *C. muris* and *C. andersoni* infect gastric mucosa. Lesions include mild mucosal hyperplasia with attachment of organisms to epithelium. Giardiasis has not been reported as a natural disease in gerbils, but gerbils are highly susceptible to infection with *Giardia* cysts of human origin (aka *Giardia lamblia*, *Giardia intestinalis*, and *Giardia duodenalis*). Trophozoites can be found in the upper small intestine, and heavy infections may occur throughout the bowel. Mild mucosal hyperplasia and increased mucin production were evident in infected gerbils. Nonpathogenic enteric protozoa that have been observed in laboratory gerbils include *Tritrichomonas caviae* and *Entamoeba* sp.

Helminth Infestations

Gerbils can become infested with several oxyurid nematodes, but none appear to cause clinical problems. *Dentostomella translucida* has been reported in a variety of gerbils (Fig. 4.7). It may inhabit both the small and large intestine, and is notably larger than other rodent pinworms. Gerbils are also susceptible to contact infestation with the mouse and rat pinworms *Syphacia obvelata*, *Aspiculuris tetraptera*, and *Syphacia muris*. Severe infestations with the "dwarf tapeworm" (*R. nana*) have been reported in pet gerbils. Debilitation, dehydration, and mucoid diarrhea were presenting signs. In another report describing an epizootic of salmonellosis in Mongolian gerbils, affected animals were also heavily parasitized with *R. nana*. At necropsy, small tapeworms are present in the small intestine. On microscopic examination of smears of intestinal mucosa, or of paraffin-embedded sections of small intestine, eggs and cysticercoids are readily identified. In view of the direct life cycle

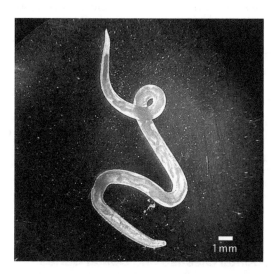

FIG. 4.7. Dentostomella translucida *pinworm from the small intestine of a Mongolian gerbil. (Source: Wilkerson et al. 2010. Reproduced with permission from American Association for Laboratory Animal Science.)*

of *R. nana*, there is a risk of transmission to human contacts. *Hymenolepis diminuta* has also been identified at necropsy in gerbils.

Arthropod Infestations
Mite Infestations: Acariasis
Gerbils can be hosts for infestation with *Demodex* spp., but clinical demodicosis is not considered to be a problem in healthy gerbils. The name *Demodex meriones* has been proposed, but it may represent *Demodex aurati* or *Demodex criceti* (hamster mites), since mites resembling both of these species have been found on the gerbil. *Demodex* mites were demonstrated in skin scrapings from a 4-year-old gerbil with diarrhea, cachexia, and rough hair coat. A lesion on the tail head was characterized by scaliness, hyperemia, and focal ulcerations. Old age and debilitation were considered to be important predisposing factors. There have been documented cases of skin lesions attributed to infestation with free-living nymphal astigmatic mites, *Acarus farris* infestations in gerbils. Copra itch mites (*Tyrophagus castellani*), probably introduced through the food, have been found incidentally on gerbils. *Liponyssoides sanguineus*, an ectoparasite occasionally seen in house mice, has also been observed in Mongolian and Egyptian gerbils. Mites were also identified on laboratory mice and wild house mice on the same premises. No manifestations of disease were observed in affected animals. Mites were also present in the bedding in the cages.

BIBLIOGRAPHY FOR PARASITIC DISEASES

Araujo, N.S., Mundim, M.J., Gomes, M.A., Amorim, R.M., Viana, J.C., Queiroz, R.P., Rossi, M.A., & Cury, M.C. (2008) *Giardia duodenalis*: pathological alterations in gerbils, *Meriones unguiculatus*, infected with different dosages of trophozoites. *Experimental Parasitology* 118:449–457.

Belosevic, M. (1983) *Giardia lamblia* infections in Mongolian gerbils: an animal model. *Journal of Infectious Diseases* 147:222–226.

Jacklin, M.R. (1997) Dermatosis associated with *Acarus farris* in gerbils. *Journal of Small Animal Practice* 38:410–411.

Kellogg, H.S. & Wagner, J.E. (1982) Experimental transmission of *Syphacia obvelata* among mice, rats, hamsters and gerbils. *Laboratory Animal Science* 32:500–501.

Kvac, M., Sak, B., Kvetonova, D., & Secor W.E. (2009) Infectivity of gastric and intestinal *Cryptosporidium* species in immunocompetent Mongolian gerbils (*Meriones unguiculatus*). *Veterinary Parasitology* 163:33–38.

Levine, J.F. & Lage, A.L. (1984) House mouse mites infesting laboratory rodents. *Laboratory Animal Science* 34:393–394.

Lussier, G. & Loew, F.M. (1970) Natural *Hymenolepis nana* infection in Mongolian gerbils (*Meriones unguiculatus*). *Canadian Veterinary Journal* 11:105–107.

Pinto, R.M., Gomes, D.C., & Noronha, D. (2003) Evaluation of coinfection with pinworms (*Aspiculuris tetraptera*, *Dentostomella translucida*, and *Syphacia obvelata*) in gerbils and mice. *Contemporary Topics in Laboratory Animal Science* 42:46–48.

Ross, C.R., Wagner, J.E., Wightman, S.R., & Dill, S.E. (1980) Experimental transmission of *Syphacia muris* among rats, mice, hamsters and gerbils. *Laboratory Animal Science* 30:35–37.

Schwartzbrott, S.S., Wagner, J.E., & Frisk, C.S. (1974) Demodicidosis in the Mongolian gerbil (*Meriones unguiculatus*): a case report. *Laboratory Animal Science* 24:666–668.

Vincent, A.L., Porter, D.D., & Ash, L.R. (1975) Spontaneous lesions and parasites of the Mongolian gerbil, *Meriones unguiculatus*. *Laboratory Animal Science* 25:711–722.

Wightman, S.R., Pilitt, P.A., & Wagner, J.E. (1978) *Dentostomella translucida* in the Mongolian gerbil (*Meriones unguiculatus*). *Laboratory Animal Science* 28:290–296.

Wightman, S.R., Wagner, J.E., & Corwin, R.M. (1978) *Syphacia obvelata* in the Mongolian gerbil (*Meriones unguiculatus*): natural occurrence and experimental transmission. *Laboratory Animal Science* 28:51–54.

Wilkerson, J.D., Brooks, D.L., Derby, M., & Griffey, S.M. (2001) Comparison of practical treatment methods to eradicate pinworm (*Dentostomella translucida*) infections from Mongolian gerbils (*Meroines unguiculatus*). *Contemporary Topics in Laboratory Animal Science* 40:31–36.

GENETIC, METABOLIC, AND OTHER DISORDERS

Epilepsy

Epileptiform seizures are common among Mongolian gerbils that are subjected to stress, which may include cage changing. Susceptibility begins at around 2 months of age and can reach an incidence of 40–80% within 6–10 months and persist throughout life. The trait is inherited as a single autosomal locus with at least 1 dominant allele, with variable penetrance. The incidence, therefore, varies with different populations or lines of gerbils. Seizure-sensitive and seizure-resistant strains have been selected for experimental purposes. Clinical signs include twitching of vibrissae and pinnae, motor arrest, myoclonic jerks, clonic–tonic seizures, vestibular aberrations, and occasionally death. The dentate gyrus is believed to be the epileptic focus. Histopathologic lesions are not obvious.

Nasal Dermatitis

"Sore nose," also known as "red nose," is a frequent problem in juvenile and adult Mongolian gerbils, appearing to be the most common in postpuberal animals. Nasal dermatitis is characterized by dermatitis and alopecia around the external nares and upper labial region. The incidence of the disease in individual colonies may be over 15%, but an incidence of around 5% is more typical. Mechanical trauma may contribute to the disease in some circumstances, but porphyrin-containing lacrimal gland secretions have been shown to be an important contributing factor. Secretions from the Harderian gland normally bathe the eye and conjunctival sac and then are transported down the nasolacrimal duct to the external nares. The secretions are mixed with saliva and spread widely over the pelage during grooming. However, if these secretions are not removed routinely from the collection site at the external nares, chemical irritation and subsequent dermatitis may occur. Marked improvement has been seen in gerbils housed on sand, allowing animals to "sand bathe." The

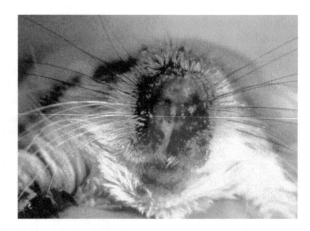

FIG. 4.8. *Nasal dermatitis in mature Mongolian gerbil. There is marked reddening with serosanguinous encrustations around the external nares. (Source: © M.E. Olson.)*

failure to groom properly results in the accumulation of protoporphyrin-containing secretions around the external nares, resulting in local irritation, scratching, hair loss, and dermatitis. Intact gerbils fitted with Elizabethan collars, which prevented self-grooming, developed nasal dermatitis, while those with bilateral Harderian gland adenectomy did not develop the disease. Secondary infection with opportunistic bacteria such as *S. xylosus* or *S. aureus* may contribute to development of the moist, ulcerative form of the disease.

There may be varying degrees of dermatitis and alopecia involving the lateral and superior nasal area and the upper and lower lips (Fig. 4.8). Lesions may progress to severe ulcerative dermatitis, with exudation and excoriation and crusting in the upper labial region. Dermatitis and hair loss may also be present on the forepaws and periocular regions. Microscopically, there is hyperkeratosis and epidermal hyperplasia, with increased melanin deposition in the dermis. Epidermal spongiosis, hyperplasia, and necrosis, with infiltration and exudation of neutrophils, may be present in acute lesions. Other changes may include ulceration and epidermal abscessation.

Barbering

Conspecific hair chewing and plucking tends to be manifest as focal alopecia over the dorsum of the tail.

Tail Slip

Inappropriate restraint of gerbils may result in degloving of the tail skin. Gerbils should never be caught and held by the tip of the tail, but rather handled at the base of the tail only.

Periodontal Disease and Dental Caries

Gerbils that are maintained on a standard laboratory pelleted diet and water may develop progressively severe periodontal disease, which is first manifested at around 6 months of age and is readily apparent by 1 year.

Advanced disease is present in gerbils over 2 years of age, often with tooth loss. They are also prone to the development of dental caries, which can be enhanced with cariogenic diets.

Malocclusion

Lack of opposing occlusal contact results in elodont tooth overgrowth in all species of rodents, including gerbils. Reported cases in gerbils are rare and have been due to loss of the upper incisors with overgrowth of the lower teeth. Molar teeth of gerbils do not grow continuously.

Ocular Proptosis

Aged gerbils may develop protrusion of the nictitating membrane and conjunctiva with bulbar proptosis. The underlying cause has not been characterized.

Aural Cholesteatoma

Aural cholesteatomas, despite their name, are not neoplasms, but are rather concentric accumulations of keratinized epithelium. Spontaneous aural cholesteatomas occur in high frequency among adult gerbils, with a prevalence of over 50% at 2 years of age. These masses of keratinized epithelium arise from the outer surface of the tympanic membrane and external auditory canal (Fig. 4.9). As keratin is accumulated, it displaces the tympanic membrane into the middle ear. Compression and secondary inflammation result in the destruction of temporal bone and inner ear structures. Clinical signs include head tilt and accumulation of keratin plugs in the external ear canal. Differential diagnosis includes otitis media/interna, but this is rare in gerbils because of the vertical configuration of their Eustachian tubes.

Spongiosis of the Caudate Nucleus

Spongiform lesions arise in the auditory system of Mongolian gerbils, increasing in size, number, and extent with age. Lesions are most severe in the posterior ventral cochlear nucleus and the ventrolateral region of the caudal anterior ventral cochlear nucleus. The spongiosis is associated with neuronal necrosis and degeneration of axons, dendrites, and glia, but neuronal loss is subtle. These lesions arise in laboratory gerbils, but are not apparent in progeny of wild-trapped gerbils. The clinical significance of these lesions is minimal.

Focal Myocardial Degeneration

Focal myocardial degeneration and fibrosis are common microscopic findings in older gerbils. In general, 50% or more of male breeders may be affected, and a smaller percentage of breeding females. Lesions are probably ischemic in origin, but the etiopathogenesis has not been elucidated. On microscopic examination, there are foci of degeneration of myofibers, with interstitial fibrosis (Fig. 4.10).

Obesity and Diabetes

Approximately 10% of gerbils maintained on a standard laboratory diet can become obese. This condition can be associated with reduced glucose tolerance, elevated insulin, and hyperplastic or degenerative changes in the endocrine pancreas.

Hyperadrenocortism/Cardiovascular Disease of Breeding Gerbils

A disease complex, attributed to hyperadrenocorticism, has been described in repeatedly bred male and female, but not virgin, gerbils. Breeding females, and to a lesser extent males, develop mild to severe plaques of intimal and medial ground substance alterations with mineralization in the aorta and mesenteric, renal, and peripheral arteries. Breeders may have grossly visible plaques of the abdominal aorta, as well as aortic arch and the entire aorta in severe cases. Breeding animals have elevated serum triglycerides, enlarged pancreatic islets, fatty

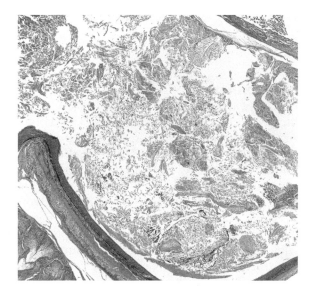

FIG. 4.9. Cholesteatoma in the external ear canal of a Mongolian gerbil. Note the keratin plug filling the canal.

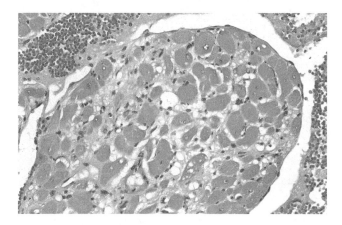

FIG. 4.10. Cardiac papillary muscle from an aged Mongolian gerbil with myocardial degeneration and interstitial fibrosis.

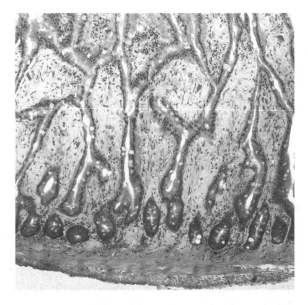

FIG. 4.11.   *Amyloid in the lamina propria of the small intestine in a Mongolian gerbil.*

livers, thymic involution, adrenal hemorrhage, and adrenal lipid depletion. Some may have pheochromocytomas. Male breeders have been found to have a high incidence of focal myocardial necrosis and fibrosis. This phenomenon is also linked to diabetes and obesity. Cause and effect relationships have not been firmly established, but it is clear that these lesions occur frequently in gerbil populations and seem to occur in higher prevalence among breeders. Spontaneously occurring stroke may be observed in aged animals.

Amyloidosis

Amyloidosis can occur in aging gerbils, and has been reported in gerbils experimentally infected with a filariid worm. Clinical signs, when present, include weight loss, dehydration, anorexia, and death. Small intestinal lamina propria, liver, spleen, and lymph nodes (Figs. 4.11 and 4.12) are common sites of amyloid deposition. In

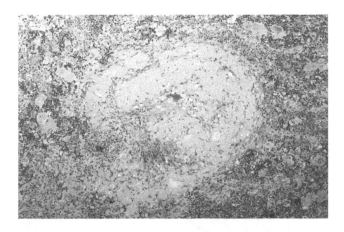

FIG 4.12.   *Amyloid in a splenic follicle of a Mongolian gerbil. Also note the prominent extramedullary hematopoiesis in the surrounding red pulp.*

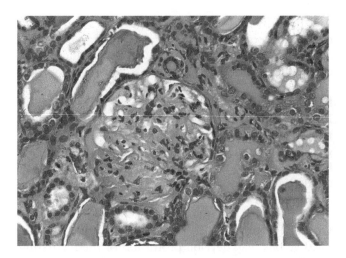

FIG. 4.13.   *Chronic progressive glomerulonephropathy in an aged Mongolian gerbil. There is thickening of glomerular and tubular basement membranes, with proteinaceous casts within tubules.*

one study, the majority of cases were secondary to chronic renal disease.

Chronic Glomerulonephropathy

Glomerular hypercellularity, thickening of glomerular basement membranes, and tubular degeneration with dilation and cast formation in tubules are changes seen in the kidneys of aging gerbils (Fig. 4.13). Mononuclear cell infiltration consistent with chronic interstitial nephritis may be present in affected kidneys.

Cystic Ovaries

Female gerbils are prone to the development of ovarian cysts. Nearly 50% of gerbils over 400 days of age may be affected. Cysts range in size from 1 to 50 mm in diameter. Microscopic descriptions suggest that they are of follicular origin. Ovulation and corpus luteum formation continue to occur in the presence of cysts, but litter sizes are reduced, and severely affected females become infertile.

Toxic Disorders
Streptomycin Toxicity

Aminoglycoside antibiotics (dihydrostreptomycin, neomycin) cause a direct neuromuscular blocking effect at excessive doses by inhibition of acetylcholine release. Although other rodents and rabbits are susceptible to this effect, they are less likely to be treated with these drugs and are, in addition, big enough to receive the proper dose. The margin of safety for streptomycin is low, and antibiotic preparations are seldom prepared so that an appropriate dose in a small volume can be administered to a rodent. Gerbils treated with these preparations have developed acute toxicity, characterized by depression, ascending flaccid paralysis, coma, and death within minutes of administration.

Lead Toxicity

Because of their urine-concentrating ability, gerbils are prone to accumulation of lead and chronic lead toxicity. Their ability to accumulate lead in their kidneys is 4–6 times greater than rats. They are used for this purpose experimentally, and there is the potential for natural toxicity because of their gnawing behavior. Chronically toxic animals become emaciated. Their livers become small and pigmented; their kidneys pale and pitted. Microscopic findings include acid-fast intranuclear inclusions in proximal convoluted tubular epithelium and chronic progressive nephropathy. Occasional intranuclear inclusions may be found in liver, but the predominant finding is lipofuscin pigment granules in hepatocytes and Kupffer's cells. Gerbils may also develop a microcytic, hypochromic anemia with basophilic stippling. Differential diagnoses should include age-related glomerulonephropathy and erythrocytic basophilic stippling, a condition that occurs normally in the gerbil, but to a lesser degree.

BIBLIOGRAPHY FOR GENETIC, METABOLIC, AND OTHER DISORDERS

Bingel, S.A. (1995) Pathologic findings in an aging Mongolian gerbil (*Meriones unguiculatus*) colony. *Laboratory Animal Science* 45:597–600.

Marston, J.H. & Chang, M.C. (1965) The breeding, management and reproductive physiology of the Mongolian gerbil, *Meriones unguiculatus*. *Laboratory Animal Care* 15:34–48.

Norris, M.L. & Adams, C.E. (1972) Incidence of cystic ovaries and reproductive performance in the Mongolian gerbil, *Meriones unguiculatus*. *Laboratory Animals* 6:337–342.

Vincent, A.L., Porter, D.D., & Ash, L.R. (1975) Spontaneous lesions and parasites of the Mongolian gerbil, *Meriones unguiculatus*. *Laboratory Animal Science* 25:711–722.

Vincent, A.L., Rodrick, G.E., & Sodeman, W.A., Jr. (1979) The pathology of the Mongolian gerbil (*Meriones unguiculatus*): a review. *Laboratory Animal Science* 29:645–651.

Epilepsy

Buckmaster, P.S. & Wong, E.H. (2002) Evoked responses of the dentate gyrus during seizures in developing gerbils with inherited epilepsy. *Journal of Neurophysiology* 88:783–793.

Loskota, W.J., Lomax, P., & Rich, S.T. (1974) The gerbil as a model for the study of the epilepsies: seizure patterns and ontogenesis. *Epilepsia* 15:109–119.

Theissen, D.D., Lindzey, G., & Friend, H.C. (1968) Spontaneous seizures in the Mongolian gerbil (*Meriones unguiculatus*). *Psychonomic Science* 11:227–228.

Nasal Dermatitis

Breshnahan, J.F., Smith, G.D., Lentsch, R.H., Barnes, W.G., & Wagner, J.E. (1983) Nasal dermatitis in the Mongolian gerbil. *Laboratory Animal Science* 33:258–263.

Donnelly, T.M. (1997) Nasal lesions in gerbils (what's your diagnosis?). *Laboratory Animals* 27(2):17–18.

Farrar, P.L., Opsomer, M.J., Kocen, J.A., & Wagner, J.E. (1988) Experimental nasal dermatitis in the Mongolian gerbil: effect of bilateral Harderian gland adenectomy on development of facial lesions. *Laboratory Animal Science* 38:72–76.

Solomon, H.F., Dixon, F.M., & Pouch, W. (1990) A survey of *staphylococci* isolated from the laboratory gerbil. *Laboratory Animal Science* 40:316–318.

Theissen, D.D. & Kittrell, E.M.W. (1980) The Harderian gland and thermoregulation in the gerbil (*Meriones unguiculatus*). *Physiology and Behavior* 24:417–424.

Theissen, D.D. & Pendergrass, M. (1982) Harderian gland involvement in facial lesions in the Mongolian gerbil. *Journal of the American Veterinary Medical Association* 181:1375–1377.

Dental/Periodontal Disease

Afonsky, D. (1957) Dental caries in the Mongolian gerbil. *New York State Dental Journal* 23:315–316.

Fitzgerald, D.B. & Fitzgerald, R.J. (1965) Induction of dental caries in gerbils. *Archives of Oral Biology* 11:139–140.

Loew, F.M. (1967) A case of overgrown mandibular incisors in a Mongolian gerbil. *Laboratory Animal Care* 17:137–139.

Moskow, B.S., Wasserman, B.H., & Rennert, M.C. (1968) Spontaneous periodontal disease in the Mongolian gerbil. *Journal of Periodontal Research* 3:69–83.

Aural Cholesteatoma

Chole, R.A., Henry, K.R., McGinn, M.D. (1981) Cholesteatoma: spontaneous occurrence in the Mongolian gerbil, *Meriones unguiculatus*. *American Journal of Otolaryngology* 2:204–210.

Henry, K.R., Chole, R.A., & McGinn, M.D. (1983) Age-related increase of spontaneous aural cholesteatoma in the Mongolian gerbil. *Archives of Otolaryngology* 109:19–21.

Spongiosis of the Caudate Nucleus

McGinn, M.D. & Faddis, B.T. (1998) Neuronal degeneration in the gerbil brainstem is associated with spongiform lesions. *Microscopy Research and Techniques* 41:187–204.

Ostapoff, E.M. & Morest, D.K. (1989) A degenerative disorder of the central auditory system of the gerbil. *Hearing Research* 37:141–162.

Statler, K.D., Chamberlin, S.C., Slepecky, N.B., & Smith, R.L. (1990) Development of mature microcystic lesions in the cochlear nuclei of the Mongolian gerbil, *Meriones unguiculatus*. *Hearing Research* 50:275–288.

Metabolic Disease

Boquist, L. (1972) Obesity and pancreatic islet hyperplasia in the Mongolian gerbil. *Diabetologia* 8:274–282.

Nakama, K. (1977) Studies on diabetic syndrome and influences of long-term tolbutamide administration in Mongolian gerbils (*Meriones unguiculatus*). *Endocrinologia japonica* 24:421–433.

Wexler, B.C., Judd, J.T., Lutmer, R.F., & Saroff, J. (1971) Spontaneous arteriosclerosis in male and female gerbils (*Meriones unguiculatus*). *Atherosclerosis* 14:107–119.

Toxic Disorders

Boquist, L. (1975) The Mongolian gerbil as a model for chronic lead toxicity. *Journal of Comparative Pathology* 85:119–131.

Port, C.D., Baxter, D.W., & Richter, W.R. (1974) The Mongolian gerbil as a model for lead toxicity. I. Studies of acute poisoning. *American Journal of Pathology* 76:79–94.

Port, C.D., Baxter, D.W., & Richter, W.R. (1975) The Mongolian gerbil as a model of chronic lead toxicity. *Journal of Comparative Pathology* 85:119–131.

Wightman, S.R., Mann, P.C., & Wagner, J.E. (1980) Dihydrostreptomycin toxicity in the Mongolian gerbil, *Meriones unguiculatus*. *Laboratory Animal Science* 30:71–75.

NEOPLASMS

In general, the incidence of spontaneous tumors in this species is relatively low, with increasing incidence in gerbils over 2 years of age, at which point the prevalence of tumors can become common. There is frequently a striking variation in the percentage and types of tumors

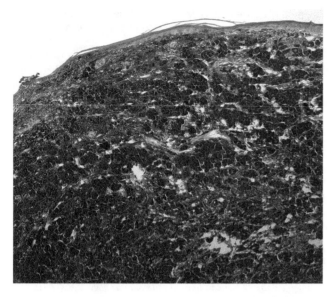

FIG. 4.14. *Cutaneous malignant melanoma from a Mongolian gerbil.*

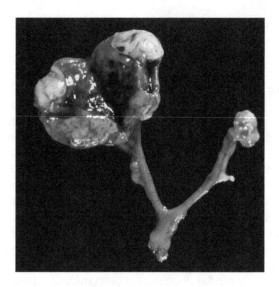

FIG. 4.16. *Ovaries and uterine horns from an aged female Mongolian gerbil. The left ovary, which contains a dark red to pale granulosa cell tumor, is markedly enlarged, fleshy, and lobulated. (Source: D. Schlafer, Cornell University, Ithaca, NY. Reproduced with permission from D. Schlafer.)*

that occur in different colonies of Mongolian gerbils. Cutaneous, ovarian, and adrenocortical tumors are the most commonly recognized neoplasms in this species. The most common cutaneous tumors are squamous cell carcinomas and melanomas. Melanomas (Figs. 4.14 and 4.15) tend to develop around the ear, nose, feet, and base of the tail. Squamous cell carcinomas, sebaceous adenomas, and adenocarcinomas of the ventral marking gland are relatively common in gerbils. In aged females, granulosa cell tumors appear to be the most common ovarian neoplasm. Granulosa cell tumors are frequently bilateral and vary from fleshy and lobulated to cystic masses (Fig. 4.16). Transformed granulosa cells are sometimes identifiable microscopically in the ovary in the absence of macroscopic change. On histopathology, vascular spaces surrounded by aggregations of granulosa cells

are the typical patterns observed (Fig. 4.17). Dysgerminomas, luteal cell tumors, leiomyomas, and, rarely, thecal cell carcinomas have been identified. Adrenal cortical adenomas and carcinomas also occur. Neoplasms of the lymphopoietic system are uncommon in gerbils. Leukemia with lymphoblastic infiltrates in spleen, liver, lymph nodes, and muscle was observed in an aged animal, and there are single case reports of primary cutaneous B-cell lymphoma and systemic mastocytosis. There is a relatively low incidence of tumors of the pituitary, mammary gland, and lung in the Mongolian gerbil. In a study involving other species of gerbillinae, neoplasms included squamous carcinoma of the ear, thymoma, Hodgkin-like lymphoma, uterine adenocarcinoma, adrenocortical tumors, and primary ovarian tumors. Gastric carcinomas have been produced experimentally in gerbils inoculated with *H. pylori*.

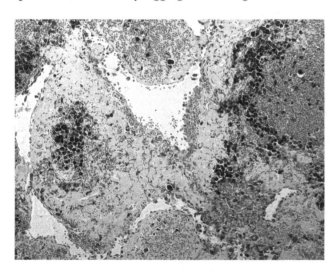

FIG. 4.15. *Renal lymph node with metastasis of malignant melanoma in a Mongolian gerbil. Also note the amyloid in interstitial areas.*

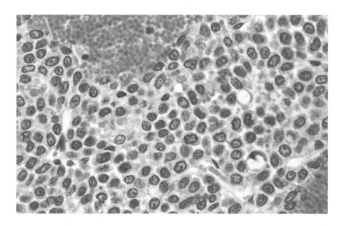

FIG. 4.17. *Granulosa cell tumor in a Mongolian gerbil. Note the prominent vascular spaces.*

BIBLIOGRAPHY FOR NEOPLASMS

Benitz, K.F. & Kramer, A.W. (1965) Spontaneous tumors in the Mongolian gerbil. *Laboratory Animal Care* 15:281–294.

Guzman-Silva, M.A. (1997) Systemic mast cell disease in a Mongolian gerbil *Meriones unguiculatus*: case report. *Laboratory Animals* 31:373–378.

Guzman-Silva, M.A. & Costa-Neves, M. (2006) Incipient spontaneous granulosa cell tumour in the gerbil, *Meriones unguiculatus*. *Laboratory Animals* 40:96–101.

Matsuoka, K. & Suzuki, J. (1995) Spontaneous tumors in the Mongolian gerbil (*Meriones unguiculatus*). *Experimental Animals* 43:755–760.

Meckley, P.E. & Zwicker, G.M. (1979) Naturally-occurring neoplasms in the Mongolian gerbil (*Meriones unguiculatus*). *Laboratory Animals* 13:203–206.

Rembert, M.S., Coleman, S.U., Klei, T.R., & Goad, M.E. (2000) Neoplastic mass in an experimental Mongolian gerbil. *Contemporary Topics in Laboratory Animal Science* 39(3):34–36.

Ringler, D.H., Lay, D.M., & Abrams, G.D. (1972) Spontaneous neoplasms in aging gerbillinae. *Laboratory Animal Science* 22:407–414.

Rowe, S.E., Simmons, J.L. Ringler, D.H., & Lay, D.M. (1974) Spontaneous neoplasms in aging Gerbillinae. *Veterinary Pathology* 11:38–51.

Shumaker, R.C., Paik, S.K., & Houser, W.D. (1974) Tumors in Gerbillinae: a literature review and report of a case. *Laboratory Animal Science* 24:688–690.

Su, Y.C., Wang, M.H., & Wu, M.F. (2001) Cutaneous B cell lymphoma in a Mongolian gerbil (*Meriones unguiculatus*). *Contemporary Topics in Laboratory Animal Science* 40(5):53- 56.

Vincent, A.L. & Ash, L.R. (1978) Further observations on spontaneous neoplasms in the Mongolian gerbil (*Meriones unguiculatus*). *Laboratory Animal Science* 28:297–300.

Vincent, A.L., Porter, D.D., & Ash, L.R. (1975) Spontaneous lesions and parasites of the Mongolian gerbil, *Meriones unguiculatus*. *Laboratory Animal Science* 25:711–722.

Vincent, A.L., Rodrick, G.E., & Sodeman, W.A., Jr. (1979) The pathology of the Mongolian gerbil (*Meriones unguiculatus*): a review. *Laboratory Animal Science* 29:645–651.

5 Guinea Pig

Guinea pigs (*Cavia porcellus*) belong to the order Rodentia, suborder Hystricomorpha, superfamily Cavioidea, and family Caviidae. For a brief period, taxonomists proposed that guinea pigs were not within the order Rodentia, but that classification has lost favor. Within Caviidae, other closely related members are capybaras, wild cavies, and Patagonian "hares" (maras). The guinea pig, also called cavy or cuy, was domesticated over 7000 years ago from wild cavies (*Cavia aperea*, *Cavia fulgida*, and *Cavia tschudii*). Initially raised for food and for use in religious ceremonies by the Incas in South America, both domesticated and free-ranging wild cavies are still found on that continent. Guinea pigs were apparently introduced into Europe by seafarers sometime in the 16th or 17th century, where they were raised as pets and, later, as laboratory animals. Guinea pigs are popular as pets because of their ease of maintenance and docile temperament. There are approximately 16 breeds of guinea pigs recognized by guinea pig fanciers in the world today, which originated from the basic hair coat varieties known as shorthair (also known as English shorthair), Abyssinian, Peruvian, and Sheltie (Silkie). The outbred albino shorthair guinea pig, which was developed by Dunkin and Hartley, is the most commonly used guinea pig for research. Other laboratory breeds have been developed, such as hairless guinea pigs and a small number of valid inbred strains, including strains 2 and 13. The use of guinea pigs as research animals in recent decades has significantly declined. Unlike some of the smaller rodents, guinea pigs have relatively few clinically significant viral infections. In general, hypovitaminosis C (either clinical or subclinical), bacterial respiratory tract infections, and enteric diseases are the major diagnostic problems seen in this species.

BEHAVIORAL, PHYSIOLOGIC, AND ANATOMIC FEATURES

Behavioral Features

Adult male guinea pigs are called "boars," females "sows," and infants "pups." Guinea pigs live in harems with a strong male dominance hierarchy and a loose female hierarchy. They tend to live in family units centered around an alpha male. Mature boars, particularly if strangers, will fight savagely, sometimes with fatal outcome. Sows will also fight on occasion. Guinea pig activity tends to be crepuscular. Vocalization is well developed and complex. They respond to sudden auditory stimulation and unfamiliar surroundings by freezing in place (immobility response), whereas sudden movement will elicit a random stampede (scatter response), which may result in injury to young animals. Guinea pigs eat frequently and unlike most rodents, do not cache their food or burrow, although wild cavies will make use of borrowed burrows. They require a constant source of water and tend to contaminate their water sources with ingesta as they drink. They do not lick sipper tubes without training, a consideration that can lead to dehydration and death. They are indiscriminate defecators and renowned for their tendency to sit in and soil their food bowls. Guinea pigs are polyestrus, with breeding activity occurring year-round. Sows do not make nests. The gestation period is 59–72 days, depending upon litter size, which generally ranges between 1 and 6 pups. Sows have a postpartum estrus within 2–10 hours after farrowing. Pups are highly precocious at birth and are fully furred and mobile, with eyes completely open. At parturition, both boars and sows assist in grooming pups and eating placentas, and lactating sows will nurse unrelated pups. Newborn pups do

Pathology of Laboratory Rodents and Rabbits, Fourth Edition. Stephen W. Barthold, Stephen M. Griffey, and Dean H. Percy.
© 2016 John Wiley & Sons, Inc. Published 2016 by John Wiley & Sons, Inc.

not receive much maternal attention, other than anogenital grooming, which stimulates defecation and urination. Cannibalism or consumption of aborted fetuses and stillborn pups does not occur. Pups are normally weaned within 3 weeks but can be weaned as early as 3–4 days if anogenital stimulation is provided. Nervous in temperament, guinea pigs may refuse to eat or drink for some time following any significant change in location, feed, or management practices.

Unique Physiologic Features

Unlike other rodents and similar to primates, guinea pigs require dietary sources of vitamin C due to deficiency in L-gulonolactone oxidase. Commercial diets that are formulated for guinea pigs are supplemented with vitamin C, but attention must be paid to the expiration date and proper storage due to instability of this vitamin. Provision of leafy green vegetables is often used to supplement guinea pig diets, which is thoroughly enjoyed, but poses a risk for introduction of pathogens to guinea pig populations. Similar to rabbits, guinea pigs absorb calcium through their intestine in proportion to the amount in the diet, and depend upon renal excretion for calcium balance (see Rabbit Chapter 6, "Physiologic Features").

Anatomic Features
External Features

Guinea pigs have 4 toes on their front feet and 3 toes on their hind feet with hairless footpads. There is a region behind the ears that normally lacks hair that can be misconstrued as alopecia. They possess a vestigial tail with a supracaudal scent gland (coccygeal gland or "grease gland"). In addition, guinea pigs have a pair of perineal scent glands (anal or perianal glands) and sebaceous glandular tissue in the penile sheath and skin of the perineal sacs. The perineal sacs, which are larger in boars, consist of bilateral skin diverticula that surround the anogenital region and secrete and accumulate a creamy substance for scent marking. Dermal sebaceous glands are abundant along the dorsum and perineal regions, particularly in boars. Old or obese guinea pigs that are incapable of suitable grooming may take on a greasy appearance. Guinea pigs have a single pair of inguinal mammary nipples, but supernumerary nipples are frequent. The external genitalia are unique, and pose a challenge for the inexperienced when attempting to sex young pups. Sex identification in pups is facilitated by gentle pressure above the prepuce, which causes partial extrusion of the penis in males. The inguinal canals are open and the scrotum of boars is represented as scrotal pouches lateral to the prepuce and anus. The urethral opening of sows is outside the vagina, and the vaginal orifice is closed by a vaginal closure membrane during anestrus and pregnancy (see "Reproductive System").

Lymphoid and Hematopoeitic Systems

The counterpart of the neutrophil in guinea pigs is the heterophil or pseudoeosinophil, due to distinct eosinophilic cytoplasmic granules. Lymphocytes are the

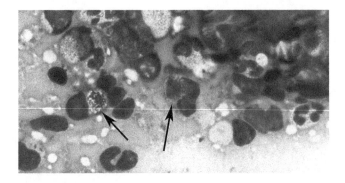

FIG. 5.1. *Impression smear of spleen from an adult female guinea pig, illustrating Kurloff cells (arrows). Note the large, finely granular Kurloff bodies within the cytoplasm of these mononuclear cells.*

predominant leukocyte in the peripheral blood, and both small and large forms are normally found. Up to 4% of circulating white blood cells may be Kurloff (Foa-Kurloff) cells. Kurloff cells are unique innate mononuclear leukocytes with natural killer (NK) cell activity that are found routinely in certain tissues in guinea pigs and have also been documented in capybaras. The cells contain a finely fibrillar to granular structure (Kurloff body) 1–8 μm in diameter within a cytoplasmic vacuole, with displacement of the nucleus (Fig. 5.1). The intracytoplasmic material is PAS positive and stains positive for fibrinoid material with the Lendrum stain. On ultrastructural examination, inclusions are membrane bound, and cytoplasmic organelles in these cells are consistent with secretory activity. In nonpregnant animals, Kurloff cells are located primarily in the sinusoids of the spleen, particularly in sows, and in stromal tissues of the bone marrow and thymus. Large numbers of Kurloff cells accumulate in pulmonary capillaries (Fig. 5.2). They are not normally found in lymph nodes.

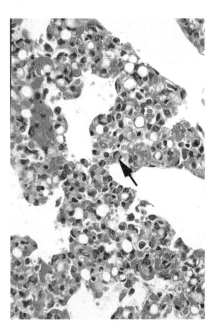

FIG. 5.2. *Kurloff cells (arrow) within pulmonary capillaries of an adult female guinea pig.*

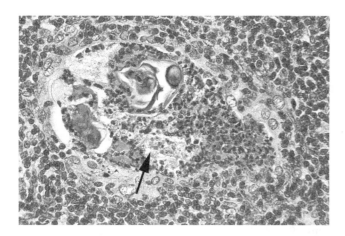

FIG. 5.3. *Thymus from a young guinea pig. Note the prominent Hassall's corpuscle (arrow) containing desquamated epithelium, cellular debris, and heterophils, which is a normal feature of the thymus in this species.*

Kurloff cells are rarely seen in newborn guinea pigs, but are present in relatively large numbers in adult sows. Their numbers fluctuate with the stage of the estrous cycle. Increased numbers are usually present in the peripheral blood during pregnancy. In addition, large numbers of these cells aggregate in the placental labyrinth in pregnant sows. Kurloff cells have been shown to release material into the trophoblast and fetal endothelium of the placental labyrinth. In vitro studies have demonstrated that this material has a toxic effect on macrophages. It has been suggested that Kurloff cells may play a role in preventing maternal rejection of the fetal placenta during pregnancy.

Thymic tissue is present in the cervical region, and accessory thymic tissue is frequently associated with the parathyroid glands. Hassall's corpuscles are very prominent in guinea pigs, with exfoliation of squamous cells and infiltration of heterophils. Degenerate thymocytes are frequently observed in close association with Hassall's corpuscles (Fig. 5.3). These areas of degeneration may evolve into small cysts. The thymus involutes with age, which is essentially complete by 1 year. Maternal antibody is transferred in utero during late gestation through the yolk sac splanchnopleure.

Respiratory System

Guinea pigs, like other rodents and rabbits, are obligate nasal breathers, so that obstruction of nasal passages with exudate may present as dyspnea. Pulmonary arteries and arterioles have well-developed smooth muscular thickening of the tunica media (Fig. 5.4), which can be misconstrued as an abnormal finding. Smooth muscle is also prominent around pulmonary veins. Furthermore, longitudinal orientation of pulmonary arteries reveals that smooth muscle is arranged in unique segmental bulges, reminiscent of sphincters (Fig. 5.5). Thus, depending upon level of section, arteries may either appear to be surrounded by a lot of smooth muscle or

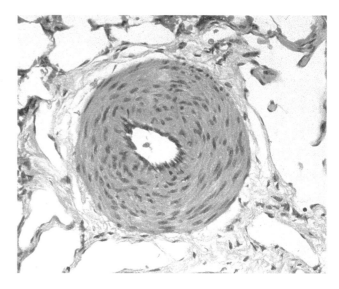

FIG. 5.4. *Pulmonary artery in the lung of a normal guinea pig, illustrating the thick smooth muscle of the tunica media.*

none at all. Unlike other rodents, cardiac muscle does not surround pulmonary veins within the lung. Larger airways are surrounded by prominent concentric bands of smooth muscle. The contraction of the peribronchial muscle may result in marked distortion, thickening, and sloughing of the respiratory epithelium that lines affected airways. Such artifacts have been interpreted to be neoplastic by the untrained observer. Clara cells are the prevalent cell type lining bronchioles, but they are absent in the trachea and larger bronchi.

Aggregations of lymphocytes in the adventitia of pulmonary vessels are a common incidental finding in guinea pigs. Microscopic foci have been observed in animals as young as 5 days of age, but nodular aggregates are more common in older animals. These perivascular changes are normally found only in the lung. At necropsy, close examination may reveal circumscribed, pale, pinpoint

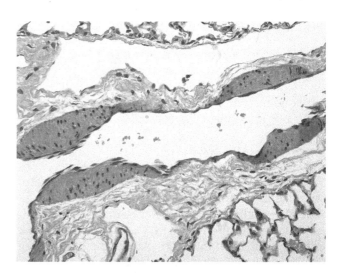

FIG. 5.5. *Longitudinal section of a pulmonary artery in a normal guinea pig, revealing the unique segmental bulges of smooth muscle, which are reminiscent of sphincters.*

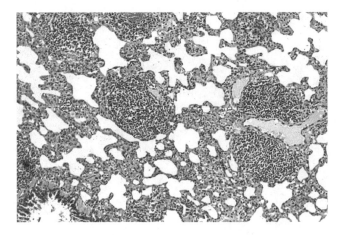

FIG. 5.6.   *Lung from an adult guinea pig with prominent perivascular lymphoid aggregates. These infiltrates are commonly present in the adventitia of small pulmonary vessels of adult guinea pigs.*

subpleural foci up to 0.5 mm in diameter. On microscopic examination, concentric to eccentric aggregations of small- to medium-size lymphocytes are oriented around small arteries and veins (Fig. 5.6). Nodules are focal to segmental in distribution in the perivascular regions. There may be focal to diffuse infiltrates of lymphocytes and thickening of the alveolar septa in some animals, but the airways and alveoli are free of exudate in the typical cases. Ultrastructural studies have revealed morphologically normal lymphocytes, and there was no evidence of viral agents associated with the cellular infiltrates. The lymphoid nodules have been ascribed to a variety of antigenic stimuli, but the pathogenesis and significance of these changes are not well understood. If the lesions are accompanied by adjacent alveolar inflammation, they are likely to be associated with a disease process.

Bony spicules (osseous metaplasia) have been observed in the lung in guinea pigs. Similar changes have been seen in other species, such as the rat and hamster. They are composed of dense, lamellar bone, with varying degrees of mineralization. There is usually no or minimal reaction in the adjacent alveolar septa. They have been interpreted as inhaled fragments of bone of dietary origin, but it is more likely that they are foci of osseous metaplasia. Large numbers of metaplastic osseous foci, including well-differentiated bone marrow, have been observed in the lungs of guinea pigs following X-irradiation.

Gastrointestinal System

Guinea pigs are monophyodont with open-rooted, continuously growing (elodont) incisors and cheek teeth. Their dental formula is I1/1, C0/0, P1/1, M3/3. Cheek teeth grow slightly inward, predisposing them to interfere with mastication if overgrown. Guinea pigs have a simple stomach without a nonglandular portion. They are hindgut fermenters with a large cecum that holds approximately 65% of the enteric digesta. The cecum has 3 linear taeniae and taeniae coli run the entire length of the colon. Unlike most other species, the guinea pig cecum is located on the left side of the abdominal cavity.

In contrast to the rabbit, the only macroscopic gut-associated lymphoid tissues are Peyer's patches. Guinea pigs engage in cecotrophy, with production of mucoid vitamin-rich cecotropes, but they do not have the more complex retropulsive system of rabbits. Guinea pigs digest 34% of crude fiber compared to only 10% by rabbits fed the same diet.

Urinary System

As with rabbits, renal excretion of calcium is the major means of calcium homeostasis in guinea pigs. Guinea pig urine, like that of rabbits, is therefore normally thick and cloudy with numerous crystals visible on microscopic examination. This material may accumulate as "sludge" in the bladder, but obstruction due to sludge is not common, whereas calculi may develop and result in obstructive uropathy. Guinea pigs enjoy alfalfa, but its high calcium content may predispose them to urolithiasis.

Reproductive System

Boars, like other rodents, are endowed with a number of accessory sex glands, including large seminal vesicles, coagulating glands, prostate, and bulbourethral glands. They produce a copulatory plug upon ejaculation. The glans penis has numerous cornified scales or spurs. The ventral aspect of the glans has an intromittent sac with additional scales and 2 horny styles that evert upon erection. Sows have a vaginal closure membrane that is unique to hystricomorph rodents (Fig. 5.7). During pregnancy and anestrus, the vaginal orifice is sealed with a membrane covered with stratified squamous epithelium on the internal and external surfaces. The

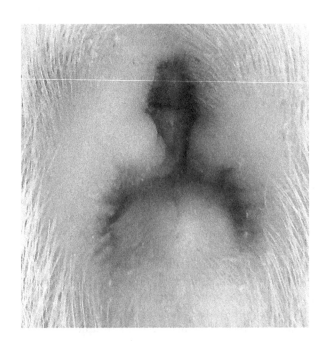

FIG. 5.7.   *Vaginal closure membrane in an anestrus guinea pig sow. During anestrus and pregnancy, the vaginal orifice is sealed with an epithelial membrane, which is unique to hystricomorph rodents. (Courtesy M. Hunrath)*

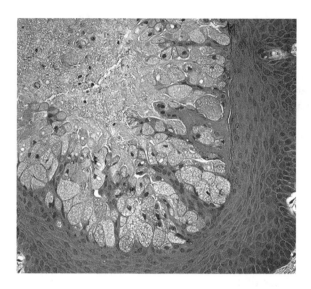

FIG. 5.8. *Vaginal mucosa of a normal guinea pig sow, illustrating mucinous metaplasia of stratified squamous epithelium.*

membrane ruptures when the vulva swells prior to parturition and during estrus. During pregnancy, the vaginal lumen fills with mucoid fluid produced by mucoid metaplasia (mucification) of the cornified epithelium (Fig. 5.8). This occurs in other rodents, but is particularly pronounced in guinea pigs. The guinea pig uterus is bicornuate, with a very short uterine body and a single cervical os. Placentation is discoidal and hemomonochorial. Its structure has favored its study as a model of human placentation. Placentation includes a subplacenta, which is unique to hystricomorph rodents. It is an extension of the chorion into the floor of the central placenta on the maternal side of the main placenta and is separated from the main placenta by a band of fetal mesenchyme.

Musculoskeletal System

The pubic symphysis generally remains fibrocartilaginous throughout life, but may completely ossify in older boars. Preparturient sows elaborate the peptide hormone relaxin, which is produced by the corpus luteum and placenta. This allows relaxation of the pubic ligament, which features leukocytic infiltration, degradation of collagen, and angiogenesis, resulting in increased weight and length of the ligament (Fig. 5.9). This allows passage of the exceptionally large and precocious fetuses. This process is less efficient in older sows, whose pubic symphyses tend to become partially ossified.

BIBLIOGRAPHY FOR BEHAVIORAL, PHYSIOLOGIC, AND ANATOMIC FEATURES

Hargaden, M. & Singer, L. (2012) Guinea pigs: anatomy, physiology, and behavior. In: *The Laboratory Rabbit, Guinea Pig, Hamster, and Other Rodents* (eds. M.A. Suckow, K.A. Stevens, & R.P. Wilson), pp. 575–602. Academic Press, London.

Lymphoid and Hematopoeitic Systems
Christensen, H.E., Wanstrup, J., & Ranlov, P. (1970) The cytology of the Foa-Kurloff reticular cells of the guinea pig. *Acta Pathologica et Microbiologica Scandinavica* (Suppl.) 212:15–24.

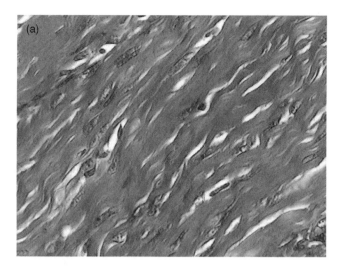

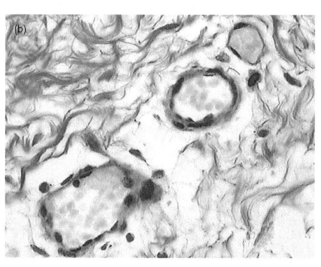

FIG. 5.9. *Pubic ligament of a nonpregnant guinea pig sow (a) compared to the pubic ligament of a preparturient sow (b). Note the diminished collagen, mild leukocytic infiltration, and prominent vascularity in the preparturient ligament, which allow relaxation of the pubic symphysis during parturition. (Source: © 2003 Rodríguez et al; licensee BioMed Central Ltd. This is an Open Access article: verbatim copying and redistribution of this article are permitted in all media for any purpose, provided this notice is preserved along with the article's original URL.)*

Debout, C., Birebent, B. Griveau, A.M., & Izard, J. (1993) In vitro cytotoxic effect of guinea pig natural killer cells (Kurloff cells) on homologous leukemic cells (L2C). *Leukemia* 7:733–735.

Debout, C., Quillec, M., & Izard, J. (1999) New data on the cytolytic effects of natural killer cells (Kurloff cells) on a leukemic cell line (guinea pig L2C). *Leukemia Research* 23:137–147.

Jara, L.F., Sanchez, J.M., Alvarado, H., & Nassar-Montoya, F. (2005) Kurloff cells in peripheral blood and organs of wild capybaras. *Journal of Wildlife Diseases* 41:431–434.

Ledingham, J.C.G. (1940) Sex hormones and the Foa-Kurloff cell. *Journal of Pathology and Bacteriology* 50:201–219.

Pouliot, N., Maghni, K., Blanchette, F., Cironi, L., Sirois, P., Stankova, J., & Rola-Pleszczynski, M. (1996) Natural killer and lectin-dependent cytotoxic activities of Kurloff cells: target cell selectivity, conjugate formation, and Ca++ dependency. *Inflammation* 20:647–671.

Revell, P.A., Vernon-Roberts, B., & Gray, A. (1971) The distribution and ultrastructure of the Kurloff cell in the guinea pig. *Journal of Anatomy* 109:187–199.

Respiratory System
Baskerville, A., Dowsett, A.B., & Baskerville, M. (1982) Ultrastructural studies of chronic pneumonia in guinea pigs. *Laboratory Animals* 16:351–355.
Best, P.V. & Heath, D. (1961) Interpretation of the appearances of the small pulmonary blood vessels in animals. *Circulation Research* 9:288–294.
Innes, J.R.M., Yevich, P.P., & Donati, E.J. (1956) Note on the origin of some fragments of bone in the lungs of laboratory animals. *Archives of Pathology* 61:401–406.
Knowles, J.F. (1984) Bone in the irradiated lung of the guinea pig. *Journal of Comparative Pathology* 94:529–533.
Kramer, A.W. & Marks, L.S. (1965) The occurrence of cardiac muscle in the pulmonary veins of rodents. *Journal of Morphology* 117:135–150.
Thompson, S.W., Hunt, R.D., Fox, M.A., & Davis, C.L. (1962) Perivascular nodules of lymphoid cells in the lungs of normal guinea pigs. *American Journal of Pathology* 40:507–517.

Gastrointestinal System
Sakaguchi, E., Itoh, H., Uchida, S., & Horigome, T. (1987) Comparison of fibre digestion and digesta retention time between rabbits, guinea pigs, and hamsters. *British Journal of Nutrition* 58:149–158.
Snipes, R.L. (1982) Anatomy of the guinea-pig cecum. *Anatomy and Embryology (Berlin)* 165:97–111.

Reproductive System
Davies, J., Dempsey, E.W., & MAmoroso, E.C. (1961) The subplacenta of the guinea pig: development, histology and histochemistry. *Journal of Anatomy (London)* 95:457–473.
Iburg, T.M., Arnbjerg, J., & Ruelokke, M.L. (2013) Gender differences in the anatomy of the perineal glands in guinea pigs and the effect of castration. *Anatomy, Histology, and Embryology* 42:65–71.
Meyer, R.K. & Allen, W.M. (1933) The production of mucified cells in the vaginal epithelium of certain rodents by oestrin and by corpus luteum extracts. *Anatomical Record* 56:321–343.
Miglino, M.A., Carter, A.M., dos Santos Ferraz, R.H., & Fernandes Machado, M.R. (2002) Placentation in the capybara (*Hydrochaerus hydrochaeris*), agouti (*Dasyprocta aguti*) and pace (*Agouti paca*). *Placenta* 23:416–428.
Stockard, C.R. & Papanicolaou, G.N. (1919) The vaginal closure membrane, copulation, and the vaginal plug in the guinea-pig, with further considerations of the oestrus rhythm. *Biological Bulletin* 37:222–245.
Weir, B.J. (1975) Reproductive characteristics of hystricomorph rodents. *Symposium of the Zoological Society of London* 34:265–301.

Musculoskeletal System
Rodriguez, H.A., Ortega, H.H., Ramos, J.G., Munoz-de-Toro, M., & Luque, E.H. (2003) Guinea-pig interpubic joint (symphysis pubica) relaxation at parturition: underlying cellular processes that resemble an inflammatory response. *Reproductive Biology and Endocrinology* 1:113.

VIRAL INFECTIONS

DNA Viral Infections
Guinea Pig Adenovirus Infection
Outbreaks of respiratory disease attributed to guinea pig adenovirus (GPAdV-1) have been recognized in Europe, North America, and Australia, and probably occur elsewhere in the world. The disease is characterized by low morbidity, but the mortality rate in clinically affected animals may reach 100%. In those cases described to date, animals have often been subjected to experimental manipulations that may have resulted in impairment of the immune response. GPAdV infections in colonies of guinea pigs are probably more prevalent than generally recognized. Clinical disease appears to occur primarily in young animals. Typical lesions have been observed in the airways of clinically normal young adults, emphasizing that subclinical infections do occur.

Pathology
Consolidation of the cranial lobes of the lung and hilus is a characteristic finding at necropsy. Microscopic changes are those of a necrotizing bronchitis and bronchiolitis, with desquamation of lining epithelial cells and leukocytic infiltration, mononuclear cells predominating. Some airways may be obliterated by cell debris, leukocytes, and fibrinous exudate. Numerous necrotic foci may be scattered throughout the lung. The nuclei of affected epithelial cells often contain round to oval basophilic inclusion bodies 7–15 μm in diameter (Fig. 5.10). The virus has not been recovered and characterized to date, but electron microscopic examination has revealed typical adenovirus particles in affected nuclei. Using homogenates of lung prepared from a spontaneous case of the disease, typical lesions have been produced in intranasally inoculated newborn guinea pigs. The incubation period was 5–10 days. Older inoculated animals were relatively refractory to the disease.

Diagnosis
The presence of necrotizing bronchitis and bronchiolitis in young guinea pigs with characteristic intranuclear basophilic inclusion bodies is consistent with adenoviral

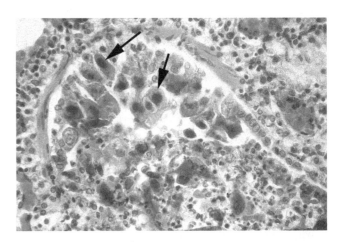

FIG. 5.10. *Lung from a natural case of adenoviral bronchoalveolitis in a young guinea pig. Note the prominent intranuclear inclusion bodies (arrows) in the exfoliating bronchial epithelial cells and peribronchial leukocyte infiltration.*

pneumonitis. The diagnosis may be confirmed by immunocytochemistry, serology, PCR, or the demonstration of adenoviral particles in affected cells by electron microscopy. In the past, mouse adenovirus was utilized as a heterotypic antigen for serologic testing of GPAdV, but was relatively insensitive. Recently, a homotypic antigen has been engineered using the GPAdV hexon gene incorporated into replication defective adenovirus vector. This assay has proven to be more specific and sensitive. Differential diagnoses include parainfluenza virus infections, cytomegalovirus infections, and bacterial infections of the lower respiratory tract, such as *Bordetella bronchiseptica*.

Guinea Pig Cytomegalovirus Infection

Members of the cytomegalovirus group are species-specific viruses of the family Herpesviridae. Guinea pig cytomegalovirus (GPCMV), also known as Caviid herpesvirus 2, is quite common among conventionally housed guinea pigs, and salivary gland lesions are typically discovered as incidental findings. Guinea pigs housed under conventional conditions seroconvert to GPCMV by a few months of age.

GPCMV is transmitted by exposure to infected saliva or urine or as a transplacental infection. The latter feature has prompted interest in GPCMV as a model of congenital CMV infection. Infection may persist as an inapparent or latent infection for years. Systemic disease, with associated lesions, has been produced in weanling guinea pigs inoculated subcutaneously with GPCMV. In the experimental disease, focal lesions with intranuclear inclusion bodies were present in salivary gland, liver, spleen, lung, and kidney. Pregnant guinea pigs developed more extensive visceral lesions when inoculated with GPCMV than did nonpregnant animals. Lymphoproliferative disease, with mononucleosis-like syndrome and lymphadenopathy, has been observed in guinea pigs following experimental inoculation with GPCMV. Infection of neonatal guinea pigs resulted in growth retardation, thymic involution due to depletion of T-lymphocytes, splenomegaly due to lymphoproliferation, and immunosuppression. However, naturally occurring GPCMV infections rarely cause detectable clinical disease in the guinea pig, a pattern similar to that observed in human CMV infections. There is 1 report of systemic CMV infection with visceral lesions in 2 young guinea pigs introduced into a conventional facility. Focal destructive lesions with large intranuclear and cytoplasmic inclusion bodies were observed in various tissues including spleen, liver, kidney, and lung. Pregnancy can precipitate acute generalized infection in sows. Both natural and experimental infections have been shown to cause abortion, stillbirth, and neonatal mortality.

Pathology

Lesions are usually confined to the ductal epithelial cells of the salivary glands. Large eosinophilic inclusion

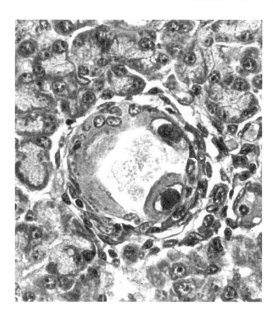

FIG. 5.11. *Submandibular salivary gland from an adult guinea pig with cytomegalovirus infection. Note the karyomegaly and large intranuclear inclusion bodies, with margination of nuclear chromatin in cells lining a duct. (Source: G.D. Hsiung.)*

bodies are associated with marked karyomegaly and margination of the nuclear chromatin in affected cells (Fig. 5.11). Intracytoplasmic inclusions are occasionally present in ductal epithelial cells. There may be a concurrent mononuclear cell infiltration around infected ducts. In the acute systemic form of the disease, interstitial pneumonitis with multifocal areas of necrosis in the lymph nodes, spleen, liver, kidney, lung, and other viscera are typical findings. Intranuclear and intracytoplasmic inclusion bodies may be present in affected foci. Congenital infection can be associated with encephalitis and labyrinthitis, features that have attracted interest in GPCMV as a model of human disease.

Other Guinea Pig Herpes Viral Infections

Guinea pig "herpes-like virus" (GPHLV, Caviid herpesvirus 1) is a lymphotropic virus that was isolated from degenerating primary kidney cell cultures prepared from strain 2 guinea pigs, but to date GPHLV has not been shown to be capable of producing natural disease in guinea pigs. Guinea pig "X virus" (GPXV, Caviid herpesvirus 3) was originally isolated from the leukocytes of strain 2 guinea pigs. Based on serologic studies and DNA analyses, GPXV is different from either GPHLV or GPCMV. Following experimental inoculation of GPXV into Hartley guinea pigs, focal hepatic necrosis and mortality was observed. GPHLV and GPXV do not appear to be important primary pathogens in the guinea pig. However, they represent a possible complicating factor, should either occur as an inapparent infection in guinea pigs under experiment in the laboratory.

Equine Herpesvirus 1 Infection

Neurologic signs, abortions, and stillbirths were observed in guinea pigs housed in a European zoo in association with an Equine herpesvirus 1 outbreak. The outbreak involved a variety of other species, some of which were cohoused in the same building as the guinea pigs. Nonsuppurative meningoencephalitis, neuronal and glial necrosis, gliosis, and intranuclear inclusions were observed.

Poxvirus Infection

There is a single report of 8-month-old guinea pigs within a colony that developed markedly swollen thighs due to fibrovascular proliferation. The tissue was grown in culture, and poxvirus-like structures were observed by electron microscopy. Anecdotal information among guinea pig fanciers in the United Kingdom has suggested that a poxvirus may be associated with cheilitis, but this has not been documented in the scientific literature.

RNA Viral Infections
Arenavirus Infection: Lymphocytic Choriomeningitis Virus Infection

Lymphocytic choriomeningitis virus (LCMV) infection is relatively rare in guinea pigs, but it does represent an infection that can complicate research projects and is of public health significance. Lesions observed in guinea pigs with LCMV infection have included lymphocytic infiltrates in the meninges, choroid plexi, ependyma, liver, adrenals, and lungs. There is a wide host range, including wild mice. Exposure may occur by inhalation or ingestion, and apparently in guinea pigs through the intact skin. Confirmation requires the demonstration of viral antigen in affected tissues, serology, and/or PCR. LCMV infection has been shown to prolong the life of guinea pigs prone to L2C leukemia, which emphasizes the potential for the virus to be an important complicating factor in certain types of research. Several species, including humans, are susceptible to LCMV infection.

Coronavirus-Like Infection

A syndrome characterized by wasting, anorexia, and diarrhea has been observed in young guinea pigs following their arrival at a research facility. The disease was characterized by low morbidity and mortality. Affected animals had an acute to subacute necrotizing enteritis involving primarily the distal ileum, with copious amounts of mucoid material present throughout the gastrointestinal tract. On microscopic examination, lesions were particularly prominent in the terminal small intestine. There was blunting and fusion of affected villi, with necrosis and sloughing of enterocytes from the tips of villi and formation of epithelia syncytia in the intestinal mucosa. Viral particles consistent with the morphology of a coronavirus were demonstrated in fecal samples examined by electron microscopy. In another study, clinically normal guinea pigs of different ages were observed to shed coronavirus-like particles in the feces for long periods of time. The importance of suspected coronavirus infections in this species is currently unknown. However, until additional information is available, it should be considered in the differential diagnoses in cases of enteritis and/or wasting in young guinea pigs.

Influenza Virus Infection

Influenza viruses belong to the family Orthomyxoviridae, and are divided into 3 antigenic types: A, B, and C. Guinea pigs are experimentally susceptible to unadapted human influenza A and B viruses, and readily transmit infection among one another under both direct and indirect contact conditions. Experimentally induced lesions tend to be mild, consisting of rhinitis, tracheitis, bronchitis, and alveolitis. A serosurvey performed among farmed guinea pigs in Ecuador revealed a high prevalence of seroconversion to both influenza A and B viruses. Although naturally occurring clinical disease has not been reported, guinea pigs appear to be susceptible to natural infection with influenza viruses.

Parainfluenza Virus Infections

The family Paramyxoviridae contains a number of viruses that infect guinea pigs, including multiple members of the subfamily Paramyxovirinae: murine parainfluenza virus-1 (Sendai virus), parainfluenza virus-2 (Simian virus-5, SV-5), human parainfluenza virus-3 (PIV-3), guinea pig parainfluenza virus-3 (GpPIV-3), Caviid parainfluenza virus-3 (CavPIV-3), and 1 member of the subfamily Pneumovirinae: Pneumonia Virus of Mice (PVM). Much of the documentation on these infections in guinea pigs is based upon natural seroconversion, but antigens are notably cross-reactive among these viruses. None of these agents are known to cause natural clinical disease in guinea pigs. Sendai virus, SV-5, and PIV-3 have all been isolated from naturally infected guinea pigs.

Based on serologic surveys, PIV-3 antibodies are relatively common in colonies of guinea pigs. Newborn animals born to PIV-3-positive sows acquire protection via maternal immunity during the first 2 weeks of life, then usually become transiently infected (based upon seroconversion) anywhere from 2 to 8 weeks of age. Two isolates of PIV-3 (GpPIV-3 and CavPIV-3) have been isolated from subclinically infected guinea pigs, genetically sequenced, and are closely related to human and bovine PIV-3s, as well as to each other. It is unclear if these viruses are of human origin. Experimental inoculation of guinea pigs with CavPIV-3 resulted in seroconversion, but there is no clinical or histological evidence of the disease. In guinea pigs inoculated experimentally with human PIV-3, animals developed a transient interstitial pneumonia and alveolitis, with pulmonary congestion and hemorrhage. Residual lesions persisted for up to 50 days. In addition to interstitial alveolitis, documented changes have included increased histamine release from basophils, and decreased phagocytic activity of heterophils. Guinea pigs infected with human PIV-3 have been used to study mechanisms of virus-induced asthma and airway hyperactivity.

Picornavirus Infection

Antibodies to murine encephalomyelitis virus (MEV) are occasionally observed when guinea pigs are tested for this virus. Weight loss and paresis have been noted in guinea pigs that were seropositive to MEV, and meningoencephalitis was observed. Clinical disease in seropositive pet guinea pigs was also attributed to MEV infection, although the animals recovered following treatment with vitamin C. The significance of seroconversion to MEV in this species has not been resolved.

Rabies Virus Infection

A single case of raccoon-variant rabies virus infection has been documented in a pet guinea pig, requiring post-exposure treatment of humans.

Other Viral Infections

Serology studies indicate that guinea pigs will seroconvert to reovirus 3.

Endogenized Viruses

Guinea pigs have an endogenous retrovirus known as guinea pig retrovirus (GPRV). GPRV has also been called guinea pig C-type virus, but it is morphologically similar to murine B-type viruses. It is serologically distinct from mouse, rat, and hamster retroviruses. Expression has been observed in cells and tissues of L2C leukemic guinea pigs and cultured cells and cell lines from other guinea pig strains. Although it is claimed to be oncogenic, its association with leukemia is coincidental and efforts to induce leukemia with GPRV have failed. Like other mammals, the genome of hystricomorph species contains a conserved endogenous retroviral syncytin-like *env-Cav1*, which is expressed at the level of the placental invasive trophoblast junctional zone. In addition to endogenous retrovirus integration, the guinea pig genome contains a number of incomplete RNA and DNA viral sequence integrations, including bornavirus-, parvovirus-, and filovirus-related sequences. None of these elements have clinical significance.

BIBLIOGRAPHY FOR VIRAL INFECTIONS

General References for Viral Infections
Brabb, T., Newsome, D., Burich, A., & Hanes, M. (2012) Infectious diseases. In: *The Laboratory Rabbit, Guinea Pig, Hamster, and Other Rodents* (eds. M.A. Suckow, K.A. Stevens, & R. P. Wilson), pp. 637–683. Elsevier, London.
Van Hoosier, G.L., Jr. & Robinette, L.R. (1976) Viral and chlamydial diseases. In: *The Biology of the Guinea Pig* (eds. J.E. Wagner& P.J. Manning), pp. 137–152. Academic Press, New York.

DNA Viral Infections

Guinea Pig Adenovirus Infection
Brennecke, L.H., Dreier, T.M., & Stokes, W.W. (1983) Naturally occurring virus-associated respiratory disease in two guinea pigs. *Veterinary Pathology* 20:488–491.
Butz, N., Ossent, P., & Homberger, F.R. (1999) Pathogenesis of guinea pig adenovirus infection. *Laboratory Animal Science* 49:600–604.
Crippa, L., Giusti, A.M., Sironi, G., Cavaletti, E., & Scanziani, E. (1997) Asymptomatic adenoviral respiratory tract infection in guinea pigs. *Laboratory Animal Science* 47:197–199.
Feldman, S.H., Richardson, J.A., & Chubb, F.J., Jr. (1990) Necrotizing viral bronchopneumonia in guinea pigs. *Laboratory Animal Science* 40:82–83.
Feldman, S.H., Sikes, R.A., & Eckhoff, G.A. (2001) Comparison of the deduced amino acid sequence of guinea pig adenovirus hexon protein with that of other mastadenoviruses. *Comparative Medicine* 51:120–126.
Finnie, J.W., Noonan, D.E., & Swift, J.G. (1999) Adenovirus pneumonia in guinea pigs. *Australian Veterinary Journal* 77:191–192.
Kaup, F.-J., Naumann, S., Kunstyr, I., & Drommer, W. (1984) Experimental viral pneumonia in guinea pigs: an ultrastructural study. *Veterinary Pathology* 21:521–527.
Kunstyr, I., Maess, J., Naumann, S., Kaup, F.-J., Kraft, V., & Knocke, K.W. (1984) Adenovirus pneumonia in guinea pigs: an experimental reproduction of the disease. *Laboratory Animals* 18:55–60.
Naumann, S., Kunstyr, I,. Langer, I., Maess, J., & Horning, R. (1981) Lethal pneumonia in guinea pigs associated with a virus. *Laboratory Animals* 15:235–242.
Pring-Akerblom, P., Blazek, K., Schramlova, J., & Kunstyr, I. (1997) Polymerase chain reaction for detection of guinea pig adenovirus. *Journal of Veterinary Diagnostic Investigation* 9:232–236.

Guinea Pig Cytomegalovirus Infection
Bia, F.J., Hastings, K., & Hsiung, G.D. (1979) Cytomegalovirus infection in guinea pigs. III. Persistent viruria, blood transmission, and viral interference. *Journal of Infectious Diseases* 140:914–920.
Connor, W.S. & Johnson, K.P. (1976) Cytomegalovirus infection in weanling guinea pigs. *Journal of Infectious Diseases* 134:442–449.
Cook, J.E. (1958) Salivary gland virus disease of guinea pigs. *Journal of the National Cancer Institute* 20:905–909.
Fong, C.K., Lucia, H., Bia, F.J., & Hsiung, G.D. (1983) Histopathologic and ultrastructural studies of disseminated cytomegalovirus infection in strain 2 guinea pigs. *Laboratory Investigation* 49:183–194.
Griffith, B.P. & Hsiung, G.D. (1980) Cytomegalovirus infection in guinea pigs. IV. Maternal infection at different stages of gestation. *Journal of Infectious Diseases* 141:787–793.
Griffith, B.P., Lucia, H.L., Bia, F.J., & Hsiung, G.D. (1981) Cytomegalovirus-induced mononucleosis in guinea pigs. *Infection and Immunity* 32:857–863.
Griffith, B.P., Lucia, H.L., & Hsiung, G.D. (1982) Brain and visceral involvement during cytomegalovirus infection of guinea pigs. *Pediatric Research* 16:455–459.
Griffith, B.P., Lucia, H.L., Tillbrook, J.L., & Hsiung, G.D. (1983) Enhancement of cytomegalovirus infection during pregnancy in guinea pigs. *Journal of Infectious Diseases* 147:990–998.
Johnson, K.P. & Connor, W.S. (1979) Guinea pig cytomegalovirus: transplacental transmission. *Archives of Virology* 59:263–267.
Lucia, H.L., Griffith, H.L., & Hsiung, G.D. (1985) Lymphadenopathy during cytomegalovirus-induced mononucleosis in guinea pigs. *Archives of Pathology and Laboratory Medicine* 109:1019–1023.
Motzel, S.L. & Wagner, J.E. (1989) Diagnostic exercise: fetal death in guinea pigs. *Laboratory Animal Science* 39:342–344.

Schleiss, MR., Bourne, N., Bravo, F.J., Jensen, N.J., & Berstein, D.I. (2003) Quantitative-competitive PCR monitoring of viral load following experimental guinea pig cytomegalovirus infection. *Journal of Virological Methods* 108:103–110.

Van Hoosier, G.L., Jr., Giddens, W.E., Jr., Gillett, C.S., & Davis, H. (1985) Disseminated cytomegalovirus in the guinea pig. *Laboratory Animal Science* 35:81–84.

Zheng, Z.M,. Lavallee, J.T., Bia, F.J., & Griffith, B.P. (1987) Thymic hypoplasia, splenomegaly and immune depression in guinea pigs with neonatal cytomegalovirus infection. *Developmental and Comparative Immunology* 11:407–418.

Other Guinea Pig Herpesviral Infections

Bhatt, P.N., Percy, D.H., Craft, J.L., & Jonas, A.M. (1971) Isolation and characterization of a herpes-like (Hsiung–Kaplow) virus from guinea pigs. *Journal of Infectious Diseases* 123:178–189.

Bia, F.J., Summers, W.C., Fong, C.K., & Hsiung, G.D. (1980) New endogenous herpesvirus of guinea pigs: biological and molecular characterization. *Journal of Virology* 36:245–253.

Dowler, K.W., McCormick, S., Armstrong, J.A., & Hsiung, G.D. (1984) Lymphoproliferative changes induced by infection with lymphotropic herpes virus of guinea pigs. *Journal of Infectious Diseases* 150:105–111.

Hsiung, G.D., Bia, F.J., & Fong, C.K.Y. (1980) Viruses of guinea pigs: considerations for biomedical research. *Microbiological Reviews* 44:468–490.

Nayak, D.P. (1971) Isolation and characterization of a herpesvirus from leukemic guinea pigs. *Journal of Virology* 8:579–588.

Equine Herpesvirus 1 Infection

Wohlstein, P., Lehmbecker, A., Spitzbarth, I., Algermissen, D., Baumgartner, W., Boer, M., Kummrow, M., Haas, L., & Grummer, B. (2011) Fatal epizootic equine herpesvirus 1 infections in new and unnatural hosts. *Veterinary Microbiology* 149:456–460.

Poxvirus Infection

Hampton, E.G., Bruce, M., & Jackson, F.L. (1968) Virus-like particles in a fibrovascular growth in guinea pigs. *Journal of General Virology* 2:205–206.

RNA Viral Infections

Lymphocytic Choriomeningitis Virus Infection

Hotchin, J. (1971) The contamination of laboratory animals with lymphocytic choriomeningitis virus. *American Journal of Pathology* 64:747–769.

Jungeblut, C.W. & Kodza, H. (1962) Interference between lymphocytic choriomeningitis virus and the leukemia transmitting agent of leukemia L2C in guinea pigs. *Arch Gesamte Virusforsch* 12:522–560.

Shaughnessy, H.J. & Zichis, J. (1940) Infection of guinea pigs by application of virus of lymphocytic choriomeningitis to their normal skins. *Journal of Experimental Medicine* 72:331–343.

Coronavirus-Like Infection

Jaax, G.P., Jaax, N.K., Petrali, J.P., Corcoran, K.D., & Vogel, A.P. (1990) Coronavirus-like virions associated with a wasting syndrome in guinea pigs. *Laboratory Animal Science* 40:375–378.

Marshall, J.A. & Doultree, J.C. (1996) Chronic excretion of coronavirus-like particles in laboratory guinea pigs. *Laboratory Animal Science* 46:104–106.

Influenza Virus Infection

Aziykat-Dupuis, E., Lambre, C.R., Soler, P., Moreau, J., & Thibon, M. (1984) Lung alterations in guinea pigs infected with influenza virus. *Journal of Comparative Pathology* 94:273–283.

Leyva-Grado, V., Mubareka, S., Krammer, F., Cardenas, W.B., & Palese, P. (2012) Influenza virus infection in guinea pigs raised as livestock, Ecuador. *Emerging Infectious Diseases* 18:1135–1138.

Lowen, A.C., Mubareka, S., Tumpey, T.M., Garcia-Sastre, A., & Palese, P. (2006) The guinea pig as a transmission model for human influenza viruses. *Proceedings of the National Academy of Science of the United States of America* 103:9988–9992.

Pica, N., Chou, Y.Y., Bouvier, N.M., & Palese, P. (2012) Transmission of influenza B viruses in the guinea pig. *Journal of Virology* 86:4279–4287.

Parainfluenza Virus Infection

Blomqvist, G.A., Martin, K., & Morein, B. (2002) Transmission of parainfluenza 3 in guinea pig breeding herds. *Contemporary Topics in Laboratory Animal Science* 41:53–57.

Ohsawa, K., Yamada, A., Takeuchi, K., Watanabe, Y., Miyata, H., & Sato, H. (1998) Genetic characterization of parainfluenza virus 3 from guinea pigs. *Journal of Veterinary Medical Science* 60:919–922.

Porter, W.P. & Kudlacz, E.M. (1992) Effects of parainfluenza virus infection in guinea pigs. *Laboratory Animals* 21:45–49.

Simmons, J.H., Purdy, G.A., Franklin, C.L., Trottier, P., Churchill, A.E., Russell, R.J., Besch-Williford, C.L., & Riley, L.K. (2002) Characterization of a novel parainfluenza virus, cavid parainfluenza virus 3, from laboratory guinea pigs (*Cavia prcellus*). *Comparative Medicine* 52:548–554.

Watanabe, Y., Sato, H., Miyata, H., & Ohsawa, K. (2001) Isolation of parainfluenza virus type 3-like agent from guinea pigs. *Acta Medica Nagasaki* 46:15–18.

Picornavirus Infection

Hansen, A.K., Thomsen, P., & Jensen, H.J. (1997) A serological indication of the existence of a guinea pig poliovirus. *Laboratory Animals* 31:212–218.

Rabies Virus Infection

Eidson, M., Matthews, S.D., Willsey, A.L., Cherry, B., Rudd, R.J., & Timarchi, C.V. (2005) Rabies virus infection in a pet guinea pig and seven pet rabbits. *Journal of the American Veterinary Medical Association* 227:932–935.

Endogenized Viruses

Belyi, V.A., Levine, A.J., & Skalka, A.M. (2010) Unexpected inheritance: multiple integrations of ancient bornavirus and Ebolavirus/Marburgvirus sequences in vertebrate genomes. *PLoS Pathogens* 6:e1001030.

Horie, M. & Tomonaga, K. (2011) Non-retroviral fossils in vertebrate genomes. *Viruses* 3:1836–1848.

Hsiung, G.D., Bia, F.J., & Fong, K.Y. (1980) Viruses of guinea pigs: considerations for biomedical research. *Microbiological Reviews* 44:468–490.

Vernochet, C., Heidmann, O., Dupressoir, A., Cornelis, G., Dessen, P., Catzeflis, F., & Heidman, T. (2011) A syncytin-like endogenous retrovirus envelope gene of the guinea pig specifically expressed in the placenta junctional zone and conserved in Caviomorpha. *Placenta* 32:885–892.

BACTERIAL INFECTIONS

Bordetella bronchiseptica Infection

Bordetella bronchiseptica is a major pathogen in guinea pigs of all ages. However, disease and mortality occur most often in young guinea pigs, particularly during winter. In some outbreaks, there may be other identifiable manipulations or environmental factors that appear to precipitate disease. Guinea pigs may harbor the organism in the upper respiratory tract and trachea as an inapparent infection. In enzootically infected colonies, the prevalence of nasal shedders may be relatively high. Infection rates are usually highest in the winter months. Most animals appear to develop solid immunity and eventually eliminate the organism, but a small percentage may remain carriers. The organism is readily transmitted as an airborne infection. It has an affinity for ciliated respiratory epithelium and has been shown to cause ciliostasis in other species. During epizootics of bordetellosis, pregnant sows may die, abort, or produce stillborn offspring. Commercial and autogenous bacterins have been used to reduce the incidence of disease. However, it is unlikely that immunization will eliminate the carrier state.

Pathology

The external nares, nasal passages, and trachea frequently contain mucopurulent or catarrhal exudate. Consolidated areas of the lung vary from dark red to gray, are cranioventral in distribution, and may involve entire lobes or individual lobules (Fig. 5.12). Mucopurulent exudate is present in affected airways, pleuritis occasionally occurs, and purulent exudate may be present in the tympanic bullae. Histologically, there is an acute to chronic suppurative bronchopneumonia, with marked infiltration by heterophils in airways and alveoli, with obliteration of the normal architecture (Fig. 5.13). *Bordetella* has also been isolated from a case of pyosalpinx in the guinea pig.

Diagnosis

The organism can usually be readily recovered on blood agar cultures from the respiratory tract, affected tympanic bullae, and in cases of metritis, the uterus. Differential diagnoses include acute *Streptococcus pneumoniae*, *Klebsiella* spp., or *Staphylococcus aureus* infections, as well as a systemic *Streptococcus equi* subsp. *zooepidemicus* infection.

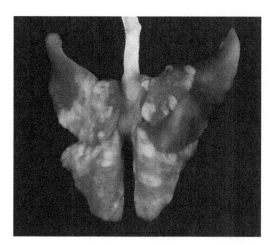

FIG. 5.12. *Cranioventral bronchopneumonia in a juvenile guinea pig with acute* Bordetella bronchiseptica *infection.*

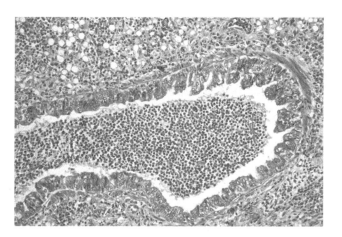

FIG. 5.13. *Chronic suppurative bronchitis associated with* Bordetella bronchiseptica *infection in an adult guinea pig.*

Brachyspira spp. Infection: Intestinal Spirochetosis

Intestinal spirochetosis due to infection with *Brachyspira* spp. (formerly *Serpulina*) has been observed on multiple occasions in guinea pigs. In 1 report that appeared to involve *Brachyspira* spp. as the primary pathogen, affected guinea pigs experienced rectal prolapse, sudden death, and diarrhea. Infection spread rapidly within the affected population. Subclinical infection was also observed. Gross findings typically included distention of the cecum and colon, and less commonly duodenum, with greenish-yellow or hemorrhagic liquid and mucus. Histopathology revealed hyperemia, variable necrosis, and mixed leukocyte infiltration in the cecal mucosa with diffuse colonization of cecal and proximal colonic surface mucosa with filamentous bacteria, typical of *Brachyspira*. Colonization of the duodenum was found in 1 guinea pig. Other reports observed *Brachyspira* in association with Tyzzer's disease. *Brachyspira* organisms densely populate end-on to the brush border of intestinal enterocytes, with displacement and reduction of microvilli. Diagnosis can be achieved by observation of the typical morphology and location of organisms or culture. Although the species of *Brachyspira* has not been identified in guinea pigs, PCR using porcine *Brachyspira pilosicoli* 16S ribosomal sequences is effective for confirming diagnosis in guinea pigs.

Brucella spp. Infection: Brucellosis

Guinea pigs are susceptible to *Brucella* spp. infection, and have been used as models of brucellosis, but natural cases are rare, since infection requires contamination of feed with animal by-products. Nevertheless, a few infections with *Brucella abortus*, *Brucella melitensis*, and *Brucella suis* have been observed in guinea pigs. In 1 report, a male guinea pig from a commercial vendor had testicular and joint swelling, and a female had abscesses of the liver and pancreas.

Campylobacter spp. Infection

Pregnant guinea pigs have been used to test the aborto-facient capacity of human and animal *Campylobacter* isolates, and experimentally infected guinea pigs have been reported to develop diarrhea. Naturally occurring subclinical infection with *Campylobacter jejuni* has been documented in laboratory guinea pigs.

Chlamydophila caviae Infection: Guinea Pig Inclusion Body Conjunctivitis

Chlamydophila caviae is relatively widespread in conventional colonies and pet guinea pigs. In enzootically infected colonies, clinical signs are absent, although the organism may be demonstrable in conjunctival smears. Guinea pigs 4–8 weeks of age are most frequently infected with the organism in such herds, and most adults are likely to be seropositive under these circumstances. Young seronegative animals, when introduced into a colony that is enzootically infected with *C. caviae*, may then develop the typical clinical disease.

Transmission is primarily by direct contact. In addition to conjunctival lesions, rhinitis and urogenital tract infections may occur. Abortions and lower respiratory tract disease have been attributed to the organism, although lung lesions may be complicated by concurrent *Streptococcus* or *Bordetella* infections. Sows with genital infections can transmit *C. caviae* to their offspring and infected boars can sexually transmit the organism to sows.

Pathology

The conjunctiva become reddened and swollen (Fig. 5.14), with serous to purulent exudate. Conjunctival smears stained with the Giemsa method will reveal sloughed epithelial cells containing intracytoplasmic inclusions (Fig. 5.15) with a scattering of heterophils and lymphocytes. Genital infections in sows involve the cervix, with minimal inflammation, and oviducts, which may develop salpingitis. Inclusions are

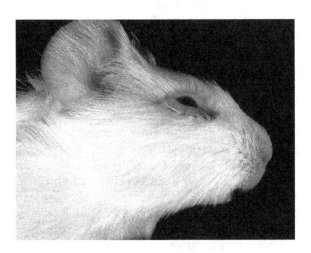

FIG. 5.14. *Guinea pig with acute Chlamydial conjunctivitis and swelling of the eyelids.*

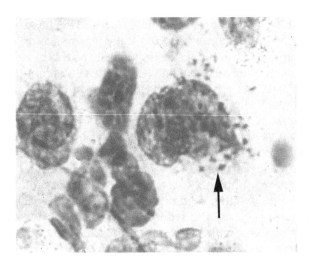

FIG. 5.15. *Conjunctival swab from a case of Chlamydial conjunctivitis. Note the intracytoplasmic inclusions (arrow).*

diagnostic, but may be difficult to demonstrate, particularly if preparations are smudged or there are numerous bacteria in the smear. The demonstration of antigen in conjunctival or cervical smears by immuno-histochemistry using specific antibody or PCR analysis are more sensitive and reliable methods. Serology has been used to detect antibody to the organism. Bacterial culture of conjunctival swabs is recommended in an effort to differentiate guinea pig inclusion body conjunctivitis from other bacterial conjunctivitides. Possible transmission of *C. caviae* to a human contact has been reported, and rabbits and other species have been found to be infected with *C. caviae*.

Citrobacter freundii Infection

On occasion, *C. freundii* has been associated with septicemia in guinea pigs. An epizootic of *C. freundii* septicemia with high mortality has been reported in guinea pigs. Pneumonia, pleuritis, and enteritis were observed, and *C. freundii* was isolated from lung, liver, spleen, and intestine at necropsy. No predisposing factors or possible sources of the infection were identified. *Citrobacter* spp. and *C. freundii* have also been isolated from various lesions in hysterectomy-derived, barrier-maintained guinea pigs.

Clostridium difficile and *Clostridium perfringens* Enterotoxemia: "Antibiotic Toxicity," Enterotoxemia

Guinea pigs are susceptible to *C. difficile* and *C. perfringens* typhlocolitis as a consequence of enteric dysbiosis, as well as Tyzzer's disease caused by *Clostridium piliforme*. *Clostridium difficile* is often associated with a syndrome known as "antibiotic toxicity," in which antibiotics perturb normal microflora, allowing overgrowth of toxin-producing Clostridia.

Following treatment of guinea pigs with certain antibiotics, up to 50% or more may develop a profuse diarrhea, with high mortality within 1–5 days. In guinea pigs, Gram-positive organisms such as streptococci and lactobacilli predominate in the small and large intestine. However, when a narrow-spectrum antibiotic with antibacterial activity against Gram-positive bacteria, such as penicillin, bacitracin, or ampicillin, is administered per os or parenterally, striking changes occur in the gut flora. Antibiotics such as ampicillin and penicillin are excreted, at least in part, in the bile, which explains their profound effects on the bacterial flora of the gut, even after parenteral administration. Following the administration of a single intramuscular dose of 50,000 units of penicillin, there was an estimated 100-fold decrease in cultivable Gram-positive bacteria within 12 hours, followed by up to a 10,000,000-fold increase in Gram-negative bacteria. A high incidence of bacteremia due to *Escherichia coli* has also been observed in treated animals. In addition, clostridial overgrowth also occurs. Following treatment with penicillin or ampicillin, large numbers of *C. difficile* have been recovered from animals with diarrhea, and *C. difficile* enterotoxin has been demonstrated in the intestinal contents following treatment with penicillin. This organism is normally not present in intestinal contents of guinea pigs. Antibiotic treatment causes sufficient disruption of the gut flora (dysbiosis) to permit the proliferation of a pathogenic organism not normally recoverable from this species. The problem can be prevented by treating with broader spectrum antibiotics.

Although antibiotic treatment is the most common precipitating factor in dysbiosis leading to clostridial enterotoxemia, *C. difficile* has also been found to cause enterotoxemia in the absence of such treatment, and enterotoxemia has also been found to be associated with *C. perfringens*, type A. Regardless of precipitating factors (antibiotic, nutritional, other stressors) of dysbiosis, the pathogenesis of enterotoxemia is the same: overgrowth of toxin-producing Clostridia. *Clostridium perfringens* has been isolated from cases of enterotoxemia in ex-germ-free guinea pigs that had incompletely stabilized gut microflora.

Pathology

The cecum is often atonic and dilated with fluid and gaseous content. The cecal mucosa is edematous and frequently hemorrhagic (Fig. 5.16). Microscopically, there may be necrosis or mucosal hyperplasia with mononuclear cell infiltration in the lamina propria of the terminal ileum. In the cecum, there is degeneration and sloughing of enterocytes, edema of the lamina propria, and leukocytic infiltration. Focal hepatic and splenic infarction has been associated with acute infection with *C. perfringens* type A.

Diagnosis

A history of recent antibiotic treatment or other causes of dysbiosis and the typical gross and microscopic changes

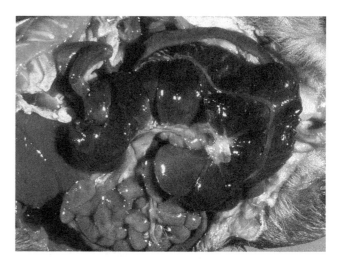

FIG. 5.16. *Acute typhlitis in a guinea pig following treatment with narrow-spectrum antibiotic treatment. The cecum is hemorrhagic and distended with liquid digesta and gas.*

should provide an accurate provisional diagnosis. Bacteriology and assay of cecal contents for clostridial toxins are recommended. Differential diagnoses include Tyzzer's disease, acute coccidiosis, cryptosporidiosis, viral enteritides, and bacterial enteritides.

Clostridium piliforme Infection: Tyzzer's Disease

Guinea pigs, like all of the other species covered in this book, are susceptible to Tyzzer's disease caused by *C. piliforme*. Although in other species Tyzzer's disease typically involves intestine, liver, and heart, some reported cases in young guinea pigs have found lesions that were confined to the intestinal tract. In young guinea pigs inoculated orally with *C. piliforme*, lesions were observed in the ileum, large intestine, and liver by 4 days post-inoculation. Bacilli were demonstrated in the gut lesions at 4–10 days and in the liver at 8–10 days postinoculation. Vertical transmission has been reported to occur in a hysterectomy-derived, gnotobiotically reared guinea pig. Necrotizing ileitis and typhlitis, frequently with transmural involvement, are typical findings in cavian Tyzzer's disease. Hepatic lesions, when present, are characterized by focal coagulation necrosis in periportal regions, with variable heterophil infiltration. Fascicles of intracellular bacilli are best demonstrated by the Warthin–Starry or Giemsa stains. *Brachyspira* sp. has been found in association with *C. piliforme* infections in guinea pigs in some outbreaks of Tyzzer's disease.

Corynebacterium spp. Infection

Corynebacteria appear to be a part of the normal flora of guinea pigs, but have also been occasionally associated with diseases, including *Corynebacterium pyogenes* septicemia in a guinea pig, and pulmonary infection by *Corynebacterium kutscheri* in a guinea pig during an epizootic of streptococcal disease. In addition,

Corynebacterium renale was a common isolate from urine or bladder in guinea pigs with urinary calculi.

Escherichia coli Infection: Colibacillosis

As in rabbits, *E. coli* is not normally present in the gut of healthy guinea pigs, but has been associated with enteritis and septicemia in poorly managed colonies. Infection may be fatal, particularly in weanling animals. Necropsy findings included intestinal distention with fluid and gas, peritoneal exudation, splenomegaly, and multifocal hepatitis. Pure cultures of *E. coli* were obtained from blood, peritoneal fluid, and other organs. This bacterium has also been isolated from cases of mastitis and cystitis. *Escherichia coli* septicemia has also been found in association with clostridial enterotoxemia.

Klebsiella pneumoniae Infection

Epizootics of acute infections due to *K. pneumoniae* have been reported on rare occasions. Patterns of disease vary from acute septicemia to acute necrotizing bronchopneumonia, with pleuritis, pericarditis, peritonitis, and splenic hyperplasia. *Klebsiella oxytoca* and *K. pneumoniae* have been isolated from miscellaneous inflammatory lesions in guinea pigs, including mastitis.

Lawsonia intracellularis Infection: Adenomatous Intestinal Hyperplasia

Multiple species of animals, including guinea pigs, are susceptible to *L. intracellularis* enteric disease, which has previously been attributed to intracellular *Campylobacter*-like organisms. Grossly visible segmental thickening with microscopic evidence of epithelial hyperplasia of the duodenum was observed in a guinea pig on steroid treatment. Cagemates of the index case had acute enteritis without hyperplasia, but all had typical intracytoplasmic *Lawsonia*-like organisms in small intestinal mucosal epithelium. An outbreak of diarrhea among 2 adults and 5 juvenile guinea pigs with weight loss, diarrhea, and mortality was also reported in Japan. Grossly, the jejunal and ileal mucosa was thickened and rugose. Histopathology revealed mucosal hyperplasia with intracellular organisms that were interpreted to be *Campylobacter* (*Lawsonia*). Organisms were observed in immature crypt epithelial cells by electron microscopy. The changes observed were similar to those seen in *Lawsonia*-associated enteritis in hamsters and rabbits. Warthin–Starry silver staining of tissue sections are diagnostic, revealing a typical distribution of intracellular *L. intracellularis* within the apical cytoplasm of infected enterocytes (see Hamster Chapter 3, "Fig. 3.16" and Rabbit Chapter 6, "Fig. 6.39").

Leptospira spp. Infection: Leptospirosis

There are approximately 20 species of saprophytic and pathogenic *Leptospira*, among which *Leptospira interrogans* is the most common pathogenic species that infects animals and humans. Within this species are approximately 200 serovars, names of which are often used as

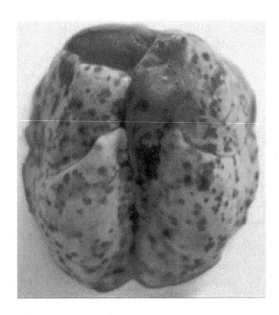

FIG. 5.17. *Multifocal pulmonary hemorrhages in a guinea pig with disseminated leptospirosis. (Source: Reprinted from Zhang, Y., et al. BMC Infectious Diseases. Zhang, Y., Lou, X.-L., Yang, H.-L., Guo, X.-Y., He, P. & Jiang, X.-C. (2012) Establishment of a leptospirosis model in guinea pigs using an epicutaneous inoculations route. BMC Infectious Diseases 12:20.)*

species names, such as *Leptospira pomona* and *Leptospira icterohemorrhagica*. The guinea pig is commonly used as a model of leptospirosis, but natural infection is rare. Wild cavies (*C. aperea*) were found to have a high prevalence of *L. pomona* infection in association with infected cattle in Argentina. Natural infection among domestic guinea pigs, presumably through exposure to wild rats, has also been documented in Europe. Affected animals were jaundiced with disseminated hemorrhages. Mucous membranes and skin are the primary modes of entry, and guinea pigs have been shown to be readily susceptible to infection through abraded skin. Regardless of the route of infection, there is a rapid bacteremia resulting in disseminated infection, with multifocal hemorrhages in the skin, lungs (Fig. 5.17), serosa, kidneys, and perirenal tissue (Fig. 5.18). Microscopic lesions, in addition to hemorrhage and edema, include focal hepatic necrosis, and renal tubular necrosis with hematuria. Bacteria with typical spirochetal morphology can be visualized in tissues with silver stains and immunohistochemistry, and confirmation can be achieved by culture or PCR.

Listeria monocytogenes Infection: Listeriosis

Guinea pigs are used as a model of maternal-fetal listeriosis because of the similarity of their placentation to that of humans. Experimental oral infection of pregnant guinea pigs has been shown to result in abortion and stillbirth as well as focal hepatic lesions, with isolation of organisms from placenta and variably from fetuses. Naturally occurring listeriosis is a rare entity in guinea pigs, but when it does occur, it has been shown to be manifest as conjunctivitis or multisystemic disease. An outbreak with up to

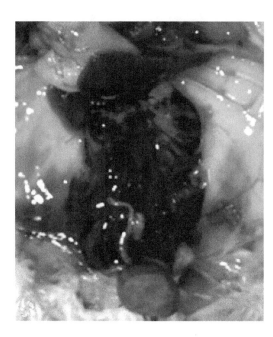

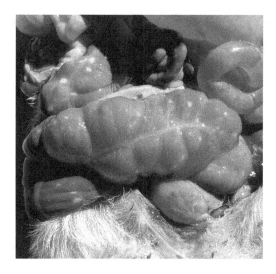

FIG. 5.19. *Natural case of listeriosis in a guinea pig. Note multifocal white nodules on the cecal wall. (Source: D. Driemeier.)*

FIG. 5.18. *Acute perirenal hemorrhage in a guinea pig with leptospirosis. (Source: Reprinted from Zhang, Y., et al. BMC Infectious Diseases. Zhang, Y., Lou, X.-L., Yang, H.-L., Guo, X.-Y., He, P. & Jiang, X.-C. (2012) Establishment of a leptospirosis model in guinea pigs using an epicutaneous inoculations route. BMC Infectious Diseases 12:20.)*

80–100% mortality has been documented following feeding of contaminated cabbage. The intestine appears to be an important site for *Listeria* colonization. Experimental studies have shown that following oral inoculation, *L. monocytogenes* rapidly colonized the liver, with a second wave of dissemination to the mesenteric lymph nodes. Intestinal mucosa was found to be a niche for bacterial replication, with shedding into the intestinal lumen, reinfection of Peyer's patches, and trafficking of infected immune cells to the liver and mesenteric lymph nodes.

Pathology
In a natural outbreak, guinea pigs had grossly visible multifocal white nodules up to 2–4 mm in the cecum (Fig. 5.19) and liver (Fig. 5.20), with smaller foci in the stomach, small intestine, mesenteric lymph node, spleen, and uterus. Focal myocarditis has also been observed following experimental infection. Microscopically, lesions in various organs consisted of focal necrosis with mixed leukocytic infiltration and numerous Gram-positive bacteria. Some of the guinea pigs had suppurative bronchopneumonia. Another report described conjunctivitis in a group of hairless guinea pigs, without systemic dissemination.

Diagnosis
Definitive diagnosis is best achieved by culture. Isolation of *Listeria* is enhanced when tissues to be cultured are held at 4°C for several days before inoculating culture plates. PCR methods have also been used for rapid diagnosis. Differential diagnoses include agents causing disseminated hepatic and enteric foci, including *Clostridium piliforme*, *Salmonella* spp., or *Yersinia pseudotuberculosis*.

Mycobacterium spp. Infection: Tuberculosis
Although guinea pigs are highly susceptible to tuberculosis experimentally, natural disease is rare. Natural infections with both *Mycobacterium tuberculosis* and *Mycobacterium bovis* have been observed in guinea pigs, presumably incurred through human exposure. Lesions included enlarged bronchial lymph nodes with central caseation, as well as disseminated tubercles in lung, spleen, liver, and other lymph nodes (cervical, portal, inguinal, and prescapular). Most lesions featured caseation necrosis and stained positive for acid-fast bacilli.

Mycoplasma spp. and *Acholeplasma* spp. Infections
A number of cell wall-deficient bacteria, known as mollicutes, infect cells of the respiratory and urogenital tracts of guinea pigs. Their taxonomy is in flux, as

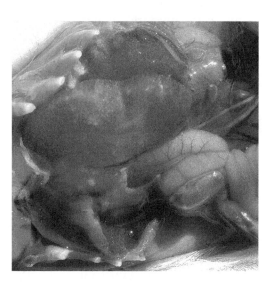

FIG. 5.20. *Natural case of listeriosis in a guinea pig. Note the multifocal hepatic nodules. (Courtesy D. Driemeier.)*

they do not appear to be a phylogenetically coherent group. Guinea pig isolates include *Mycoplasma caviae*, *Mycoplasma cavipharyngis*, *Mycoplasma pulmonis*, *Acholeplasma granularum*, *Acholeplasma laidlawii*, and *Acholeplasma cavigenitalium*. Although some have been recovered coincidentally from diseased tissue, their pathogenicity is questionable.

Pasteurella multocida Infection: Pasteurellosis

Disease associated with *P. multocida* is rare in guinea pigs. It has been reported to cause sporadic mortality in a colony of guinea pigs, with fibrinopurulent pneumonia, pleuritis, pericarditis, peritonitis, and conjunctivitis. Disease manifestations resembled those of *S. pneumoniae*.

Pseudomonas and *Aeromonas* Infection

In a single report, pulmonary botryomycosis in 2 guinea pigs was attributed to *Pseudomonas aeruginosa* infection. Sulfur granules were present within the focal suppurative pulmonary lesions. An outbreak of septicemic disease in which *Aeromonas* (formerly *Pseudomonas*) *caviae* was isolated has been documented, and Koch's postulates were fulfilled with this isolate.

Salmonella spp. Infection: Salmonellosis

Salmonellosis in guinea pigs was once very common, but is now rare among laboratory guinea pigs due to current standards of husbandry and hygiene. It continues to be a threat to pet guinea pigs that are fed contaminated greens. There are 2 major species of *Salmonella*—*Salmonella enterica* and *Salmonella bongeri*—and numerous serotypes. *Salmonella enterica* serotype Typhimurium and *S. enterica* serotype Enteritidis are the most common isolates from guinea pigs, but a number of other serotypes have been documented to infect guinea pigs. Outbreaks of salmonellosis spread rapidly within a population. Guinea pigs of all ages and strains are susceptible, but young weanlings and sows around farrowing time are particularly at risk. Inapparent carriers may occur. Recovered animals may shed the organism intermittently in the feces. Ingestion of contaminated feces or feed is considered to be the usual source of infection, but the conjunctiva has been shown to be an important portal of entry as well.

Aside from the dangers of interspecies spread, the zoonotic potential must be emphasized. A recent outbreak of salmonellosis occurred in the United States among humans consuming contaminated guinea pig meat. Strict hygienic measures and the culling of all contact animals have been used to eliminate the organism from an infected colony.

Pathology

Clinical signs include depression, conjunctivitis, abortions, and sudden death in young guinea pigs. Diarrhea is often not experienced. A mortality rate of 50% is common, but has been known to reach 100%. Gross lesions include pinpoint to several millimeter diameter pale foci on the liver and spleen. Mesenteric lymph nodes may be enlarged and splenomegaly frequently occurs. Necrotic miliary foci may also be present in other viscera, including lung, pleura, peritoneum, and uterus. Lesions may be absent in peracute cases. Histopathologic lesions feature multifocal granulomatous hepatitis, splenitis, and lymphadenitis, with infiltration by histiocytic cells and heterophils. Focal suppurative lesions may also occur in lymphoid tissues of the intestinal tract.

Diagnosis

Culture of the organism from heart blood, spleen, and feces is best accomplished with media selective for *Salmonella*. In the absence of bacteriology, the characteristic paratyphoid nodules seen in organs such as liver and spleen are useful morphologic criteria. Differential diagnoses include *C. piliforme*, *S. pneumoniae*, *Yersinia enterocolitica*, and *L. monocytogenes*.

Staphylococcus aureus Infections: Staphylococcosis

Staphylococcus aureus is largely an opportunistic pathogen in guinea pigs. Guinea pigs are known to have a high prevalence of subclinical nasal colonization with *S. aureus*, which also readily contaminates the animals' environment. Guinea pigs have been found to be carriers of the same phage types as their human handlers. Diseases that are related to *S. aureus* include pododermatitis, exfoliative dermatitis, pneumonia, mastitis, and conjunctivitis.

Pododermatitis

Pododermatitis (bumble foot) is frequently associated with coagulase-positive *S. aureus* infections in a number of species, including guinea pigs. Predisposing factors include trauma due to defective or rusty cage wire, and poor sanitation. The plantar surfaces of the forefeet typically are swollen, painful, and encrusted with necrotic tissue and clotted blood. In some advanced cases, amyloid deposition has been observed in the spleen, liver, adrenals, and islets.

Staphylococcal Dermatitis: Exfoliative Dermatitis

Staphylococcal dermatitis (exfoliative dermatitis) has been observed in guinea pigs infected with coagulase-positive *S. aureus*, characterized by alopecia and erythema in the ventral abdominal region, with exfoliation of the epidermis. There was an age-related variation in mortality that was negligible in adults and relatively high in young animals, particularly those born to affected dams. Skin lesions usually regressed in survivors within 2 weeks, with subsequent new hair growth. At necropsy, there was erythema and hair loss, with dull red scabs and cracks in the epidermis, particularly along the ventral abdomen and the medial aspect of the extremities. On microscopic examination, there was marked epidermal cleavage, with parakeratotic hyperkeratosis and minimal inflammatory response. *Staphylococcus aureus* was isolated from the lesions in the majority of affected animals, and the disease was reproduced in young guinea pigs inoculated with *S. aureus* isolated from an affected animal. The organism was also isolated from the upper respiratory tract and pharynx of many of the affected animals and from clinically normal guinea pigs. Abrasions of the skin may have been an important predisposing factor, resulting in colonization and invasion of the epidermis. This condition was reported to occur most frequently in strain 13 guinea pigs.

Streptobacillus moniliformis Infection

Streptobacillus moniliformis, the agent of rat bite fever, has been isolated from a few cases of cervical lymphadenitis, abscesses, and from a young guinea pig with pyogranulomatous bronchopneumonia. Suppurative lesions contained caseous to creamy exudate and were similar to those associated with streptococcal infections.

Streptococcal Infections

A number of different *Streptococcus* spp. are important pathogens in guinea pigs, particularly *S. equi* subsp. *zooepidemicus*, and *S. pneumoniae*. In addition, *Streptococcus pyogenes* has been reported as a pathogen in guinea pigs. *Streptococcus* spp. are termed alpha-hemolytic when grown on blood agar and colonies turn the underlying agar dark or greenish, as is the case with *S. pneumoniae*. When termed beta-hemolytic, the colonies completely lyse the surrounding agar, as is the case with *S. equi*, *Streptococcus equisimilis*, and *S. pyogenes*. Furthermore, beta-hemolytic streptococci are differentiated by their cell wall carbohydrate antigens into Lancefield groups. Guinea pigs are known to be infected with Lancefield group A (*S. pyogenes*) and group C (*S. equi*, *S. equisimilis*) streptococci.

Streptococcus equi *subsp.* Zooepidemicus Infections: Cervical Lymphadenitis, Septicemia

The lay term for this infection is "lumps," since this organism commonly causes cervical lymphadenitis. The organism may be carried in the nasopharynx and conjunctiva as an inapparent infection. Sows have been shown to be more susceptible to disease than males, and there is a strain-related variation in susceptibility. Steroid treatment does not appear to increase susceptibility to the disease. Lymphadenitis has been produced consistently in guinea pigs inoculated sublingually with *S. equi* subsp. *zooepidemicus*. The usual route of invasion appears to be via abrasions in the oral mucosa, but inhalation, skin abrasions, and invasion of the genital tract at farrowing are other possible portals of entry. The disease has also been produced in young guinea pigs by inoculation of the intact nasal and conjunctival mucous membranes. Following penetration of the oral mucosa and invasion of the underlying tissue, the organism is likely transported to the draining cervical lymph nodes via the lymphatics. The pyogenic organisms then proliferate, producing a chronic suppurative inflammatory process.

Pathology

Affected adults usually have lesions confined to the regional lymph nodes. In the localized form of the disease, there is bilateral enlargement of the cervical lymph nodes. The nodes are freely movable, firm to soft, and frequently nonfluctuant, and they contain thick purulent exudate (Fig. 5.21). Localized abscessation involving other sites such as mesenteric lymph nodes is an infrequent finding. Retroorbital abscessation, accompanied by exophthalmus, is another possible manifestation of the disease. Otitis media may also occur. Occasionally, there is an acute systemic form of the disease, particularly in younger animals. In this case, fibrinopurulent bronchopneumonia, pleuritis, and pericarditis may be present at necropsy. On rare occasions, arthritis and abortions have been attributed to *S. equi* subsp. *zooepidemicus* infections. Microscopically, changes present in the cervical lymph nodes are those of a chronic suppurative lymphadenitis with central necrosis, peripheral fibrosis, and marked infiltration with heterophils. In the acute systemic form, fibrinopurulent pericarditis, focal myocardial degeneration, focal hepatitis, and acute lymphadenitis may be evident on histologic examination.

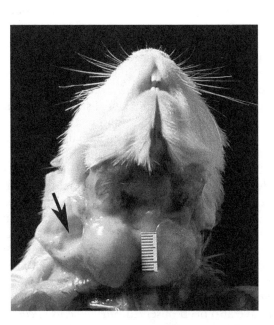

FIG. 5.21. *Bilateral suppurative cervical lymphadenitis in a guinea pig infected with* Streptococcus equi *subsp.* zooepidemicus. *Note the purulent exudate (arrow) in the incised lymph node.*

Diagnosis

The typical beta-hemolytic streptococci can usually be recovered from affected tissues, except in some cases of chronic lymphadenitis of some duration. Differential diagnoses in the acute systemic form of the disease include *S. pneumoniae*, *S. pyogenes*, and acute *B. bronchiseptica* infection. Cervical lymphadenopathy must also be differentiated from lymphoma, which frequently involves the cervical lymph nodes.

Streptococcus pneumoniae *Infection: Diplococcal or Pneumococcal Infection*

Pneumococcus (aka diplococcus) infections can be an important cause of disease and mortality in enzootically infected guinea pig colonies. *Streptococcus pneumoniae* is a lancet-shaped, Gram-positive encapsulated coccus that occurs in pairs and short chains. Capsular polysaccharide type 19 is most frequently isolated from guinea pigs. Type 4 has also been identified. Serotypes isolated from guinea pigs are identical to human isolates. The possibility of interspecies transmission is, therefore, feasible, but not proven.

Pneumococcal infections have been recognized to occur in guinea pigs for decades. In enzootically infected colonies, up to 50% of the animals may be subclinical carriers, with colonization of the upper respiratory tract. Transmission is primarily by aerosols. Epizootics occur most often during winter months, and younger animals and pregnant sows are particularly at risk. Other predisposing factors include changes in environmental temperature, poor husbandry, experimental procedures, and inadequate nutrition. During epizootics, high mortality, abortions, and stillbirths may occur. The organisms do not produce toxins but are protected from phagocytosis primarily through their abundant polysaccharide capsules. Many pneumococci can activate the alternate complement pathway; thus complement activation may be the important stimulus for the early tissue changes.

Pathology

Clinical signs are varied, including listlessness, nasal and ocular discharge, torticollis, dyspnea, abortions, and stillbirth. At necropsy, lesions include upper respiratory exudation, otitis media, fibrinopurulent pleuritis, pericarditis, peritonitis (Fig. 5.22), and marked consolidation of affected lobes of lung. Microscopic changes are those of an acute bronchopneumonia with fibrinous exudation and polymorphonuclear cell infiltration. Thrombosis of pulmonary vessels may occur in acute cases. Infiltrating cells may be elongated and fusiform, forming pallisading patterns within affected airways and alveoli. Splenitis, fibrinopurulent meningitis, metritis, focal hepatic necrosis, lymphadenitis, and ovarian abscessation have also been observed. *Streptococcus pneumoniae*-associated suppurative arthritis and osteomyelitis have also been reported to occur in guinea pigs with borderline vitamin C deficiency.

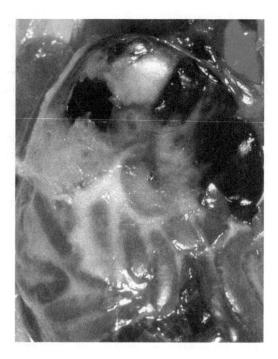

FIG. 5.22. *Acute fibrinopurulent peritonitis in a young guinea pig infected with* Streptococcus pneumoniae.

Diagnosis

Direct smears of Gram-stained inflammatory exudate should reveal the typical Gram-positive diplococci. Using blood agar or enrichment media, the organism should be recoverable from affected tissues (*S. pneumoniae* is more fastidious in growth requirements than are most other streptococci). Differential diagnoses include acute septicemia due to *S. equi* subsp. *zooepidemicus*, and acute *B. bronchiseptica* infections.

Streptococcus *spp. Infections: Hemorrhagic Septicemia*

Septicemic *S. pyogenes* infection has been reported to cause high mortality in a colony of adult, suckling, and weanling guinea pigs. The disease particularly involved adults. Animals were seen to bleed from the nose, mouth, and vagina. Necropsy revealed necrohemorrhagic and fibrinopurulent pneumonia with abscessation, hemopericardium, hemothorax, petechiation of heart and kidneys, and suppurative metritis. Culture of lung and other organs yielded *S. pyogenes*. A nearly identical syndrome, which also featured gastrointestinal hemorrhages, was associated with a beta-hemolytic group C streptococcus. The authors suggested that the organism was related to *S. equisimilis*. Differential diagnoses for disseminated hemorrhagic lesions include leptospirosis and hypovitaminosis C.

Yersinia pseudotuberculosis *Infection: Pseudotuberculosis, Yersiniosis*

Spontaneous outbreaks of disease and mortality due to *Y. pseudotuberculosis* are relatively rare. Inapparent carriers may occur. In the acute form of the disease, miliary, cream-colored nodules are present in the intestinal wall and liver

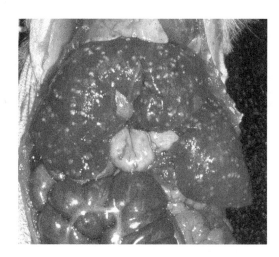

FIG. 5.23. Yersinia pseudotuberculosis *infection. Note the multiple pale nodules in the wall of the cecum and throughout the liver. (Source: D. Agnew, Michigan State University, East Lansing, Michigan. Reproduced with permission from D. Agnew.)*

(Fig. 5.23), with enteritis and mucosal ulceration, particularly in the terminal ileum and cecum. Pulmonary involvement may result in acute pneumonia. In the subacute and chronic forms of the disease, miliary to caseous lesions may be present in mesenteric lymph nodes, spleen, liver, and lung. Recovery and identification of the organism are necessary to confirm the diagnosis. Infection arises through contamination of feed (especially greens) by infected wild birds and rodents.

Miscellaneous Bacterial Syndromes
Otitis Media
Middle ear infections frequently go undetected clinically in the guinea pig. Careful examination of the tympanic bullae should be performed as a routine procedure at necropsy in order to detect subclinical cases. The otosclerosis associated with chronic middle ear infection may be detected antemortem by radiographic examination. Otitis media appears to be more common in colonies harboring pathogens in their upper respiratory tract. Organisms isolated from these cases include *S. pneumoniae*, *S. equi* subsp. *zooepidemicus*, *B. bronchiseptica*, and *P. aeruginosa*, among others.

Bacterial Mastitis
Mastitis occurs sporadically in colonies of guinea pigs, particularly in sows during early lactation. Cases are usually sporadic and are not particularly contagious. The offspring may be unaffected. Affected glands are red to purple, enlarged, firm, congested, and edematous on the cut surface. In sows with acute mastitis, lesions are characterized microscopically by mild degeneration to necrosis of ductal epithelium, with marked heterophil infiltration in ducts and alveoli, with a scattering of inflammatory cells in the interstitium. In chronic cases, there may be marked interstitial fibrosis, with

mononuclear cell infiltration and obliteration of the normal architecture in severely affected areas. In 1 study, bacteria most frequently isolated (in decreasing order of frequency) were *E. coli*, *K. pneumoniae*, and *S. equi* subsp. *zooepidemicus*.

Bacterial Conjunctivitis
Aside from *Chlamydophila*, organisms isolated from cases of bacterial conjunctivitis include *S. equi* subsp. *zooepidemicus*, *S. pneumonia*, *Salmonella* spp., *E. coli*, *S. aureus*, *P. multocida*, *Corynebacterium* spp., and *Actinobacillus* spp, among others. In addition to culture, conjunctival smears should always be examined to ensure that there is not a concurrent chlamydial infection.

BIBLIOGRAPHY FOR BACTERIAL INFECTIONS

General References
Boot, R. & Walvoort, H.C. (1986) Opportunistic infections in hysterectomy-derived, barrier-maintained guinea pigs. *Laboratory Animals* 20:51–56.

Brabb, T., Newsome, D., Burich, A., & Hanes, M. (2012) Infectious diseases. In: *The Laboratory Rabbit, Guinea Pig, Hamster, and Other Rodents* (eds. M. A. Suckow, K. A. Stevens, & R. P. Wilson), pp. 637–683. Elsievier, London.

Ganaway, J.R. (1976) Bacterial, mycoplasma, and rickettsial diseases. In: *The Biology of the Guinea Pig* (eds. J.E. Wagner& P.J. Manning), pp. 121–135. Academic Press, New York.

Harkness, J.E., Murray, K.A., & Wagner, J.E. (2002) Biology and diseases of guinea pigs. In: *Laboratory Animal Medicine* (eds. J.G. Fox, L.C. Anderson, F.M. Loew, & F.W. Quimby), pp. 203–246. Academic Press, New York.

Rigby, C. (1976) Natural infections of guinea-pigs. *Laboratory Animals* 10:119–142.

***Bordetella bronchiseptica* Infection**
Baskerville, M., Baskerville, A., & Wood, M. (1982) A study of chronic pneumonia in a guinea pig colony with enzootic *Bordetella bronchiseptica* infection. *Laboratory Animals* 16:290–296.

Bemis, D.A. & Wilson, S.A. (1985) Influence of potential virulence determinants on *Bordetella bronchiseptica*-induced ciliostasis. *Infection and Immunity* 50:35–42.

Ganaway, J.R., et al. (1965) Prevention of acute *Bordetella bronchiseptica* pneumonia in a guinea pig colony. *Laboratory Animal Care* 15:156–162.

Nakagawa, M., Muto, T., Yoda, H., Nakano, T., & Imaizumi, K. (1971) Experimental *Bordetella bronchiseptica* infection in guinea pigs. *Japanese Journal of Veterinary Science* 33:53–60.

Sinka, D.P. & Sleight, S.D. (1968) Bilateral pyosalpinx in guinea pig. *Journal of the American Veterinary Medical Association* 153:830–831.

Traham, C.J. (1987) Airborne-induced experimental *Bordetella bronchiseptica* pneumonia in strain 13 guinea pigs. *Laboratory Animals* 21:226–232.

Yoda, H., Nakagawa, M., Muto, T., & Imaizumi, K. (1972) Development of resistance to reinfection of *Bordetella bronchiseptica* in guinea pigs recovered from natural infection. *Japanese Journal of Veterinary Science* 34:191–196.

***Brachyspira* spp. Infection**
Helie, P. (2000) Intestinal spirochetosis in a guinea pig with colorectal prolapse. *Canadian Veterinary Journal* 41:134.

McLeod, C.G., Stookey, J.L., Harrington, D.G., & White, J.D. (1977) Intestinal Tyzzer's disease and spirochetosis in a guinea pig. *Veterinary Pathology* 14:229–235.

Muniappa, N., Mathiesen, M.R., & Duhamel, G.E. (1997) Laboratory identification and enteropathogenicity testing of *Serpulina pilisicoli* associated with porcine colonic spirochetosis. *Journal of Veterinary Diagnostic Investigation* 9:165–171.

Vanrobaeys, M., de Herdt, P., Ducatelle, R., Devriese, L.A., Charlier, G., & Haesebrouck, F. (1998) Typhlitis caused by intestinal *Sepulina*-like bacteria in domestic guinea pigs (*Cavia porcellus*). *Journal of Clinical Microbiology* 36:690–694.

Zwicker, G.M., Dagle, G.E., & Adee, R.R. (1978) Naturally occurring Tyzzer's disease and intestinal spirochetosis in guinea pigs. *Laboratory Animal Science* 28:193–198.

Campylobacter spp. Infection

Batza, H.J., Rubsamen, S., & Schliesser, T. (1983) Occurrence of *Campylobacter fetus* subsp. *jejuni* in mice and guinea pigs from experimental animal establishments. *Zentralblatt fur Veterinarmedizin B* 30:455–461.

Meanger, J.D. & Marshall, R.B. (1989) *Campylobacter jejuni* infection within a laboratory animal production unit. *Laboratory Animals* 23:126–132.

Chlamydophila caviae Infection

Barron, A.L., White, H.J., Rank, R.G., & Soloff, B.L. (1979) Target tissue associated with genital infection of female guinea pigs by the chlamydial agent of guinea pig inclusion conjunctivitis. *Journal of Infectious Diseases* 139:60–68.

Deeb, B.J., DiGiacomo, R.F., & Wang, S.P. (1989) Guinea pig inclusion conjunctivitis (GPIC) in a commercial colony. *Laboratory Animals* 23:103–106.

Lutz-Wohlgroth, L., Becker, A., Brugnera, E., Huat, Z.L., Zimmermann, D., Grimm, F., Haessig, M., Greub, G., Kaps, S., Spiess, B., Pospischil, A., & Vaughan, L. (2006) Chlamydiales in guinea pigs and their zoonotic potential. *Journal of Veterinary Medicine A: Physiology, Pathology and Clinical Medicine* 53:185–193.

Mount, D.T., Bigazzi, P.E., & Barron, A.L. (1972) Infection of genital tract and transmission of ocular infection to newborns by the agent of guinea pig inclusion conjunctivitis. *Infection and Immunity* 5:921–926.

Murray, E.S. (1964) Guinea pig inclusion conjunctivitis virus. I. Isolation and identification as a member of the psittacosis-lymphogranuloma-trachoma group. *Journal of Infectious Diseases* 114:1–12.

Pantchev, A., Sting, R., Bauerfeind, R., Tyczka, J., & Sachse, K. (2010) Detection of all *Chlamydophila* and *Chlamydia* spp. of veterinary interest using species-specific real-time PCR assays. *Comparative Immunology, Microbiology and Infectious Diseases* 33:473–484.

Strik, N.I., Alleman, A.R., & Wellehan, J.F. (2005) Conjunctival swab cytology from a guinea pig: It's elementary! *Veterinary Clinical Pathology* 34:169–171.

Citrobacter freundii Infection

Ocholi, R.A., Chima, J.C., Uche, E.M., & Oyetunde, I.L. (1988) An epizootic of *Citrobacter freundii* in a guinea pig colony: short communication. *Laboratory Animals* 22:335–336.

Clostridium difficile and *Clostridium perfringens* Enterotoxemia

Boot, R., Angulo, A.F., & Walvoort, H.C. (1989) *Clostridium difficile*-associated typhlitis in specific pathogen free guinea pigs in the absence of antimicrobial treatment. *Laboratory Animals* 23:203–207.

Eyssen, H., De Somer, P., & Van Dijck, P. 1957. Further studies on antibiotic toxicity of guinea pigs. *Antibiotics and Chemotherapy* 7:55–64.

Farrar, W.E. & Kent, T.H. (1965) Enteritis and coliform bacteremia in guinea pigs given penicillin. *American Journal of Pathology* 47:629–642.

Feldman, S.H., Songer, J.G., Bueschel, D., Weisbroth, S.P., & Weisbroth, S.H. (1997) Multifocal necrotizing enteritis with hepatic and splenic infarction associated with *Clostridium perfringens* type A in a guinea pig raised in a conventional environment. *Laboratory Animal Science* 47:540–544.

Keel, M.K. & Sanger, J.G. (2006) The comparative pathology of *Clostridium difficile*-associated disease. *Veterinary Pathology* 43:225–240.

Lowe, B.R., Fox, J.G., & Bartlett, J.G. (1980) *Clostridium difficile*-associated cecitis in guinea pigs exposed to penicillin. *American Journal of Veterinary Research* 41:1277–1279.

Maddon, D.L., Horton, R.E., & McCullough, N.B. (1970) Spontaneous infection in ex-germ-free guinea pigs due to *Clostridium perfringens*. *Laboratory Animal Care* 20:454–455.

Rehg, J. & Pakes, S.P. (1981) *Clostridium difficile* antitoxin neutralization and penicillin-associated colitis. *Laboratory Animal Science* 31:156–160.

Young, J.D., Hurst, W.J., White, W.J., & Lang, C.M. (1987) An evaluation of ampicillin pharmacokinetics and toxicity in guinea pigs. *Laboratory Animal Science* 37:652–656.

Clostridium piliforme Infection: Tyzzer's Disease

Boot, R. & Walvoort, H.C. (1984) Vertical transmission of *Bacillus piliformis* infection (Tyzzer's disease) in a guinea pig: case report. *Laboratory Animals* 18:195–199.

McLeod, C.G., Stookey, J.L., Harrington, D.G., & White, J.D. (1977) Intestinal Tyzzer's disease and spirochetosis in a guinea pig. *Veterinary Pathology* 14:229–235.

Waggie, K.S., Thornburg, L.P., Grove, K.J., & Wagner, J.E. (1987) Lesions of experimentally induced Tyzzer's disease in Syrian hamsters, guinea pigs, mice and rats. *Laboratory Animals* 21:155–160.

Zwicker, G.M., Dagle, G.E., & Adee, R.R. (1978) Naturally occurring Tyzzer's disease and spirochetosis in guinea pigs. *Laboratory Animal Science* 28:193–198.

Corynebacterium spp. Infection

Hawkins, M.G., Ruby, A.L., Drazenovich, T.L., & Westropp, J.L. (2009) Composition and characteristics of urinary calculi from guinea pigs. *Journal of the American Veterinary Medical Association* 234:214–220.

Klebsiella pneumoniae Infection

Branch, A. (1927) Spontaneous infections of guinea pigs. Pneumococcus, Friedlander bacillus and pseudotuberculosis (*Eberthella caviae*). *Journal of Infectious Diseases* 40:533–548.

Dennig, H.K. & Eidmann, E. (1960) Klebsielleninfektionen bein meerschweinchen. *Berliner Tierarztliche Wochensschrift* 73:273–274.

Perkins, R.G. (1901) Report of a laboratory epizootic among guinea pigs associated with gaseous emphysema of the liver, spleen and kidneys due to *Bacillus mucosus capsulatus*. *Journal of Experimental Medicine* 5:389–396.

Lawsonia intracellularis Infection

Elwell, M.R., Chapman, A.L., & Frenkel, J.K. (1981) Duodenal hyperplasia in a guinea pig. *Veterinary Pathology* 18:136–139.

Muto, T., Noguchi, Y., Suzuki, K., & Zaw, K.M. (1983) Adenomatous intestinal hyperplasia in guinea pigs associated with *Campylobacter*-like bacteria. *Japanese Journal of Medical Science and Biology* 36:337–342.

Leptospira spp. Infection

Blood, B.D., Szyfres, B., & Moya, V. (1963) Natural *Leptospira pomona* infection in the pampas cavy. *Public Health Reports* 78:537–542.

Mason, N. (1937) Leptospiral jaundice occurring naturally in guinea pigs. *Lancet* 232:564–565.

Zhang, Y., Lou, X.-L., Yang, H.-L., Guo, X.-Y., He, P., & Jiang, X.-C. (2012) Establishment of a leptospirosis model in guinea pigs using an epicutaneous inoculations route. *BMC Infectious Diseases* 12:20.

Listeria monocytogenes Infection

Chukwu, C.O., Ogo, N.I., Antiabong, J.F., Muhammad, M.J., Ogbonna, C.I., & Chukwukere, S.C. (2006) Epidemiological evidence of listeriosis in guinea pigs fed with cabbage (*Brassica oleracea*) in Nigeria. *Animal Production Research Advances* 2:248–252.

Colgin, L.M., Nielsen, R.E., Tucker, F.S., & Okerberg, C.V. (1995) Case report of listerial keratoconjunctivitis in hairless guinea pigs. *Laboratory Animal Science* 45:435–436.

Dustoor, M., Croft, W., Fulton, A., & Blazkovec, A. (1977) Bacteriological and histopathological evaluation of guinea pigs after infection with *Listeria monocytogenes. Infection and Immunity* 15:916–924.

Ferreira, H.H., Zlotowski, P., Watanabe, T.T.N., Gomes, D.C., Cardoso, M.R.I., & Driemeier, D. (2011) Natural infection by *Listeria monocytogenes* in guinea pigs (*Cavia porcellus*). *Ciencia Rural* 41:682–685.

Irvin, E.A., Williams, D., Voss, K.A., & Smith, M.A. (2008) *Listeria monocytogenes* infection in pregnant guinea pigs is associated with maternal liver necrosis, a decrease in maternal serum TNF-alpha concentrations, and an increase in placental apoptosis. *Reproductive Toxicology* 26:123–129.

Melton-Witt, J.A., Rafelski, S.M., Portnoy, D.A., & Bakardjiev, A.I. (2012) Oral infection with signature-tagged *Listeria monocytogenes* reveals organ-specific growth and dissemination routes in guinea pigs. *Infection and Immunity* 80:720–732.

Mycobacterium spp. Infection

Vink, H.H. (1955) Spontaneous tuberculosis in the guinea pig. *Antonie Van Leeuwenhoek* 21:446–448.

Mycoplasma spp. Infection

Hill, A.C. (1971) *Mycoplasma caviae,* a new species. *Journal of General Microbiology* 65:109–113.

Hill, A. (1971) The isolation of two further species of mycoplasma from guinea pigs. *Veterinary Record* 83:225.

Hill, A. (1984) *Mycoplasma cavipharyngis,* a new species isolated from the nasopharynx of guinea pigs. *Journal of General Microbiology* 130:3183–3188.

Hill, A.C. (1992) *Acholeplasma cavigenitalium* sp. nov., isolated from the vagina of guinea pigs. *International Journal of Systematic Bacteriology* 42:589–592.

Johansson, K.E., Tully, J.G., Bolske, G., & Pettersson, B. (1999) *Mycoplasma cavipharyngis* and *Mycoplasma fastidiosum,* the closest relatives to *Eperythrozoon* spp. and *Haemobartonella* spp. *FEMS Microbiology Letters* 174:321–326.

Juhr, N.C. & Obi, S. (1970) Uterusinfektionen beim Meerschweinchen. *Zeitschrift fur Versuchstierkunde* 12:383–387.

Stalheim, O.H. & Matthews, P.J. (1975) Mycoplasmosis in specific-pathogen-free and conventional guinea pigs. *Laboratory Animal Science* 25:70–73.

Pseudomonas spp. Infection

Bostrum, R.E., Huckins, J.G., Kroe, D.J., Lawson, N.S., Martin, J.E., Ferrell, J.F., & Whitney, R.A., Jr. (1969) A typical fatal pulmonary botryomycosis in two guinea pigs due to *Pseudomonas aeruginosa. Journal of the American Veterinary Medical Association* 115:1195–1199.

Salmonella spp. Infection

Iijima, O.T., Saito, M., Nakayama, K., Kobayashi, S., Matsuno, K., & Nakagawa, M. (1987) Epizootiological studies of *Salmonella typhimurium* infection in guinea pigs. *Jikken Dobutsu* 36:39–49.

Moore, B. (1957) Observations pointing to the conjunctiva as the portal of entry in *Salmonella* infection of guinea pigs. *Journal of Hygiene (London)* 55:414–433.

Nelson, J.B. & Smith, T. (1927) Studies on paratyphoid infection in guinea pigs: I. Report of a natural outbreak of paratyphoid in a guinea pig population. *Journal of Experimental Medicine* 45:353–363.

Olfert, E.D., Ward, G.E., & Stevenson, D. (1976) *Salmonella typhimurium* infection in guinea pigs: observations on monitoring and control. *Laboratory Animal Science* 26:78–80.

Onyekaba, C.O. (1983) Clinical salmonellosis in a guinea pig colony caused by a new *Salmonella* serotype *S. ochiogu. Laboratory Animals* 17:213–216.

Staphylococcus aureus Infection

Blackmore, D.K. & Francis, R.A. (1970) The apparent transmission of staphylococci of human origin to laboratory animals. *Journal of Comparative Pathology* 80:645–651.

Ishihara, C. (1980) An exfoliative skin disease in guinea pigs due to *Staphylococcus aureus. Laboratory Animal Science* 30:552–557.

Markham, N.P. & Markham, J.G. 1966. *Staphylococci* in man and animals: distribution and characteristics of strains. *Journal of Comparative Pathology* 76:49–56.

Taylor, J.L., Wagner, J.E., Owens, D.R., & Stuhlman, R.A. (1971) Chronic pododermatitis in guinea pigs: a case report. *Laboratory Animal Science* 21:944–945.

Streptobacillus moniliformis Infection

Aldred, P., Hill, A.C., & Young, C. (1974) The isolation of *Streptobacillus moniliformis* from cervical abscesses of guinea pigs. *Laboratory Animals* 8:275–277.

Kirchner, B.K., Lake, S.G., & Wightman, S.R. (1992) Isolation of *Streptobacillus moniliformis* from a guinea pig with granulomatous pneumonia. *Laboratory Animal Science* 42:519–521.

Streptococcus equi subsp. *zooepidemicus* Infection

Fraunfelter, F.C., Schmidt, R.E., Beattie, R.J., & Garner, F.M. (1971) Lancefield type C streptococcal infections in strain 2 guinea pigs. *Laboratory Animals* 5:1–13.

Mayora, J., Soave, O., & Doak, R. (1978) Prevention of cervical lymphadenitis in guinea pigs by vaccination. *Laboratory Animal Science* 28:686–690.

Murphy, J.C., Ackerman, J.I., Marini, R.P., & Fox, J.G. (1991) Cervical lymphadenitis in guinea pigs: infection via intact ocular and nasal mucosa by *Streptococcus zooepidemicus. Laboratory Animal Science* 41:251–254.

Olson, L.D., Schueler, R.L., Riley, G.M., & Morehouse, L.G. (1976) Experimental induction of cervical lymphadenitis in guinea pigs with group C *Streptococci. Laboratory Animals* 10:223–231.

Rae, V. (1936) Epizootic streptococcal myocarditis in guinea pigs. *Journal of Infectious Diseases* 59:236–241.

Streptococcus pneumoniae Infection

Branch, A. (1927) Spontaneous infection in guinea pigs: Pneumococcus, Friedlander bacillus and pseudotuberculosis. *Journal of Infectious Diseases* 40:533–548.

Homburger, F., Wilcox, C. Barnes, M.W., & Finland, M. (1945) An epizootic of *Pneumococcus* type 19 infections in guinea pigs. *Science* 102:449–450.

Keyhani, M. & Naghshineh, R. (1974) Spontaneous epizootic of pneumococcus infection in guinea pigs. *Laboratory Animals* 8:47–49.

Parker, G.A., Russel, R.J., & De Paoli, A. (1977) Extrapulmonary lesions of *Streptococcus pneumoniae* infection in guinea pigs. *Veterinary Pathology* 14:332–337.

Petrie, G.F. (1933) The pneumococcal disease of the guinea pig. *Veterinary Journal* 89:25–30.

Witt, W.M., Hubbard, G.B., & Fanton, J.W. (1988) *Streptococcus pneumoniae* arthritis and osteomyelitis with vitamin C deficiency in guinea pigs. *Laboratory Animal Science* 38:192–194.

Streptococcus spp. Infection

Adams, M.R., Hawkins, P., & Schrire, L. (1986) An unusual outbreak of a streptococcal infection in a colony of guinea pigs. *Animal Technology* 37:105–108.

Okewole, P.A., Odeyemi, P.S., Oladunmade, M.A., Ajagbonna, B.O., Onah, J., & Spencer, T. (1991) An outbreak of *Streptococcus pyogenes* infection associated with calcium oxalate urolithiasis in guinea pigs (*Cavia porcellus*). *Laboratory Animals* 25:184–186.

Yersinia enterocolitica Infection

Obwolo, M.J. (1977) The pathology of experimental yersiniosis in guinea pigs. *Journal of Comparative Pathology* 87:213–221.

Miscellaneous Bacterial Infection

Boot, R. & Walvoort, H.C. (1986) Otitis media in guinea pigs: pathology and bacteriology. *Laboratory Animals* 20:242–248.

Kinkler, R.J., Jr., Wagner, J.E., Doyle, R.E., & Owens, D.R. (1976) Bacterial mastitis in guinea pigs. *Laboratory Animal Science* 26:214–217.

Kohn, D.F. (1974) Bacterial otitis media in the guinea pig. *Laboratory Animals* 24:823–825.

Wagner, J.E., Owens, D.R., Kusewitt, D.F., & Corley, E.A. (1976) Otitis media in guinea pigs. *Laboratory Animal Science* 26:902–907.

FUNGAL INFECTIONS

Encephalitozoon cuniculi Infection: Microsporidiosis

Subclinical *E. cuniculi* infections have been recognized in the guinea pig. Multifocal nonsuppurative meningoencephalitis and interstitial nephritis occur. Lesions and diagnostic methods are similar to those seen in other species (see Rabbit Chapter 6, "*Encephalitozoon cuniculi* Infection"). Guinea pigs have also been found to be subclinical enteric carriers of *Enterocytozoon bienusi*, an opportunistic pathogen in immunosuppressed humans.

Pneumocystis spp. Infection: Pneumocystosis

Mortality among weanling athymic guinea pigs has been noted to be due to *Pneumocystis* sp. pneumonia. Lesions were not described and the species of *Pneumocystis* was not identified.

Dermatophyte Infection: Dermatophytosis

Dermatophytosis (ringworm) in guinea pigs is usually due to *Trichophyton mentagrophytes*, and less commonly *Microsporum canis*. In a survey of laboratory animals in Europe, over half of the guinea pigs sampled were positive for either *T. mentagrophytes* or *M. canis*. The majority of the guinea pigs were subclinically infected. There appears to be a strain-related variation in susceptibility to the disease. Epizootics that arise in guinea pig populations are usually associated with *T. mentagrophytes*. In 1 recorded outbreak, the mortality rate among guinea pigs during the first week after birth was up to 50%.

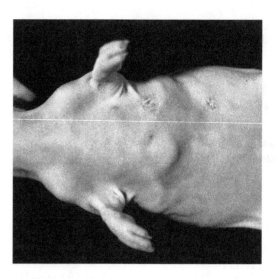

FIG. 5.24. *Circumscribed, scaling lesions of the skin of a hairless guinea pig with dermatophytosis.*

Spontaneous regression of lesions may occur, particularly in adults. However, in sows where skin lesions had disappeared, the clinical signs frequently recurred at parturition. High environmental temperatures and humidity may be predisposing factors in outbreaks of the disease. Pathogenic dermatophytes are readily transmitted from infected guinea pigs to human contacts as well as other animals, including rabbits.

Pathology

Circumscribed, scaly, pruritic lesions with raised, erythematous borders (Fig. 5.24) and localized alopecia arise in clinically affected animals. Lesions often initially appear on the nose, but other regions of the head, as well as neck, sides, and back, may become involved. Frequently, there may be pustule formations due to secondary bacterial infections. On microscopic examination, there is hyperkeratosis, epidermal hyperplasia, and polymorphonuclear cell infiltration. Pustules may be present in the superficial epidermis and hair follicles. Arthrospores can usually be observed microscopically in H & E-stained tissue sections, particularly in hair follicles. PAS or methenamine silver staining procedures are best for optimal visualization of the fungi in sections. Hyphae and arthrospores usually can also be readily demonstrated in wet mount preparations of hair shafts collected from lesions that are cleared in 10% KOH. Culture of skin scrapings or hair shafts on appropriate media, such as Sabouraud's dextrose, is recommended for positive identification.

Cryptococcus neoformans Infection: Cryptococcosis

A number of case reports have documented *C. neoformans* infection in guinea pigs. One report involved a group of subclinically infected laboratory guinea pigs from an accredited vendor in the United Kingdom. Affected animals had multifocal granulomatous lesions in the meninges with fibrosis. Both fungal filaments and typical thick-walled yeast forms could be visualized in tissue sections of brain, but not other organs. Focal cutaneous lesions have also been described. Diagnosis can be confirmed by silver staining or staining with mucicarmine, PAS, or Alcian blue, which reveal the thick mucinous capsules.

Histoplasma capsulatum Infection: Histoplasmosis

An outbreak of histoplasmosis in laboratory guinea pigs was described in which affected animals developed progressive emaciation and posterior paresis. At necropsy, lesions included ulcerative gastritis, mucohemorrhagic enteritis, splenomegaly, and enlarged mesenteric lymph nodes. Less commonly, lesions were found in lung, liver, mediastinal lymph nodes, and other organs. Lesions contained histiocytes with basophilic round or ellipsoid cytoplasmic bodies, consistent with *H. capsulatum*, which was confirmed by culture on Sabouraud agar. Infection was suspected to be introduced through contaminated wild grass.

BIBLIOGRAPHY FOR FUNGAL INFECTIONS

Dermatophyte Infections

Kraemer, A., Mueller, R.S., Werckenthin, C., Straubinger, R.K., & Hein, J. (2012) Dermatophytes in pet guinea pigs and rabbits. *Veterinary Microbiology* 157:208–213.

McAleer, R. (1980) An epizootic in laboratory guinea pigs due to *Trichophyton mentagrophytes*. *Australian Veterinary Journal* 56:234–236.

Papini, R., Gazzano, R., & Mancianti, F. (1997) Survey of dermatophytes isolated from the coats of laboratory animals in Italy. *Laboratory Animal Science* 47:75–77.

Pombier, E.C. & Kim, J.C.S. (1975) An epizootic outbreak of ringworm in a guinea pig colony caused by *Trichophyton mentagrophytes*. *Laboratory Animals* 9:215–221.

Vangeel, I., Pasmans, F., Vanrobaeys, M., De Herdt, P., & Haesebrouck, F. (2000) Prevalence of dermatophytes in asymptomatic guinea pigs and rabbits. *Veterinary Record* 146:440–441.

Other Fungal Infections

Betty, M.J. (1977) Spontaneous cryptococcal meningitis in a group of guinea pigs caused by a hyphae-producing strain. *Journal of Comparative Pathology* 87:377–382.

Correa, W.M. & Pacheco, A.C. 1967. Naturally occurring histoplasmosis in guinea pigs. *Canadian Journal of Comparative Medicine* 31:203–206.

Moffat, R.E. & Schiefer, B. (1973) Microsporidiosis (encephalitozoonosis) in the guinea pig. *Laboratory Animal Science* 23:282–283.

Reed, C. & O'Donoghue, J.L. (1979) A new guinea pig mutant with abnormal hair production and immunodeficiency. *Laboratory Animal Science* 29:744–748.

Van Herck, H., Van Den Ingh, T.S.G.A.M., Van Der Hage, M.H., & Zwart, P. (1988) Dermal cryptococcosis in a guinea pig. *Laboratory Animals* 22:88–91.

Wan, C.-H., Franklin, C., Riley, L.K., Hook, R.R., Jr., & Besch-Williford, C. (1996) Diagnostic exercise: granulomatous encephalitis in guinea pigs. *Laboratory Animal Science* 46:228–230.

PARASITIC DISEASES

Protozoal Infections
Cryptosporidium wrairi *Infection: Cryptosporidiosis*

Infection rates with *C. wrairi* of 30–40% are considered to be typical in conventional colonies. Clinical signs are often absent in adults, but include diarrhea, weight loss, and emaciation in young animals. In outbreaks of the disease, morbidity and mortality rates among young animals range from negligible to up to 50%. Infection in adults is transient, whereas infection in young animals is of longer duration. Recovered animals are immune to reinfection.

Pathology

Affected animals may be thin and potbellied, with fecal staining of the perineum. The small and large intestine usually contain watery material. Microscopically, acute lesions are usually concentrated in the small intestine. There is hyperplasia of the crypt epithelium, edema of the lamina propria with leukocytic infiltration, and frequently marked dilation of lacteals (Fig. 5.25). Necrosis, sloughing, and flattening of enterocytes occur at the tips of the villi. In chronic lesions, villus attenuation and fusion and crypt hyperplasia commonly occur. Cryptosporidia are most numerous in acute cases. They are present within the brush border along the apices of enterocytes (Fig. 5.26), with the number of cryptosporidia progressively increasing distally from duodenum to ileum. Infections with *E. coli* have been associated with clinical cases of cryptosporidiosis.

Diagnosis

Identification of the parasite by mucosal scrapings and examination by phase contrast microscopy is recommended. The organism may also be demonstrated in embedded sections of affected gut prepared for light or electron microscopy. PCR can also be used for detection and speciation.

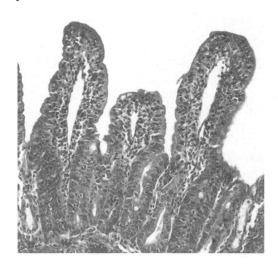

FIG. 5.25. *Ileum from a young guinea pig with cryptosporidiosis. There is marked dilation of lacteals, blunting of villi, leukocytic infiltration of the lamina propria, and crypt hyperplasia.*

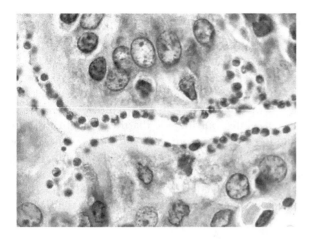

FIG. 5.26.   Cryptosporidium wrairi *organisms attached to the brush border of enterocytes in an infected guinea pig. (Source: R. Feinstein, The National Veterinary Institute, Sweden. Reproduced with permission from R. Feinstein.)*

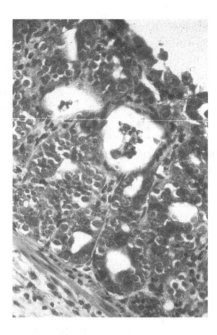

FIG. 5.27.   *Large intestinal mucosa of a young guinea pig with coccidiosis due to* Eimeria caviae. *Note the large numbers of micro- and macrogametocytes.*

Eimeria caviae *Infection: Intestinal Coccidiosis*

Intestinal coccidiosis in the guinea pig is associated with *E. caviae*. Clinical outbreaks of diarrhea occur predominantly in weanling animals. Seasonal fluctuations may occur, peaking in the spring and fall. Mortality rates are variable but are usually relatively low, although they may reach 30%. Improved sanitation and husbandry are essential steps in the control of the disease. Following ingestion of the sporulated oocysts, sporozoites penetrate the intestinal mucosa, and schizogony is detectable by 7–8 days postinfection. Endogenous stages occur primarily in the cryptal cells of the anterior colon, although the cecum may also be involved. Diarrhea usually occurs at 10–13 days. The prepatent period is around 11 days, but severely affected animals may succumb with profuse diarrhea before oocysts are evident on fecal flotation. The time required for sporulation of oocysts is from 2–3 days to up to 10 days.

Pathology

At necropsy, the colon may be thickened and often contains fluid, fetid material, and sometimes brown flecks of blood. The mucosa and peritoneal serosa are congested and edematous, with variable petechial hemorrhages and serosanguinous fluid within the peritoneal cavity. Microscopic changes are characterized by mucosal hyperplasia, sloughing of enterocytes, edema of the lamina propria, and infiltration with mixed leukocytes. Micro- and macrogametocytes are usually present in large numbers in the colonic, and to a lesser extent, cecal mucosa (Fig. 5.27).

Diagnosis

Demonstration of the organisms by mucosal scrapings, histopathology, and fecal flotation will confirm the diagnosis. Deaths may occur before oocysts are evident

on fecal flotation. Differential diagnoses include cryptosporidiosis, clostridial enteropathies, and other infectious enteritides.

Klossiella cobayae *Infection: Renal Coccidiosis*

Sporadic cases of renal coccidiosis apparently occurred on a global basis in the early to mid-20th century. However, it is a rare occurrence under current laboratory conditions. The organism is shed in the urine, and following ingestion, the sporozoites of *K. cobayae* invade the intestinal mucosa and enter adjacent capillaries or lymphatics. Sporozoites reaching the kidney undergo schizogony in endothelial cells of the glomerular capillaries. Infected endothelial cells rupture, releasing merozoites, and schizogony is repeated in epithelial cells lining convoluted tubules. Gametogony occurs in epithelial cells of Henle's loop, and sporulated sporocysts are eventually released in the urine, to repeat the cycle. Clinical signs are normally absent, and the diagnosis is usually based on the demonstration of the schizogonous stage in glomerular capillaries or, more commonly, schizonts or the gametogenous stages in the cytoplasm of epithelial cells lining renal tubules (see Mouse Chapter 1, "*Klossiella muris* Infection").

Toxoplasma gondii *Infection: Toxoplasmosis*

Naturally occurring infections with *T. gondii* have been reported in this species, but they rarely occur, particularly under current housing practices. Infections are frequently subclinical, although multifocal hepatitis and pneumonitis have been noted in active infections. Cysts may be present in tissues such as myocardium and central nervous system in subclinical chronic infections. Animals may become infected through ingestion of material contaminated with oocysts from felids or via the accidental injection of contaminated biological material.

Miscellaneous Commensal and Opportunistic Protozoa

The enteric microbiome of the guinea pig is embellished with a panoply of protozoa that are often listed as parasitic pathogens, although they are rarely, if ever, associated with disease. These include the amoeba species *Endolimax caviae* and *Entamoeba caviae*, *Tritrichomonas caviae*, *Giardia duodenalis* (formerly *G. caviae*), and *Balantidium caviae*. The latter 2 organisms may act as opportunistic pathogens in immunodeficient guinea pigs (such as athymic guinea pigs) and as coinfections. Their presence should signal a search for the primary cause of disease.

Helminth Infestations
Nematode Larval Migrans

Following ingestion of wood shaving bedding contaminated with raccoon feces, a colony of guinea pigs was reported to develop *Baylisascaris procyonis* larval migrans. Affected guinea pigs manifested cachexia, stupor, hyperexcitability, lateral recumbency, and opisthotonos. They had multifocal malacia and eosinophilic granulomatous inflammation in the brain associated with the presence of nematode larvae, which feature diagnostic lateral alae. Eosinophilic granulomata containing nematode larvae were also found in the lungs of some animals. The raccoon is the primary host for this nematode. Another report described a guinea pig with neurologic signs due to *Paralaphosostrongylus tenuis*. Worms were found in the meninges, with nonsuppurative and eosinophilic leptomeningitis. The natural host for this nematode is the white-tailed deer, and the adult worms reside in the subdural space in that species. Worms within the affected guinea pig brain included mature males and females, as in the natural host. The guinea pig was fed grass from a lawn grazed by deer.

Paraspidodera uncinata Infestation

The most common helminth of guinea pigs is the cecal worm, *P. uncinata*. These small worms measure up to approximately 25 mm in length. The life cycle is direct and is complete in around 65 days. Microscopic findings may include larval invasion of mucosa. No migration beyond the intestinal mucosa occurs, and infestations are usually subclinical.

Peloderma strongyloides Infestation

Alopecia and dermatitis has been described in a colony of guinea pigs infested with the saprophytic nematode, *Peloderma* (formerly *Rhabditis*) *strongyloides*. Microscopic examination of skin revealed the presence of small larvae within hair follicles and inflammation of the surrounding dermis. These nematodes live in moist decaying organic material, and were likely acquired through substandard husbandry conditions. They are known to cause similar dermal disease in many species of animals.

Fasciola spp. Infestation

Guinea pigs have been known to become naturally infested with *Fasciola hepatica* as well as *Fasciola gigantia*. Domestic guinea pigs in Peru were seen to have a high prevalence of *F. hepatica* infestation, which appeared to be an important factor in the life cycle of this trematode in cattle, when guinea pig feces is spread upon fields. An outbreak of illness was reported in a colony of guinea pigs in Malaya infected with *F. gigantia*. Necropsy revealed fibrotic cysts containing dark brown fluid and flukes in multiple tissues, ectopic flukes in the pelvic region, and lesions in kidneys, liver, and lungs. Fascioliasis in guinea pigs is another example of an unexpected infestation acquired through feeding contaminated grass or hay.

Miscellaneous Other Helminth Infections

The reader is referred to Flynn's Parasites of Laboratory Animals for a more comprehensive list of helminths found in wild and domestic guinea pigs.

Arthropod Infestations
Chirodiscoides caviae Infestation: Fur Mites

These fur mites have been identified in guinea pigs from commercial suppliers, in laboratory facilities, and in pet animals. The parasite tends to be concentrated in the lumbar region and lateral aspect of the hindquarters. Even parasite loads of up to 200/cm^2 appear to evoke minimal or no clinical evidence of pruritus or damage to the skin. Other predisposing factors, including concurrent disease, may have a significant influence on the parasite load in infested animals. Microscopic examination of the adult mite is necessary for positive identification.

Trixacarus caviae Infestation: Mange Mites

Mange in guinea pigs is primarily associated with *T. caviae* infestation. This pathogenic sarcoptid mite appears to be widespread in some conventional colonies of guinea pigs, and is capable of causing urticaria in human contacts. Lesions are usually distributed over the neck, shoulders, inner thighs, and abdomen. Changes in the skin seen grossly are keratosis with scaling, crusting, and alopecia (Fig. 5.28). Marked pruritis may occur, and in severe cases, animals become emaciated. Hematological changes include heterophilia, monocytosis, eosinophilia, and basophilia. Vigorous scratching may precipitate convulsive seizures. Some affected animals have exhibited flaccid paralysis. Untreated animals with extensive lesions may die. On

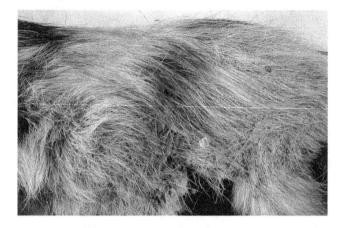

FIG. 5.28. *Hyperkeratotic dermatitis in a guinea pig with mange due to* Trixacarus caviae *infestation. (Source: R.O. Zavodovskaya, University of California, Davis, CA.)*

microscopic examination, there is epidermal hyperplasia and spongiosis, with orthokeratotic and parakeratotic hyperkeratosis. Irregular burrows in the stratum corneum contain mites and eggs (Fig. 5.29). There is usually leukocytic infiltration in the underlying dermis. Hair follicles are normally not invaded by the parasite.

Skin scrapings of hair and scale cleared with 10% KOH and examined microscopically should reveal the typical mites and eggs. The parasites can also be demonstrated in paraffin-embedded sections of affected skin. Differential diagnoses include pediculosis, dermatophytosis, trauma, and idiopathic alopecia.

Demodex caviae *Infestation*

Demodex caviae has been noted in guinea pigs in the absence of clinical signs. The prevalence and significance of these infestations in the laboratory guinea pigs is currently unknown.

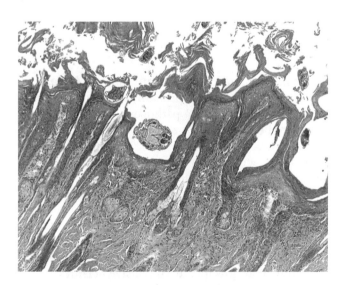

FIG. 5.29. *Skin from the guinea pig depicted in the previous figure. Note the marked hyperkeratosis and mites embedded within the keratin.*

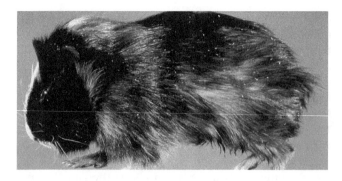

FIG. 5.30. *Pediculosis in a guinea pig infested with* Gliricola porcelli. *Multiple lice are visible on the ends of hair shafts.*

Other Mite Infestations

Infestations with other mites such as *Myocoptes musculinus*, *Sarcoptes scabei*, and *Notoedres muris* are rare and may be due to interspecies contact. Anecdotal reports of *Psoroptes equi* (*P. cuniculi*) otitis exist in the pet guinea pig population. There is a single report of alopecia due to infestation of guinea pigs with free-living nymphal astigmatic mites, *Acarus farris*, which were introduced through contaminated hay. The infestation caused minimal inflammatory response.

Pediculosis

Gliricola porcelli and *Gyropus ovalis* are large biting lice that are associated with pediculosis in guinea pigs. Both species of lice are common among guinea pigs and coinfestations may occur. Frequently, moderate infestations are not accompanied by clinical signs. Pruritus, rough hair coat, and alopecia may occur in heavy infestations (Figs. 5.30 and 5.31). *Trimenopon hispidium* is an exceedingly rare louse that may also infest guinea pigs. Diagnosis of pediculosis is accomplished by identification of lice and nits within the pelage, and enhanced at necropsy when the carcass has cooled and lice tend to accumulate at the end of hair shafts.

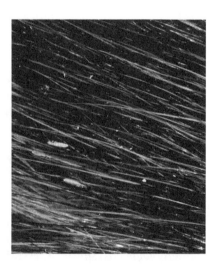

FIG. 5.31. *Magnified view of pelage from the guinea pig depicted in the previous figure.*

BIBLIOGRAPHY FOR PARASITIC DISEASES

General References
Baker, D.G. (2008) *Flynn's Parasites of Laboratory Animals*, 2nd edn. Wiley-Blackwell Publishing, Ames.

Brabb, T., Newsome, D., Burich, A., & Hanes, M. (2012) Infectious diseases. In: *The Laboratory Rabbit, Guinea Pig, Hamster, and Other Rodents* (eds. M.A. Suckow, K.A. Stevens, & R.P. Wilson), pp. 637–683. Elsievier, London.

Vetterling, J.M. (1976) Protozoan parasites. In: *The Biology of the Guinea Pig* (eds. J.E. Wagner & P.J. Manning), pp. 163–196. Academic Press, New York.

Protozoal Infections

Cryptosporidium wrairi Infection
Chrisp, C.E. & LeGendre, M. (1994) Similarities and differences between DNA of *Cryptosporidium parvum* and *C. wrairi* detected by the polymerase chain reaction. *Folia Parasitologica (Praha)* 41:97–100.

Chrisp, C.E., Reid, W.C., Rush, H.G., Suckow, M.A., Bush, A., & Thomann, M.J. (1990) Cryptosporidiosis in guinea pigs: an animal model. *Infection and Immunity* 58:674–679.

Gibson, S.V. & Wagner, J.E. (1986) Cryptosporidiosis in guinea pigs: a retrospective study. *Journal of the American Veterinary Medical Association* 189:1033–1034.

Vetterling, J.M., Jervis, H.R., Merrill, T.G., & Sprinz, H. (1971) *Cryptosporidium wrairi* sp. n. from the guinea pig *Cavia procellus*, with an emendation of the genus. *Journal of Protozoology* 18:243–247.

Eimeria caviae Infection
Ellis, P.A. & Wright, A.E. (1961) Coccidiosis in guinea pigs. *Journal of Clinical Pathology* 14:394–396.

Muto, T., Sugisaki, M., Yusa, T., & Noguchi, Y. (1985) Studies on coccidiosis in guinea pigs. 1. Clinico-pathological observation. *Jikken Dobutsu* 34:23–30.

Muto, T., Yusa, T., Sugisaki, M., Tanaka, K., Noguchi, Y., & Taguchi, K. (1985) Studies on coccidiosis in guinea pigs. 2. Epizootiological survey. *Jikken Dobutsu* 34:31–39.

Klossiella cobayae Infection
Cossel, L. (1958) Renal findings in guinea pigs with *Klossiella* infection (*Klossiella cobayae*): study of special pathology in experimental animals. *Schweizer Zeitschrift fur Pathologie und Bakteriologie* 21:62–73.

Pearce, L. (1916) Klossiella infection of the guinea pig. *Journal of Experimental Medicine* 23:431–442.

Toxoplasma gondii Infection
Henry, L. & Beverly, J.K.A. (1976) Toxoplasmosis in rats and guinea pigs. *Journal of Comparative Pathology* 87:97–102.

Markham, F.S. (1937) Spontaneous toxoplasma encephalitis in the guinea pig. *American Journal of Hygiene* 26:193–196.

Helminth Infestations
Coman, S., Bacescu, B., Coman, T., Petrut, T., Coman, C., & Vlase, E. (2009) Aspects of the parasitary infestations of guinea pigs reared in intensive system. *Revista Scientia Parasitologica* 10:97–100.

Gamarra, R.G. (1966) Fasciola infection in guinea pigs in the Peruvian highlands. *Tropical Animal Health Production* 28:143–144.

Southard, T., Bender, H., Wade, S.E., Grunenwald, C., & Gerhold, R.W. (2012) Naturally occurring *Paraelaphostrongylus tenuis*-associated choriomeningitis in a guinea pig with neurologic signs. *Veterinary Pathology* 50:560–562.

Strauss, J.M. & Heyneman, D. (1966) Fatal ectopic fascioliasis in a guinea pig breeding colony. *Journal of Parasitology* 52:413.

Todd, K.S., Jr., Seaman, W.J., & Gretschmann, K.W. (1982) *Pelodermastrongyloides* dermatitis in a guinea pig. *Veterinary Medicine and Small Animal Clinician* 77:1400–1402.

Van Andel, R.A., Franklin, C.L., Besch-Williford, C., Riley, L.K., Hook, R.R., Jr., & Kazacos, K.R. (1995) Cerebrospinal larva migrans due to *Baylisascaris procyanis* in a guinea pig colony. *Laboratory Animal Science* 45:27–30.

Arthropod infestations
Dorrestein, G.M. & Van Bronswijk, J.E.M.H. (1979) *Trixacarus caviae* as a cause of mange in guinea pigs and papular urticaria in man. *Veterinary Parasitology* 5:389–398.

Fuentealbea, C. & Hanna, P. (1996) Mange induced by *Trixacarus caviae* in the guinea pig. *Canadian Veterinary Journal* 37:749–750.

Hirsjarvi, P. & Phyala, L. (1995) Ivermectin treatment of a colony of guinea pigs infested with fur mite (*Chirodiscoides caviae*). *Laboratory Animals* 29:200–203.

Kummel, B.A., Estes, S.A., & Arlian, L.G. (1980) *Trixacarus caviae* infestation of guinea pigs. *Journal of the American Veterinary Medical Association* 177:903–908.

Linek, M. & Bourdeau, P. (2005) Alopecia in two guinea pigs due to hypopodes of *Acarus farris* (Acaridae: Astigmata). *Veterinary Record* 157:58–60.

Rothwell, T.L., Pope, S.E., Rajczyk, Z.K., & Collins, G.H. (1991) Haematological and pathological responses to experimental *Trixacarus caviae* infection in guinea pigs. *Journal of Comparative Pathology* 104:179–185.

Wagner, J.E., Al-Rabae, S., & Rings, R.W. (1972) *Chirodiscoides caviae* infestation in guinea pigs. *Laboratory Animal Science* 22:750–752.

NUTRITIONAL, METABOLIC, AND TOXIC DISORDERS

Hypovitaminosis C: Scurvy

Deficiency of dietary vitamin C is a significant clinical entity in guinea pigs that may manifest itself in a number of ways. Ascorbic acid-dependent species are genetically deficient in the enzyme L-gulonolactone oxidase, which is involved in the conversion of L-gulonolactone to L-ascorbic acid. This biosynthetic activity occurs in the liver in mammals, but the synthesis of vitamin C occurs in the kidney in amphibians and reptiles. In addition to the inability of simian and human primates and guinea pigs to synthesize endogenous vitamin C, certain bats (e.g., Indian fruit bat), some birds (e.g., red-vented bulbul bird, northern shrike), some fish (e.g., channel catfish), and cetaceans also require dietary sources of vitamin C. Ascorbic acid is essential in the hydroxylase reactions necessary for the formation of hydroxyproline and hydroxylysine in the collagen molecule. Thus, connective tissue cells are unable to synthesize collagen at a normal rate, resulting in deficient and defective production of interstitial osseous matrix. Vitamin C is also necessary for the catabolism of cholesterol to bile acids. In scurvy, cartilage produced in the physeal plates persists and lengthens, but it is not replaced by bone. This calcified cartilage scaffolding is relatively susceptible to mechanical forces; thus multiple microfractures occur in the epiphyseal region. Immobilization of the limb in a

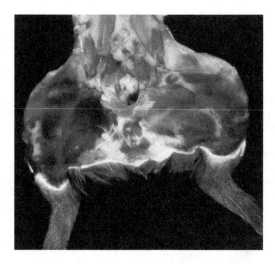

FIG. 5.32. *Hypovitaminosis C (scurvy) in a young guinea pig. Note the periarticular hemorrhages in the region of the knees.*

plaster cast will prevent the occurrence of microfractures, emphasizing the effect of the normal stresses and strains of limb movement on the development of lesions. There is increased capillary fragility, with widening of intercellular spaces between endothelial cells, vacuolar degeneration of endothelium, and depletion of subendothelial collagenous tissue. There is also increased prothrombin time in animals with scurvy. The increased susceptibility of scorbutic guinea pigs to bacterial infections such as *S. pneumoniae* is probably due, at least in part, to impaired macrophage migration and depressed phagocytic activity of heterophils.

Pathology

Hemorrhages are present in the periarticular regions, particularly in the hind limbs (Fig. 5.32), but may also appear randomly in other tissues. There may be enlargement of the costochondral junctions (scorbutic rosary, Fig. 5.33), with hemorrhages into the regional soft tissues. Animals may be thin and appear unkempt. Evidence of diarrhea is a variable finding. Occasionally,

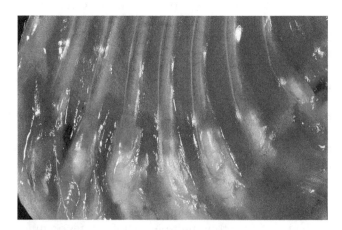

FIG. 5.33. *Enlarged costochondral junctions (scorbutic rosary) and regional hemorrhages in a young guinea pig with hypovitaminosis C.*

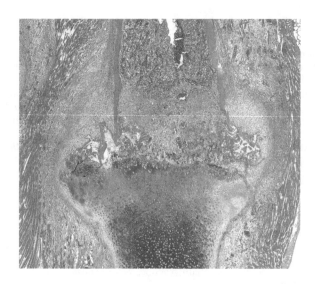

FIG. 5.34. *Costochondral junction from a case of scurvy in a guinea pig. Note the callus formation of the junctional periostieum, persistence of cartilage with failure of ossification, microfractures of bone, and marked proliferation of fusiform mesenchymal cells in the periosteal and medullary regions.*

blood-tinged gut contents are observed, and there may be ecchymoses in the urinary bladder. Adrenal glands are frequently markedly enlarged. Microscopically, persistence and irregularities of the physeal cartilage is evident in young growing animals. Microfractures of the cartilaginous spicules and hemorrhage are common findings. In bones including ribs, there is marked proliferation of poorly differentiated fusiform mesenchymal cells in the periosteal regions (Figs. 5.34 and 5.35) and medullary cavity, with displacement of normal hematopoietic cells. Frequently, there are aggregations of eosinophilic material interspersed between the mesenchymal cells. Dental abnormalities also occur. Fibrosis of the pulp and derangement of odontoblasts have been observed during the early stages of the disease. Hemosiderin-laden

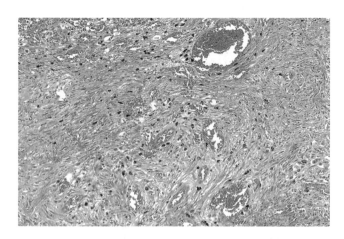

FIG. 5.35. *Higher magnification of mesenchymal proliferation from the case depicted in the previous figure. Note the hemorrhage and numerous hemosiderin-laden cells throughout the proliferating mesenchyma.*

macrophages that are commonly present in the lamina propria of the intestine have been considered by some to be due to subclinical hypovitaminosis C.

Myopathies
Nutritional Myopathy

Guinea pigs are prone to development of degenerative and necrotizing myopathy. The etiology may not be determined in many cases. However, there is a clear relationship to selenium/vitamin E deficiency. Myopathy can be readily induced in guinea pigs with selenium/vitamin E deficient diets, and natural cases of myopathy have been reversed by dietary change and treatment with selenium and alphatocopherol. Experimental studies have shown that combined selenium and vitamin E deficiency causes a fatal myopathy that is more severe than the myopathy that arises with vitamin E alone. Furthermore, combined selenium and vitamin C deficiency causes more severe myopathy than selenium alone.

Depression and conjunctivitis may be present on clinical examination. In 1 report, spontaneous hind limb weakness was a prominent clinical feature of the disease. Severely affected animals may die within 1 week of the onset of clinical signs. Elevated serum creatine phosphokinase (CPK) is a feature of the disease. At necropsy, there is a marked pallor of the affected muscles. Microscopic changes are characterized by coagulative necrosis and hyalinization of cardiac and skeletal myofibers, fragmentation of sarcoplasm, increased basophilia of the sarcoplasm, and rowing of nuclei in regenerating myofibers (Fig. 5.36). Multinucleated muscle fibers may be present in regenerating myofibers. Mineralization of myofibers is apparently not an important feature of the disease. There may be marked reduction in reproductive performance in affected sows, and fetuses of vitamin E-deficient sows may develop encephalomalacia. Testicular degeneration is a later development seen in vitamin E-deficient boars.

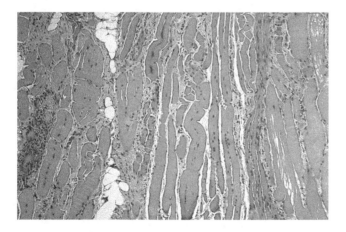

FIG. 5.36. *Myocardium from an adult guinea pig with multiphasic degeneration and regeneration of myofibers.*

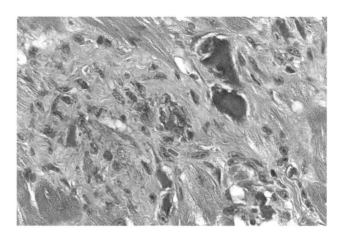

FIG. 5.37. *Focal myocardial degeneration and fibrosis with mineralization in an aged guinea pig.*

Myocardial and Skeletal Muscle Degeneration with Mineralization

This is a poorly understood syndrome, and the contributing factors have not been clearly identified. Multifocal mineralization/calcification of individual muscle fibers may be seen as an incidental finding, particularly in the major muscles of the hind limbs. Affected animals frequently are subclinical. On microscopic examination, there may be multifocal mineralization of skeletal myofibers, and less commonly cardiac myofibers. Changes are characterized by degeneration of myofibers, with variable mineralization and minimal mononuclear cell infiltration. In chronic lesions of longer duration, there may be concurrent mineralization with fibrosis (Fig. 5.37). In 1 report, myocardial lesions were observed in crossbred Abyssinian/Hartley guinea pigs. Vitamin E and selenium levels were within normal limits, and genetic factors were implicated in the disease.

Cardiac Glycogenosis: Rhabdomyomatosis

This condition is observed as an incidental finding in guinea pigs of various ages. It has been interpreted to be a degenerative condition and a congenital tissue malformation with "blastemoid" characteristics. It has been speculated but not proven that rhabdomyomatosis occurs more frequently in animals with scurvy. The current assessment is that rhabdomyomatosis is related to a disorder of glycogen metabolism.

Smaller lesions are not visible on macroscopic examination. Occasionally, larger areas appear as pale pink, poorly delineated foci or streaks. These changes have been observed in various regions of the heart, including ventricles, atria, interventricular septa, and papillary muscles. Lesions are most frequently found in the left ventricle. Microscopic examination reveals a spongy network of vacuolated myofibers composed of finely fibrillar to granular, eosinophilic cytoplasm (Fig. 5.38). Vacuoles are rounded to polygonal in shape and usually fill the sarcolemmal sheath. Vacuoles contain large quantities of glycogen, which is washed out in the

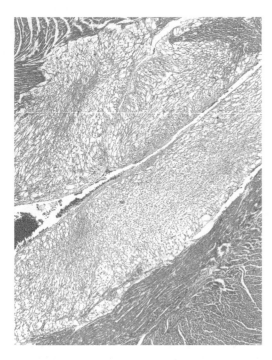

FIG. 5.38. *Heart from an adult guinea pig with focal myocardial rhabdomyomatosis, in which foci of myofibers are pale staining due to distention of sarcoplasm with glycogen, which is lost during histologic processing.*

fixation and processing procedures (Fig. 5.39). Glycogen is readily demonstrated in PAS-stained, alcohol-fixed specimens. There may be displacement and flattening of myocyte nuclei in some affected fibers. In other fibers, there may be a cytoplasmic marginal rim with a round nucleus projecting into the vacuole. Myofibers with centrally located nuclei and radiating fibrillar processes have been called "spider cells." Interspersed within the affected myofibers, there may be poorly differentiated fibers with identifiable cross-striations.

Metastatic Mineralization

Metastatic mineralization occurs most often in guinea pigs over 1 year of age. Muscle stiffness and unthriftiness are variable findings. In some cases, mineral deposition

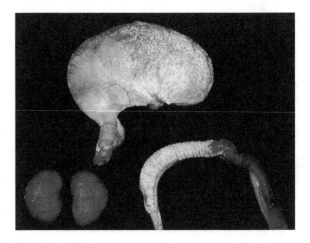

FIG. 5.40. *Metastatic mineralization of the gastric and intestinal walls in an aged guinea pig with chronic kidney disease (lower left). There are chalky deposits on the serosal surface of the stomach and intestine.*

may be confined to soft tissues around the elbows and ribs. There may be more widespread mineralization of tissues, such as lung, trachea, heart, aorta, liver, kidney, stomach, uterus, and sclera (Figs. 5.40 and 5.41). Dietary factors such as low magnesium and high phosphorus have been implicated in this syndrome. High-calcium or high-phosphorus diets appear to interfere with magnesium absorption and metabolism. Therefore, this syndrome may not be the result of a deficiency of a single component but rather may be due to a dietary imbalance of 2 or more nutrients. As with the rabbit, renal excretion of calcium is an important regulator of serum calcium levels, so metastatic mineralization may be associated with renal disease.

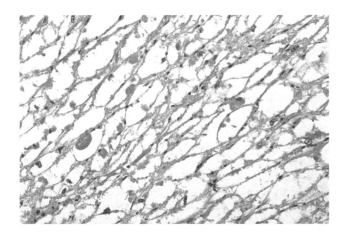

FIG. 5.39. *Higher magnification of affected myocardium with rhabdomyomatosis.*

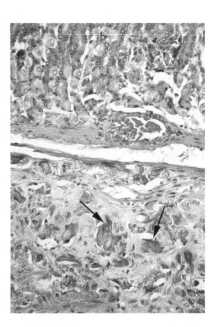

FIG. 5.41. *Gastric wall with metastatic mineralization of the smooth muscle (arrows).*

Pregnancy Toxemia

Although the clinical signs are similar in many respects, there are 2 different patterns of disease associated with pregnancy toxemia in the guinea pig: the fasting or metabolic form and the circulatory or toxic form. Both forms normally occur in advanced pregnancy. Depression, acidosis, ketosis, proteinuria, ketonuria, and a lowered urinary pH from around 9 (normal) to 5–6 are frequent manifestations in both forms of pregnancy toxemia.

Metabolic Form

This form of pregnancy toxemia occurs in obese sows during the last 2–3 weeks of pregnancy, particularly in sows during their first or second pregnancy. The uterine contents of guinea pigs in advanced pregnancy may represent up to 50% of the weight of the nonpregnant dam. Stress factors such as shipping or changes in feeding routines may be sufficient to precipitate the disease. In 1 study, withholding the usual supplemental cabbage ration resulted in a mortality rate of approximately 5% in obese dams. The syndrome has also been produced in obese, nonpregnant animals subjected to the stress of cabbage deprivation. Lowered blood glucose, ketosis, and hyperlipidemia are typical findings. Animals usually become comatose and die within 5–6 days after the onset of the disease. It appears to be triggered by high-energy feeding followed by subsequent withdrawal, resulting in mobilization of fat as a source of energy, with disastrous results. At necropsy, animals usually have abundant fat reserves, with marked hepatic lipidosis. Microscopically, marked lipidosis is evident in hepatocytes (Fig. 5.42), as well as in kidney and adrenals. Lipid may also be demonstrable in vessels with fat stains.

Circulatory/Toxic Form: Preeclampsia

In this form of pregnancy toxemia, uteroplacental ischemia may occur due to compression of the aorta caudal to the renal vessels by the gravid uterus. This results in a significant reduction in blood pressure in the uterine vessels, with subsequent placental necrosis and hemorrhage,

thrombocytopenia, ketosis, and death. On microscopic examination, there is uterine and placental hemorrhage, necrosis, and leukocytic infiltration. Multifocal periportal liver necrosis, nephrosis, and adrenocortical hemorrhage are typical findings. The disease has been reproduced in female guinea pigs by banding and transection of uterine and ovarian vessels.

Diabetes Mellitus

Spontaneous diabetes mellitus can arise in guinea pigs. Affected animals frequently show no clinical signs during the early stages of the disease. In 1 report, animals were usually affected by 6 months of age, and the average age of onset was 3 months. Both sexes were affected. Changes evident by clinical chemistry were hyperglycemia, glycosuria, and rarely ketonuria. There was a marked reduction in fertility in affected sows. Animals introduced into the affected colony subsequently became diabetic. An unidentified infectious agent was suspected to be involved. On microscopic examination, there was vacuolation of and degranulation of the beta islet cells with fatty vacuolation of exocrine cells and fibrosis of the vascular stroma. The exocrine component was found to result in reduced overall secretion, bicarbonate concentration, and enzyme production. In advanced cases, there was thickening of basement membranes of the glomerular tufts, sometimes with sclerosis and scarring of Bowman's capsule.

Systemic Amyloidosis

Amyloidosis is occasionally found in guinea pigs as an incidental finding at necropsy. It typically involves deposition of hyaline AA amyloid in the periphery of splenic follicles, between hepatic cords and sinusoids, kidney (Figs. 5.43 and 5.44), and adrenal cortex. Other organs

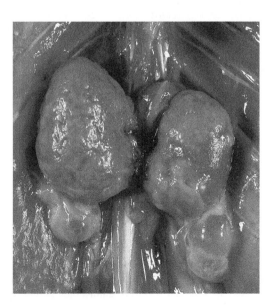

FIG. 5.43. *Renal amyloidosis in an aged guinea pig. Also note the bilateral cystic rete ovarii below the kidneys. (Source: R. Burns, University of Connecticut, Mansfield, Connecticut. Reproduced with permission from R. Burns.)*

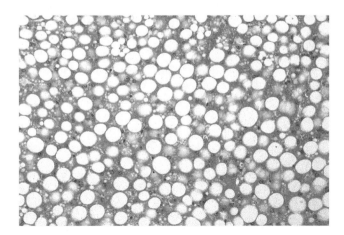

FIG. 5.42. *Hepatic lipidosis in a sow with the metabolic form of pregnancy toxemia.*

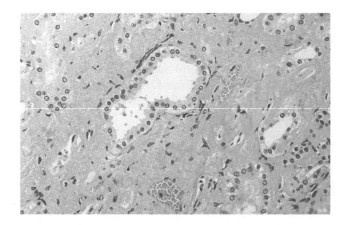

FIG. 5.44. *Amyloid deposition in the renal cortical intersitium in the aged guinea pig depicted in the previous figure.*

may be involved less commonly. It tends to occur in immunized guinea pigs and in animals with chronic bacterial infections, such as pododermatitis.

Toxic Disorders

Guinea pigs are subject to a number of ingested toxins, similar to rabbits. Their chewing behavior makes them prone to chronic lead poisoning from lead-containing environmental surfaces. A large number of poisonous plants pose a risk to guinea pigs, including philodendron and peace lily, which contain oxylates that result in renal failure.

BIBLIOGRAPHY FOR NUTRITIONAL, METABOLIC, AND TOXIC DISORDERS

General Reference
Williams, B. (2012) Non-infectious diseases. In: *The Laboratory Rabbit, Guinea Pig, Hamster, and Other Rodents* (eds. M. A. Suckow, K. A. Stevens, & R. P. Wilson), pp. 685–704. Elsievier, London.

Hypovitaminosis C: Scurvy
Clarke, G.L., Allen, A.M. Small, J.D., & Lock, A. (1980) Subclinical scurvy in the guinea pig. *Veterinary Pathology* 17:40–44.
Eva, J.K., Fifield, R., & Rickett, M. (1976) Decomposition of supplementary vitamin C in diets compounded for laboratory animals. *Laboratory Animals* 10:157–159.
Follis, R.H. (1943) Effect of mechanical force on the skeletal lesions in acute scurvy in guinea pigs. *Archives of Pathology* 35:579–582.
Ganguly, R., Durieux, M.F., & Waldman, R.H. (1976) Macrophage function in vitamin C-deficient guinea pigs. *American Journal of Clinical Nutrition* 29:762–765.
Gillespie, D.S. (1980) An overview of species needing vitamin C. *Journal of Zoo Animal Medicine* 11:88–91.
Gore, I., Fujinami, T., & Shirahama, T. (1965) Endothelial changes produced by ascorbic acid deficiency in guinea pigs. *Archives of Pathology* 80:371–376.
Kim, J.C.S. (1977) Ultrastructural studies of vascular and muscular changes in ascorbic acid–deficient guinea pigs. *Laboratory Animals* 11:113–117.
Nungester, W.J. & Ames, A.M. 1948. The relationship between ascorbic acid and phagocytic activity. *Journal of Infectious Diseases* 83:50–54.

Myopathies
Griffith, J.W. & Lang, C.M. (1987) Vitamin E and selenium status of guinea pigs with myocardial necrosis. *Laboratory Animal Science* 37:776–779.
Hill, K.E., Motley, A.K., Li, X., May, J.M., & Burk, R.F. (2001) Combined selenium and vitamin E deficiency causes fatal myopathy in guinea pigs. *Journal of Nutrition* 131:1798–1802.
Hill, K.E., Motley, A.K., May, J.M., & Burk, R.F. (2009) Combined selenium and vitamin C deficiency causes cell death in guinea pig skeletal muscle. *Nutritional Research* 29:213–219.
Howell, J.M. & Buxton, P.H. (1975) Alpha tocopherol responsive muscular dystrophy in guinea pigs. *Neuropathology and Applied Neurobiology* 1:49–58.
Hueper, W.C. (1941) Rhabdomyomatosis of the heart in a guinea pig. *American Journal of Pathology* 17:121–126.
Pappenheimer, A.M. & Schogoleff, C. (1944) The testis in vitamin E deficiency in guinea pigs. *American Journal of Pathology* 20:239–244.
Saunders, L.Z. (1958) Myositis in guinea pigs. *Journal of the National Cancer Institute* 20:899–903.
Takahashi, M., Iwata, S., Matsuzawa, H., & Fujiwara, H. (1985) Pathological findings of cardiac rhabdomyomatosis in the guinea pig. *Jikken Dobutsu* 34:417–424.
Vink, H. (1969) Rhabdomyomatosis of the heart in guinea pigs. *Journal of Pathology* 97:331–334.
Ward, G.S., Johnsen, D.O., Kovatch, R.M., & Peace, T. (1977) Myopathy in guinea pigs. *Journal of the American Veterinary Medical Association* 171:837–838.
Webb, J.N. (1970) Naturally occurring myopathy in guinea pigs. *Journal of Pathology* 100:155–162.

Metastatic Mineralization
Galloway, J.H., Glover, D., & Fox, W.C. (1964) Relationship of diet and age to metastatic calcification in guinea pigs. *Laboratory Animal Care* 14:6–12.
Sparschu, G.L. & Christie, R.J. (1968) Metastatic calcification in a guinea pig colony: a pathological survey. *Laboratory Animal Care* 18:520–526.

Pregnancy Toxemia
Bergman, E.N. & Sellers, E.F. (1960) Comparison of fasting ketosis in pregnant and nonpregnant guinea pigs. *American Journal of Physiology* 198:1083–1086.
Ganaway, J.R. & Allen, A.M. (1971) Obesity predisposes to pregnancy toxemia (ketosis) of guinea pigs. *Laboratory Animal Science* 21:40–44.
Golden, J.G., Hughes, H.C., & Lang, C.M. (1980) Experimental toxemia in the pregnant guinea pig (*Cavia porcellus*). *Laboratory Animal Science* 30:174–179.
Lachmann, G., Hamel, I., Holdt, J., & Furll, M. (1989) The fat mobilization syndrome of guinea pigs (*Cavia porcellus* L.). *Archiv fur Experimentelle Veterinarmedizin* 43:231–240.
Seidl, D.C., Hughes, H.C., Bertolet, R., & Lang, C.M. (1979) True pregnancy toxemia (preeclampsia) in the guinea pig (*Cavia porcellus*). *Laboratory Animal Science* 29:472–478.

Diabetes Mellitus
Balk, M.W., Lang, C.M., White, W.J., & Munger, B.L. (1975) Exocrine pancreatic dysfunction in guinea pigs with diabetes mellitus. *Laboratory Investigation* 32:28–32.
Lang, C.M., Munder, R.L., & Rapp, F. (1977) The guinea pig as a model of diabetes mellitus. *Laboratory Animal Science* 27:789–805.
Langner, P.H., Lang, C.M., Singh, S.B., Munger, B.L., & Abt, A.B. (1981) Glomerular basement membrane changes in aging nondiabetic and diabetic guinea pigs. *Experimental Aging Research* 7:93–105.

Munger, B.L. & Lang, C.M. (1973) Spontaneous diabetes mellitus in guinea pigs: the acute cytopathology of the islets of Langerhans. *Laboratory Investigation* 29:685–702.

Systemic Amyloidosis
Pirani, C.L., Bly, C.G., Sutherland, K., & Chereso, F. (1949) Experimental amyloidosis in the guinea pig. *Science* 110:145–146.
Taylor, J.L., Wagner, J. E., Owens, D.R., & Shulman, R.A. (1971) Chronic pododermatitis in guinea pigs. *Laboratory Animal Science* 21:944–945.

Toxic Disorders
Gfeller, R.W. & Messonnier, S.P. (2004) *Handbook of Small Animal Toxicology and Poisonings*, 2nd edn. Mosby, St. Louis, MO.
Holowaychuk, M.K. (2006) Renal failure in a guinea pig (*Cavia porcellus*) following ingestion of oxalate containing plants. *Canadian Veterinary Journal* 47:787–789.

MISCELLANEOUS DISORDERS

Behavioral Diseases

Hair pulling, chewing (barbering), and trichophagia are common behavior patterns among guinea pigs in a group and can become an excessive activity once it is in vogue. As noted under Alopecia (below), trichophagy may reflect a nutritional disorder. An extension of this behavior is ear chewing, which can result in notching or severe trauma and amputation of the ear pinnae (Fig. 5.45). Frequently, sexually mature boars fight when placed together, and severe lacerations or death may result. Very young guinea pigs in communal housing may be trampled by older animals in group stampedes.

Alopecia

Alopecia may arise in guinea pigs for a variety of reasons, including endocrine dysfunction, nutrition, behavior vices, general illness, ringworm, and parasitism. Bilateral

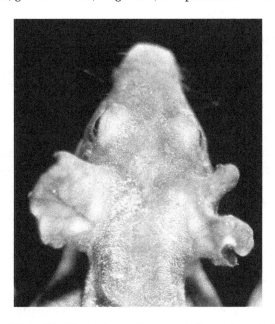

FIG. 5.45. *Notching of the ear pinnae of a hairless guinea pig due to chewing by conspecifics.*

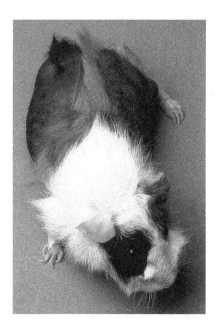

FIG. 5.46. *Bilateral alopecia in an aged guinea pig sow with cystic rete ovarii. (Source: N.J. Schoemaker, University of Utrecht, Netherlands. Reproduced with permission from N.J. Schoemaker.)*

alopecia commonly occurs in sows in advanced pregnancy and during lactation, particularly in older animals. In pregnant animals, hair loss may be due to reduced anabolism of maternal skin during fetal growth. The hair loss frequently occurs over the back, flanks, and rump, and the pelage will return to normal in due course in the typical case. Similar bilateral alopecia is very common in older sows with cystic rete ovarii (Fig. 5.46), and less common in guinea pigs with Cushing's syndrome related to adrenal cortical adenomas. Guinea pigs require crude fiber in their diet, which may not be met with formulated diets. Supplementation with hay has been shown to ameliorate alopecia among breeding guinea pigs. The mechanism for alopecia in guinea pigs without hay supplementation was apparently due to trichophagia among cage mates. Barbering as a behavioral vice may also occur among conspecifics. Chronic illness due to *Salmonella* infection has also been shown to cause bilateral alopecia, which responded to vitamin C supplementation. Dermatitis with hair loss may occur with urine scalding and contact dermatitis. These conditions have characteristic patterns that assist with diagnosis. Acariasis, pediculosis, and dermatophytosis are also associated with alopecia.

Foreign Body Pneumonia: Pneumoconiosis

Focal pulmonary lesions associated with aspirated food or bedding occur as an incidental finding, particularly in young guinea pigs. This has been observed in guinea pigs on various bedding materials, including wood products and rice straw. At necropsy, there may be foci of atelectasis or circumscribed nodules in the parenchyma of the lung, but frequently lesions are not detected on gross examination. On microscopic examination, plant fibers may be found lodged within small airways, with heterophilic and mononuclear cell infiltration. In lesions of some duration there may be focal granulomatous bronchiolitis and/or interstitial alveolitis, with mononuclear cell infiltration and foreign body multinucleated giant cell formation. Differential diagnoses include osseous metaplasia, lesions of primary bacterial or viral origin, focal mycotic lesions (e.g., *Aspergillus* spp.), and granulomatous pulmonary lesions associated with the subcutaneous administration of Freund's adjuvant.

Adjuvant-Associated Pulmonary Granulomas

Pulmonary granulomas may occur in guinea pigs and other rodents or rabbits following subcutaneous injection with complete Freund's adjuvant. Microscopic changes are characterized by multifocal granulomatous inflammatory response. Posterior paresis and osteolysis was observed in guinea pigs immunized subcutaneously with Freund's adjuvant. It was presumed that this condition resulted from inadvertent injection into epaxial muscles, with tracking of granulomatous inflammation into the spinal canal and bone. Pulmonary granulomata were also found. Differential diagnoses include perivascular lymphoid nodules, pneumoconiosis, and focal pneumonia due to infectious agents.

Osteoarthritis

Laboratory-housed Dunkin–Hartley guinea pigs are prone to development of osteoarthritis involving the femorotibial joints. Lesions become apparent by 3 months of age, and progress with age. Lesions involve focal degeneration of hyaline cartilage, osteophyte formation, and synovial proliferation and fibrosis. High levels of ascorbic acid accentuated the disease, apparently through activation of TGF-beta. Wild guinea pigs have been shown to have no osteoarthritis in the knee joints, and it is unknown what the prevalence may be in the pet population.

Gastrointestinal Diseases
Chelitis

Inflammation of the oral labia and rhinarium is common in guinea pigs, and appears to be associated with acidic diets. The lesions manifest as serous excoriations, and may become secondarily infected with *S. aureus* or other opportunistic organisms.

Malocclusion: "Slobbers"

This condition may involve the incisors, as well as the molar and premolar teeth in guinea pigs. As elodont teeth, they grow continuously throughout life, and good opposition is required to prevent overgrowth. If the alignment is defective, maxillary teeth may overgrow labially and the mandibular teeth overgrow medially. Excessive salivation, inanition, and wasting occur in severely affected animals. Nutritional factors have

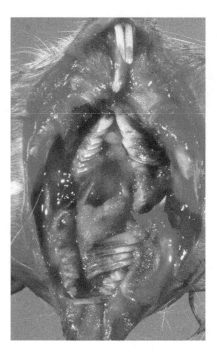

FIG. 5.47. *Malocclusion and overgrowth of cheek teeth.*

been implicated, and fluorosis has been associated with this condition. However, there is evidence that genetic factors play an important role in this disease. There may be a single gene involved, or more than 1 gene with incomplete penetrance. The incidence is higher in some inbred strains. At necropsy, cheek teeth have irregular contours and sharp edges on their occlusal surfaces (Fig. 5.47). In tooth abnormalities attributed to fluorosis, lesions were characterized by impairment of dentin and enamel formation and by excessive wear. Abnormalities of this type are not evident in typical cases of malocclusion.

Gastric Dilatation and Volvulus

Multiple cases of acute gastric dilatation associated with gastric volvulus have been recognized in a colony of guinea pigs, and it occurs sporadically in other facilities. Frequently, affected animals were found dead, with no previous indication of disease. Typical cases had a 180° rotation along the mesenteric axis, and stomachs are distended with fluid and gas. Death has been attributed to respiratory impairment and possibly vascular shock.

Gastric Ulcers

Gastric ulceration is common in guinea pigs, and appear to be precipitated by a number of infectious and other nonspecific stressors.

Intestinal Hemosiderosis

Accumulations of hemosiderin-laden macrophages in the lamina propria of the intestine, particularly large bowel, are a common finding in the guinea pig. There is speculation that this is due to subclinical scurvy, but

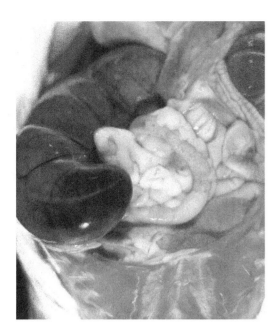

FIG. 5.48.   *Cecal volvulus in an adult guinea pig. The cecum is hemorrhagic and infarcted due to torsion of vascular supply.*

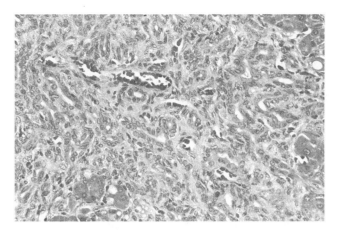

FIG. 5.49.   *Liver from an adult guinea pig with marked bile ductular proliferation and portal fibrosis.*

some believe that it is due to the normally zealous iron-uptake and binding of herbivores with diets containing excess iron.

Cecal Volvulus

Deaths due to cecal torsion are occasionally observed in this species. At necropsy, the displaced organ is edematous, hemorrhagic, and distended with fluid and gas (Fig. 5.48). Cecal volvulus has been known to occur in association with impaction and may be precipitated by typhlitis of various causes.

Anorectal Impaction

Impaction of the perineal sac region with feces, sebaceous secretions, and bedding material is common in older boars, resulting in occlusion of the anus and inability to defecate. It has been claimed to be related to muscle atony.

Prolapsed Rectum

As with other species, rectal prolapse may occasionally occur in association with inflammatory conditions of the large intestine.

Focal Hepatic Necrosis

Multifocal coagulation necrosis of the liver is occasionally seen at necropsy. Affected areas tend to be subcapsular in distribution, with minimal or no inflammatory response. They are frequently interpreted to be a terminal event and may be due to hypoxic change secondary to impaired blood flow in the region. Differential diagnoses include bacterial hepatitis (e.g., Tyzzer's disease) and toxic change.

Chronic Idiopathic Cholangiofibrosis

Periportal fibrosis with bile ductular proliferation is occasionally seen in adult guinea pigs as an enzootic problem in individual colonies. Lesions are characterized by hepatocyte degeneration, proliferation of cholangioles, and interstitial fibrosis (Fig. 5.49). The changes are suggestive of a toxin-induced change, but the etiopathogenesis has not been resolved.

Hepatic Contusions

Capsular rupture of the liver, with hemorrhage into the peritoneal cavity, is occasionally observed at necropsy. Traumatic lesions of this type may be caused by events such as mishandling or falls. Multiple simultaneous cases of hepatic contusions should alert investigation into inappropriate restraint of struggling guinea pigs by an inexperienced handler.

Fatty Infiltration of the Pancreas

Interstitial infiltration of adipose tissue occurs in the pancreas in older guinea pigs as a normal part of the aging process. The proportion of the exocrine pancreas decreases with age, with no apparent impairment of function. Histologically, there are large areas of adipose tissue interposed between normal pancreatic tissue. Fatty infiltration can also occur within the islets (Fig. 5.50).

Urogenital Diseases
Nephrosclerosis: Chronic Renal Disease

Irregularly pitted, granular renal cortices are a common finding at necropsy, particularly in guinea pigs that are at least a year of age. It is usually an incidental finding, but lesions may be extensive enough to result in renal insufficiency. Pathogenesis has not been resolved. The renal lesions have been interpreted to be the result of a general vascular disturbance, resulting in focal areas of ischemia and fibrosis. Using immunohistochemical techniques, glomerular changes were evaluated in guinea pigs collected from several sources. Spontaneous

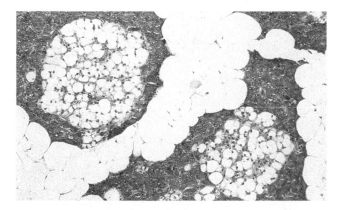

FIG. 5.50. *Pancreas of an adult guinea pig with fatty infiltration of the interstitium and lipidosis of islet cells. These common changes can occur independently or together in individual animals.*

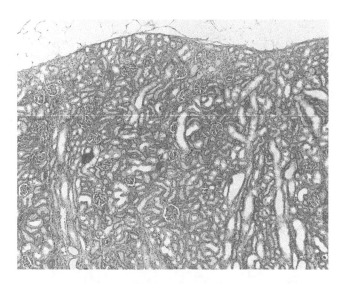

FIG. 5.52. *Early nephrosclerosis in a guinea pig. Note the segmental distribution of tubular degeneration with depression of the renal capsule.*

deposits of IgG and complement (C3) were demonstrated along the mesangial and peripheral glomerular basement membranes. It was suggested that the antigen–antibody complexes might be due to an infectious agent or endogenous tissue antigen. An accelerated disease process (and an increased incidence) has been observed in guinea pigs fed an unusually high protein diet. Mild hypertension has been recorded in affected guinea pigs.

Pathology

Multiple, granular, pitted areas may be visible on the surface of the kidney, resulting in irregular contours in severely affected animals (Fig. 5.51). On cut surface, pale linear streaks extend into the cortex, with some involvement of the medulla in advanced lesions. On microscopic examination, there is segmental to diffuse-tubular degeneration and interstitial fibrosis, with distortion and obliteration of the normal architecture (Fig. 5.52). Tubular lesions are concentrated primarily in the convoluted tubules and Henle's loop. Scattered tubules are dilated and lined with poorly differentiated, cuboidal to squamous epithelial cells. Some nephrons, interpreted to be nonfunctional, consist of tubular remnants lined by poorly differentiated cuboidal epithelium with lightly

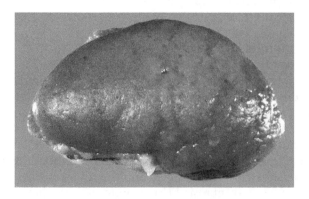

FIG. 5.51. *Kidney from an aged guinea pig with chronic nephrosclerosis. The cortical surface is finely granular and pitted.*

eosinophilic to amphophilic cytoplasm. Tubules are occasionally dilated and contain proteinaceous material and cellular debris. In nephrons interpreted to be fully functional, convoluted tubules are lined by hypertrophied epithelial cells with abundant, eosinophilic cytoplasm. Most glomeruli are essentially normal histologically. Occasionally, there is atrophy of individual glomeruli, with regional fibrosis. In advanced lesions, there is diffuse to segmental infiltration with fibroblasts and collagenous tissue formation. There are minimal focal aggregations of mononuclear cells consisting mainly of lymphocytes. Arterioles and arteries may have moderate medial hypertrophy, sometimes with prominent endothelial lining cells. High BUN and serum creatinine, nonregenerative anemia, and low urinary-specific gravity are clinical findings in animals with advanced nephrosclerosis.

Cystitis and Urolithiasis

Urinary tract infections occur occasionally, particularly in older sows. This may be due to the proximity of the urethral orifice to the anus in females, with fecal contaminants such as *E. coli*. At necropsy, changes may vary from thickening of the bladder mucosa with congestion in chronic cases to intramural and/or intraluminal hemorrhage in animals with acute cystitis. Microscopic changes seen in chronic cases are characterized by leukocytic infiltration in the lamina propria, and occasionally fibroblast proliferation. In acute cases, there may be ulceration, hemorrhage, and infiltration with heterophils. Most cases have some degree of accompanying pyelonephritis. Cystitis often occurs in concert with urolithiasis. Urinary calculi occur frequently in older sows, and less commonly in older boars. They vary from sand-like crystals to large concentric stones. They are typically composed of calcium carbonate.

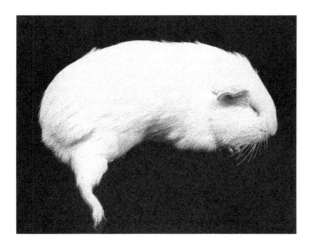

FIG. 5.53. *Unilateral posterior paresis in a postpartum sow due to obturator nerve damage during parturition.*

Urolithiasis may cause obstructive uropathy, with urethral plugging in males, hydroureter, and hydronephrosis.

Male Genitourinary Diseases
In addition to obstructive uropathy and nephrosclerosis, boars are prone to accumulation of detritus in their prepuce, resulting in balanoposthitis. Older boars are prone to impaction of perineal gland secretions and other debris. Seminal vesiculitis also occasionally occurs. Guinea pigs, like other rodents, ejaculate a copulatory plug, which may cause urethral obstruction.

Disorders of Pregnancy
In addition to pregnancy toxemia, the exceptionally large fetuses at term may result in dystocia, particularly in older sows with incomplete relaxation of the pubic ligament. Obturator nerve paralysis can be a consequence of dystocia (Fig. 5.53). The large gravid uterus is prone to torsion, and ectopic pregnancies have been rarely observed in sows, which in some cases were related to uterine rupture. Stillbirth is common in guinea pigs, and the incidence may be particularly high among inbred strains, which has been shown to occur at a rate of 28.4% in strain 13 guinea pigs.

Ovarian Cysts
Cystic rete ovarii are extremely common in older sows, with 1 report documenting a prevalence of 75% in sows over 18 months of age. Bilateral ovarian involvement is very frequent (Fig. 5.54), but when unilateral, the right ovary appears to be more commonly involved. Small ovarian cysts less than 1 mm in diameter may be present on the ovaries of younger females, but they are frequently missed at necropsy. In older sows, thin-walled, fluid-filled, fluctuant cysts up to 2 cm in diameter may be present on the ovaries. Cysts may be much larger, and present clinically as abdominal distention. Smaller cysts are usually concentrated in the cephalic pole near the

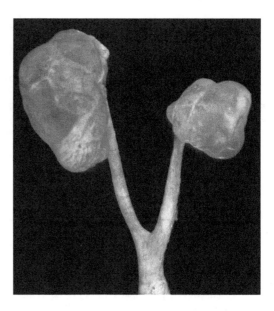

FIG. 5.54. *Reproductive tract from an aged guinea pig sow, illustrating bilateral cystic rete ovarii. Large, fluid-filled cysts are on the surface of both ovaries.*

hilus of the ovary. Occasionally, there is a single large cyst, with no recognizable ovarian tissue. Cysts contain clear, serous fluid. On microscopic examination, cysts are of variable size and are lined by low cuboidal to columnar epithelial cells. Solitary cilia or tufts of cilia are present on the luminal surface of some cells. Depending on the size of the cysts, there may be marked compression of the ovarian tissue, and in advanced cases only remnants of the ovary remain. Serial sections have revealed continuity between rete ovarii, follicles, and ovarian mesothelium, and the large serous cysts appear to develop from the rete ovarii.

Cystic rete ovarii have been associated with reduced reproductive performance in sows at 15 months of age and older. The most common clinical sign is bilateral symmetrical alopecia over the flank region (see "Fig. 5.46"), and there may be crusting of the skin around the nipples. Sows may manifest atypical sexual behavior. Cystic endometrial hyperplasia, mucometra, endometritis, and leiomyomas are the other changes associated with cystic rete ovarii.

Considerably less common, follicular cysts may also occur in sows. Cysts develop from preovulatory follicles, and can be differentiated from cystic rete by their lining of granulosa cells. The rarest form of ovarian cysts are paraovarian cysts, which consist of tubules arising from remnants of the mesonephric duct.

BIBLIOGRAPHY FOR MISCELLANEOUS DISORDERS

Gerold, S., Huisinga, E., Iglauer, F., Kurzawa, A., Morankic, A., & Reimers, S. (1997) Influence of feeding hay on the alopecia of breeding guinea pigs. *Zentralblatt fur Veterinarmedizin A* 44:341–348.

Hill, W.A., Boyd, K.L., Ober, D.P., Farrar, P.L., & Mandrell, T.D. (2006) Posterior paresis and osteolysis in guinea pigs (*Cavia porcellus*) secondary to Freund's adjuvant immunization. *Journal of the American Veterinary Medical Association* 45:53–56.

Muto, T. (1984) Spontaneous organic dust pneumoconiosis in guinea pigs. *Japanese Journal of Veterinary Science* 46:925–927.

Schiefer, B. & Stunzi, H. 1979. Pulmonary lesions in guinea pigs and rats after subcutaneous injection of complete Freund's adjuvant or homologous pulmonary tissue. *Zentralblatt fur Veterinarmedizin A* 26:1–10.

Singh, B.R., Alam, J., & Hansda, D. (2005) Alopecia induced by salmonellosis in guinea pigs. *Veterinary Record* 156:516–518.

Osteoarthritis
Bendele, A.M. & Hulman, J.F. (1989) Spontaneous cartilage degeneration in guinea pigs. *Arthritis and Rheumatism* 31:561–565.

Bendele, A.M., White, S.L., & Hulman, J.F. (1988) Osteoarthritis in guinea pigs: histopathologic and scanning electron microscopic features. *Laboratory Animal Science* 39:115–121.

Jimenez, P.A., Glasson, S.S., Trubestskoy, O.V., & Haimes, H.B. (1997) Spontaneous osteoarthritis in Dunkin Hartley guinea pigs: histologic, radiologic, and biochemical changes. *Laboratory Animal Science* 47:598–601.

Kraus, V.B., Huebner, J.L., Stabler, T., Flahiff, C.M., Setton, L.A., Fink, C., Vilim, V., & Clark, A.G. (2004) Ascorbic acid increases the severity of spontaneous knee osteoarthritis in a guinea pig model. *Arthritis and Rheumatism* 50:1822–1831.

Gastrointestinal Diseases
Hard, G.C. & Atkinson, F.F.V. (1967) "Slobbers" in laboratory guinea pigs as a form of chronic fluorosis. *Journal of Pathology and Bacteriology* 94:95–104.

Lee, K.J., Johnson, W.D., & Lang, C.M. (1977) Acute gastric dilatation associated with gastric volvulus in the guinea pig. *Laboratory Animal Science* 27:685–686.

Rest, J.R., Richards, T., & Ball, S.E. (1982) Malocclusion in inbred strain-2 weanling guineapigs. *Laboratory Animals* 16:84–87.

Smith, M.W. (1977) Staphylococcus cheilitis in the guinea-pig. *Journal of Small Animal Practice* 18:47–50.

Urogenital Diseases
Alves, D.A. (2012) Pathology in Practice. *Journal of the American Veterinary Medical Association* 241:185–187.

Araujo, P. (1964) A case of ectopic abdominal pregnancy in guinea pig. *Laboratory Animal Care* 14:1–5.

Bean, A.D. (2013) Ovarian cysts in the guinea pig (*Cavia porcellus*). *Veterinary Clinics of North America Exotic Animal Practice* 16:757–776.

Doyle, R.E., Sharp, G.C., Irvin, W.S., & Berck, K. (1976) Reproductive performance and fertility testing in strain 13 and Hartley guinea pigs. *Laboratory Animal Science* 25:573–580.

Hawkins, M.G., Ruby, A.L., Drazenovich, T.L., & Westropp, J.L. (2009) Composition and characteristics of urinary calculi from guinea pigs. *Journal of the American Veterinary Medical Association* 234:214–220.

Hong, C.C. & Armstrong, M.L. (1978) Ectopic pregnancy in 2 guinea pigs. *Laboratory Animals* 12:243–244.

Keller, L.S.F. & Lang, C.M. (1987) Reproductive failure associated with cystic rete ovarii in guinea pigs. *Veterinary Pathology* 24:335–339.

Kunstyr, I. (1981) Torsion of the uterus and the stomach of guinea pigs. *Zeitschrift fur Versuchstierkunde* 23:67–69.

Nielsen, T.D., Holt, S., Ruelokke, M.L., & McEvoy, F.J. (2003) Ovarian cysts in guinea pigs: influence of age and reproductive status on prevalence and size. *Journal of Small Animal Practice* 44:257–260.

Peng, X., Griffith, J.W., & Lang, C.M. (1990) Cystitis, urolithiasis and cystic calculi in aging guinea pigs. *Laboratory Animals* 24:159–163.

Pliny, A. (2014) Ovarian cystic disease in guinea pigs. *Veterinary Clinics of North America Exotic Animal Practice* 17:69–75.

Quattropani, S.L. (1977) Serous cysts in aging guinea pig ovary: light microscopy and origin. *Anatomical Record* 188:351–360.

Steblay, R.W. & Rudofsky, U. (1971) Spontaneous renal lesions and glomerular deposits of IgG and complement in guinea pigs. *Journal of Immunology* 107:1192–1196.

Takeda, T. & Grollman, A. (1970) Spontaneously occurring renal disease in the guinea pig. *American Journal of Pathology* 40:103–117.

Wood, M. (1981) Cystitis in female guinea pigs. *Laboratory Animal Science* 15:141–143.

NEOPLASMS

Spontaneous tumors are rare in guinea pigs under 3 years of age and uncommon even in older animals. There appear to be variations in genetic susceptibility to spontaneous neoplasia. A thorough review of neoplastic diseases of the guinea pig was provided by Manning (1976).

Cutaneous Neoplasia

Trichoepitheliomas/trichofolliculomas are the most common tumors of the skin (Fig. 5.55). These tumors contain multiple discrete epithelial structures reminiscent of hair bulbs and keratinized structures reminiscent of hair sheaths. Cutaneous papillomas, sebaceous gland adenomas, penile papillomas, lipomas, fibrosarcomas, fibromas, and carcinomas have also been described.

Mammary Neoplasia

Mammary adenocarcinomas occur in both male and female guinea pigs. The majority are interpreted to be of ductal origin. Metastases may occur to regional lymph nodes. Some are of low-grade malignancy and remain localized to the original site. Other mammary tumors

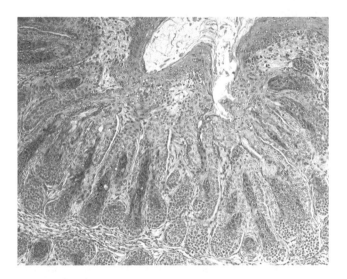

FIG. 5.55.   *Trichofolliculoma in the skin of an aged guinea pig. Note the aggregations of follicular structures that are typical of these tumors.*

include mammary gland adenoma and malignant mixed mammary tumor.

Pseudo-odontoma: Odontoma
Pseudo-odontomas arise rarely from the elodont tooth roots of rabbits and rodents, including guinea pigs (see Rabbit Chapter 6, "Pseudo-odontoma"). They consist of disorganized epithelial and mesenchymal elements of tooth origin that are well differentiated. They are not true neoplasms, but are rather believed to be hamartomas.

Cavian Leukemia
On rare occasions, lymphoid leukemia occurs as a spontaneous disease in various inbred and noninbred strains of guinea pigs. Cases are most frequently seen in young adult animals. Leukocyte counts in the peripheral blood are relatively high, varying from 50,000 to over 200,000/mm^3. Leukemia has been produced experimentally with transplanted cells and cell-free filtrates. Leukocytosis (up to 180,000 mm^3 or greater) with a preponderance of lymphoblastic cells is the typical picture seen in blood samples. At necropsy, lymph nodes, such as cervical (Fig. 5.56), axillary, mesenteric, and inguinal, are enlarged and firm, homogeneous, and tan on the cut surface. There is marked splenomegaly and hepatomegaly. Microscopically, there is usually moderate to marked infiltration of lymphoblastic cells in the spleen, liver, bone marrow, interstitium of the lung, thymus, alimentary tract lymphoid tissue, heart, eyes, and adrenals. Guinea pig leukemia is associated with, but not necessarily caused by, an endogenous retrovirus. The primary differential diagnosis for cervical lymphadenomegaly is *S. equi* subsp. *zooepidemicus*.

Respiratory Tract Neoplasia
Pulmonary tumors represented approximately 35% of reported tumors in 1 survey. The majority were benign papillary adenomas, and most were interpreted to be of bronchogenic origin. The changes were similar to those produced by certain infectious agents, and it was suggested that there may be hyperplastic and adenomatous changes in airways and alveoli in response to various stimuli, not bona fide primary pulmonary tumors. Small, white, circumscribed nodules, visible macroscopically, on microscopic examination consist of papillary structures lined by a single layer of hyperchromatic cuboidal epithelium. Primary malignant tumors of the lung are rare in guinea pigs. Nasal adenocarcinoma is another malignancy reported to occur in this species.

Reproductive Tract Neoplasia
Tumors of the reproductive tract represent approximately 25% of spontaneous tumors in this species. Of the ovarian tumors, granulosa cell tumors occur, but the majority are teratomas. A variety of tissue types may be evident in teratomas, including ciliated and mucous epithelial cells, striated muscle, and cells of ectodermal origin. These tumors should not be confused with cystic rete ovarii seen commonly in older sows. Uterine tumors are primarily benign and of mesenchymal origin. Most are leiomyomas (Fig. 5.57) or fibromas. Rarely, malignant uterine tumors such as myxosarcomas or leiomyosarcomas have been described. Primary malignant uterine tumors consist of poorly differentiated mesenchymal cells, with extension into the peritoneal cavity. Tumors of the male reproductive system are very rare.

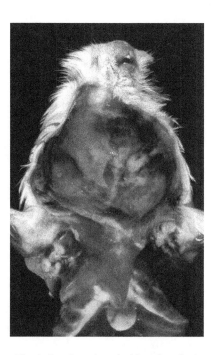

FIG. 5.56. *Massively enlarged cervical lymph nodes in a guinea pig with lymphoid leukemia.*

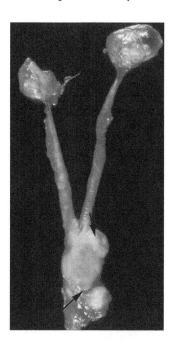

FIG. 5.57. *Uterine leiomyoma (arrows) in an aged guinea pig sow with concomitant cystic rete ovarii. The leiomyoma consists of a multilobulated mass at the uterocervical junction with extension into the vaginal area.*

Endocrine and Cardiovascular Neoplasia

Tumors of the endocrine system in guinea pigs include benign adrenocortical tumors and insulinomas. Neurologic signs were observed in animals with insulinomas, and Cushing's syndrome has been observed in guinea pigs with adrenocortical adenomas. Although rarely observed in laboratory guinea pigs, thyroid adenomas and carcinomas have been reported to be common among pet guinea pigs. Benign mixed tumors (myxomas) are the most commonly reported tumors of the cardiovascular system. They may include well-differentiated mesenchymal components, such as cartilage, bone, and fat. Primary myocardial tumors should not be confused with rhabdomyomatosis.

Other Neoplasms

Other neoplasms include bile duct tumors, undifferentiated carcinoma, lipomas, fibrosarcoma, and histiocytic lymphosarcoma.

BIBLIOGRAPHY FOR NEOPLASMS

Andrews, E.J. (1976) Mammary neoplasia in the guinea pig (*Cavia porcellus*). *Cornell Veterinarian* 66:82–96.

Field, K.J., Griffith, J.W., & Lang, C.M. (1989) Spontaneous reproductive tract leiomyomas in aged guinea pigs. *Journal of Comparative Pathology* 101:287–294.

Franks, L.M. & Chesterman, F.C. (1962) The pathology of tumours and other lesions of the guinea pig lung. *British Journal of Cancer* 16:696–700.

Gibbons, P.M., Garner, M.M., & Kiupel, M. (2013) Morphological and immunohistochemical characterization of spontaneous thyroid gland neoplasms in guinea pigs (*Cavia porcellus*). *Veterinary Pathology* 50:334–342.

Hong, C.C., Liu, P.I., & Poon, K.C. (1980) Naturally occurring lymphoblastic leukemia in guinea pigs. *Laboratory Animal Science* 30:222–226.

Jungeblut, C.W. & Opler, S.R. (1967) On the pathogenesis of cavian leukemia. *American Journal of Pathology* 51:1153–1160.

Kitchen, D.N., Carlton, W.W., & Bickford, A. (1975) A report of fourteen spontaneous tumors of the guinea pig. *Laboratory Animal Science* 25:92–102.

Manning, P.J. (1976) Neoplastic diseases. In: *The Biology of the Guinea Pig* (eds. J. E. Wagner & P. J. Manning), pp. 211–225. Academic Press, San Diego.

Opler, S.R. (1967) Pathology of cavian leukemia. *American Journal of Pathology* 51:1135–1147.

Suarez-Bonnet, A., de las Mulas, M., Millan, M.Y., Herraez, P., Rodriguez, F., & de los Monteros, A.E. (2010) Morphological and immunohistochemical characterization of spontaneous mammary gland tumors in the guinea pig (*Cavia porcellus*). *Veterinary Pathology* 47 (2): 298–305.

Williams, B. (2012) Non-infectious diseases. In: *The Laboratory Rabbit, Guinea Pig, Hamster, and Other Rodents* (eds. M. A. Suckow, K. A. Stevens, & R. P. Wilson), pp. 685–704. Elsievier, London.

Zwart, P., van der Hage, M.H., Mullink, W.M.A., & Cooper, J.E. (1981) Cutaneous tumors in the guinea pig. *Laboratory Animals* 15:375–377.

6 Rabbit

INTRODUCTION

This chapter is focused not only on laboratory rabbits but also on commercially raised rabbits and pet rabbits. It is difficult to draw the line on what diseases to cover, since many institutions obtain laboratory rabbits from commercial vendors that raise rabbits for other purposes. In addition, many sources of rabbits are raised out of doors, which increases the potential for infectious disease transmission from wild rabbits. If a disease has been documented in laboratory rabbits, or if there is a potential for encountering a particular disease in laboratory rabbits, it is covered herein.

Members of the order Lagomorpha have a worldwide distribution, and consist of 2 living families, including Ochotonidae (pikas) and Leporidae (rabbits and hares). There are several species of New World rabbits, including *Sylvilagus* spp. In addition, several species of hares (*Lepus* spp.) occupy both the New and the Old World. *Sylvilagus* and *Lepus* are not covered in this text, except when they relate to *Oryctolagus*. The only species of this order to have been domesticated is *Oryctolagus cuniculus*, which originated from wild European progenitors whose native range is the Iberian peninsula. This region is populated by 2 subspecies of wild rabbits, *O. cuniculus* ssp. *algirus* and *O. cuniculus* ssp. *cuniculus*. Domestic rabbits are genetically derived from *O. cuniculus* ssp. *cuniculus*. The exceptional phenotypic variation and ease with which to create new breeds of domestic rabbits exemplifies the limited gene pool among domestic rabbits. Recent genetic analysis of several rabbit breeds suggest a single origin of domestication in France approximately 1,500 years ago, which correlates with historical evidence of domestication within French monasteries. Two successive genetic bottlenecks appear to have taken place, with development of most modern breeds 200 years ago. Rabbits are raised extensively for meat production, which is estimated to yield over 1 million tons per year worldwide, and they are also popular as pets. The American Rabbit Breeders Association recognizes 47 breeds and the British Rabbit Council recognizes 50 breeds, with numerous varieties. It is estimated that there are over 200 breeds worldwide. One such breed is the Belgian hare, which is an *O. cuniculus* bred to phenotypically resemble hares. A small number of nondomesticated European hares are bred in captivity in different parts of Europe. Laboratory rabbits are most often albino New Zealand White (NZW) and Dutch (Dutch Belted) breeds. There are a small number of inbred rabbit strains (which are difficult to maintain due to inbreeding depression), several rabbit lines with unique genetic traits that lend themselves to research such as the Watanabe rabbit (heritable hypercholesterolemia), and growing numbers of transgenic rabbits. Rabbits are used extensively for cardiovascular research, as well as production of polyclonal antiserum.

BEHAVIORAL, PHYSIOLOGIC, AND ANATOMIC FEATURES

Behavioral Features

Adult male rabbits are called "bucks," females "does," and infants "kits." Bucks must be kept separately, as they will fight to the death. Aggressive bucks may also traumatize does when breeding. Does are induced ovulators, and do not have overt estrus cycles, although they have periodic intervals of receptivity. These periods can be detected by reddened vulvas, and conception rate is highest during this time. Following parturition (kindling), does leave their nest and return to nurse their altricial kits only once or twice daily. Prior to parturition, does create nests lined with fur plucked from their dewlaps, causing prepartum alopecia. Does can conceive almost immediately following kindling. Pseudopregnancy is common, and can be induced by a variety

Pathology of Laboratory Rodents and Rabbits, Fourth Edition. Stephen W. Barthold, Stephen M. Griffey, and Dean H. Percy.
© 2016 John Wiley & Sons, Inc. Published 2016 by John Wiley & Sons, Inc.

of stimuli, including mounting by other does, sterile matings by bucks, or bucks housed nearby. Female rabbits may be aggressive to unrelated litters of kits. Does, particularly nervous primiparous does, are prone to infant cannibalism. Rabbits engage in cecotrophy, or reingestion of soft mucus-coated "night feces." Cecotrophs are relatively high in protein and B complex vitamins. Rabbits are frequently nervous and easily frightened. When alarmed, rabbits may freeze (tonic immobility), run to shelter, or thump their hind feet as a group warning. Careful, firm handling, including support of the hind legs, is essential to avoid unrestrained kicking, which may result in accidental fracture of the vertebral column. Confined rabbits may exhibit various patterns of stereotypic behavior, barbering, obesity, and compulsive self-mutilation, particularly of digits. Rabbits mark their territory with urine, feces, scent glands, and by rubbing their chins (mental glands) on surfaces. The primary means of thermoregulation is through countercurrent blood exchange of ear vessels, panting, and salivation, all of which are inefficient. Thus, heat stroke is a significant problem for rabbits in hot climates. Wild rabbits effectively thermoregulate by living in burrows (warrens).

Physiologic Features

Serum calcium levels up to 16 mg/dl are normal in rabbits. In contrast to most mammals in which intestinal calcium absorption is regulated according to metabolic needs, calcium is absorbed by rabbits in proportion to the amount in the diet, and intestinal uptake is not influenced by vitamin D. Serum calcium regulation is achieved through renal excretion. In rabbits, the renal fractional calcium excretion is 45%, compared to 2% in most mammals. Renal disease can, therefore, directly result in hypercalcemia, as well as through secondary hyperparathyroidism. Rabbits are very sensitive to hypercholesterolemia, since they are unable to increase sterol excretion in response to excess cholesterol in their diet. They exhibit hypercholesterolemia within days of being fed high-cholesterol diets, which has contributed to the use of rabbits for atherosclerosis research.

The rabbit gastrointestinal system is unique among herbivores. Their system is designed for maximal utilization of protein and vitamin-rich products of cecal fermentation while differentially eliminating indigestible fibrous waste. This is accomplished by a complex process that allows elimination of fibrous feces and reingestion of nutrient-rich cecotrophs. During the digestive process, fine digestible materials are retropulsed from the upper colon back into the cecum, while larger indigestible material is directed into the colon and passed as feces. This is facilitated by the spiral valve of the cecum, the taeniae of the haustrated upper colon, and the fusus coli, a ganglionic structure that separates the upper and lower colon. The fusus coli is known as the "pacemaker" of the rabbit intestine, and orchestrates the complex motility of the

hind gut that is critical to cecotrophy. This separation of digestible from nondigestible material facilitates the act of cecotrophy. Soft, mucous-covered cecotrophs (night feces) are selectively passed from the cecum to the anus during the act of coprophagy. Cecotrophs are major sources of B vitamins and protein, which are absorbed in the small intestine. Their mucous coating protects them as they pass through the acidic environment of the stomach.

The major driving force of the rabbit digestive process is the presence of indigestible fiber, and lack thereof is a common cause of gastrointestinal disorders in rabbits. Intensive commercial production of rabbits has contributed to many of the gastrointestinal disorders in them. High-carbohydrate/low-fiber diets are deleterious to the digestive process. Pelleted diets should be supplemented with a source of fiber (hay). Perturbation of the microbiome by dietary and husbandry practices arises in a number of conditions, which precipitate severe and difficult to reverse dysbiosis. A stable enteric microbiome is essential to the health of the rabbit. Enteric microflora are minimal in the small intestine. The large bowel is populated by strict anaerobic bacteria, particularly *Bacteroides* spp. and facultative anaerobic bacteria such as *Streptococcus spp.* and *Clostridium* spp. are sometimes present in low numbers. Suckling and weanling rabbits are particularly prone to gastrointestinal disease. The cecal microbiota evolves from a simple and unstable microbiome after birth into a complex and stable community in sub-adult rabbits. The microbiome is a critical determinant of susceptibility to pathogens. For example, colonization of the ileum with segmented filamentous bacteria significantly inhibits colonization by enteropathogenic *Escherichia coli*. An understanding of rabbit gastrointestinal disease is best approached with an understanding of rabbit gastrointestinal physiology. An excellent review of rabbit gastrointestinal physiology is available (see R. & J.A.E Rees Davies).

Anatomic Features
External Features

Rabbits have 5 toes on their front feet and 4 toes on their rear feet, with dense fur on their rear foot pads. They may shed the fur 3 or 4 times a year, with hair growth cycles generally starting at the ventrum, growing dorsally and posteriorly, but regrowth may occur in irregular patchy configurations, which are obvious when the fur is clipped (Fig. 6.1). Rabbits develop folds of skin beneath their chins, known as dewlaps, which are especially prominent in mature does. The ear represents approximately 12% of the body surface area in domestic rabbits. Their size and accessible vessels make them ideal for venipuncture from the lateral veins, or collecting arterial blood from the central artery. Rabbits have inguinal and anal scent glands, as well as mental (chin) scent glands for territorial marking.

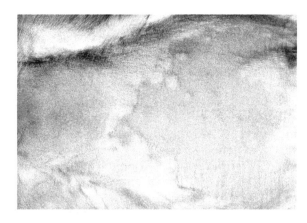

FIG. 6.1. Hair growth cycles generally start at the ventrum, progressing dorsally and posteriorly, but regrowth may often occur in irregular patchy configurations following clipping of the fur.

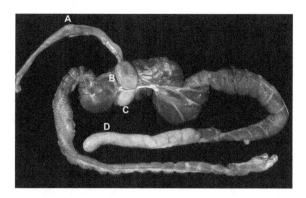

FIG. 6.2. Alimentary tract from a mature rabbit, illustrating the prominent gut-associated lymphoid tissue (GALT), including a Peyer's patch (A) in the wall of the ileum, the sacculus rotundus (B) at the terminal ileum, the cecal tonsil (C) in wall of the proximal cecum, and the cecal appendix (D) at the terminus of the cecum.

Central Nervous System

An incidental finding in normal rabbits is the presence of adipocytes in the interstitium of the choroid plexus.

Hematology/Clinical Chemistry

Erythrocytes are approximately 6.5–7.5 μm in diameter, and tend to be smaller in young rabbits. Polychromasia and anisocytosis are common, with 2–5% reticulocytosis. The mean life span for erythrocytes is relatively short, ranging from 57 to 67 days. The counterpart of the neutrophil in rabbits is termed the heterophil. Heterophils are 9–15 μm in diameter and have distinct, acidophilic cytoplasmic granules. Experts have suggested that the neutrophil name should be retained in rabbits, since the characteristics of this cell resemble neutrophils more closely than the true heterophils that are seen in avian species. Eosinophils are 12–16 μm in diameter, with large cytoplasmic granules that stain a dull pink-orange with conventional hematology stains. Basophils may be relatively numerous and occasionally represent up to 30% of circulating leukocytes. Lymphocytes are usually the predominant leukocyte in the peripheral blood. Small lymphocytes are approximately 7–10 μm in diameter; large lymphocytes vary from 10 to 15 μm in diameter and may have a few azurophilic cytoplasmic granules. Normal hemogram and clinical chemistry ranges are published elsewhere. However, it is notable that rabbits tend not to develop leukocytosis, even with chronic bacterial infections.

Lymphoid System

Rabbits have a unique immunoglobulin repertoire. There is no evidence of IgD in rabbits. They possess a single IgG class that can activate complement as well as bind to Fcγ receptors, and the rabbit germline encodes 13 IgA isotypes, 2 of which are not expressed because of defective promoter regions. The thymus does not regress with age. Development of the primary antibody repertoire of rabbits occurs between 4 and 8 weeks of age, during which the VDJ genes of nearly all B cells undergo

somatic diversification within the gut associated lymphoid tissue (GALT). Thus, rabbit GALT functions in a manner similar to the Bursa of Fabricius in birds. In addition, this process is dependent upon select species of normal intestinal microflora, which drive gene diversification in a nonantigen-dependent manner.

The GALT represents over 50% of the total mass of lymphoid tissue in the body, which accounts for the relatively small spleen in this species. The GALT includes Peyer's patches of the small intestine, as well as structures that are unique to the rabbit. The *sacculus rotundus* is a spherical, thick-walled enlargement of the terminal ileum at the ileocecal junction (Fig. 6.2). The adjacent cecum has a round patch of lymphoid tissue called the *cecal tonsil*. The tip of the cecum contains the prominent thick-walled cecal appendix. These lymphoid structures contain aggregates of organized lymphoid tissue in the lamina propria and submucosa. A common incidental finding in rabbits is the presence of large histiocytes filled with particulate debris in the follicular centers of the GALT (Fig. 6.3).

Transfer of maternal immunoglobulins from dam to kit is mediated predominantly in utero through yolk sac receptors, although postnatal transfer also occurs from birth to 12 days of age. Passively transferred immunoglobulin begins to wane around 3 weeks of age.

Cardiovascular System

The right chambers of the heart are relatively thin-walled, and a frequent postmortem finding is a quantity of clotted blood in the right ventricle, with no evidence of postmortem contraction. The right atrioventricular valve, which is tricuspid in most mammals, is bicuspid in rabbits.

Respiratory System

Rabbits are obligate nasal breathers, and exhibit marked dyspnea when nasal passages are obstructed. The rabbit lung does not contain respiratory bronchioles. Airways

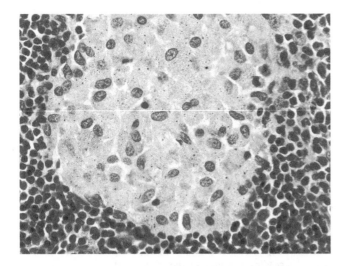

FIG. 6.3.   *GALT from a normal mature rabbit, depicting the common presence of histiocytes filled with refractile particulate debris within the follicular center.*

terminate in vestibules that contain alveoli. Pulmonary arteries are enveloped in a prominent smooth muscle layer, which can be misinterpreted as hypertrophy (Fig. 6.4).

Gastrointestinal System

Rabbits have a dental formula of I2/1, C0/0, P3/2, M3/3, with continuously growing (elodont) incisors as well as cheek teeth. Lagomorphs have 4 upper incisors, including peg teeth aligned directly behind the upper front incisors. Rarely, rabbits may congenitally lack peg teeth, but can function well as long as there is not malocclusion. Although not generally noticed, rabbits have diphyodont dentition (deciduous and permanent teeth). Deciduous teeth are shed around birth, including a third pair of incisors, lateral to the upper incisors. As

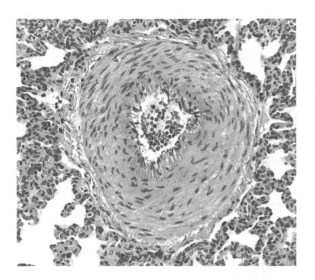

FIG. 6.4.   *Pulmonary artery of a normal rabbit. Pulmonary arteries are highly muscular, which can be misinterpreted as muscular hypertrophy.*

with other herbivores, rabbits have a large and relatively complex digestive system, which is a challenge to dissect at necropsy. The stomach is thin-walled and typically contains approximately 15% of the ingesta present in the alimentary tract. The small intestine is short compared to that in many species, representing roughly 12% of the total volume of the gastrointestinal tract. Brunner's glands are distributed throughout the length of the duodenum. The bile and pancreatic ducts have separate openings into the duodenum. The cecum typically holds around 40% of the ingesta present in the digestive system. The colon consists of 2 major segments, the craniad portion being haustrated with prominent muscular taeniae. The mucosal surface of the proximal upper colon has multiple wart-like projections (warzen) that increase surface area. The lower colon lacks haustra and taeniae. These regions of the colon are divided by a region known as the fusus coli, which is 4–5 times thicker than the lower colonic wall, and contains aggregates of ganglia, which are involved in the highly coordinated digestive process.

The intestinal mucosa is endowed with copious numbers of goblet cells, which occupy the depths of crypts to the tips of villi. This is often misdiagnosed as goblet cell hyperplasia. In the liver, hepatocytic vacuolation associated with glycogen accumulation is a variable finding in rabbits fed with commercial diets. As in rodents, aged rabbit livers may feature polykarya, anisokarya, and intranuclear invagination of cytoplasm. The rabbit liver secretes biliverdin, rather than papilla, and rabbits produce copious amounts of bile compared to other species. The pancreas is a poorly defined collection of lobules adjacent to the duodenum.

Urogenital System

Once rabbits begin eating solid rations, the alkaline urine normally contains large quantities of dull yellow to brown ammonium magnesium phosphate and calcium carbonate monohydrate crystals. Occasionally, normal rabbit urine may be dark red to orange, which is due to porphyrins. Hyperpigmented urine has also been associated with elevated levels of urobilin, the oxidative product of urobilinogen. Pigmented urine must be differentiated from hematuria, which may arise due to uterine adenocarcinoma, uterine polyps, endometrial venous aneurysms, cystitis, urinary bladder polyps or tumors, pyelonephritis, and renal infarction with hemorrhage. Rabbit kidneys have a single papilla, and ectopic glomeruli can be frequently found in the medulla and peripelvic regions.

The rabbit has a bicornuate uterus comprised of 2 separate uterine horns and 2 cervices (Fig. 6.5). Placentation is hemochorial and bidiscoidal. Neonatal rabbits receive most of their maternal antibody via transplacental transfer during pregnancy. Both anterior and breach deliveries are normal. The testes of bucks descend at around 12 weeks of age, but inguinal canals remain

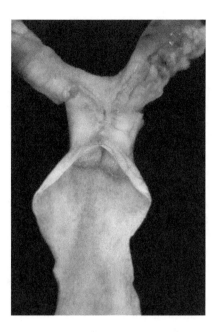

FIG. 6.5. *Female reproductive tract of a normal doe, depicting the 2 separate cervices, which is typical for this species. The uterus is bicornuate, with 2 separate horns.*

open and testes can be retracted abdominally. Scrotums are hairless. Testes may undergo seasonal involution, which may involve abdominal retraction, with testicular size reduced up to one-half their normal size. During this phase, spermatid giant cells and atrophic changes may be apparent microscopically. Seasonal infertility may occur in bucks in hot climates.

Musculoskeletal System

In the domestic rabbit, bones are relatively fragile. The skeleton of New Zealand White rabbits represents approximately 6–7% of the total body weight. On the other hand, skeletal muscle constitutes over 50% of the body weight in this species. Fractures, particularly those of the vertebral column, readily occur, particularly when the hind legs are not restrained properly during handling.

BIBLIOGRAPHY FOR BEHAVIORAL, PHYSIOLOGIC, AND ANATOMIC FEATURES

Carneiro, M., Alfonso, S., Geraldes, A., Garreau, H., Bolet, G., Boucher, S., Tircazes, A., Queney, G., Nachman, M., & Ferrand, N. (2011) The genetic structure of domestic rabbits. *Molecular Biology and Evolution* 28:1801–1816.
Christensen, N.D. & Peng, X. (2012) Rabbit genetics and transgenic models. In: *The Laboratory Rabbit, Guinea Pig, Hamster, and Other Rodents* (eds. M.A. Suckow, K.A. Stevens, & R.P. Wilson), pp. 165–193. Academic Press, London.
Clark, M.R. (1997) IgG effector mechanisms. *Chemical Immunology* 65:88–110.
Clauss, M., Burger, B., Liesegang, A., Del Chicca, F., Kaufmann-Bart, M., Riond, B., Hassig, M., & Hatt, J.-M. (2011) Influence of diet on calcium metabolism, tissue calcification and urinary sludge in rabbits (*Oryctolagus cuniculus*). *Journal of Animal Physiology and Animal Nutrition* 96:798–807.
Combes, S., Michelland, R.J., Monteils, V., Cauquil, L., Soulie, V., Tran, N.U., Gidenne, T., & Fortun-Lamothe, L. (2011) Postnatal development of the rabbit caecal microbiota composition and activity. *FEMS Microbiology and Ecology* 77:680–689.
Crossley, D.A. (1995) Clinical aspects of lagomorph dental anatomy: The rabbit (*Oryctolagus cuniculus*). *Journal of Veterinary Dentistry* 12:137–140.
Heczko, U., Abe, A., & Finlay, B.B. (2000) Segmented filamentous bacteria prevent colonization of enteropathogenic *Escherichia coli* O103 in rabbits. *Journal of Infectious Diseases* 181:1027–1033.
Mage, R. G., Lanning, D., & Knight, K.L. (2006) B cell and antibody repertoire development in rabbits: the requirement of gut-associated lymphoid tissues. *Developmental and Comparative Immunology* 30:137–153. MediRabbit.com
Naff, K.A. & Craig, S. (2012) The domestic rabbit, *Oryctolagus cuniculus*: origins and history. In: *The Laboratory Rabbit, Guinea Pig, Hamster, and Other Rodents* (eds. M.A. Suckow, K.A. Stevens, & R.P. Wilson), pp. 157–163. Academic Press, London.
Peri, B.A. & Rothberg, R.M. (1996) Transmission of maternal antibody prenatally and from milk into serum of neonatal rabbits. *Immunology* 57:49–53.
Rees Davies, R. & Rees Davies, J.A.E. (2003) Rabbit gastrointestinal physiology. *Veterinary Clinics of North America Exotic Animal Practice* 6:139–153.
Sohn, J. & Couto, M.A. (2012) Anatomy, physiology, and behavior. In: *The Laboratory Rabbit, Guinea Pig, Hamster, and Other Rodents* (eds. M.A. Suckow, K.A. Stevens, & R.P. Wilson), pp. 195–215. Academic Press, New York.
Suckow, M.A., Brammer, D.W., Rush, H.G., & Chrisp, C. (2002) Biology and diseases of rabbits. In: *Laboratory Animal Medicine*, 2nd edn (eds. J.G. Fox, L.C. Anderson, F.M. Loew, & F.W. Quimby), pp. 329–364. Academic Press, New York.
Suckow, M.A. & Schroeder, V. (2010) *The Laboratory Rabbit*, Laboratory Animal Pocket References. CRC Press, Boca Raton, FL.
Tsunenari, I. & Kast, A. (1992) Developmental and regressive changes in the testes of the Himalayan rabbit. *Laboratory Animals* 26:167–179.
Washington, I.M. & Van Hoosier, G. (2012) Clinical biochemistry and hematology. In: *The Laboratory Rabbit, Guinea Pig, Hamster, and Other Rodents* (eds. M.A. Suckow, K.A. Stevens, & R.P. Wilson), pp. 57–116. Academic Press, London.
Wells, M.Y., Weisbrode, S.E., Maurer, J.K., Capen, C.C., & Bruce, R.D. (1988) Variable hepatocellular vacuolization associated with glycogen in rabbits. *Toxicologic Pathology* 16:360–365.

DNA VIRAL INFECTIONS

Adenovirus Infection

Adenoviral enteritis has been documented in commercial rabbits in Hungary. Peak losses occurred at 6–8 weeks of age. Profuse diarrhea was observed in severely affected animals, with low mortality. There was a dramatic increase in the numbers of *E. coli* in the small intestine and cecum in rabbits that succumbed to the disease, suggesting a contributing role in pathogenesis. Severely affected animals were dehydrated, with fluid contents in the cecum. The adenovirus was isolated from the intestinal wall and gut contents, spleen, kidney, and lung when inoculated onto rabbit kidney cell cultures. A significant rise in adenoviral antibody levels was detected in convalescent sera. To date, confirmed cases of adenoviral enteritis in rabbits appear to be confined to Europe, although naturally occurring seroconversion to bovine adenovirus (type 1) antigen has been detected in meat rabbits from multiple commercial colonies in Quebec, Canada.

Herpesvirus Infections

There are 4 known herpesviruses of rabbits, known as leporid herpesvirus (LHV) -1, -2, -3, and -4. LHV-1, -2, and -3 belong to the subfamily Gammaherpesvirinae, whereas LHV-4 belongs to the genus Simplex of the subfamily Alphaherpesvirinae. In addition, rabbits are naturally susceptible to *Human herpesvirus* 1 (*Herpes simplex* 1). Among the 4 rabbit herpesviruses, LHV-1 (cottontail herpesvirus) and LHV-3 (*Herpesvirus sylvilagus*) are indigenous to *Sylvilagus* rabbits and do not infect *Oryctolagus* rabbits. They are covered in this chapter because they are traditionally listed among rabbit viruses. LHV-2 and LHV-4 naturally infect domestic rabbits, but only LHV-4 has clinical significance.

Leporid Herpesvirus 1 and 3 Infection

Both LHV-1 and LHV-3 were isolated from primary kidney cell cultures of weanling cottontail (*Sylvilagus*) rabbits. LHV-3 enjoyed a brief period of interest as a model of human Epstein-Barr virus infection. Inoculation of young cottontail rabbits with *H. sylvilagus* (LHV-3) by the parenteral route produces a chronic infection with persistent viremia and atypical lymphocytosis. Within 6–8 weeks following inoculation, changes consistent with a lymphoproliferative disease are observed grossly and microscopically. Histological examination reveals alterations that vary from lymphoid hyperplasia to lymphoma. Other lesions include myocarditis, interstitial pneumonia, and myositis. In the malignant form of the disease, diffuse infiltration of various tissues with immature lymphocytes commonly occurs. Although *H. sylvilagus* replicates in kidney cells prepared from the domestic rabbit, attempts to infect New Zealand White rabbits with the virus have been unsuccessful. No disease has been reported in cottontail rabbits naturally infected with LHV-1, and no attempts to infect domestic rabbits with LHV-1 have been reported.

Leporid Herpesvirus 2 Infection

LHV-2 has also been termed "Virus III" and *Herpesvirus cuniculi*. The virus was originally discovered during serial testicular transfer following inoculation of blood from a human varicella patient, and subsequently isolated from rabbit cell kidney cultures. It appears to be a subclinical infection among seropositive rabbits under natural conditions, but experimental intracerebral inoculation results in nonsuppurative encephalitis with intranuclear inclusion bodies.

Leporid Herpesvirus 4 Infection

Systemic infections with a LHV-4 have been observed in several commercial rabbitries in Canada. Outbreaks have mysteriously occurred among isolated rabbit populations, as well as following introduction of outside rabbits to rabbitries. The disease, which affects animals of various ages, is characterized by sudden onset with mortality up to 30%, with highest mortality among young rabbits.

Animals are frequently found dead, with no previous evidence of illness. Clinical signs include anorexia, conjunctivitis, periocular and facial swelling, subcutaneous swellings, respiratory distress, diarrhea, and abortion. Additional gross findings include disseminated cutaneous hemorrhagic macules, pulmonary congestion and edema, hydrothorax, hydropericardium, and multifocal hemorrhage in spleen, kidney, stomach, and intestine. Microscopic findings include multifocal necrohemorrhagic lesions in skin (Fig. 6.6), spleen, adrenals, stomach, intestine, heart, kidney, uterus, and liver. Pulmonary hemorrhage and edema are prominent. Intranuclear eosinophilic and amphophilic inclusions are present in multiple tissues, particularly respiratory epithelium, and multinucleate syncytia are present in some affected tissues (Fig. 6.7). Experimental intranasal inoculation resulted in periocular swelling, facial dermatitis, oculonasal discharge, and severe necrohemorrhagic bronchopneumonia. Inclusion bodies and syncytia were noted in multiple tissues. Notably, encephalitis has not been found in affected rabbits. Differential diagnosis must rule out caliciviral infection (rabbit hemorrhagic disease), but LHV-4 can be readily differentiated by the presence of characteristic intranuclear inclusion bodies and syncytia. Periocular swelling and acute death may also mimic myxomatosis, which is associated with intracytoplasmic pox viral inclusions. The sporadic incidence and severity of the disease suggest that rabbits may not be the natural host for this virus. LHV-4 is closely related to bovine herpesvirus 2, which infects a variety of ruminant species. No serosurveys have been performed among domestic rabbits.

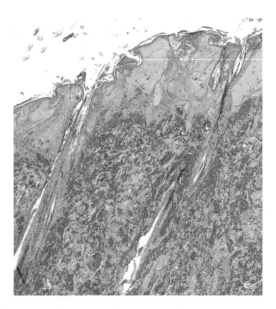

FIG. 6.6. *Integument from a rabbit with leporid herpesvirus 4 infection, depicting necrosis of the epidermis and papillary dermis with underlying dermal hemorrhage. (Source: Brash et al. 2010. Reproduced with permission from Canadian Veterinary Medical Association.)*

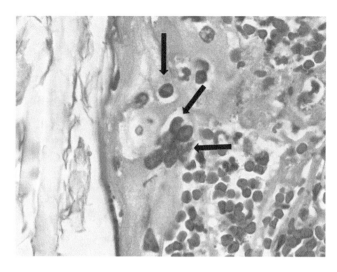

FIG. 6.7. *Leporid herpesvirus 4 infection of the skin from a rabbit, depicting a multinucleate syncytium and intranuclear inclusion bodies (arrows) in the follicular epithelium. (Source: Brash et al. 2010. Reproduced with permission from Canadian Veterinary Medical Association.)*

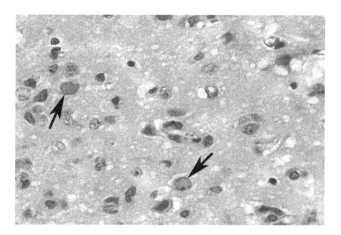

FIG. 6.9. *Cerebrum from a rabbit with naturally acquired herpes simplex virus encephalitis. Note the prominent intranuclear inclusion bodies in neurons (arrows) and astroglia.*

Herpes Simplex Virus Infection

For decades, domestic rabbits have served as an animal model for experimental *Human herpesvirus-1* (*Herpes simplex*-1 virus) encephalitis. Sporadic naturally occurring cases of fatal encephalitis due to *H. simplex* virus infection have been observed in pet rabbits. Affected rabbits may present with conjunctivitis (Fig. 6.8) and neurologic signs. Necropsy reveals nonsuppurative meningoencephalitis with neuronal necrosis and prominent amphophilic intranuclear inclusion bodies in neurons and astroglial cells (Fig. 6.9). Lesions in other organs have not been described. Typical herpesvirus particles have been observed in affected cells by electron microscopy, and *H. simplex*-1 has been confirmed as the

causative agent. Contact with humans infected with *H. simplex* virus has been documented in most reported cases in rabbits.

Lapine Parvovirus Infection

A parvovirus has been isolated from clinically normal rabbits in Japan. In a serological survey of commercial rabbits, approximately 60% of animals evaluated had antibody to lapine parvovirus. Oral or intravenous inoculation of 1 month old rabbits with lapine parvovirus resulted in transient depression and anorexia, with no mortality. The virus could be isolated from a variety of organs for up to 2 weeks postinoculation and from the small intestine on day 30 postinoculation. On microscopic examination, a mild to moderate enteritis was present in the small intestine, with exfoliation of enterocytes. In a survey of laboratory rabbits from commercial and private sources in the United States, the majority had relatively high antibody titers to lapine parvovirus. In addition, lapine parvovirus has been isolated from the kidneys of neonatal rabbits. The role (if any) of lapine parvovirus in the enteritis complex is currently unknown.

Necrotic hepatitis associated with a parvovirus was reported in Mexico in 1989. Rabbits also had splenic necrosis, and microinfarctions in the myocardium, kidney, and lung believed to be associated with intravascular coagulation. These lesions were reminiscent of rabbit hemorrhagic disease (RHD), but affected rabbits also had severe segmental necrosis of the small intestinal crypts and villi, which is not a feature of RHD. Furthermore, liver lesions contained intranuclear paracrystalline arrays of parvoviral-like virions by electron microscopy, and intranuclear staining with monoclonal antibodies against porcine parvovirus and murine parvovirus (MVM) was present. No other reports of this syndrome have been published, and this case may have been due to activation of parvovirus during the course of an RHD epizootic.

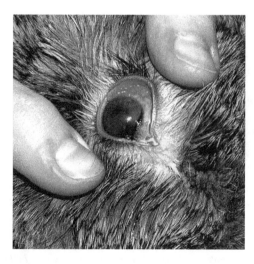

FIG. 6.8. *Acute conjunctivitis in a rabbit naturally infected with herpes simplex virus infection following transmission from an infected human. (Source: Muller et al. 2009. Reproduced with permission from the American Veterinary Medical Association.)*

Papillomavirus Infections

Papilloma viruses were once classified as members of the family Papoviridae that included 2 genera, *Papillomaviruses* and *Polyomaviruses*, which differ in size, biology, and DNA sequence. That family has been eliminated and papilloma viruses are now classified within the family Papillomaviridae. Rabbits can be infected with 2 papilloma viruses, cottontail rabbit papillomavirus (CRPV) and rabbit oral papilloma virus (ROPV), both of which belong to the genus *Kappapapillomavirus*. Both of these viruses are used as experimental models of papilloma virus pathogenesis and immunity in the laboratory rabbit.

Cottontail Rabbit Papillomavirus (CRPV) Infection

CRPV, which is also known as Shope papilloma virus, is native to New World *Sylvilagus* spp. rabbits, although *Oryctolagus* is experimentally and naturally susceptible to infection. Papillomaviruses cannot be propagated in cell culture, but infectious clones of viral DNA are extensively used to induce experimental infection of laboratory rabbits.

Epizootiology and Pathogenesis

Primarily a benign disease of cottontail rabbits, papillomatosis due to CRPV has occurred in spontaneous outbreaks among domestic rabbits. Insect vectors are the usual means of mechanical spread of the virus from cottontail rabbits to domestic rabbits, and ticks are important for infection among *Sylvilagus* rabbits. When the CRPV is inoculated into *Oryctolagus* rabbits, it produces papillomas with a high incidence (75%) of progression to squamous cell carcinomas. Transformation to carcinomas also occurs in *Sylvilagus*, but to a lesser degree. Papillomas induced by this virus in *Oryctolagus* rabbits produce minimal or no infectious virus, in contrast to papillomas induced in the natural *Sylvilagus* host or in hares (*Lepus* spp.). Papillomas typically undergo immune-mediated resolution if they do not progress to carcinomas. Host immunity has been shown to have 2 distinct targets: virus structural antigens, invoking protection against virus reinfection, and tumor antigens, invoking papilloma regression. If rabbits are immunized against the virus, viral immunity does not affect papilloma status, and rabbits remain susceptible to induction of papillomas with infectious DNA. Once tumors have undergone immune-mediated regression, rabbits resist both virus and DNA challenge. Virus DNA can remain latent, with no histologic changes in the epidermis, until nonspecific irritants activate the formation of papillomas.

Pathology

Naturally occurring papillomas on *Orycolagus* rabbits occur most frequently on the eyelids and ears, which are sites most often accessed by insects. Papillomas

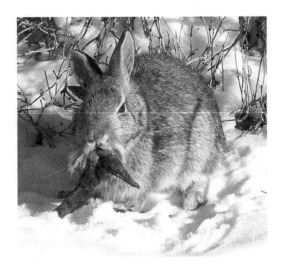

FIG. 6.10. *Multiple cutaneous papillomas (horns) projecting from the lips of a* Sylvilagus *rabbit naturally infected with cottontail rabbit papilloma virus (CRPV). (Source: Flicker © C Forry wd45/364229280.)*

consist of a pedunculated, cornified surface overlying a fleshy central core. Papillomas in *Sylvilagus* rabbits vary in size and number, up to numerous large cutaneous horns that debilitate the host (Fig. 6.10). Papillomas due to CRPV, which arise in naturally infected *Oryctolagus* rabbits, tend to be small and few in number (Fig. 6.11). Histologic findings are consistent with squamous papilloma. In those tumors that progress to malignancy, squamous cell carcinomas are locally invasive as well as metastatic to regional lymph nodes and lung. Differential diagnosis must discriminate from spontaneous nonviral papillomas, which tend to arise in haired skin.

Rabbit Oral Papillomavirus (ROPV) Infection

ROPV is distinct from CRPV. The natural host of ROPV is the *Oryctolagus* rabbit. Like CRPV, ROPV is also used as an experimental model for papilloma virus pathogenesis

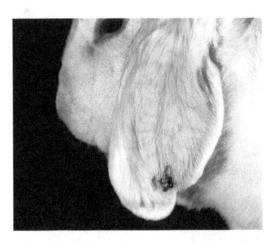

FIG. 6.11. *Solitary papilloma on the ear of a laboratory rabbit naturally infected with cottontail rabbit papilloma virus (CRPV). Since CRPV papillomas arise in an abnormal host (domestic rabbit), these tumors do not support virus replication and are prone to malignant transformation.*

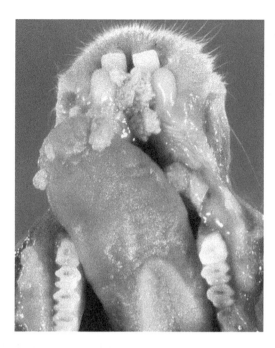

FIG. 6.12. *Oral papillomas involving the tongue and gingiva of a juvenile New Zealand White rabbit naturally infected with rabbit oral papilloma virus. These lesions undergo regression with no tendency toward malignancy.*

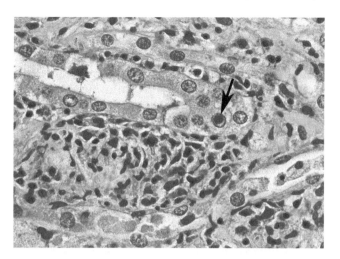

FIG. 6.13. *Intranuclear inclusion body (arrow), found as an incidental finding in the renal tubular epithelium of an adult New Zealand White rabbit. These inclusions are suspected to be due to an uncharacterized polyomavirus.*

and immunity. Natural infection is common among domestic rabbits, and infection is spread by direct contact, including from does to their kits.

Lesions most frequently occur in rabbits between 2 and 18 months of age. Pedunculated and sessile lesions are most commonly found along the ventral aspect of the tongue (Fig. 6.12), but may also involve other areas of oral and labial mucosa. These papillomas usually regress spontaneously within a few weeks. They are typical squamous papillomas on microscopic examination. Persistent papillomas of the conjunctiva have also been attributed to ROPV. Basophilic intranuclear inclusions and viral antigen may be present in the stratum spinosum. There are no reports of malignant transformation of oral papillomas in rabbits. Viral DNA can be detected in oral swabs in rabbits without lesions, latent virus remains in epithelium following papilloma regression, and latent virus can be activated by nonspecific injury.

Polyomavirus Infection

Cottontail rabbits are frequently subclinically infected with rabbit kidney vacuolating virus, a nononcogenic member of the Polyomaviridae family. The virus was isolated from CRPV papillomas inoculated into primary kidney cultures derived from *Sylvilagus* rabbits. This virus has no known pathogenic effect in cottontail or domestic rabbits but can be a contaminant of papilloma virus stocks. Seroconversion to the virus has been found in *Sylvilagus* rabbits, but antibodies have not been detected against the virus in domestic rabbits. Intranuclear inclusions in renal tubular epithelium, consistent with

polyomavirus-like inclusions, may be seen as an incidental finding in domestic rabbits (Fig. 6.13), but their etiology has not been defined.

Poxvirus Infections

Rabbits are host to several poxviruses with considerable clinical significance. The family Poxviridae is divided into 2 subfamilies, Entomopoxvirinae (which infect insects) and Chordopoxvirinae (which infect mammals). The latter contains the *Leporipoxvirus* genus, which includes the lagomorph pathogens known as myxoma, rabbit fibroma, and hare fibroma viruses. These viruses, particularly myxoma and rabbit fibroma viruses, are closely related and are represented by a number of strains with an overlapping spectrum of virulence. Another *Leporipoxvirus* is squirrel fibroma virus, which is antigenically and genetically closely related to, but distinct from myxoma and rabbit fibroma viruses. Finally, rabbitpox virus is closely related to vaccinia virus in the *Orthopox* genus. A comprehensive review of poxviral infections of rabbits is available in Brabb and DiGiacomo (2012).

Myxoma Virus Infection: Myxomatosis

Myxomatosis was first recognized in laboratory *Oryctolagus* rabbits acquired for experiments in a South American laboratory in the late 19th century. The name "infectious myxomatosis" was used to denote the myxoid appearance of the subcutaneous masses associated with the disease. In the original cases described, the virus was believed to have been transmitted by insect vectors from the relatively resistant tropical forest rabbit (*S. braziliensis*). Myxomatosis was also recognized in North America in 1930, where outbreaks of the disease occurred in rabbitries in southern California. The brush rabbit (*S. bachmani*) has been implicated as the reservoir host in that area. Myxomatosis is enzootic in the western

United States, with sporadic cases spreading into domestic rabbits, and is also endemic in wild *Sylvilagus* and feral *Oryctolagus* rabbits in South and Central America. Around 1950, a highly virulent South American strain of myxoma virus was introduced into Australia in an effort to reduce (or eliminate) the overpopulation of feral *Oryctolagus cuniculus*, which had become a major economic problem in that country. Mortality rates of up to 99% subsequently dropped to around 25% within a few years. The dramatic reduction in mortality was related to natural selection for genetically resistant rabbits and the emergence of attenuated strains of the virus. In 1953, myxoma virus was released into France by a citizen who was disenchanted with the wild rabbit problem. The virus subsequently spread to other countries in western Europe, including England, where it is now a well-established enzootic among wild *Oryctolagus* rabbits. Transmission of the virus is usually mechanical and by arthropod vectors, primarily mosquitoes in the Americas and Australia and fleas in Europe, but also by direct contact and fomites. There is considerable variation in virulence among myxoma virus strains that have evolved from these events. Attenuated strains of myxoma virus and rabbit fibroma virus are used as live vaccines in Europe to protect commercially raised rabbits.

Pathology

Disease severity is highly variable, depending upon virus strain and host species. *Sylvilagus* rabbits (natural hosts) tend to be resistant, and develop localized cutaneous lesions similar to those induced by fibroma viruses. Following inoculation of *Oryctolagus* rabbits by an arthropod vector, viral replication results in the development of a primary subcutaneous myxoid mass, usually within 3–4 days. Within 6–8 days, mucopurulent conjunctivitis, facial edema, and multiple cutaneous skin masses (myxomas) are usually observed (Fig. 6.14), often involving the base of the ears. Swelling of the anogenital region is also common, with scrotal edema. In rabbits that die with a peracute form of the disease, the animal may be found dead, and other than redness of the conjunctiva, there may be no other

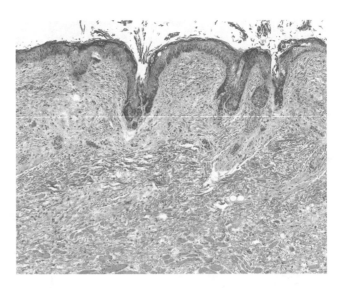

FIG. 6.15.   *Skin of a rabbit with myxomatosis. Note the blue-staining mucoid material in the superficial dermis.*

evidence of disease. Microscopically, there is dermal and subcutaneous proliferation of large, stellate mesenchymal cells (myxoma cells) interspersed within a homogeneous mucinoid matrix (Fig. 6.15), with a sprinkling of inflammatory cells. Hypertrophy and proliferation of endothelial cells occur, and changes in the epithelium overlying the lesions may vary from hyperplasia to degeneration. Intracytoplasmic inclusions are often present in the affected epidermis and in epithelial cells of the conjunctiva (Fig. 6.16), and in some cases may be found in respiratory epithelium. Remarkably, systemic changes are minimal, except lymphoid tissue. These include proliferation of alveolar epithelium, pulmonary hemorrhage, and orchitis in bucks. Myxoma virus is T lymphocytotropic, and viremic dissemination involves lymphocytes and monocytes, as well as rapid local dissemination to draining lymph nodes. Lymph nodes are initially enlarged with formation of syncytia

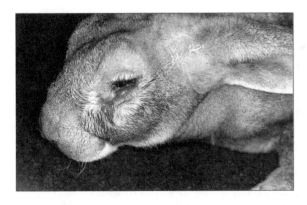

FIG. 6.14.   *Mucopurulent conjunctivitis, periocular swelling, and facial edema in a rabbit with myxomatosis.*

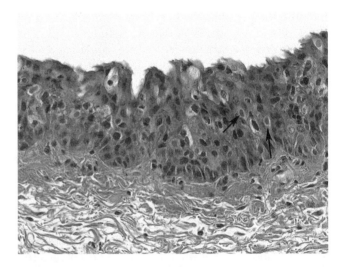

FIG. 6.16.   *Intracytoplasmic inclusion bodies (arrows) in the conjunctival epithelium of a rabbit with myxomatosis.*

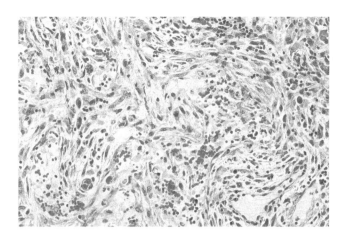

FIG. 6.17. *Lymph node of a rabbit with myxomatosis, depicting hypertrophy and hyperplasia of stellate myxoma cells and severe lymphocytic depletion.*

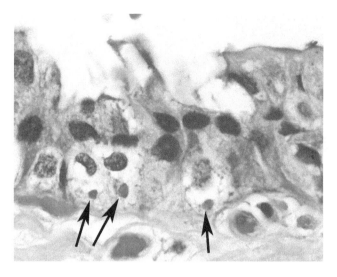

FIG. 6.18. *Intracytoplasmic inclusion bodies (arrows) in the respiratory epithelium of a rabbit with "amyxomatous" myxomatosis. (Source: S. Diab, University of California, Davis, CA. Reproduced with permission from S. Diab.)*

among apoptotic lymphoid cells, followed by marked lymphocytic depletion, particularly the T-cell zones. Affected lymph nodes, and to a lesser extent spleen, have hypertrophy and hyperplasia of stellate myxoma cells (Fig. 6.17), as well as focal necrosis, hemorrhage, and proliferative vasculitis. The cause of death in myxomatosis has never been fully defined, and suggested to be related to cytokine-mediated shock. Limited analysis of natural cases suggests that acute sepsis may contribute to mortality due to massive immunodeficiency. Mild disease may occur in rabbits inoculated with live attenuated vaccine strains, or partially immune-vaccinated rabbits exposed to myxoma virus. Under these circumstances, rabbits may develop nodular fibromatous masses of the conjunctiva.

"Amyxomatous" myxomatosis is also recognized, in which rabbits have minimal or small skin nodules, and present with respiratory signs. Rabbits develop pneumonia, and pox inclusions may be visualized in respiratory epithelium (Fig. 6.18). Presumably, this form of myxomatosis is spread through respiratory contact.

Rabbit Fibroma Virus Infection

Rabbit fibroma virus, also known as Shope fibroma virus, is closely related antigenically to myxoma virus and to the hare and squirrel fibroma viruses. Shope fibroma virus was first isolated from a cottontail rabbit (*S. floridanus*) in the United States in 1932. The virus is transmissible to *Oryctolagus* rabbits, producing localized fibromas. Shope fibroma virus infections are relatively widespread in wild cottontail rabbits in the eastern United States and Canada. Infection is usually a benign, self-limiting disease in the wildlife population. The virus may persist for several months within lesions, and mechanical transmission by arthropod vectors appears to be the primary means of spread. In rare occasions, fibromatosis has been diagnosed in commercial rabbitries. Wild cottontail rabbits in the area are the likely

reservoir host, with spread by insect vectors. In naturally infected cottontail and European rabbits, firm, flattened tumors occur on the legs and feet (Fig. 6.19), sometimes with involvement of the muzzle, periorbital, and perineal regions. These cutaneous tumors may be up to 7 cm in diameter, are usually freely movable, and may persist for several months, and then undergo spontaneous resolution. In young rabbits, fibromatous lesions may arise in abdominal viscera and bone marrow. There is localized fibroblast proliferation, with mononuclear and polymorphonuclear cell infiltration. Affected fibroblasts are characteristically fusiform to polygonal. In European domestic rabbits, subcutaneous masses may vary from myxoid in type to typical fibromas. Large, intracytoplasmic, eosinophilic inclusion bodies may be present in fibromatous cells (Fig. 6.20) and in epidermal cells overlying the tumors. The typical gross and histological appearance of the circumscribed masses should

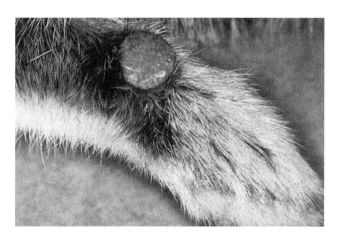

FIG. 6.19. *Nodular fibroma on the forelimb of a* Sylvilagus *rabbit naturally infected with Shope rabbit fibroma virus.*

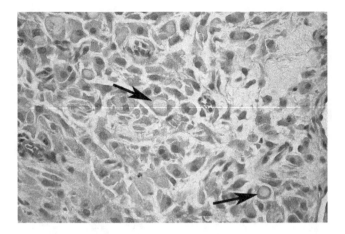

FIG. 6.20. *Skin of a* Sylvilagus *rabbit infected with Shope fibroma virus. There is a dense network of fusiform to polyhedral fibroblasts in the dermis, many of which contain prominent intracytoplasmic inclusion bodies (arrows).*

facilitate the differentiation of rabbit fibromatosis from myxomatosis and from the raised, horny, epidermal growths seen in papillomatosis. However, the myxoid forms sometimes seen histologically can be confused with myxomatosis. Considerable variation in microscopic appearance may occur.

Hare Fibroma Virus Infection
Hare fibroma virus is closely related to rabbit fibroma virus and myxoma virus and is an infection of European hares. Hare fibroma virus has been documented in European hares prior to the introduction of myxoma virus to Europe, and outbreaks have been documented in captive-bred European hares. Fibromatous lesions, 1–3 cm in diameter, typically arise on the ears and legs of affected hares, and spontaneously regress in adult hares. Lesions consist of large spindle and stellate cells with prominent intracytoplasmic inclusions. Virus is transmitted by insects and contact. Myxoma virus can also infect hares, resulting in formation of firm nodular cutaneous masses of the head, back, and limbs, which resemble hare fibroma virus-induced lesions.

Rabbitpox (Vaccinia) Virus Infection
Rabbit pox is relatively rare and has generally been associated with inadvertent exposure to vaccinia virus. Recent sequence analysis of rabbitpox virus has confirmed its close relationship to vaccinia virus. During outbreaks of rabbit pox, virus is highly contagious. It is readily transmitted by aerosol, with the respiratory tract being the primary site of replication, followed by viremic dissemination. Papular lesions may occur in the oropharynx, respiratory tract, spleen, and liver. In the "pockless" form, a few pocks were present in the oral cavity, and focal hepatic necrosis, pleuritis, and splenomegaly were observed. Histologic changes include disseminated focal necrosis with leukocytic infiltration in the skin and affected viscera, as well as necrosis of

lymphoid tissue. Because of the similarity to smallpox, rabbitpox virus has been used as a model of variola virus infection, thereby emphasizing the possibility of future outbreaks due to the marked ability of natural spread among susceptible rabbits.

RNA VIRAL INFECTIONS
Astrovirus Infection
Astroviruses are associated with gastroenteritis in children and a variety of mammals and birds. Astrovirus infection has been documented by PCR and gene sequencing in association with enteritis and mortality in young rabbits in the United States and Italy. It remains to be determined if astrovirus can be a primary pathogen in rabbits, as it is usually associated with other pathogens of the rabbit enteritis complex.

Borna Virus Infection: Borna Disease
Borna virus has a wide host range, and is particularly known to cause meningitis and encephalomyelitis in horses and sheep. Natural infection of rabbits has been documented in Europe, with demonstration of viral antigen in the brain. Experimental infection of laboratory rabbits results in encephalitic lesions with multifocal retinopathy preferentially involving the posterior pole of the eye.

Calicivirus Infections
Caliciviruses are highly significant pathogens of lagomorphs. Pathogenic caliciviruses encompass the *Lagovirus* genus (rabbit hemorrhagic disease virus and European Brown Hare syndrome virus) and the *Vesivirus* genus (rabbit *vesivirus*).

Rabbit Hemorrhagic Disease Virus Infection
RHD virus specifically infects *Oryctolagus* rabbits. *Sylvilagus* rabbits and hares are resistant to RHD virus infection, although European hares are afflicted with a closely related virus, European Brown Hare Syndrome (EBHS) virus. RHD was first recognized among rabbits imported from Germany into China in 1984. Within months, RHD virus killed over 140 million domestic rabbits in China, and subsequently spread to Korea. By the 1990s, RHD was reported in over 40 countries. RHD virus is endemic in wild rabbit populations throughout Europe, and RHD virus was iatrogenically introduced to Australia and New Zealand in the 1990s, where it is now endemic among wild rabbits. Sporadic outbreaks of RHD, often of unknown origin, have occurred among domestic rabbits in the Americas and northern Africa. RHD virus is believed to have emerged from avirulent endemic viruses circulating subclinically among European rabbit populations. Although rabbits appear to be specifically susceptible to RHD virus, viral RNA has been documented in small mammal species sympatric to wild rabbits.

RHD is a reportable disease in the United States. Aggressive depopulation of affected colonies is required. In Europe and other areas of the world where RHD virus is enzootic, vaccination is effective at protecting susceptible populations of rabbits, although new variants of the virus have been shown to cause RHD in vaccinated populations. Various types of vaccines are available, including heat-killed liver extracts, VP60 protein, and a recombinant myxoma-RHD live virus.

Epizootiology and Pathogenesis

RHD virus is highly contagious, and is spread through oro-fecal exposure, as well as environmental contamination and mechanical transmission by blood-feeding insects. RHD virus is highly resistant and stable in the environment. Rabbits that survive RHD may persistently shed virus, and subclinically infected carriers may exist. There are several genogroups of RHD virus, including many nonpathogenic strains that are endemic among wild rabbits. Serologic surveys of RHD-free domestic and wild rabbit populations in Europe have revealed a high frequency of RHD virus-seropositive rabbits, suggesting enzootic infection with nonpathogenic strains of the virus. Contact experiments with seropositive rabbits exposed to nonpathogenic RHD virus have also revealed seroconversion in the absence of clinical signs, whereas exposure of rabbits to pathogenic RHD virus-infected rabbits resulted in clinical disease. It is generally believed that pathogenic RHD virus arose from enzootically circulating nonpathogenic strains of the virus. New pathogenic variants of RHD virus, which are genetically closely related to nonpathogenic strains, have been documented. For example, an outbreak of disease resembling RHD was reported in Michigan, and the agent was found by sequence analysis to be related to "nonpathogenic" RHD strains.

RHD virus binds to carbohydrate moieties of host-cell histo-blood group antigens (HBGAs) that are expressed on the surface of upper respiratory and intestinal epithelium. Young rabbits weakly express one of these HBGAs, which is believed to be a possible mechanism by which rabbits less than 2 months of age are remarkably resistant to infection. Other susceptibility factors are involved, as hepatocytes are a major cellular target for RHD virus, but do not express HBGAs. The age-related resistance of young rabbits is also not absolute. Variant RHD virus strains have been associated with outbreaks in young rabbits on farms in Spain and Portugal where rabbits had been vaccinated, suggesting that these virus strains are antigenically distinct, but also have evolved to target alternate receptors. Furthermore, field strains of RHD virus in Australia have been shown to be more virulent than the original released strain, thereby overcoming host genetic resistance, and there is evidence that HBGA specificities have progressively shifted in virus strains that have evolved in France. Thus, RHD virus poses considerable challenges for control and prevention.

Pathology

The incubation period of RHD ranges between 1 and 3 days, and rabbits are typically moribund within 12–36 hours after onset of fever. Mortality may reach greater than 80% of adult rabbits. In peracute infections, no clinical signs may be apparent. Acute infections are manifest as anorexia, depression, conjunctival congestion, and neurologic signs. Tracheitis, dyspnea, and cyanosis, with foamy hemorrhagic epistaxis and ocular hemorrhage may be present. Subacute infections are milder, with some rabbits surviving, and a small percentage of rabbits may develop chronic disease that features anorexia, lethargy, and jaundice. Chronically infected rabbits usually succumb within 1–3 weeks, but may survive. At necropsy, there may be blood-stained nasal discharge, pulmonary hemorrhage and edema (Fig. 6.21), hepatomegaly with accentuated lobular pattern (Fig. 6.22), splenomegaly, perirenal hemorrhage, and serosal ecchymoses on areas such as pericardium and intestine. The major histopathologic lesion of RHD is acute necrotizing hepatitis (Fig. 6.23). Viral antigen can be found in hepatocytes within hours of infection. Viral antigen can also be demonstrated in Kupffer cells, macrophages of the spleen, pulmonary macrophages, kidney, and small intestine. Segmental necrotizing enteritis of the small intestine is a primary lesion, but is relatively minor compared to pathology in other

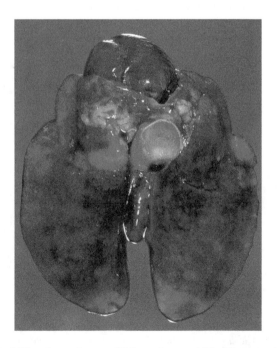

FIG. 6.21. *Lungs from a wild* Oryctolagus *rabbit with acute rabbit hemorrhagic disease (RHD) virus infection. There is marked pulmonary edema with multifocal ecchymoses.*

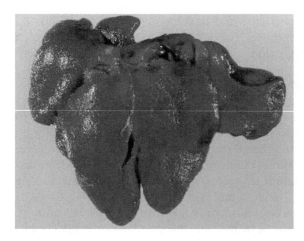

FIG. 6.22. *Liver from a domestic rabbit naturally infected with RHD virus. Note the granular texture of the hepatic capsule and accentuated lobular pattern. (Source: Bergin, I.L., et al. 2009. Reproduced from Centers for Disease Control and Prevention, a U.S. Government agency. http://wwwnc.cdc.gov/eid/page/copyright-and-disclaimers)*

organs. There is generalized lymphocytic depletion with immunosuppression. The major cause of death in RHD is massive disseminated intravascular coagulation (DIC). Fibrin thrombi are present in small vessels of multiple organs, including kidney, brain, adrenals, heart, testes, and lung (Fig. 6.24).

Diagnosis

Aside from the characteristic clinical signs and lesions, infection can be confirmed by PCR. RHD virus cannot be successfully grown in cell culture. The presence of calicivirus within rabbit populations can be evaluated by serology.

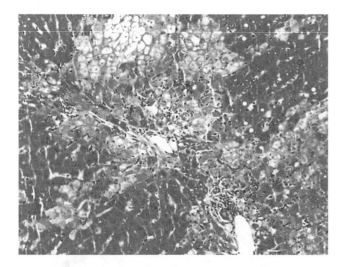

FIG. 6.23. *Liver from a rabbit experimentally infected with rabbit hemorrhagic disease virus. Note the acute periportal and midzonal hepatocellular necrosis. (Source: Bergin, I.L., et al. 2009. Reproduced from Centers for Disease Control and Prevention, a U.S. Government agency. http://wwwnc.cdc.gov/eid/page/copyright-and-disclaimers)*

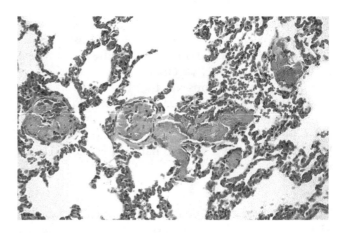

FIG. 6.24. *Lung from a case of RHD in a feral Oryctolagus rabbit from Australia. Note multiple intravascular thromboses (Source: M. Kabay.)*

European Brown Hare Syndrome Virus Infection

European Brown Hare Syndrome (EBHS) is caused by a virus that is closely related to RHD virus. The first outbreak of disease occurred in 1980 among hares in Sweden, and is now prevalent throughout Europe. EBHS virus is not infectious to *Oryctolagus* or *Sylvilagus* rabbits. The virus has been associated with outbreaks of high morbidity and mortality among farmed hares in Europe, as well as among multiple species of free-ranging hares in Europe. Adult animals experience the highest mortality, and animals less than 40 days of age are unaffected. Disease is characterized as acute necrotizing hepatitis and pulmonary hemorrhages, with DIC, reminiscent of RHD in rabbits. There is no vaccine available for EBHS prevention.

Rabbit Vesivirus Infection

Rabbit vesivirus has been observed in a small Oregon rabbitry. Its etiology was confirmed by electron microscopy and cultivated from the intestine of juvenile domestic rabbits with severe diarrhea and enteritis. Genetic analysis of the virus grouped it within a clade that contained a number of marine caliciviruses and a nonhuman primate calicivirus. As with most cases of rabbit enteritis, other agents including *E. coli* and coccidia likely contributed to disease severity. Oral inoculation of susceptible rabbits with cell culture (Vero cells)-grown virus resulted in subclinical seroconversion.

Coronavirus Infections

Coronaviruses are now divided into 4 genera: *Alpha-, Beta-, Gamma-,* and *Deltacoronavirus.* Based upon serologic evidence and recent genetic sequence analysis, rabbits have been shown to be infected with a member of the *Alphacoronavirus* genus (pleural effusion disease virus) and *Betacoronavirus* genus (rabbit enteric coronavirus). The family Coronaviridae also includes the subfamily Torovirinae. Toroviruses infect a variety of mammals, and have been associated with gastroenteritis in horses and cattle. Neutralizing antibodies against the equine torovirus, Berne virus, have been detected in clinically normal laboratory rabbits. The role of toroviruses in rabbit enteric disease is unknown.

Rabbit Enteric Coronavirus Infection

Enteritis has been reported in young rabbits from commercial rabbitries, as well as barrier-maintained laboratory rabbits in Europe and Canada. Serosurveys suggest that coronavirus infection is also present among rabbits in the United States, and recent studies have shown that infection is widespread among rabbits in China. Young rabbits 3–10 weeks of age appear to be most susceptible to enteritis, with mortality reaching 60% of affected rabbits. Experimental infection of susceptible rabbits resulted in transient and mild diarrhea. In natural outbreaks, animals are thin and dehydrated, with fecal staining of the perineal region. The cecum may be distended, containing watery, off-white to tan feces. Microscopic changes are confined to the small and large intestine. Villus blunting, vacuolation, and necrosis of enterocytes, mucosal edema, and polymorphonuclear and mononuclear leukocyte infiltration are characteristic findings. Coronaviral infection is likely to be complicated by other pathogens of the rabbit enteritis complex. The presence of typical coronaviral particles in the feces of young diarrheic rabbits is confirmatory. However, coronaviral particles have also been observed in the gut contents of subclinically infected animals. Although coronaviral enteritis may occur in the absence of identifiable copathogens, careful screening for concurrent infections with other pathogens is recommended.

Pleural Effusion Disease Virus: Coronaviral Cardiomyopathy

Pleural effusion disease and cardiomyopathy have been associated with coronaviral infections in laboratory rabbits in the United States and Europe. In the Scandinavian reports, pleural effusion was recognized in rabbits following inoculation with a coronavirus-contaminated stock of the Nichols strain of *Treponema pallidum*. The virus was related antigenically to human coronavirus strain 229E. Fatal infections were characterized by lymphoid depletion of the splenic follicles, focal degenerative changes in the thymus and lymph nodes, proliferative changes in glomerular tufts, and uveitis. In rabbits inoculated with material containing the same strain of *T. pallidum* in the United States, multifocal myocardial degeneration and necrosis were observed. Viral particles were demonstrated in the sera of infected rabbits postinoculation. Antibodies to 2 human strains of coronavirus were demonstrated in convalescent rabbit sera, and antigen was detected in myocardial lesions using antisera to human 229E coronavirus. There is no evidence that the causative agent occurs as a natural pathogen of rabbits.

Hepatitis E Virus Infection

Hepatitis E virus (HEV) is associated with acute hepatitis in humans. Five genotypes, consisting of a single serotype, have been identified in a variety of mammals: genotypes 1 and 2 are restricted to humans, and genotypes 3 and 4 are zoonotic, particularly in swine. HEVs closely related to genotype 3 have been isolated from commercially raised rabbits in China and the United States. The rabbit HEVs were infectious to other rabbits, swine, and macaques. HEV could be detected in serum, tissues and feces of inoculated rabbits, and acute necrotizing hepatitis was found in infected rabbits and macaques. In addition, rabbits are experimentally susceptible to infection with HEV genotypes 1 and 4. Although HEV is not likely to be associated with clinical disease in rabbits under natural conditions, these findings emphasize the potential zoonotic risk of HEV-infection in rabbits.

Paramyxovirus Infection

During the mid-1980s, a survey of laboratory rabbits in Japan revealed seroconversion to Sendai virus in over 50% of rabbits from a number of different colonies. Laboratory rabbits are susceptible to experimental Sendai virus infection, although viral replication appeared to be confined to the upper respiratory tract. Following intranasal inoculation with the MN strain of Sendai virus, there was transient viral shedding postinoculation, and animals seroconverted. Viral antigen was detected in the nasal epithelium for up to 10 days. Infected rabbits remained clinically normal throughout the study. Sendai virus is now rare or nonexistent among laboratory animals, but other paramyxoviruses may arise in the future. Acute fatal pneumonia was reported in a single dwarf rabbit from a small colony in Europe in which a paramyxovirus was incriminated, based upon ultrastructural findings. The rabbit developed acute interstitial pneumonia in which alveoli were filled with exfoliated lining cells, macrophages, and cellular debris. Rare multinucleate syncytia and eosinophilic inclusions were observed among detached alveolar lining cells.

Rabies Virus Infection

Rabies has been documented in several domestic rabbits in the United States, and both raccoon and skunk variants have been documented in infected rabbits. These cases serve to emphasize the importance of adequate protection for any pet animals with access to an outdoor environment.

Rotavirus Infection

Rotaviruses are divided into 5 species: A, B, C, D, and E. Group A rotaviruses are the most significant pathogens for both humans and animals, including rabbits. Within each rotavirus species, rotaviruses are classified based upon nucleotide sequences of 2 outer capsid proteins, VP7 (glycoprotein) and VP4 (protease-sensitive), which define the "G" and "P" genotypes. Rabbits rotaviruses are typically G3P[14] and G3P[22], although a bovine-like G6P[11] genotype rotavirus was recently found in a laboratory rabbit colony, but rabbits had no clinical signs of disease. Rotaviruses have been associated with diarrheal disease in domestic rabbits in Europe, Japan, and the United States.

Epizootiology and Pathogenesis
Rotavirus typically causes diarrhea among infant rabbits, since virus targets terminally differentiated enterocytes lining the tips of villi of the jejunum and ileum. Since neonatal bowels have a high number of terminally differentiated enterocytes with slow epithelial turnover kinetics, young rabbits are most susceptible to clinical disease. However, maternal antibody, if present, is protective at this early age. Serosurveys have confirmed that rotaviral infections are commonly endemic within domestic *Oryctolagus* rabbits, as well as among wild *Sylvilagus* and *Lepus* lagomorphs in Europe, Asia, and North America. Epidemiologic studies have indicated that protection may be afforded by transplacentally derived maternal antibodies, which subsequently decline to low levels in kits by 1 month of age. However, on exposure to the virus at 30–45 days of age, there may be sufficient residual antibody to protect kits from overt disease. Based on serological surveys, clinically healthy rabbits may have a subclinical infection at around 4 weeks, with subsequent rise in antibodies to rotavirus. In 1 epizootic of rotaviral enteritis in a specific-pathogen-free rabbitry, sucklings 1–3 weeks of age were affected. The disease was characterized by rapid spread, with high morbidity and mortality. This was consistent with the introduction of virus into a colony not previously exposed, thus with no maternal immunity to afford protection during the neonatal period. Virus shedding in diarrheic rabbits is frequently seen at 35–42 days of age. In addition to relatively mild lytic effects of virus infection, which may not be microscopically apparent, virus NSP4 induces a number of physiologic effects upon enterocytes, including chloride secretion, disruption of water reabsorption, disruption of disaccharidases, and activation of secretory reflexes of the enteric nervous system. Due to perturbation of disaccharidases, lactose and other disaccharides remain in the gut lumen, causing an osmotic drain and attracting fluid into the lumen. Viral infections of enterocytes may also facilitate bacterial adhesion to damaged cells. In weanling rabbits inoculated with an enteropathogenic strain of *E. coli*, superimposed rotaviral infections have been shown to have an additive effect, resulting in increased morbidity and mortality.

Pathology
On gross examination, animals may be dehydrated, and fluid contents are present in the cecum. Other organs are usually grossly normal. In the small intestine, lesions are generally mild, although there may be moderate to severe villus blunting, villus fusion, and vacuolation to flattening of apical enterocytes in the jejunum and

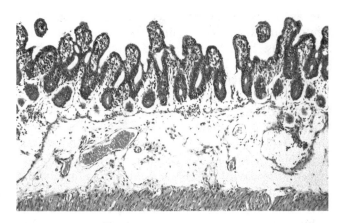

FIG. 6.25. *Small intestine from a juvenile rabbit with a natural case of epizootic rotaviral enteritis. There is submucosal edema, with blunting and fusion of villi. Enterocytes within crypts and on villi are immature, indicative of regeneration. (Source: Schoeb et al. 1986. Reproduced with permission from American Association for Laboratory Animal Science.)*

ileum, variable epithelial exfoliation, and edema of the submucosa (Fig. 6.25). There may be focal areas of exfoliation of surface epithelium in the cecum.

Diagnosis
Demonstration of the virus (usually by examination of intestinal contents for viral particles by electron microscopy), virus isolation, and serology enable incrimination of rotavirus as the causative viral agent. ELISA kits, marketed for detection of human rotavirus antigen in feces, are available from commercial suppliers and work well for testing fecal samples for group A rotaviral antigen. Fecal flotation and/or microscopic examination of the small and large intestines are essential steps to determine whether coccidia or copathogenic bacteria are playing a role in the disease. Differential diagnoses include coronaviral enteritis, coliform enteritis, salmonellosis, clostridial enteropathies, and coccidiosis. Demonstration of rotaviral particles or antigen in the feces does not constitute a definitive diagnosis but should be confirmed by microscopic examination of the gastrointestinal tract for characteristic lesions.

Endogenized Viruses
Genomic sequencing has demonstrated a number of viruses that have been integrated (endogenized) into the genome of lagomorphs. The best known of these viruses are endogenous retroviruses. Although rabbit endogenous retrovirus has been shown to be expressed in lymphoma cell cultures, its role as an etiologic agent of lymphoma has not been demonstrated. Notably, a rabbit endogenous retrovirus DNA has been found to contaminate human DNA samples from a number of sources, and was until recently believed to be a human retrovirus known as HRV-5. As with other placental mammals, lagomorphs have "domesticated" the envelope sequence of an ancient retrovirus, known as

syncytin (*syncytin-Ory1*). Rabbit syncytin is genetically distinct from syncytin genes of rodents and primates, suggesting a separate origin but similar evolutionary advantage. Syncytins are selectively expressed in the placenta, and are essential for syncytiotrophoblast formation. Perhaps the most interesting rabbit endogenized retrovirus is rabbit endogenous lentivirus type K (RELIK). RELIK is defective, but it represents evidence of the ancient origins of lentiviruses, and is the first lentivirus to be shown that integrated into a mammalian genome. Endogenized DNA parvovirus-like elements have also been found in the rabbit genome. These virus-like genetic sequences are incomplete (defective) and not replication-competent.

BIBLIOGRAPHY FOR VIRAL INFECTIONS

General References for Virus Diseases
Boucher, S. & Nouaille, L. (2013) *Maladies des Lapins*, 3rd edn. Editions France Agricole.
Brabb, T. & DiGiacomo, R.F. (2012) Viral diseases. In: *The Laboratory Rabbit, Guinea Pig, Hamster, and Other Rodents* (eds. M.A. Suckow, K.A. Stevens, & R.P. Wilson), pp. 365–413. Elsevier.
Kerr, P.J. & Donnelly, T.M. (2013) Viral infections of rabbits. *Veterinary Clinics of North America Exotic Animal Practice* 16:437–468.
MacLachlan, N.J. & Dubovi, E.J. (2011) *Fenner's Veterinary Virology*, 4th edn. Academic Press, New York.

DNA Viral Infections

Adenovirus Infection
Bodon, L. & Prohaska, P. (1980) Isolation of adenovirus from rabbits with diarrhoea. *Acta Veterinaria Academiae Scientiarum Hungarica* 28:247–255.
Descoteaux, J., Whissel, K., & Assaf, R. (1980) Detection of antibody titers to bovine adenoviruses in rabbit sera. *Laboratory Animal Science* 30:581–582.

Herpesvirus Infections
Brash, M.L., Nagy, E., Pei, Y., Carman, S., Emery, S., Smith, A.E., & Turner, P.V. (2010) Acute hemorrhagic and necrotizing pneumonia, splenitis, and dermatitis in a pet rabbit caused by a novel herpesvirus (leporid herpesvirus-4). *Canadian Veterinary Journal* 51:1383–1386.
de Matos, R., Russell, D., Van Alstine, W., & Miller, A. (2014) Spontaneous fatal human herpesvirus 1 encephalitis in two domestic rabbits (*Oryctolagus cuniculus*). *Journal of Veterinary Diagnostic Investigation* 26 I (5): 689–694.
Grest, P., Albicker, P., Hoelzle, L., Wild, P., & Pospischil, A. (2002) Herpes simplex encephalitis in a domestic rabbit (*Oryctolagus cuniculus*). *Journal of Comparative Pathology* 126:308–311.
Hesselton, R.M., Yang, W.C., Medveczky, P., & Sullivan, J.L. (1988) Pathogenesis of *Herpesvirus sylvilagus* infection in cottontail rabbits. *American Journal of Pathology* 133:639–647.
Hinze, H.C. (1971) Induction of lymphoid hyperplasia and lymphoma-like disease in rabbits by *Herpesvirus sylvilagus*. *International Journal of Cancer* 8:514–522.
Hinze, H.C. (1971) A new member of the herpesvirus group isolated from wild cottontail rabbits. *Infection and Immunity* 3:350–354.
Jin, L., Lohr, C.V., Vanarsdall, A.L., Baker, R.J., Moerdyk-Schauwecker, M., Levine, C., Gerlach, R.F., Cohen, S.A., Alvarado, D.E., & Rohrmann, G.F. (2008) Characterization of a novel alphaherpesvirus associated with fatal infections of domestic rabbits. *Virology* 378:13–20.
Jin, L., Valentine, B.A., Baker, R.J., Lohr, C.V., Gerlach, R.F., Bildfell, R.J., & Moerdyk-Schauwecker, M. (2008) An outbreak of fatal herpesvirus infection in domestic rabbits in Alaska. *Veterinary Pathology* 45:369–374.
Muller, K., Fuchs, W., Heblinski, N., Teifke, J.P., Brunnberg, L., Gruber, A.D., & Klopfleisch, R. (2009) Encephalitis in a rabbit caused by human herpesvirus-1. *Journal of the American Veterinary Medical Association* 235:66–69.
Onderka, D.F., Papp-Vid, G., & Perry, A.W. (1992) Fatal herpesvirus infection in commercial rabbits. *Canadian Veterinary Journal* 33:539–543.
Rivers, T.M. & Tillett, W.S. (1923) Further observations on the phenomena encountered in attempting to transmit varicella to rabbits. *Journal of Experimental Medicine* 39:777–802.
Sekulin, K., Jankova, J., Kolodziejek, J. Huemer, H.P., Gruber, A., Meyer, J., & Nowotny, N. (2010) Natural zoonotic infections in two marmosets and one domestic rabbit with herpes simplex virus type 1 did not reveal a correlation with a certain gG-, gI- or gE genotype. *Clinical Microbiology and Infection* 16:1669–1672.
Sunohara-Neilson, J.R., Brash, M. Carman, S., Nagy, E., & Turner, P.V. (2013) Experimental infection of New Zealand White rabbits (*Oryctolagus cuniculi*) with leporid herpesvirus 4. *Comparative Medicine* 63:422–431.
Swan, C., Perry, A., & Papp-Vid, G. (1991) Herpesvirus-like viral infection in a rabbit. *Canadian Veterinary Journal* 32:627–628.
Weissenbock, J.A., Hainfellner, J.A., Berger, J., & Budka, H. (1997) Naturally-occurring herpes simplex encephalitis in a domestic rabbit. *Veterinary Pathology* 34:44–47.
Zygraich, N., Berge, E., Brucher, J.M., Hoorens, J., & Huygelen, C. (1972) Experimental infection of rabbits and monkeys with *Herpesvirus cuniculi*. *Research in Veterinary Science* 13:241–244.

Papillomavirus Infections
Krieder, J.W. & Bartlett, G.L. (1981) The Shope papilloma-carcinoma complex of rabbits: a model system of neoplastic progression and spontaneous regression. *Advances in Cancer Research* 35:81–110.
Maglennon, G.A., McIntosh, P., & Doorbar, J. (2011) Persistence of viral DNA in the epithelial basal layer suggests a model for papillomavirus latency following immune regression. *Virology* 414:153–163.
Munday, J.S., Aberdein, D., Squires, R.A., Alfaras, A., & Wilson, A.M. (2007) Persistent conjunctival papilloma due to oral papillomavirus infection in a rabbit in New Zealand. *Journal of the American Association for Laboratory Animal Science*. 46:69–71.
Shope, R.E. (1937) Immunization of rabbits to infectious papillomatosis. *Journal of Experimental Medicine* 65:607–624.
Weisbroth, S.H. & Scher, S. (1970) Spontaneous oral papillomatosis in rabbits. *Journal of the American Veterinary Medical Association* 157:1940–1944.

Parvovirus Infection
Matsunaga, Y. & Chino, I. (1981) Experimental infection of young rabbits with rabbit parvovirus. *Archives of Virology* 68:257–264.
Matsunaga, Y., Matsumo, S., & Mukoyama, J. (1977) Isolation and characterization of a parvovirus of rabbits. *Infection and Immunity* 18:495–500.
Metcalf, J.B., Lederman, M., Stout, E.R., & Bates, R.C. (1989) Natural parvovirus infection in laboratory rabbits. *American Journal of Veterinary Research* 50:1048–1051.

Polyomavirus Infection
Hartley, J.W. & Rowe, W.P. (1966) New papovavirus contaminating Shope papillomata. *Science* 143:258–261.

Poxvirus Infections
Adams, M.M., Rice, A.D., & Moyer, R.W. (2007) Rabbitpox virus and vaccinia virus infection of rabbits as a model for human smallpox. *Journal of Virology* 81:11084–11095.

Bedson, H.S. & Duckworth, M.J. (1963) Rabbit pox: an experimental study of the pathways of infection in rabbits. *Journal of Pathology and Bacteriology* 85:1–20.

Best, S.M., Collins, S.V., & Kerr, P.J. (2000) Coevolution of host and virus: cellular localization of virus in myxoma virus infection of resistant and susceptible European rabbits. *Virology* 277:76–91.

Fenner, F. (1990) Poxviruses of laboratory animals. *Laboratory Animal Science* 40:469–480.

Fenner, F. & Radcliffe, F.N. (1965) *Myxomatosis*. Cambridge University Press, London and New York.

Green, H.S.N. (1934) Rabbit pox. I. Clinical manifestations and course of the disease. *Journal of Experimental Medicine* 60:427–440.

Green, H.S.N. (1934) Rabbit pox. II. Pathology of the epidemic disease. *Journal of Experimental Medicine* 60:441–457.

Grilli, G., Piccirillo, A., Pisoni, A.M., Cerioli, M., Gallazzi, D., & Lavazza, A. (2003) Re-emergence of fibromatosis in farmed game hares (*Lepus europaeus*) in Italy. *Veterinary Record* 153:152–153.

Hurst, E.W. (1937) Myxoma and Shope fibroma. 1. The histology of myxoma. *British Journal of Experimental Pathology* 18:1–15.

Joiner, G.N., Jardine, J.H., & Gleiser, C.A. (1971) An epizootic of Shope fibromatosis in a commercial rabbitry. *Journal of the American Veterinary Medical Association* 159:1583–1587.

Marcato, P.S. & Simoni, P. (1977) Ultrastructural researches on rabbit myxomatosis: lymphnodal lesions. *Veterinary Pathology* 14:361–367.

Patton, N.M. & Holmes, H.T. (1977) Myxomatosis in domestic rabbits in Oregon. *Journal of the American Veterinary Medical Association* 171:560–562.

Silvers, L., Inglis, B., Labudovic, A., Janssens, P.A., van Leeuwen, B.H., & Kerr, P.J. (2006) Virulence and pathogenesis of the MSW and MSD strains of California myxoma virus in European rabbits with genetic resistance to myxomatosis compared to rabbits with no genetic resistance. *Virology* 348:72–83.

Wibbelt, G. & Frolich, K. (2005) Infectious diseases in European brown hare (*Lepus europaeus*). *Wildlife Biology in Practice* 1:86–93.

RNA Viral Infections

Astrovirus Infection

Martella, V., Moschidou, P., Pinto, P., Catella, C., Desario, C., Larocca, V., Circella, E., Banyal, K., Lavazza, A., Magistrali, C., Decaro, N., & Buonavoglia, C. (2011) Astroviruses in rabbits. *Emerging Infectious Diseases* 12:2287–2293.

Stenglein, M.D., Velazquez, E., Greenacre, C., Wilkes, R.P., Ruby, J.G., Lankton, J.S., Ganem, D., Kennedy, M.A., & DeRisi, J.L. (2012) Complete genome sequence of an astrovirus identified in a domestic rabbit (*Oryctolagus cuniculus*) with gastroenteritis. *Virology Journal* 9:216.

Borna Virus Infection

Krey, H., Ludwig, H., & Rott, R. (1979) Spread of infectious virus along the optic nerve into the retina in Borna disease virus-infected rabbits. *Archives of Virology* 61:283–288.

Metzler, A., Ehrensperger, F., & Wyler, R. (1978) Natural borna virus infection in rabbits. *Zentralblatt fur Veterinarmedizen B* 25:161–164.

Roddendorf, W., Sasaki, S., & Ludwig, H. (1983) Light microscope and immunohistochemical investigations on the brain of Borna disease virus-infected rabbits. *Neuropathology and Applied Neurobiology* 9:287–296.

Calicivirus Infections

Abrantes, J., Lopes, A.M., Dalton, K.P., Melo, P., Correia, J.J., Ramada, M., Alves, P.C., Parra, F., & Esteves, P.J. (2013) New variant of rabbit hemorrhagic disease virus, Portugal, 2012–2013. *Emerging Infectious Diseases* 19:1900–1902.

Abrantes, J., van der Loo, W., Le Pendu, J., & Esteves, P.J. (2012) Rabbit hemorrhagic disease (RHD) and rabbit hemorrhagic disease virus (RHDV): a review. *Veterinary Research* 43:12–19.

Bergin, I.L., Wise, A.G., Bolin, S.R., Mullaney, T.P., Kiupel, M., & Maes, R.K. (2009) Novel calicivirus identified in rabbits, Michigan, USA. *Emerging Infectious Diseases* 15:1955–1962. (Abrantes, J. & Esteves, P.J. (2010) Not-so-novel Michigan rabbit calicivirus. *Emerging Infectious Diseases* 16:1331–1332.)

Dalton, K.P., Nicieza, I., Balseiro, A., Muguerza, M.A., Rosell, J.M., Casais, R., Alvarez, A.L., & Parra, F. (2012) Variant rabbit hemorrhagic disease virus in young rabbits, Spain. *Emerging Infectious Diseases* 18:2009–2012.

Marcato, P.S., Benazzi, C., Vecchi, G., Galeotti, M., Della Salda, L., Sarli, G., & Lucidi, P. (1991) Clinical and pathological features of viral hemorrhagic disease of rabbits and the European brown hare syndrome. *Revue Scientifique et Technique (International Office of Epizootics)* 10:371–392.

Martin-Alonso, J.M., Skilling, D.E., Gonzalez-Molleda, L., del Barrio, G., Machin, A., Keefer, N.K., Matson, D.O., Iversen, P.L., Smith, A.W., & Parra, F. (2005) Isolation and characterization of a new vesivirus from rabbits. *Virology* 337:373–383.

Wibbelt, G. & Frolich, K. (2005) Infectious diseases in European brown hare (*Lepus europaeus*). *Wildlife Biology in Practice* 1:86–93.

Coronavirus Infections

Christensen, N., Fennestad, K.L., & Brunn, L. (1978) Pleural effusion disease in rabbits: histopathological observations. *Acta Pathologica et Microbiologica Scandinavica (A)* 86:251–256.

Deeb, B.J., DiGiacomo, R.E., Evermann, J.E., & Thouless, M.E. (1993) Prevalence of coronavirus antibodies in rabbits. *Laboratory Animal Science* 43:431–433.

Descoteaux, J.-P. & Lussier, G. (1990) Experimental infection of young rabbits with a rabbit enteric coronavirus. *Canadian Journal of Veterinary Research* 54:473–476.

Eaton, P. (1984) Preliminary observations on enteritis associated with a coronavirus-like agent in rabbits. *Laboratory Animals* 18:71–74.

Edwards, S., Small, J., Geratz, J. Alexander, L., & Baric, R. (1992) An experimental model for myocarditis and congestive heart failure after rabbit coronavirus infection. *Journal of Infectious Diseases* 165:134–140.

LaPierre, J., Marsolais, G., Pilon, P., & Descoteaux, J.P. (1980) Preliminary report of a coronavirus in the intestine of the laboratory rabbit. *Canadian Journal of Microbiology* 26:1204–1208.

Lau, S.K.P., Woo, P.C.Y., Yip, C.C.Y., Fan, R.Y.Y., Huang, Y., Wang, M., Guo, R., Lam, C.S.F., Tsang, A.K.L., Lai, K.K.Y., Chan, K.-H., Che, X.-Y., & Zheng, B.-J. (2012) Isolation and characterization of a novel *Betacoronavirus* subgroup A coronavirus, rabbit coronavirus HKU14, from domestic rabbits. *Journal of Virology* 86:5481–5496.

Osterhaus, A.D.M.E., Teppema, J.S., & Van Steenis, G. (1982) Coronavirus-like particles in laboratory rabbits with different syndromes in the Netherlands. *Laboratory Animal Science* 32:663–665.

Peeters, J.E., Pohl, Pl, & Charlier, G. (1984) Infectious agents associated with diarrhea in commercial rabbits: a field study. *Annales de Recherches Veterinaraires* 15:335–340.

Small, J.D., Aurelian, L. Squire, R.A., Strandberg, J.D., Melby, E.C., Turner, T.B., & Newman, B. (1979) Rabbit cardiomyopathy associated with a virus antigenically related to human coronavirus strain 229E. *American Journal of Pathology* 95:709–729.

Hepatitis E Virus Infection

Cossaboom, C.M., Cordoba, L., Dryman, B.A., & Meng, X-J. (2011) Hepatitis E virus in rabbits, Virginia, USA. *Emerging Infectious Diseases* 17:2047–2049.

Liu, P., Bu, Q.-N., Wang, L., Han, J., Du, R.-J., Lei, Y.-X., Ouyang, Y.-Q., Li, J., Zhu, Y.-H., Lu, F.-M., & Zhuang, H. (2013) Transmission of hepatitis E virus from rabbits to cynomolgus macaques. *Emerging Infectious Diseases* 19:559–565

Ma, H., Zheng, L., Liu, Y., Zhao, C., Harrison, T.J., Ma, Y., Sun, S., Zhang, J., & Wang, Y. (2010) Experimental infection of rabbits with rabbit and genotypes 1 and 4 hepatitis E viruses. *PLoS One* 5:e9160.

Paramyxovirus Infection

Ducatelle, R., Vanrompay, D., & Charlier, G. (2010) Paramyxovirus associated with pneumonia in a dwarf rabbit. *World Rabbit Science* 2:47–52.

Iwai, H., Machii, K., Ohtsuka, Y., Ueda, K., Inoue, S., Matsumoto, T., & Satoh, Z. (1986) Prevalence of antibodies to Sendai virus and rotavirus in laboratory rabbits. *Experimental Animals* 35:491–494.

Machii, K., Otsuka, Y., Iwai, H., & Ueda, K. (1989) Infection in rabbits with Sendai virus. *Laboratory Animal Science* 39:334–337.

Rabies Virus Infection

Childs, J.E., Colby, L., Krebs, J.W., Strine, T., Feller, M., Noah, D., Drenzek, C., Smith, J.S., & Rupprecht, C.E. (1997) Surveillance and spatiotemporal associations of rabies in rodents and lagomorphs in the United States, 1985–1994. *Journal of Wildlife Diseases* 33:20–27.

Eidson, M., Matthews, S.D., Willsey, A.L., Cherry, B., Rudd, R.J., & Trimarchi, C.V. (2005) Rabies virus infection in a pet guinea pig and seven pet rabbits. *Journal of the American Veterinary Medical Association* 227:932–935.

Karp, B.E. (1999) Rabies in two privately owned domestic rabbits. *Journal of the American Veterinary Medical Association* 215:1824–1827.

Rotavirus Infection

Banyai, K., Forgach, P., Erdelyi, K., Martella, V., Bogdan, A., Hocsak, E., Havasi, V., Melegh, B., & Szucs, G. (2005) Identification of the novel lapine rotavirus genotype P[22] from an outbreak of enteritis in a Hungarian rabbitry. *Virus Research* 113:73–80.

Ciarlet, M., Gilger, M.A., Barone, C., McArthur, M., Estes, M.K., & Conner, M.E. (1998) Rotavirus disease, but not infection and development of intestinal histopathological lesions, is age restricted in rabbits. *Virology* 251:343–360.

Conner, M.E., Estes, M.K., & Graham, D.Y. (1988) Rabbit model of rotavirus infection. *Journal of Virology* 62:1625–1633.

DiGiacomo, R.F. & Thouless, M.E. (1986) Epidemiology of naturally occurring rotavirus infection in rabbits. *Laboratory Animal Science* 36:153–156.

Petric, M., Middleton, P.J., Grant, C., Tam, J.S., & Hewitt, C.M. (1978) Lapine rotavirus: preliminary studies on epizootiology and transmission. *Canadian Journal of Comparative Medicine* 42:143–147.

Schoeb, T.R., Casebolt, D.B., Walker, V.E., Potgieter, L.N., Thouless, M.E., & DiGiacomo, R.F. (1986) Rotavirus-associated diarrhea in a commercial rabbitry. *Laboratory Animal Science* 36:149–152.

Schoondermark-van de Ven, E., Van Ranst, M., de Bruin, W., van den Hurk, P., Zeller, M., Matthijnssens, J., & Heylen, E. (2013) Rabbit colony infected with a bovine-like G6P[11] rotavirus strain. *Veterinary Microbiology* 166:154–164.

Thouless, M.E., DiGiacomo, R.F., Deeb, B.J., & Howard, H. (1988) Pathogenicity of rotavirus in rabbits. *Journal of Clinical Microbiology* 26:943–947.

Thouless, M.E., et al. (1996) The effect of combined rotavirus and *Escherichia coli* infections in rabbits. *Laboratory Animal Science* 46:381–385.

Endogenized Viruses

Bedigian, H.G., Fox, R.R., & Meier, H. (1978) Induction of type C RNA virus from cultured rabbit lymphosarcoma cells. *Journal of Virology* 27:313–319.

Griffiths, D.J., Voisset, C., Venables, P.J.W., & Weiss, R.A. (2002) Novel endogenous retrovirus in rabbits previously reported as human retrovirus 5. *Journal of Virology* 76:7094–7102.

Heidmann, O., Vernochet, C., Dupressoir, A., & Heidman, T. (2009) Identification of an endogenous retroviral envelope gene with fusogenic activity and placenta-specific expression in the rabbit: a new "syncytin" in a third order of mammals. *Retrovirology* 6:107.

Horie, M. & Tomonaga, K. (2011) Non-retroviral fossils in vertebrate genomes. *Viruses* 3:1836–1848.

Katzourakis, A., Tristem, M., Pybus, O.G., & Gifford, R.J. (2007) Discovery and analysis of the first endogenous lentivirus. *Proceedings of the National Academy of Sciences* 104:6261–6265.

BACTERIAL INFECTIONS

Bacteria play a significant role in clinical disease in the rabbit. The authors have struggled with how to organize this section, and concluded that an alphabetical approach, as with viruses, would be best. Various bacteria may be sporadically involved in infections of rabbits, such as tooth abscesses and wounds, but those covered herein are pathogens associated with syndromes that may be encountered by the pathologist.

Acinetobacter calcoaceticus Infection

A single report in Germany has documented laboratory rabbits with bronchopneumonia in association with *Acinetobacter calcoacetis*, which was also isolated from other organs.

Actinobacillus spp. Infection

Septicemic disease caused by different *Actinobacillus* spp. has been reported sporadically in domestic rabbits, and infection among North American hares is common. One case involved isolation of *A. equuli* from the liver and lung of a rabbit with Tyzzer's disease in Europe. Another case involved a rabbit in the United States infected with *A. capsulatus*, which caused multifocal necrohemorrhagic pneumonia in which bacterial colonies were observed. Tarsal abscesses with emaciation and death has been reported in Sri Lanka among laboratory rabbits infected with *A. capsulatus*.

Actinomyces spp. Infection

Granulomatous osteitis of the head, spinal column, and limbs has been associated with *Actinomyces* spp. in domestic rabbits. This bacterium is one of many that can cause tooth-related abscesses, and one case of tooth abscess was associated with pulmonary abscessation. Histopathology revealed Gram-positive branching filamentous and beaded bacteria, which elicited a Splendore-Hoeppli response with formation of sulfur granules.

Bordetella bronchiseptica Infection

Bordetella bronchiseptica may be recovered from the upper and lower respiratory tracts in both clinically normal and diseased animals, suggesting that it is relatively

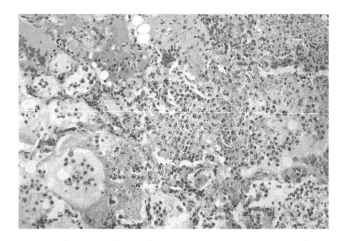

FIG. 6.26. *Acute fibrinopurulent bronchopneumonia in a young rabbit infected with* Bordetella bronchiseptica. *The terminal airway and alveoli are flooded with fibrin-rich exudate.*

nonpathogenic in rabbits. A high percentage of conventional commercial rabbits have detectable antibodies to *B. bronchiseptica*. *Bordetella bronchiseptica* tends to localize along the cilia of the respiratory epithelial cells of rabbits, and infections have been demonstrated to cause ciliostasis in the canine trachea. It is likely that initial or coinfections with *Bordetella* in airways may impair clearance mechanisms and thus facilitate *Pasteurella multocida* infection of the lower respiratory tract. Occasionally, outbreaks of respiratory disease occur among young rabbits that are attributed to primary *B. bronchiseptica* infections. Rabbits can serve as a source of infection for guinea pigs, a species particularly susceptible to *B. bronchiseptica*. Lesions associated with *B. bronchiseptica* infections, when present, are fibrinopurulent bronchopneumonia (Fig. 6.26) and interstitial pneumonia. In chronic infections, there may be prominent peribronchial and perivascular cuffing with lymphocytes. The organism can be recovered in large numbers from respiratory tract lesions.

Brucella spp. Infection: Brucellosis
Brucellosis in domestic rabbits is rare, but infection with *B. intermedia* has been observed in rabbits purchased at a market in Tunisia. No gross lesions were reported.

Brucellosis is primarily a disease of wild hares, and has been reported in both European and North American hares. In Europe, hares are believed to be important reservoir hosts for *B. suis*, but *B. melitensis* and *B. abortus* have also been isolated. In North American jackrabbits (hares), *B. suis* and *B. melitensis* were isolated. In hares, pyogranulomatous lesions have been found to arise primarily in reproductive organs of both sexes, with inconsistent involvement of liver and spleen.

Campylobacter spp. Infection
Campylobacter has been inaccurately blamed as the etiology of proliferative enteritis associated with

intracellular "*Campylobacter*-like organisms" in a number of species (rabbit, guinea pig, hamster, rat, and mouse). *Lawsonia intracellularis* is now recognized as the cause of that disease. The enteric pathogens *Vibrio coli* and *V. jejuni* have been reclassified as *Campylobacter*. An older report described "Vibrio-like organisms" in associated with enteritis among weanling rabbits. In retrospect, the morphologic features of the bacteria described in that report were consistent with *Campylobacter* spp. In the cecum, submucosal edema with polymorphonuclear cell infiltration was observed. Enterocytes were flattened and irregular, with focal ulceration. Cecal crypts were hyperplastic, and some crypts were distended with bacteria and cell debris. In Levaditi-stained tissue sections, "Vibrio-like organisms" were demonstrated on the surface and within the cytoplasm of damaged mucosal cells. Similar organisms were rarely observed in the ceca of controls, and when present, there was no evidence of invasion. Recently, a high prevalence of *Campylobacter* infection was found among commercially raised rabbits in Italy. It appears to be a novel species identified as *C. cuniculorum*. Its clinical significance is not known. A low prevalence of *C. coli* and *C. jejuni* was also detected. Healthy and diarrheic rabbits, as well as rabbit meat, have been found to be infected with *C. jejuni*. The role of *Campylobacter* spp. as primary pathogens in rabbit enteritis remains to be determined.

Chlamydophila spp. Infection
Chlamydophila species include *C. psittaci* and *C. pneumoniae*, both of which can infect domestic rabbits. The prevalence of natural infection and infecting species among domestic rabbits is unknown, since infection is usually subclinical. However, natural infections with an unspeciated *Chlamydophila* sp. have been reported to cause conjunctivitis and interstitial pneumonia. Giemsa stains have revealed inclusion bodies in conjunctiva, liver, lung, and intestine of naturally infected rabbits. Experimental intranasal or intravenous inoculation of laboratory rabbits with *C. pneumoniae* has been shown to induce arterial intimal thickening and acceleration of atherosclerosis in mildly hyperlipidemic rabbits. Species-specific PCR assays are available for detecting *Chlamydophila* spp. in rabbits.

Cilia-Associated Respiratory (CAR) Bacillus Infection
Colonization of the apices of ciliated epithelial cells lining the larynx, trachea, and bronchi with CAR bacillus has been observed in laboratory rabbits (Fig 6.27). The bacilli have been demonstrated both in silver-stained preparations and by electron microscopy, in which bacteria were aligned perpendicularly within the surface of ciliated bronchial epithelium. The animals were without clinical signs. 16S rRNA analysis indicated that the rabbit isolate belongs to a different genus than

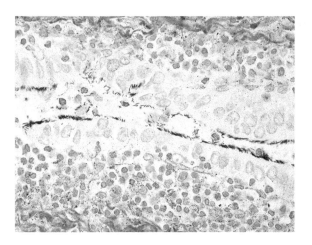

FIG. 6.27. *Lung of a rabbit naturally infected with cilia-associated respiratory (CAR) bacillus. This organism colonizes the epithelium of the larynx, trachea, and bronchi in the rabbit. Note the prominent peribronchiolar lymphocytic infiltration (Warthin-Starry stain). (Source: D. Imai, University of California, Davis, CA. Reproduced with permission from D. Imai.)*

the rat CAR bacillus. Furthermore, rabbits developed rhinitis following inoculation with a rabbit isolate, but not with a rat isolate. Mild to moderate peribronchial lymphoid hyperplasia and hyperplasia of epithelial cells lining airways were described. One study examined 3-month-old rabbits raised for meat production, and found that 30–100% of rabbits from different rabbitries were infected, based upon Warthin–Starry-stained tissues. No gross lesions were found, but a significant number of rabbits had mild inflammatory lesions in the respiratory tract, particularly bronchi, in association with CAR bacillus.

Corynebacterium bovis Infection
Testicular and pulmonary abscesses were observed in a laboratory rabbit, and *C. bovis* was isolated from both sites. Experimental infection of another rabbit reproduced a similar disease.

Clostridial Diseases
Rabbits are subject to several significant clostridial diseases, including enterotoxemia (*C. difficile, C. perfringens,* and *C. spiroforme*), Tyzzer's disease (*C. piliforme*), dysautonomia (*C. botulinum*), and epizootic rabbit enteropathy (ERE) (*C. perfringens* alpha toxin). Clostridia are Gram-positive bacilli that reside in the gut and grow under anaerobic conditions. Several Clostridial species may be present in low numbers among the enteric microflora of normal rabbits, so that isolation of *Clostridium* does not necessarily implicate the etiology of the disease. Lesion distribution and morphology, histochemical stains, or toxin assays are needed to confirm the diagnosis. A number of nonpathogenic *Clostridium* spp. may also inhabit the rabbit intestine, which can affect accuracy of diagnosis based on culture or PCR.

Clostridium difficile, Clostridium perfringens, *and* Clostridium spiroforme: *Clostridial Enteropathy*
For years, *C. perfringens* was regarded as the likely etiology of enterotoxemia in domestic rabbits. Type E iota toxin was demonstrated in fatal cases of enterotoxemia, and the disease was, therefore, attributed to *C. perfringens*. Some of these diseases associated with *C. perfringens* may have been due to *C. spiroforme*, since antitoxin prepared against *C. perfringens* type E iota toxin will also neutralize similar toxins produced by *C. spiroforme*. Fatal colitis and enterotoxemia associated with overgrowth of *C. difficile* has occurred following prolonged treatment with penicillin or ampicillin. Subsequent experimental reproduction of the disease following treatment with lincomycin was attributed to *C. difficile* or *C. perfringens*. Spontaneous enterotoxemia due to *C. difficile* infection, with identification of A and B toxins, has been reported in specific-pathogen-free rabbits in the absence of prior antibiotic treatment. Clostridial enterotoxemia has similar features in rabbits, regardless of causative *Clostridium* spp.

Epizootiology and Pathogenesis
Clostridium spiroforme is now recognized as the most common clostridial pathogen associated with enterotoxemia in young rabbits. In 1 survey of diarrheic rabbits, *C. spiroforme* was isolated from over 50% at necropsy, and 90% of the strains isolated were toxigenic. Although this organism is not a normal inhabitant of the alimentary tract in rabbits, it is often difficult to produce disease experimentally in healthy rabbits inoculated orally with *C. spiroforme*. The normal gut microbiome acts as a microbial barrier, and disruption of the normal gut microflora is an important predisposing factor. Changes in feed, weaning, previous antibiotic treatment, and concurrent infections appear to permit colonization with *C. spiroforme* and thus trigger an epizootic of enteric disease. The term "carbohydrate overload" has been associated with the syndrome. Rabbits ingesting high-energy feed may fail to digest the majority of carbohydrates in the small intestine. Significant amounts of carbohydrate may then reach the level of the large intestine, promoting the overgrowth of organisms such as Clostridia. In outbreaks of the disease, the organism may be the sole identified pathogen. However, concurrent infections with other pathogens, such as rotavirus, *E. coli, Eimeria* spp., and *Cryptosporidium* spp. are often present. Following the multiplication of pathogenic strains of *Clostridium* spp. in the large intestine, enterotoxins may be produced, resulting in damage to enterocytes, impaired function, profuse diarrhea, subsequent depression, dehydration, and death.

Pathology
In peracute cases, the carcass is usually in good condition, and perineal soiling with diarrheic feces is a

variable finding. In subacute to chronic cases, carcasses are frequently thin and dehydrated. Staining of the perineum, belly, and rear legs with watery green to tarry brown feces is common. Internally, straw-colored fluid may be present in the peritoneal cavity. Extensive ecchymoses are usually present in the cecal serosa, sometimes with involvement of the distal ileum and proximal colon. Epicardial and thymic ecchymoses may also occur. The cecum and adjacent areas are frequently dilated, with watery to mucoid, green to dark brown contents, and with gas formation. There may be marked thickening of affected areas due to submucosal edema, and mucosal changes vary from hemorrhage to ulceration and fibrinous exudation (Fig. 6.28).

Typical microscopic changes in the cecum of affected animals are those of a necrotizing typhlitis, with irregular denuding of the mucosa, ulceration, fibrinous exudation, and leukocytic infiltration, with heterophils predominating (Fig. 6.29). Changes observed in enterocytes vary, including swelling, vacuolation, flattening, denuding, and proliferation. The mucosa and submucosa are congested and edematous, frequently with focal hemorrhage, and thrombi may be present in adjacent vessels. Gram-positive bacilli may be present in large numbers on the surface of affected areas of gut mucosa. The optimal lesion (for diagnosis) is selective necrosis of mucosal epithelium, with relative sparing of the crypt bases and lamina propria, submucosal edema, and mucosal/submucosal/serosal hemorrhage. All of these features relate to the effects of luminal toxin penetrating to various depths of the intestinal wall. In subacute to chronic lesions, necrotizing changes are replaced by hyperplasia as the mucosa undergoes repair.

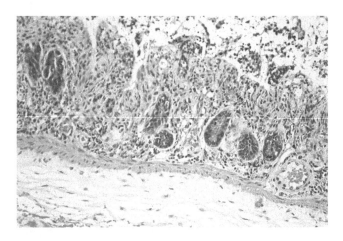

FIG. 6.29.   *Necrotizing typhlitis from a case of clostridial enteropathy due to* Clostridium spiroforme. *Note the selective loss of mucosal epithelium with relative sparing of crypts and submucosal edema.*

In this stage, clinical signs of malabsorption and diarrhea continue. Clinical support of the rabbit has often been stopped at this stage, under the erroneous assumption that the rabbit was not improving. When rabbits are presented for necropsy following death, autolysis and postmortem bacterial overgrowth can obscure mucosal lesions. However, clostridial enteropathy would be a likely candidate based on the presence of submucosal edema and hemorrhage.

Diagnosis

The typical age (usually juvenile) and history of a change in feed, management, or environment may be helpful, particularly if coinciding with an explosive outbreak of diarrhea. The microscopic examination of Gram-stained smears from the terminal ileum and cecum is a useful procedure to make a provisional diagnosis. Typical curved and coiled Gram-positive organisms are associated with *C. spiroforme* infections (Fig. 6.30). Anaerobic cultures are recommended for positive identification of

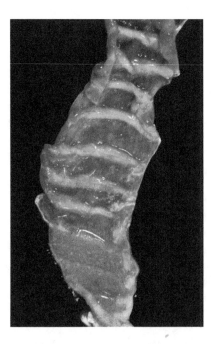

FIG. 6.28.   *Cecum from a rabbit with clostridial enteropathy. Note the hemorrhage and the fibrinous exudate on the mucosal surface.*

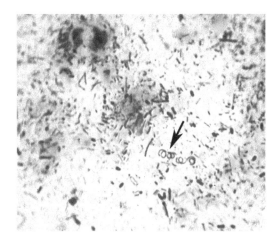

FIG. 6.30.   *Gram-stained smear of intestinal contents from a rabbit with clostridial enteropathy, demonstrating the typical coiled appearance of* Clostridium spiroforme *organisms (arrow).*

the organism, and PCR protocols have been developed that identify the organism and its toxin-encoding genes. Several procedures are available for the identification of the clostridial toxin recovered from gut contents or bacterial culture. Semiquantitative aerobic bacterial cultures of small intestine and cecum provide a useful index of dysbiosis, since aerobic bacteria should be absent or minimal in the normal intestine. Fecal flotation and virology screening are procedures recommended in order to search for possible concurrent infections. Differential diagnoses include coccidiosis, *E. coli* infections, and Tyzzer's disease.

Clostridium piliforme *Infection: Tyzzer's Disease*

Since Ernest Tyzzer's original description of disease in laboratory mice, Tyzzer's disease has now been recognized in a variety of wildlife, laboratory animals, and domestic species, including the domestic rabbit, *Sylvilagus* rabbit, mouse, rat, hamster, gerbil, guinea pig, rhesus monkey, horse, ox, dog, and cat. Formerly named *Bacillus piliformis*, it is now classified as *C. piliforme*, based upon 16S rRNA. It is relatively labile in the vegetative phase and replicates only in embryonated chick eggs and selected cell lines. Antigenic differences have been demonstrated in strains of *C. piliforme* isolated from different species. The antigenic differences observed may be due to host-associated bacterial antigens, not because of the distinctly different host organisms. It is likely that interspecies infections can occur. Typical lesions have been produced in laboratory animals inoculated orally with isolates from other species, but some isolates appear to have a limited host range.

Epizootiology and Pathogenesis

The organism may survive for long periods in the spore state and can remain infectious in contaminated bedding for at least 1 year. The organism is passed in the feces, and the infection usually occurs by ingestion. There has been speculation, but no proof, that intrauterine transmission may occur in rabbits. In rabbits, "stress factors" include shipping, changes in diet, high environmental temperatures, and poor sanitation may be important in disease outbreaks. Alterations in the gut flora may enhance susceptibility to the disease. Following oral exposure, *C. piliforme* multiplies in the intestinal mucosa, with tissue damage, followed by dissemination to the liver by the portal circulation with bacteremia, hepatitis, and on occasion, myocarditis. All ages may be affected during epizootics in domestic rabbits, but young weanlings are most frequently affected. Morbidity may vary from 10% to over 50%. The mortality rate in affected animals is high.

Pathology

The disease is characterized by a sudden onset of profuse, watery diarrhea, a short course, and high mortality in

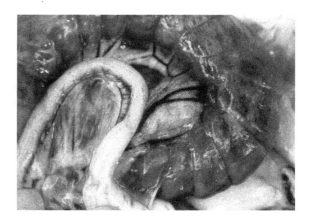

FIG. 6.31. *Acute necrohemorrhagic typhlitis in a rabbit with Tyzzer's disease. Note ecchymotic hemorrhages on the serosa.*

affected animals. Rabbits may be found dead with no prior clinical signs. On external examination, dehydration and fecal staining in the perineal region are typical findings. There are usually extensive ecchymoses and occasionally fibrinous exudate on the serosal surface of the cecum and colon (Fig. 6.31). The walls of affected areas, particularly the cecum, are markedly thickened and edematous. The cecum and colon contain dirty brown, watery contents, and the mucosal surface is discolored and dull, frequently with an irregular, granular appearance. Fibrinous strands and debris often adhere to the mucosa. Disseminated pale miliary foci up to 2 mm in diameter are frequently present in the liver (Fig. 6.32). Myocardial lesions, when present, occur as pale, linear streaks, particularly near the apex of the left ventricle. In affected rabbits that survive, carcasses are thin, usually with identifiable circumferential regions of fibrosis and stenosis in the terminal ileum or large intestine.

Microscopic changes are found consistently in the intestinal tract, usually in the liver, and infrequently in the myocardium. In rabbits examined during the acute

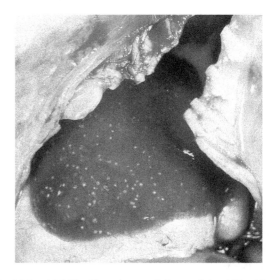

FIG. 6.32. *Multifocal hepatic necrosis in an adult rabbit with Tyzzer's disease.*

stages of the disease, variable numbers of intracellular bacilli are usually demonstrable in the cytoplasm of hepatocytes at the periphery of the focal lesions, more frequently in enterocytes, and sometimes in the adjacent smooth muscle of the gut. Occasionally bacilli are also visible in myofibers associated with myocardial lesions. Fascicles of eosinophilic intracytoplasmic bacilli should be evident in H & E-stained sections. However, Warthin–Starry silver or Giemsa stains are optimal procedures to demonstrate the characteristic bundles of filamentous bacilli (see Gerbil Chapter 4, "Fig. 4.4"). In the rabbit, a thorough search may be required in order to locate the organisms.

In the intestine, there may be focal to segmental necrosis of the cecal mucosa, with variable involvement of distal ileum and proximal colon. There is sloughing of enterocytes, and large numbers of opportunistic bacteria are often present on the surface of the damaged mucosa. Lesions are frequently transmural. There is extensive submucosal edema, necrosis of muscular layers, and concurrent leukocytic infiltration, consisting predominantly of heterophils. In the liver, focal lesions are most often adjacent to the periportal areas. Multifocal areas of coagulation to caseous necrosis contain variable numbers of heterophils, macrophages, and cell debris. In the myocardium, focal to linear areas of coagulation necrosis may be present, usually accompanied by minimal inflammatory response. Microscopic changes seen in the livers of rabbits that survive the acute stages of the disease include focal fibrosis, with infiltrating macrophages and the presence of multinucleated giant cells and mineralized debris. Focal to segmental fibrosis, with disruption of the architecture, occurs in the large intestine, and occasionally in the myocardium, in surviving animals. Tyzzer's bacilli are not present in lesions examined during the convalescent stages of the disease.

Diagnosis

Differential diagnoses include listeriosis, staphylococcosis (liver lesions), Clostridial enteropathies, and coccidiosis, among others. The presence of the extensive transmural cecal damage, together with the multifocal hepatic and myocardial lesions, should enable the pathologist to differentiate Tyzzer's disease from other infectious diseases. The demonstration of the typical bacilli in tissue sections is required to confirm the diagnosis. PCR assays have been developed, but there is significant nucleotide diversity among *C. piliforme* isolates, and some sequences may cross-react with nonpathogenic Clostridia that can inhabit the rabbit intestine. Based on serological studies of commercial rabbitries, subclinical infections with *C. piliforme* may be relatively common. However, serology can be problematic as a diagnostic assay. In 1 study, 20 rabbits with positive serology could not be confirmed by PCR or histology.

Clostridium botulinum *Dysautonomia: Grass Sickness*

Domestic rabbits, wild rabbits, and hares may spontaneously develop sudden acute gastrointestinal hypomotility and dysphagia with mortality. At necropsy, the large intestine is impacted with variable small intestinal firmness. Mucoid enteropathy may also be present. Such cases warrant examination of pre- and postsympathetic and parasympathetic neurons of the myenteric and submucosal plexes, as well as somatic and autonomic lower motor neurons in the brain stem and spinal cord. Neurons reveal neuronolysis and neuronal central chromatolysis. Lesions are similar to those of equine dysautonomia, or "grass sickness" caused by *Clostridium botulinum* toxin. Botulinum toxin has been confirmed in the gastrointestinal content of 1 case in a wild rabbit.

Clostridium perfringens: *Epizootic Rabbit Enteropathy*

Epizootic rabbit enteropathy is a major economically important disease in European rabbit farms. It was initially observed in 1996 among rabbitries in France, but has since become endemic in most European countries. ERE frequently affects rabbits that are 6–14 weeks of age, but sporadic cases can affect suckling rabbits prior to weaning. Mortality at the onset of epizootics may reach 80%. Affected rabbits stop drinking, then later stop eating, and develop a distended abdomen with mild diarrhea. Diagnosis is based upon clinical signs and gross lesions, which typically include gastric and small intestinal dilation with liquid and gas (Fig. 6.33). The cecum may be impacted or contain watery material and the colon may contain copious mucous (mucoid enteropathy). Microscopically, lesions are mild or absent. Mild villus attenuation and low-grade inflammation have been variably found in the jejunum, and some rabbits may have coccobacillary bacteria attached to the brush border. In many cases, no histologic lesions can be

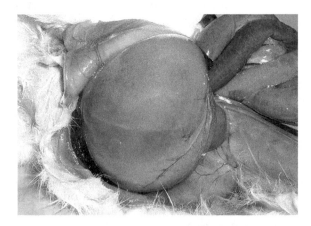

FIG. 6.33. *Acute gastric and intestinal tympany in a rabbit that died acutely with epizootic rabbit enteropathy. The stomach and intestine are distended with gas and fluid, but histologic lesions are minimal or absent in this syndrome. (Source: Licois et al 2005. Reproduced with permission from EPD Sciences.)*

found. Nonenteropathogenic (*eae*-negative) *E. coli* and *C. perfringens* in large numbers are typically isolated from feces of affected rabbits. A significant correlation has been found between gross lesions of ERE and the presence of *C. perfringens* alpha toxin. ERE can be readily reproduced in SPF rabbits inoculated with cecal contents from affected rabbits. Although the role of *C. perfringens* and its toxin in ERE pathogenesis remain to be confirmed, a notable lesion (to the authors of this book) is degeneration of neurons in the myenteric plexus, similar to dysautonomia.

Escherichia coli Infection: Colibacillosis

Escherichia coli is a Gram-negative facultative anaerobic bacterium that commonly inhabits the intestine as part of the microbiome in many species, but is present in very small numbers, if at all, in the normal rabbit intestine. In contrast, many strains of *E. coli* may be pathogenic in the rabbit. Most pathogenic strains in the rabbit are termed enteropathogenic *E. coli* (EPEC), but enterohemorrhagic *E. coli* (EHEC) has also been described. EHEC infection involves elaboration of Shiga toxin, which has local and systemic effects. A commonly used serotype classification system is based on major lipopolysaccharide surface antigens (O), flagellin antigen (H). Many serotypes of *E. coli* have been isolated from rabbits, and different serotypes appear to dominate in Europe and North America. Rabbit *E. coli* strains that attach to mucosal epithelium are known as attaching and effacing *E. coli* (AEEC) strains. Both EPEC and EHEC rabbit isolates are AEEC strains. AEECs attach intimately to the microvillus brush border, typically with pedestal or cup formation and rearrangement of the underlying cytoskeleton. AEEC strains possess a pathogenicity island within their chromosome that encodes the gene products involved in attachment, including the *eaeA* gene, which is often used to identify AEECs.

The absence or rarity of *E. coli* in the alimentary tract of suckling and weanling rabbits has been attributed to the low pH of the stomach so that the stomach and small intestine are relatively free from all bacteria. In addition, maternal milk contains (non-EPEC antibody) antimicrobial factors that can protect suckling kits from infection by *E. coli*. Under certain conditions, there may be a marked proliferation of the *E. coli*, with up to 30 million colony-forming units of *E. coli* per gram of feces in diarrheic rabbits. For example, in intestinal coccidiosis, there is a rise in cecal pH, with a striking concurrent rise in fecal output of *E. coli*. Similarly, diets with a high digestive hydrochloride may promote the dissociation of volatile cecal fatty acids, which normally exert an antibacterial effect in the gut. The rise of *E. coli* in the enteric digesta does not necessarily indicate the presence of a pathogenic *E. coli*, but it is a clear and useful indicator of dysbiosis, whatever the cause. Isolates of *E. coli* from clinically normal rabbits usually failed to produce detectable disease.

Enteropathogenic Escherichia coli

Most *E. coli* isolates recovered from diarrheic rabbits are EPEC strains, which characteristically are found attached to the surface of enterocytes. They produce minimal or no Shiga toxin and are not considered to be enteroinvasive. There are significant variations in the pathogenicity of EPEC isolates. Strains of low virulence cause problems primarily in rabbitries with poor sanitation and are usually responsive to antibiotic treatment and improved hygiene. On the other hand, highly virulent strains are often refractory to antibiotic therapy. A large number of strains have been isolated from suckling and weanling rabbits with diarrhea, serotyped, and characterized. In general, these strains of *E. coli* isolated from naturally occurring diarrheas in suckling or weanling animals produce disease experimentally only in the same age group. For example, strain RDEC-1, isolated from weanling rabbits, attaches only to the enterocytes of weanling rabbits and produces disease in this age group but not in sucklings. This may be due to the absence of the sucrose–isomaltose enzyme complex on the enterocyte brush border of suckling rabbits. The enzyme complex develops after weaning and has been shown to permit binding of this strain to enterocytes. In studies of the virulence of strains of *E. coli* isolated from suckling rabbits, the organism is attached to the enterocytes in both the large and small intestine. In weaned rabbits with experimental coliform enteritis, bacterial attachment occurred in the ileum, cecum, and colon. In rabbits, the adhesins responsible for the attachment of the EPEC strains to enterocytes are an antigenically diverse group.

Pathology

The carcass may be dehydrated, and the perineal region is frequently stained with watery yellow to brown fecal material. The cecum and colon are often distended with watery yellow to gray-brown contents. There may be serosal ecchymoses, edema of the walls of the cecum and colon, edematous mesenteric lymph nodes, and prominent lymphoid tissue in the Peyer's patches and sacculus rotundus. Depending on the strain of *E. coli*, fluid contents may also be present in the small intestine (Fig. 6.34). Microscopically, large numbers of coccobacilli are attached to enterocytes in both the small and large intestine. Microscopic changes are normally more extensive in weanlings with the disease. In the small intestine, ileal villi are often blunted, and the lamina propria of affected intestine is edematous, with leukocytic infiltration. Enterocytes at the tips of villi are swollen, and bacteria may be attached to these cells, with effacement of the microvillus brush border. In the cecum and colon, there is bacterial attachment (Fig. 6.35), with variable swelling of affected enterocytes, and frequently with detachment and erosion involving the tips of the cecal folds. Rabbit EPEC isolates appear to have a predilection for enterocytes overlying Peyer's patches.

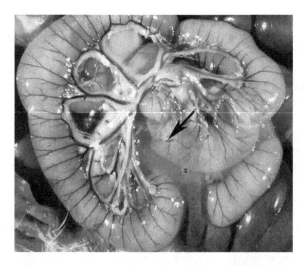

FIG. 6.34.   *Intestine from a weanling rabbit with profuse diarrhea associated with acute infection with an attaching and effacing enteropathogenic* Escherichia coli *(EPEC). Note the fluid content that has leaked from an incision in the small intestine (arrow).*

Diagnosis

The age, history, clinical signs, and gross and microscopic findings are useful criteria in making the diagnosis. The presence of EPEC is often found as a copathogen in cases of enterotoxemia and other enteritides of the rabbit. The characterization of the isolate of *E. coli* is recommended in order to determine whether the strain is likely to be a primary pathogen. Isolates of *E. coli* have been divided into biotypes according to their carbohydrate fermentation patterns. There is a good correlation between biotype and serotype in identified pathogenic strains. Differential diagnoses include clostridial enterotoxemia, Tyzzer's disease, viral enteritides, and acute coccidiosis. Concurrent infection of *E. coli* and *Lawsonia intracellularis* has been associated with proliferative enterocolitis.

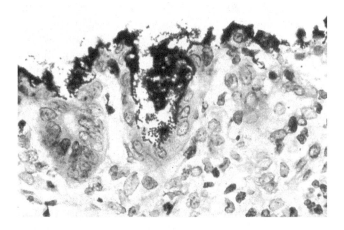

FIG. 6.35.   *Cecum from a case of acute coliform enteritis in a weanling rabbit. The surface mucosa is densely populated with attaching* Escherichia coli *(Warthin–Starry stain).*

Enterohemorrhagic Escherichia coli

Escherichia coli O157:H7 is the notorious and prototypic enterohemorrhagic *E. coli* (EHEC) that causes severe disease in humans. Dutch Belted and New Zealand White rabbits are experimentally susceptible to O157:H7 *E. coli* infection and disease and natural infections in wild rabbits have been documented. Dutch Belted rabbits have also been found to be naturally infected with an EHEC strains O145:H(-) and O153:H(-). EHEC strains are attaching and effacing, while also producing Shiga toxins, and are thus termed Shiga-toxin-producing *E. coli* (STEC).

Pathology

Clinical signs among affected rabbits varied from profuse diarrhea to acute hemorrhagic diarrhea. Anorexia, lethargy, and dehydration were other presenting signs. Petechiae and ecchymoses may be present on the serosal surface of the cecum and colon, with edema of colonic and cecal walls. On histopathology, sloughing of enterocytes, vasculitis, marked edema in the lamina propria and submucosa, and polymorphonuclear cell infiltration are present. Changes in the cecal mucosa vary from erosion to ulceration, with progression to a fibrinonecrotic typhlitis in severely affected animals.

Dutch Belted rabbits naturally infected with EHEC O153 or experimentally infected with the O157:H7 strain develop renal disease similar to the hemolytic–uremic syndrome seen in human subjects. Fibrinoedematous vasculitis and constriction of vascular lumina were typical changes seen in interlobular blood vessels on microscopic examination. There was swelling of glomerular tufts with leukocytic infiltration, and subendothelial deposition of fibrinous exudate in glomerular capillaries. Fibrin thrombi were present in some other renal vessels. Intravenous injection of Shiga toxin (Stx2) induced similar severe enteritis and renal injury. New Zealand White rabbits experimentally infected with 0157:H7 develop similar intestinal disease as Dutch Belted rabbits, but did not develop hemolytic uremic syndrome.

Francisella tularensis Infection: Tularemia, "Rabbit Fever"

The agent of tularemia, *F. tularensis*, has a broad host range, including a number of lagomorph species. In the New World, *Sylvilagus* spp. and *Lepus* spp. are commonly infected, and in Europe and Japan, *Lepus* spp. are known to be infected. Notably, wild and domestic *O. cuniculus* rabbits are resistant to infection. Lesions in susceptible lagomorphs include disseminated pinpoint necrosis and granulomatous inflammation of liver, spleen, and lymph nodes. Infections of humans can be acquired by skin abrasions during skinning and bites from infected ticks.

Fusobacterium necrophorum Infection: Schmorl's Disease, Necrobacillosis

Rabbits may develop sporadic infection of the skin and subcutis, and rarely septicemia when infected with

F. necrophorum. Infection is essentially opportunistic, and takes advantage of moist dermatitis. Dermatitis can occur in does with large dewlaps subjected to excessive moisture due to salivation. Other predisposing factors include panting associated with high environmental temperatures, as well as malocclusion. The inflammatory process in the subcutaneous tissue may progress to suppuration with ulceration of the overlying skin. Systemic infection, with embolic abscessation and necrosis of the jugular vein, lungs, and brain arising from acute inflammation and abscessation of the oropharyngeal region, has also been described as a rare entity in rabbits.

Helicobacter spp. Infection

Using PCR and 16S rRNA sequence analysis, gastric biopsy specimens were evaluated for the presence of *Helicobacter* spp. among pet, laboratory, and commercial rabbits. Rabbits from all sources tested positive for *Helicobacter* spp. Most of the positive specimens proved to be closely related to *H. heilmannii*, type II, including *H. felis* and *H. salomonis*, but a *H. pullorum/H. rappini*-like organism was detected in 1 rabbit. In a study of laboratory rabbits, *H. canadensis/H. pullorum* and *H. felis* were detected. Mild inflammatory lesions were present in the gastric mucosa of some of the rabbits. The prevalence and significance of *Helicobacter* spp. infections in domestic rabbits is currently unknown.

Klebsiella spp. Infection

There have been reports of isolated outbreaks of enterotyphlitis associated with *Klebsiella pneumoniae* and *K. oxytoca* among commercial rabbitries in Europe. Young kits and weanlings were particularly at risk, although diarrhea with mortality was occasionally seen in does. Mortality rates of up to 100% occurred in affected suckling kits, with reduced mortality in older rabbits. In suckling kits, hemorrhagic enterotyphlitis with serosal hemorrhages was a typical finding at necropsy (Fig. 6.36). In affected weaned animals,

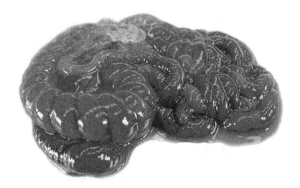

FIG. 6.36. *Hemorrhagic enterotyphlocolitis in a suckling rabbit kit due to* Klebsiella oxytoca. *(Source: Nemet et al. 2011. Reproduced with permission from BMJ Publishing Group Ltd.)*

catarrhal enteritis with serosal ecchymoses, and occasionally constipation, were observed at necropsy. On microscopic examination, hemorrhagic enterotyphlitis with marked submucosal edema was observed. Necrotic enteritis was frequently present in adults that succumbed to klebsiellosis. The organism was recoverable from a variety of tissues including intestine, liver, spleen, and lung. Possible predisposing factors that have been identified included the use of suboptimal concentrations of certain disinfectants, prior administration of antibiotics, and the emergence of antibiotic-resistant strains.

Lawsonia intracellularis Infection: Proliferative Enterocolitis/Histiocytic Enteritis

Lawsonia intracellularis is an obligate intracellular bacterium that does not grow in cell-free medium, although some success has been achieved with growth in cell cultures. Colonization of enterocytes by this organism has been identified in several species, including mice, rats, hamsters, guinea pigs, rabbits, and rhesus macaques as well as numerous other species. It is a significant pathogen in pigs and an emerging pathogen in horses. Proliferative and histiocytic lesions of the small intestine are the typical changes associated with *L. intracellularis* infections. For a number of years, the causative agent was called an intracellular *Campylobacter*-like organism. Based upon 16S rRNA sequencing, there appears to be little genetic variation among organisms from different host species, but interspecies susceptibility varies with different isolates. Transmission is likely to be by ingestion of fecal material, and experimental transmission has been achieved in this manner. There is no evidence that the organism infects tissue other than enteric mucosa. Location of lesions (gut segment) varies with species. In the rabbit, the jejunum and proximal ileum are typically affected. The fact that the location of lesions is typical for each host species suggests that intestinal microenvironment or host receptors may be critical to pathogenesis. The means of cellular invasion is not known, but in vitro studies indicate that it involves receptor–ligand mechanisms. Regardless of host species, *L. intracellularis* organisms grow to large numbers within the apical cytoplasm of enterocytes.

Pathology

In acute infections, diarrhea with mortality occurs in suckling, weanling, and young adult domestic rabbits. In animals necropsied during the acute disease, semifluid mucinous contents are frequently present, particularly in the colon and rectum. Animals with more chronic lesions have thickened opaque loops of small intestine (Fig. 6.37). The mucosal surfaces are rugose in character. Microscopically, mucosal lesions vary from suppurative and erosive to primarily proliferative in nature. Lesions of the erosive type range from focal denuding to segmental loss of enterocytes, with polymorphonuclear cell

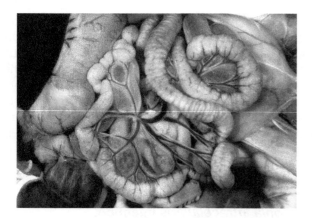

FIG. 6.37. *Histiocytic enteritis in a laboratory rabbit associated with* Lawsonia intracellularis *infection. Note the marked thickening and rugose appearance of the serosal surface of the small intestine.*

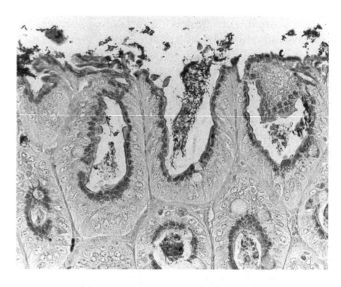

FIG. 6.39. *Intestinal mucosa from a rabbit infected with* Lawsonia intracellularis. *Note the dense argyrophilic populations of bacteria within the apical cytoplasm of enterocytes (Warthin–Starry stain).*

infiltration in the underlying areas. Proliferative lesions are characterized by multifocal to diffuse hyperplasia of enterocytes lining crypts and villi, with mononuclear cell infiltration. Histiocytes with abundant granular cytoplasm, and occasionally multinucleated giant cells, are often prominent in the lamina propria (Fig. 6.38). Lacteals are often dilated. Silver- and PAS-stained sections of affected mucosa reveal typical intracytoplasmic clusters of small bacteria in the apical cytoplasm of the crypt-villus column (Fig. 6.39). Histiocytes within the lamina propria have PAS-positive granular material in their cytoplasm. Electron microscopy reveals typical organisms in enterocytes, and histiocytes contain

degenerating bacterial debris. Marginal subclinical infections are common in enzootically infected rabbit colonies, with identification of lesions as incidental findings at necropsy. Coinfection with enteropathogenic *E. coli* has been documented in rabbits.

Diagnosis

The identification of the typical proliferative mucosal lesions and the demonstration of the intracellular organisms within the apices of enterocytes with the appropriate silver stains are confirmatory. The organism can be grown in cell culture. Other procedures described include the demonstration of the organism in fecal samples using immunomagnetic beads or PCR, the identification of bacterial surface antigen in tissue sections by immunohistochemistry, and the detection of antibodies to *L. intracellularis* in sera.

Listeria monocytogenes Infection: Listeriosis

Listeriosis was originally described in 1926 by Murray et al. in young rabbits and guinea pigs. At that time, the agent was named *Bacterium monocytogenes*. *Listeria monocytogenes* is a small Gram-positive, nonspore-forming rod with zoonotic potential. Recently, analysis of rabbit meat in Europe revealed it to be a significant source of food-borne Listeria. Listeriosis in rabbits is characterized by abortions and sudden deaths, particularly in does during advanced pregnancy.

Epizootiology and Pathogenesis

Listeria is a soil-borne organism. In sporadic outbreaks of the disease, the source of the organism is frequently attributed to contamination of feed or water. Inapparent

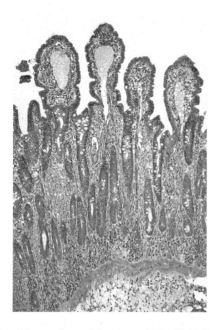

FIG. 6.38. *Jejunum from a laboratory rabbit with histiocytic enteritis due to* Lawsonia intracellularis *infection. Villi are shortened, lacteals are dilated, crypts are hyperplastic, and the lamina propria and submucosa are infiltrated with histiocytes and focal accumulations of lymphocytes. Source: © R J Hampson*

carriers and shedders may also occur. *Listeria monocytogenes* has a specific predilection for the gravid uterus in advanced pregnancy. Adult, nonpregnant does and bucks are usually resistant to the infection. Following oral or conjunctival inoculation of females in advanced pregnancy, abortions, stillbirths, and mortality in the dam usually occur. Pregnancy may be interrupted as early as 24 hours postinoculation. However, inoculation of females by the intravaginal, oral, or conjunctival route either prior to mating or early in pregnancy failed to produce disease. The organism can cross the placental barrier in advanced pregnancy. Uterine infections may persist postkindling and may serve as the source of infection for the next pregnancy. On the other hand, young rabbits may shed *Listeria* as an inapparent infection for several weeks postkindling.

Pathology

Deaths typically occur in does in advanced pregnancy. Straw-colored fluid is frequently present in the peritoneal cavity, occasionally with fibrinous exudate and ecchymoses on the serosal surface of the uterus. Disseminated pale, miliary foci of necrosis in the liver, edema of regional lymph nodes, splenomegaly, and visceral congestion are the usual macroscopic findings. The uterus may contain relatively intact, near-term kits (Fig. 6.40) or fetuses in various stages of decomposition or mummification. In acute cases, the placenta may be edematous and hemorrhagic, but in an infection of longer duration, the placenta is usually thickened, friable, and dull dirty gray, with an irregular surface. Characteristic microscopic changes seen in adult cases of listeriosis include focal hepatitis

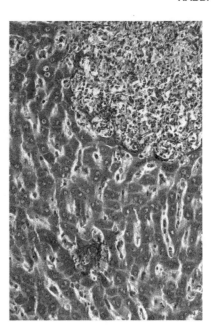

FIG. 6.41. *Focal hepatitis from a case of listeriosis in a pregnant doe. Note colonies of Gram-positive bacteria (Brown and Brenn stain).*

(Fig. 6.41). There may be focal inflammatory lesions in the adrenal cortices, congestion and thromboses in the splenic sinusoids and blood vessels, and acute necrotizing to chronic suppurative metritis and placentitis. In rabbits that die with the acute form of the disease, large numbers of Gram-positive bacilli are usually visible, particularly in the placenta. Focal hepatitis and occasionally meningitis have been observed in newborn kits that succumb within a few days of birth. Kits that survive may subsequently develop systemic listeriosis, or may present with stunting and meningoencephalitis.

Diagnosis

In acute cases of listeriosis, the organism can usually be readily recovered from the uterine wall, placenta, and fetuses. Blood, liver, and spleen are other likely sources of the organism at necropsy. Recovery of the organism by culture is considered to be a much more satisfactory method to confirm the diagnosis than are serological techniques. Isolation is enhanced when tissues to be cultured are held at 4°C for several days before inoculating culture plates. PCR methods have also been used for rapid diagnosis. Differential diagnoses include diseases causing disseminated foci of hepatic necrosis such as Tyzzer's disease, tularemia, and salmonellosis. In perinatal deaths seen in does with acute pasteurellosis and metritis, there may be acute necrotizing uterine lesions, but liver lesions are normally absent.

Moraxella bovis Infection

A rabbit that was housed in close proximity to cattle was described with suppurative metritis, pleuritis, pneumonia, and focal hepatic necrosis. Lesions were confirmed to be positive for *Moraxella bovis*.

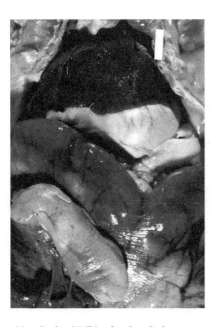

FIG. 6.40. *New Zealand White doe that died near-term with acute listeriosis. There are pinpoint-size foci of hepatitis. The externalized kit (lower left) is intact, with no evidence of maceration (Courtesy R.J. Hampson.)*

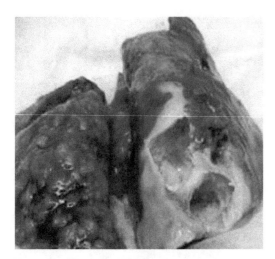

FIG. 6.42. *Pulmonary tuberculosis in a rabbit infected with* Mycobacterium tuberculosis. *Rabbits develop cavitary pulmonary lesions with frequent dissemination to other organs. (Source: Nedeltchev et al, 2009. Reproduced with permission from American Society for Microbiology.)*

Mycobacterium spp. Infection: Tuberculosis, Paratuberculosis
Tuberculosis

Rabbits are quite susceptible to experimental infection with *Mycobacterium bovis* and *M. tuberculosis*, but natural infection of domestic rabbits is now rare. Natural cases of tuberculosis in wild rabbits and hares have been reported, but are also rare. In the early 1900s, infection among domestic rabbits was relatively common due to feeding unpasteurized milk as a supplement to young rabbits. Laboratory rabbits are valued as models of tuberculosis, since they are prone to develop cavitary pulmonary lesions (Fig 6.42), as well as dissemination to other organs. Extrapulmonary dissemination is particularly common when rabbits are infected with *M. bovis*. Lesions are typical of tuberculosis, consisting of granulomas with giant cell formation and large numbers of acid-fast bacilli. Rabbits with generalized thoracic and abdominal tuberculosis have been reported, which were naturally infected with *M. avium*. In a single report, a dwarf rabbit was found to have pleural effusion and pale foci in the lungs due to infection with *M. genavense*. Microscopic findings included severe intra-alveolar infiltration with foamy macrophages and mild to moderate nonsuppurative interstitial pneumonia. Rare acid-fast organisms were observed with the Ziehl–Neelsen stain. Speciation was performed by PCR, since *M. genavense* is difficult to culture.

Paratuberculosis

Wild European rabbits are commonly infected with *Mycobacterium avium paratuberculosis* and are a significant reservoir for infection of livestock. Mild to severe histiocytic and granulomatous enteritis has been documented in wild rabbits involving primarily the small intestine, GALT, and mesenteric lymph nodes, as well as

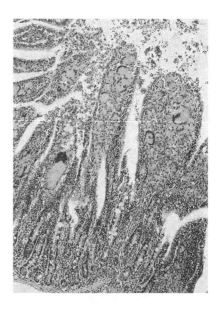

FIG. 6.43. *Small intestine of a wild* Oryctolagus *rabbit naturally infected with* Mycobacterium avium *spp.* paratuberculosis. *The lamina propria is densely infiltrated with histiocytes and multinucleated giant cells. (Source: Beard et al. 2001. Reproduced with permission from Elsevier.).*

periportal granulomas in the liver. The villus lamina propria and submucosa of affected areas were densely infiltrated with epithelioid macrophages and giant cells were prominent (Fig. 6.43). Foci of epithelioid macrophages were also present in the sacculus rotundus and appendix in the interfollicular zones at the base of lymphoid follicles. Acid-fast organisms were abundant in all lesions when tissues were stained with the Ziehl–Neelsen method (Fig. 6.44). Differential diagnosis includes *Lawsonia intracellularis* infection and accumulation of histiocytes in GALT lymphoid follicles. Definitive diagnosis can be achieved with acid-fast stains, culture, and PCR. Serology can be used for surveillance.

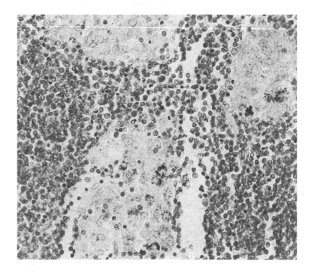

FIG. 6.44. *Acid-fast organisms within histiocytes of the GALT of a wild rabbit naturally infected with* Mycobacterium avium *spp.* paratuberculosis. *(Source: Beard et al. 2001. Reproduced with permission from Elsevier.)*

Pasteurella multocida Infection: Pasteurellosis; "Snuffles"

Pasteurella multocida is the most common bacterial pathogen of laboratory rabbits, and is a major cause of disease and mortality among pet rabbits and in many commercial rabbitries. Patterns of disease include purulent rhinitis, atrophic rhinitis, otitis media/interna, conjunctivitis, bronchopneumonia, abscessation, genital tract infections, abortions, neonatal mortality, and septicemia. For many years, *P. multocida* has been classified into a number of serotypes, based upon 5 capsular antigens (A, B, D, E, and F) and 16 serovars (formerly serotypes) based upon lipopolysaccharide (LPS) antigens. Historically, serovars 12:A, 3:A, and occasionally 3:D were the usual types found in rabbits with pasteurellosis, but serotype F originating from fowl cholera was recently discovered in rabbits in the Czech Republic. A variety of molecular genetic approaches can now be used to detect and classify *P. multocida*.

Epizootiology and Pathogenesis

The upper respiratory tract is the primary nidus of infection in affected rabbits. The organism can be spread by various routes from this site: to the lower respiratory tract by the aerogenous route; to the middle ear by the eustachian tube, hematogenously, or by local extension; to the external genital tract by venereal spread or nasal inoculation; and to other areas of the body by the hematogenous route or by local spread. In addition, infections of the upper and lower respiratory tract have been produced experimentally by subcutaneous or intravenous inoculations. Inapparent carriers of *P. multocida* are frequent, and even deep nasal swabs may fail to detect all animals carrying the organism in the nasal passages and nasopharynx on culture. Rabbits negative on nasal culture may be harboring *P. multocida* in the tympanic bullae, and the organism may be as readily recoverable from the middle ear as from the nasopharynx. Subclinical infections involving the tympanic bullae are relatively common. The organism may be acquired through various sources, including direct nasal contact with a shedder animal and contact with infected vaginal secretions. The vagina may serve as an important means of venereal spread to breeding males. Similarly, bucks may harbor *P. multocida* in their genital tract, and the organism may be transmitted to the does at mating. In young rabbits born to infected does, colonization with *P. multocida* may occur as early as 3 weeks of age. We have seen acute bronchopneumonia in kits as early as 3–4 weeks of age.

Aerosols do not appear to play a major role in the spread of infection in facilities with adequate air exchange. Housing and husbandry practices undoubtedly have a significant influence on the incidence of pasteurellosis in commercial and laboratory facilities. The reduction of air changes during colder months, poor sanitation, and overcrowding are all conditions that promote the elevation of the ammonia levels above a critical level of 25 ppm, increasing the likelihood of respiratory disease. The role of fomites in transmission under field conditions is not known. *Pasteurella* is often recoverable from the watering nipples used by rabbits with snuffles. In view of the demonstrated adherence of type A *P. multocida* to rabbit pharyngeal cells, this may be one means of spread. The possibility of interspecies transmission is an important consideration. Strains of *P. multocida* from other species (bovine and avian isolates) have been passed in mice and rabbits. Following conjunctival inoculation of New Zealand White rabbits with either of the strains, acute pasteurellosis occurred. Experimental inoculation of serotype F (fowl cholera) resulted in fibrinopurulent or hemorrhagic pneumonia by intranasal route in 3–6 days and septicemia by subcutaneous route in 2–3 days. Peroral challenge showed no clinical signs of disease or macroscopic lesions. In the laboratory setting, experimental manipulations may enhance susceptibility to the disease, particularly procedures that may have an impact on the immune system. Conversely, it is often difficult to consistently produce significant lesions in unmanipulated "healthy" rabbits inoculated intranasally with virulent strains of *P. multocida*.

Pathology

The most common clinical manifestations of pasteurellosis are rhinitis and vestibular syndrome. Chronic rhinitis, with catarrhal to mucopurulent exudate, is associated with the typical upper respiratory tract form of the disease. When performing a necropsy, it is essential that the nasal bones overlying the turbinates be removed to provide adequate exposure for a thorough examination of this area. Turbinate atrophy has been observed in rabbits naturally or experimentally infected with a 12:A serotype of *P. multocida* (Fig. 6.45). The prevalence of this manifestation has not been determined. Upper respiratory infections are often accompanied by conjunctivitis and otitis media, involving one or both tympanic bullae. In many cases, there may be no clinical evidence of middle ear infection; thus, it is essential that the tympanic bullae be opened and examined at necropsy. Grossly, the affected middle ears contain a white or dull yellow to gray, thick, viscid exudate (Fig. 6.46). The lining of the tympanic bullae is light tan and opaque. On microscopic examination, there is often squamous metaplasia of the epithelium lining the tympanic bulla, with leukocytic infiltration into the submucosa and tympanic cavity. Rupture of the tympanic membrane may also occur, with extension into the inner ear and occasionally the brain.

Pulmonary lesions arise from extension of upper respiratory infections or by the hematogenous route. Bronchopneumonia may vary from localized cranioventral involvement to acute necrotizing fibrinopurulent or fibrinohemorrhagic bronchopneumonia (Fig. 6.47).

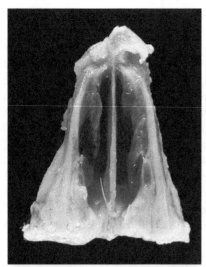

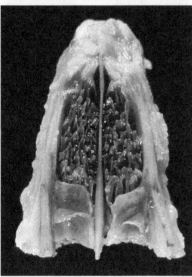

FIG. 6.45.   *Turbinate atrophy associated with chronic rhinitis due to* Pasteurella multocida *infection. Note the loss of turbinates in the affected (top) compared to the normal control rabbit (bottom). (Source: DiGiacomo et al., 1989, reprinted with permission from American Veterinary Medical Association.)*

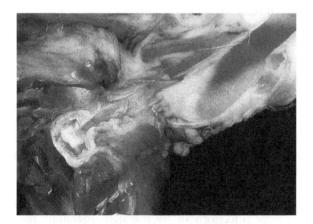

FIG. 6.46.   *Suppurative otitis media in a rabbit with chronic* Pasteurella multocida *infection. Purulent material is present within the opened tympanic bulla and the wall of the bulla is thickened.*

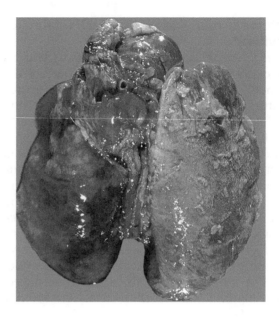

FIG. 6.47.   *Fibrinohemorrhagic bronchopneumonia and pleuritis in a rabbit with peracute pulmonary pasteurellosis. Fibrinous exudate is present on the pleural surface.*

Affected lung tissue in the acute necrotizing form is swollen and moderately firm, frequently with concurrent fibrinous pleuritis and pericarditis. In some cases, pulmonary lesions may be confined to one lung lobe. Chronic disease may encompass an entire lung lobe, with fibrinopurulent pleuritis, pericarditis, and empyema. Microscopically, in animals with localized lower respiratory tract disease, the lesions may vary from chronic bronchitis with peribronchial lymphocytic infiltration to alveolitis with infiltrating leukocytes, heterophils predominating. In the acute, necrotizing form of the disease, destruction of alveoli and small airways, alveolar flooding with fibrinous exudate and erythrocytes, and infiltration with heterophils are typical findings. Multinucleated giant cells may be present in affected alveoli. Hematogenous infection of the lung may also occur, with formation of single or multiple abscesses.

Macroscopic findings in the female reproductive tract may include pyometra, with chronic suppurative salpingitis and perioophoritis or localized suppurative lesions. Acute, transmural, necrotizing metritis has been associated with peracute pasteurellosis. This form occurs during the perinatal period, presumably due to invasion via the dilated cervices. Abortions and stillbirths may precede the death of the doe. Affected does usually die within a few hours after showing signs of disease. At necropsy, fibrinous exudate may be adherent to the uterine serosa, with ecchymoses. The uterine wall is thickened and contains necrotic material. Microscopically, there is acute, necrotizing transmural metritis and serositis, with changes in other organs consistent with a bacterial septicemia. In addition, chronic suppurative metritis and pyometra may also occur (Fig. 6.48). In

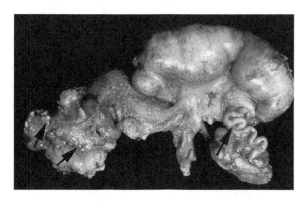

FIG. 6.48. *Pyometra in an adult doe associated with chronic* Pasteurella multocida *infection. There is asymmetric distention of the uterine horns, and the fallopian tubes are distended with purulent exudate (right arrow). Small abscesses are scattered on the serosa (left arrows).*

bucks with genital tract lesions, there may be suppurative orchitis with abscessation.

Circumscribed abscesses containing thick, yellowgray exudate may involve various sites, including subcutaneous tissue, mammary glands, brain, lung, visceral organs, and bone. Abscesses involving the jaw are particularly difficult to treat, since they tend to excavate bone and are difficult to drain because of the viscid nature of pus in this species. Localized infections may spread to other sites, resulting in manifestations such as vegetative endocarditis.

Acute septicemia is another possible manifestation of the disease. Affected animals may be found dead, with no previous evidence of disease. There may be a concurrent rhinitis and/or otitis media evident at necropsy, but frequently there is no gross evidence of lesions at necropsy. Microscopically, there should be changes consistent with an acute bacterial septicemia, including hemorrhage and variable thromboses of small vessels. Acute suppurative meningoencephalomyelitis may also occur, occasionally with concomitant optic neuritis and iritis.

Diagnosis
Definitive diagnosis is best achieved with bacterial culture. In cases of suspected septicemic pasteurellosis, the organism should be recoverable from a variety of parenchymatous organs and heart blood. Nasal cultures, although useful in identifying carriers/shedders of the organism, will not necessarily detect all infected animals. ELISA has been used to serologically identify animals that were consistently negative for *Pasteurella* on deep nasal culture. PCR can be used for detection, but molecular methods are more useful for characterizing isolates. Differential diagnoses of suppurative lesions or respiratory infections include other pyogenic infections, such as *Staphylococcus*, *Bordetella*, and rarely *Klebsiella*.

Pseudomonas aeruginosa Infection
Under conditions of chronic moisture, such as wet dewlaps, *P. aeruginosa* may be associated with exudative dermatitis. Chronically wet fur may also foster growth of *P. aeruginosa*, resulting in "green fur syndrome." In addition, an outbreak of pneumonia and diarrhea has been associated with *P. aeruginosa*. These are environmental conditions that can be managed with chlorination of the water.

Salmonella spp. Infection: Salmonellosis
Although once common in the early 1900s, salmonellosis is relatively rare in domestic rabbits housed in wellmanaged facilities. Infection with *Salmonella enterica* serotypes Typhimurium and Enteritidis, as well as other serotypes, can result in explosive epizootics of septicemia, abortion, and rapid death. Diarrhea is inconsistently present. Salmonellosis has been identified in specific-pathogen-free rabbits infected with *S. enterica* serotype Mbandaka following experimental surgery and irradiation. Pathologic changes included polyserositis, focal hepatic necrosis, splenomegaly, acute enteritis with fibrinous exudation, and suppurative metritis. In view of the public health aspects, and the dangers of interspecies spread, the diagnosis of salmonellosis warrants thorough investigation and eradication.

Staphylococcus aureus Infections: Staphylococcosis
Staphylococcus aureus is a common cause of subcutaneous abscesses, dermatitis, mastitis, pododermatitis, and septicemia in rabbits. Genital and respiratory tract infections may also occur. Within a population of rabbits, 2 patterns of infection are apparent. A low level of sporadic lesions is associated with low-virulence strains of *S. aureus*, whereas high-virulence strains may cause epizootic outbreaks with high morbidity. Following the initial epizootic, high-virulence *S. aureus* subsequently becomes enzootically entrenched within the herd, with chronic decline in production. Low- and high-virulence strains of *S. aureus* can be somewhat differentiated by biotyping (culture and beta hemolysin characteristics), but other typing methods have included phage typing, and more recently genotyping. Low-virulence strains typically belong to the poultry or human biotype, whereas high-virulence strains have a different biotype–phage type known as "mixed CV-C-3A/3C/55/71." Genetic analysis suggests that there was a single clonal origin of the most common high-virulence strain, which has become widespread in many European countries. High-density commercial production has contributed to the spread of this strain.

Epizootiology and Pathogenesis
Transmission of *S. aureus* can occur through environmental contamination, direct and indirect contact, from does to kits, among littermates and cagemates, and

through semen. Introduction of new breeding stock to the herd has been a major source of contamination with high-virulence strains. Traumatic lesions through wire cage floors and fighting, as well as the neonatal umbilicus are important conduits of *S. aureus*. In some outbreaks, the same phage type isolated from the rabbits has been isolated from the nares of human contacts. Virulent strains of the organism may be harbored as an inapparent infection in the upper respiratory tract. Such infections may spread by direct contact, but the organism has also been recovered from the air in contaminated facilities. Neonatal staphylococcal infections are a recognized cause of neonatal mortality in domestic rabbits in Europe, the United States, and Canada. In France, it is considered to be an important cause of mortality in suckling rabbits in commercial rabbitries. Disseminated staphylococcal infections have also been observed in wild rabbits and hares.

Pathology

In mature animals, chronic suppurative lesions may occur in the skin, mammary glands, genital tract, conjunctiva, footpads (see "Pododermatitis: Sore Hocks"), and upper and lower respiratory tract. In neonatal infections, lesions may be confined to the skin and manifest as multiple raised suppurative lesions a few millimeters in diameter. These may involve a variety of areas, including the extremities, head, back, and sides (Fig. 6.49). The acute septicemic form of the disease usually occurs only in suckling kits during the first week of life, frequently with high mortality in affected litters. At necropsy, multifocal suppurative lesions may be present in the subcutaneous tissue and in viscera, including lung, kidney, spleen, heart, and liver (Fig. 6.50). Occasionally, systemic staphylococcosis with focal suppurative lesions occurs in adult rabbits (Fig. 6.51). Microscopically, focal suppurative lesions are present in affected organs. Gram-

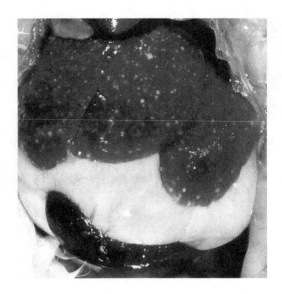

FIG. 6.50. *Multifocal suppurative hepatitis in a 10-day-old rabbit kit with fatal* Staphylococcus aureus *septicemia.*

positive bacterial colonies are typically associated with the lesions. In staphylococcal mastitis, affected glands may vary in appearance from swollen, red areas with induration of the overlying skin to chronic abscessation. Lesions in the respiratory tract, when present, vary from mucopurulent rhinitis to localized bronchopneumonia and/or abscessation of the lung. Differential diagnoses include pasteurellosis, Tyzzer's disease, and listeriosis.

Streptococcus spp. Infection

Septicemic infections of young rabbits were once associated with *Streptococcus* spp., but such infections appear to be rare among contemporary rabbit populations. Recently, an outbreak of disease with high mortality was reported in China among young commercially raised rabbits. Rabbits presented with acute respiratory distress, fever, paddling and convulsions. Necropsy revealed congestion and hemorrhage in multiple organs, particularly the lungs. Lesions consistent with diffuse intravascular coagulation were widespread. Gram-positive cocci were present in multiple tissues, and culture revealed *S. agalactiae*, which was confirmed by sequence analysis. The disease resembled streptococcal toxic shock

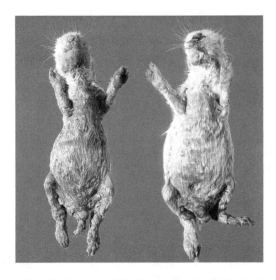

FIG. 6.49. *Pyoderma in rabbit kits associated with* Staphylococcus aureus *infection.*

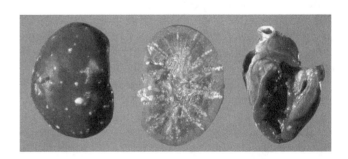

FIG. 6.51. *Multifocal suppurative nephritis and myocarditis in an adult New Zealand White rabbit with systemic* Staphylococcus aureus *infection. Source: D. Imai, University of California, Davis, CA. Reproduced with permission from D. Imai.*

syndrome. Differential diagnosis must rule out rabbit hemorrhagic disease, which presents with similar gross and microscopic lesions.

Treponema paraluis-cuniculi Infection: Rabbit Syphilis

Treponema paraluis-cuniculi (formerly *T. cuniculi*) is a spirochete that has not been successfully grown in artificial media or cell culture. Based on serological surveys, treponematosis occurs occasionally in laboratory rabbits. However, the disease is seldom detected on cursory examination. The venereal route is the most important means of spread, although extragenital contact transmission may also occur. Young animals may develop the disease following contact with an infected dam. Young rabbits have been shown to be relatively resistant to the infection, either by natural exposure or experimental inoculation. There is no evidence of intrauterine transmission. There appears to be a strain-related resistance/susceptibility to clinical disease postexposure. Infection has also been diagnosed in wild rabbits in Britain.

Pathology

Lesions associated with treponematosis may occur in the vulva, prepuce, anal region, muzzle (Fig 6.52), and periorbital region. Initially, changes are characterized by edema, erythema, and papules at the mucocutaneous junctions. Syphilitic lesions later progress to ulceration and crusting. On microscopic examination, hyperplasia of the epidermis, necrosis of epithelial cells, and erosions and ulcerations, with infiltration by plasma cells, macrophages, and heterophils, are typical changes (Fig. 6.53). The infection is confined primarily to the epithelium, and other than hyperplasia of the regional lymph nodes, visceral involvement does not occur.

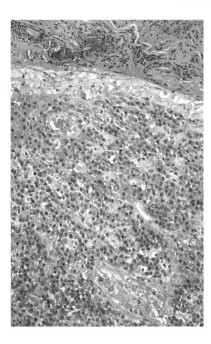

FIG. 6.53. *Skin from the muzzle of a laboratory rabbit with rabbit syphilis. There is dense infiltration of the dermis with mixed leukocytes, degeneration of epidermis, and serous exudation on the surface. Source: A. Strom, University of California, Davis, CA. Reproduced with permission from A. Strom.*

Diagnosis

Scrapings from lesions, with wet mount preparation and dark-field examination, is the recommended method for confirming the diagnosis. Demonstration of the spirochetes by silver staining of lesions in histology sections may be used (Fig. 6.54). Serology is a reliable diagnostic procedure. Tests available include the demonstration of plasma reagin antibody and the fluorescent treponemal antigen test. Differential diagnoses include moist dermatitis, *Pasteurella* infections of the external genitalia, and traumatic lesions.

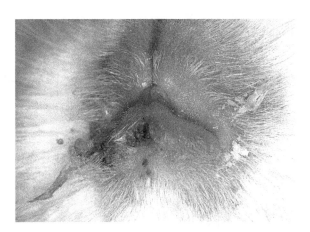

FIG. 6.52. *Erosive chelitis in a laboratory rabbit infected with* Treponema paraluis-cuniculi. *The muzzle region is a frequent site for rabbit syphilis lesions.*

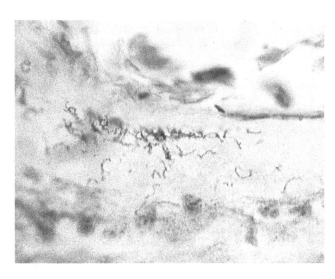

FIG. 6.54. *Rabbit syphilis lesion, depicting numerous spirochetes within the surface exudate (Warthin–Starry stain).*

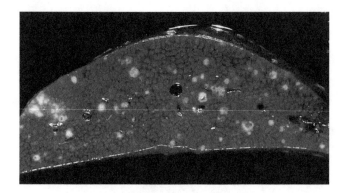

FIG. 6.55. *Multifocal caseation necrosis in the liver of a rabbit naturally infected with* Yersinia pseudotuberculosis. *(Courtesy D. Imai.)*

Yersinia pestis Infection: Plague

Wild rabbits are among many wild species that may become infected with *Yersinia pestis*, and transmission to humans from infected *Sylvilagus* spp. rabbits has been documented on multiple occasions. Infection of domestic rabbits is exceedingly rare. The bacterium causes septicemic disease in infected animals.

Yersinia pseudotuberculosis Infection: Pseudotuberculosis, Yersiniosis

Infection of domestic rabbits with *Y. pseudotuberculosis* is rare, but infection may be common in some populations of hares. It is among the most important lethal infections in wild hares in Europe. The bacterium is usually transmitted by the ingestion of food or water contaminated by birds and rodents. Lesions are characterized by focal granulomatous lesions in the intestine, with foci of caseation necrosis in the liver (Fig 6.55), spleen, lymph nodes, and reproductive tract.

BIBLIOGRAPHY FOR BACTERIAL INFECTIONS

General Reference for Bacterial Diseases of the Rabbit
Boucher, S. & Nouaille, L. (2013) *Maladies des Lapins*, 3rd edn. Editions France Agricole.
DeLong, D. (2012) Bacterial diseases. In: *The Laboratory Rabbit, Guinea Pig, Hamster, and Other Rodents* (eds. M.A. Suckow, K.A. Stevens, & R.P. Wilson), pp. 301–363. Elsevier.
Wibbelt, G. & Frolich, K. (2005) Infectious diseases in European brown hares (*Lepus europaeus*). *Wildlife Biology in Practice* 1:86–93.

Acinetobacter calcoaceticus Infection
Kunstyr, I. & Hansen, H. (1978) *Acinetobacter calcoaceticus* as the possible cause of bronchopneumonia in rabbits. *Deutsche Tier-arztliche Wochenschrift* 85:293–295.

Actinobacillus spp. Infection
Arseculeratne, S.N. (1962) Actinobacillosis in joints of rabbits. *Journal of Comparative Pathology* 72:33–39.
Meyerholz, D.K. & Haynes, J.S. (2005) *Actinobacillus capsulatus* septicemia in a domestic rabbit (*Oryctolagus cuniculus*). *Journal of Veterinary Diagnostic Investigation* 17:83–85.

Moyaert, H., Decostere, A., Baele, M., Hermans, K., Tavernier, P., Chiers, K., & Haesebrouck, F. (2007) An unusual *Actinobacillus equuli* strain isolated from a rabbit with Tyzzer's disease. *Veterinary Microbiology* 124:184–186.

Actinomyces spp. Infection
Hong, I.H., Lee, H.S., Park, J.K., Goo, M.J., Yuan, D.W., Hwang, O.K., Hong, K.S., Han, J.Y., Ji, A.R., Ki, M.R., & Jeong, K.S. (2009) Actinomycosis in a pet rabbit. *Journal of Veterinary Dentistry* 26:110–111.
Sorenson, B. & Saliba, A.M. (1961) Actinomycose espontanea em coelhos. *Biologico* 27:131–135.
Tyrrell, K.L., Citron, D.M., Jenkins, J.R., Goldstein, E.J.C., et al. (2002) Periodontal bacteria in rabbit mandibular and maxillary abscesses. *Journal of Clinical Microbiology* 40:1044–1047.

Bordetella bronchiseptica Infection
Bemis, D.A. & Wilson, S.A. (1985) Influence of potential virulence determinants on *Bordetella bronchiseptica*-induced ciliostasis. *Infection and Immunity* 50:35–42.
Deeb, B.J., DiGiacomo, R.F., Bernard, B.L., & Silbernagel, S.M. (1990) *Pasteurella multocida* and *Bordetella bronchiseptica* infection in rabbits. *Journal of Clinical Microbiology* 28:70–75.
Glass, L.S. & Beasley, J.N. (1990) Infection with and antibody response to *Pasteurella multocida* and *Bordetella bronchiseptica* in immature rabbits. *Laboratory Animal Science* 39:406–410.
Matsuyama, T. & Taking, T. (1980) Scanning electron microscopic studies of *Bordetella bronchiseptica* on the rabbit tracheal mucosa. *Journal of Medical Microbiology* 13:159–161.
Percy, D.H., Karrow, N., & Bhasin, J.L. (1988) Incidence of *Pasteurella* and *Bordetella* infections in fryer rabbits: an abattoir survey. *Journal of Applied Rabbit Research* 11:245–246.
Watson, W.T., Goldsboro, J.A., Willimans, F.P., & Sueur, R. (1975) Experimental respiratory infections with *Pasteurella multocida* and *Bordetella bronchiseptica* in rabbits. *Laboratory Animal Science* 25:459–464.

Brucella spp. Infection: Brucellosis
Renoux, G. & Sacquet, E. (1957) Brucellose spontanee du lapin domestique. *Archives de l' Institut Pasteur de Tunis* 34:231–232.
Sterba, F. (1983) Differential pathognomonic diagnosis of brucellosis in hares. *Veterinarni Medicina-Praha* 28:293–308.
Vitovec, J., Vladik, P., Zahor, Z., & Slaby, V. (1976) Morphological study of 70 cases of brucellosis in rabbits caused by *Brucella suis*. *Veterinarni Medicina-Praha* 21:359–368.

Campylobacter spp. Infection
Moon, H.W., Cutlip, R.C., Amtower, W.C., & Matthews, P.J. (1974) Intraepithelial vibrio associated with acute typhlitis of young rabbits. *Veterinary Pathology* 11:313–326.
Revez, J., Rossi, M., Piva, S., Florio, D., Lucchi, A., Parisi, A., Manfreda, G., & Zanoni, R.G. (2013) Occurrence of (ε-proteo-bacterial species in rabbits (*Oryctolagus cuniculus*) reared in intensive and rural farms. *Veterinary Microbiology* 162:288–292.
Zanoni, R.G., Debruyne, L., Rossi, M., Revez, J., & Vandamme, P. (2009) *Campylobacter cuniculorum* sp. Nov., from rabbits. *International Journal of Systematic and Evolutionary Microbiology* 59:1666–1671.

Chlamydophila spp. Infection
Flatt, R.E. & Dungworth, D.L. (1971) Enzootic pneumonia in rabbits: microbiology and comparison with lesions experimentally produced by *Pasteurella multocida* and a chlamydial organism. *American Journal of Veterinary Research* 32:627–637.
Krishna, L. & Gupta, V.K. (1989) Chlamydial pneumonia in an angora rabbit: a case report. *Journal of Applied Rabbit Research* 12:83.
Krishna, L. & Kulshrestha, L. (1985) Spontaneous cases of chlamydial conjunctivitis in rabbits. *Journal of Applied Rabbit Research* 8:75.

Mousa, H.A.A., Mahmoud, A.H., & Ibrahim, A.M. (2010) Detection of chlamydia in rabbit using traditional methods and electron microscopy. *Global Veterinaria* 4:74–77.

Muhlestein, J.B. (2000) *Chlamydia pneumoniae*-induced atherosclerosis in a rabbit model. *Journal of Infectious Diseases* 181 (Suppl. 3): S505–S507.

Pantchev, A., Sting, R., Bauerfeind, R., Tyczka, J., & Sachse, K. (2010) Detection of *Chlamydophila* and *Chlamydia* spp. of veterinary interest using species-specific real-time PCR assays. *Comparative Immunology, Microbiology and Infectious Diseases* 33:473–484.

CAR Bacillus Infection

Caniatti, M., Crippa, L., Giusti, M., Mattiello, S., Grill, G., Orsenigo, R., & Scanziani, E. (1998) Cilia-associated respiratory (CAR) bacillus infection in conventionally reared rabbits. *Zentralblatt fur Veterinarmedizin B* 45:363–371.

Cundiff, D.D., Besch-Williford, C.L., Hook, R.R., Jr, Franklin, C.L., & Riley, L.K. (1995) Characterization of cilia-associated respiratory bacillus in rabbits and analysis of the 16s rRNA gene sequence. *Laboratory Animal Science* 45:22–26.

Kurisu, K., Kyo, S., Shiomoto, Y., & Matsushita, S. (1990) Cilia-associated respiratory bacillus infection in rabbits. *Laboratory Animal Science* 40:413–415.

Oros, J., Poveda, J.B., Rodriguez, J.L., Franklin, C.L., & Fernandez, A. (1997) Natural cilia-associated respiratory bacillus infection in rabbits used for elaboration of hyperimmune serum against *Mycoplasma* sp. *Zentralblatt fur Veterinarmedizin B* 44:313–317.

Corynebacterium bovis Infection

Arseculeratne, S.N. & Navaratnam, C. (1975) *Corynebacterium bovis* as a pathogen in rabbits. *Research in Veterinary Science* 18:216–217.

Clostridial Diseases

Clostridial Enteropathy/Enterotoxemia

Butt, M.T., Papendick, R.E., Carbone, L.G., & Quimby, F.W. (1994) A cytotoxicity assay for *Clostridium spiroforme* enterotoxin in cecal fluid of rabbits. *Laboratory Animal Science* 44:52–54.

Carman, R.J. & Borriello, S.P. (1984) Infectious nature of *Clostridium spiroforme*-mediated rabbit enterotoxaemia. *Veterinary Microbiology* 9:497–502.

Carman, R.J. & Evans, R.H. (1984) Experimental and spontaneous clostridial enteropathies of laboratory and free living lagomorphs. *Laboratory Animal Science* 34:443–452.

Cheeke, P.R. & Patton, N.M. (1978) Effect of alfalfa and dietary fiber on the growth performance of weanling rabbits. *Laboratory Animal Science* 28:167–172.

Drigo, I., Bacchin, C., Cocchi, M., Bano, L. & Agnoletti, F. (2008) Development of PCR protocols for specific identification of *Clostridium spiroforme* and detection of sas and sbs genes. *Veterinary Microbiology* 131:414–418.

Holmes, H.T., et al. (1988) Isolation of *Clostridium spiroforme* from rabbits. *Laboratory Animal Science* 39:167–168.

Keel, M.K. & Sanger, J.G. (2006) The comparative pathology of *Clostridium difficile*-associated disease. *Veterinary Pathology* 43:225–240.

Lee, W.K., Fujisawa, T., Kawamura, S., Itoh, K., & Mitsuoka, T. (1991) Isolation and identification of clostridia from the intestine of laboratory animals. *Laboratory Animals* 25:9–15.

Patton, N.M., Holmes, H.T., Riggs, R.J., & Cheeke, P.R. (1978) Enterotoxemia in rabbits. *Laboratory Animal Science* 28:536–540.

Peeters, J.E., Geeroms, R., Carman, R.J., & Wilkins, T.D. (1986) Significance of *Clostridium spiroforme* in the enteritis-complex of commercial rabbits. *Veterinary Microbiology* 12:25–31.

Perkins, S.E., et al. (1995) Detection of *Clostridium difficile* toxins from small intestine and cecum of rabbits with naturally acquired enterotoxemia. *Laboratory Animal Science* 45:379–385.

Rehg, J.E. & Lu, Y.-S. (1981) *Clostridium difficile* colitis in a rabbit following antibiotic therapy for pasteurellosis. *Journal of the American Veterinary Medical Association* 179:1296–1297.

Rehg, J.E. & Pakes, S.P. (1982) Implication of *Clostridium difficile* and *Clostridium perfringens* iota toxins in experimental lincomycin-associated colitis of rabbits. *Laboratory Animal Science* 32:253–257.

Clostridium piliforme Infection: Tyzzer's Disease

Allen, A.M., Ganaway, J.R., Moore, T.D., & Kinard, R.F. (1965) Tyzzer's disease syndrome in laboratory rabbits. *American Journal of Pathology* 46:859–882.

Duncan, A.J. (1993) Assignment of the agent of Tyzzer's disease to *Clostridium piliforme* comb. nov. on the basis of 16S rRNA sequence analysis. *International Journal of Systematic Bacteriology* 43:314–318.

Feldman, S.H., Kiavand, A., Seidelin, M., & Reiske, H.R. (2006) Ribosomal RNA sequences of *Clostridium piliforme* isolated from rodent and rabbit: re-examining the phylogeny of the Tyzzer's disease agent and development of a diagnostic polymerase chain reaction assay. *Journal of the American Association for Laboratory Animal Science* 45:65–73.

Franklin, C.L., Motzel, S.L., Besch-Williford, C.L., Hook, R.R., Jr, & Riley, L.K. (1994) Tyzzer's infection: host specificity of *Clostridium piliforme* isolates. *Laboratory Animal Science* 44:568–571.

Fries, A.S. (1977) Studies on Tyzzer's disease: application of immunofluorescence for detection of *Bacillus piliformis* and for demonstration and determination of antibodies to it in sera from mice and rabbits. *Laboratory Animals* 11:69–73.

Ganaway, J.R., McReynolds, R.S., & Allen, A.M. (1976) Tyzzer's disease in free-living cottontail rabbits (*Sylvilagus floridanus*) in Maryland. *Journal of Wildlife Diseases* 12:545–549.

Motzel, S.L. & Riley, L.K. (1991) *Bacillus piliformis* flagellar antigens for serodiagnosis of Tyzzer's disease. *Journal of Clinical Microbiology* 29:2566–2570.

Niepceron, A. & Licois, D. (2010) Development of a high-sensitivity nested PCR assay for detection of *Clostridium piliforme* in clinical samples. *The Veterinary Journal* 185:222–224.

Peeters, J.E., Charlier, G., Halen, P., Geeroms, R., & Raeymaekers, R. (1985) Naturally-occurring Tyzzer's disease (*Bacillus piliformis* infection) in commercial rabbits: a clinical and pathological study. *Annalles de Recherches Veterinaires* 16:69–79.

Spencer, T.H., Ganaway, J.R., & Waggie, K.S. (1990) Cultivation of *Bacillus piliformis* (Tyzzer) in mouse fibroblasts (3T3) cells. *Veterinary Microbiology* 29:291–297.

Clostridium botulinum Dysautonomia

Hahn, C.N., Whitwell, K.E., & Mayhew, G. (2001) Central nervous system pathology in cases of leporine dysautonomia. *Veterinary Record* 149:745–746.

Hahn, C.N., Whitwell, K.E., & Mayhew, I.G. (2005) Neuropathological lesions resembling equine grass sickness in rabbits. *Veterinary Record* 156:778–779.

Van der Hage, M.H. & Dorrestein, G.M. (1996) Caecal impaction in the rabbit: relationships with dysautonomia. Proceedings of the 6th World Rabbit Congress, Toulouse, France, pp. 77–80.

Whitwell, K.E. (1991) Do hares suffer from grass sickness? *Veterinary Record* 128:395–396.

Whitwell, K. & Needham, J. (1996) Mucoid enteropathy in UK rabbits: dysautonomia confirmed. *Veterinary Record* 139:323–333.

Clostridium perfringens Epizootic Rabbit Enteropathy

Coudert, P. & Licois, D. (2005) Epizootic rabbit enteropathy: Study of early phenomena with fresh inoculum and attempt at inactivation. *World Rabbit Science* 13:229–238.

Dewree, R., Meulemans, L., Lassence, C., Desmecht, D., Ducatelle, R., Mast, J., Licois, D., Vindevogel, H., & Marlier, D. (2007)

Experimentally induced epizootic rabbit enteropathy: clinical, histopathological, ultrastructural, bacteriological and haematological findings. *World Rabbit Science* 15:91–102.

Licois, D., Wyers, M., & Coudert, P. (2005) Epizootic rabbit enteropathy: experimental transmission and clinical characterization. *Veterinary Research* 36:601–613.

Marlier, D., Dewree, R., Lassence, C., Licois, D., Mainil, J., Coudert, P., Meulemans, L., Ducatelle, R., & Vindevogel, H. (2006) Infectious agents associated with epizootic rabbit enteropathy: isolation and attempts to reproduce the syndrome. *The Veterinary Journal* 172:493–500.

Romero, C., Nicodemus, N., Jarava, M.L., Menoyo, D., & de Blas, C. (2011) Characterization of *Clostridium perfringens* presence and concentration of its alpha-toxin in the caecal contents of fattening rabbits suffering from digestive diseases. *World Rabbit Science* 19:177–189.

Escherichia coli Infection

Enteropathogenic *Escherichia coli*

Blanco, J.E., Blanco, M., Blanco, J., Mora, A., Balaguer, L., Mourino, M., Juarez, A., & Jansen, W.H. (1996) O serogroups, biotypes, and *eae* genes in *Escherichia coli* strains isolated from diarrheic and healthy rabbits. *Journal of Clinical Microbiology* 34:3104–3107.

Coussement, W., Ducatelle, R., Charlier, G., Okerman, L., & Hoorens, J. (1984) Pathology of experimental colibacillosis in rabbits. *Zentralblatt fur Veterinarmedizin B* 31:64–72.

Gallois, M., Gidenne, T., Tasca, C., Caubet, C., Coudert, C., Milon, A., & Boulier, S. (2007) Maternal milk contains antimicrobial factors that protect young rabbits from enteropathogenic *Escherichia coli* infection. *Clinical and Vaccine Immunology* 14:585–592.

Heczko, U., Abe, A., & Finlay, B.B. (2000) In vivo interactions of rabbit enteropathogenic *Escherichia coli* O103 with its host: an electron microscopic and histopathologic study. *Microbes and Infection* 2:5–16.

Peeters, J.E., Charlier, G.J., & Halen, P.H. (1984) Pathogenicity of attaching and effacing enteropathogenic *Escherichia coli* isolated from diarrheic suckling and weanling rabbits for newborn rabbits. *Infection and Immunity* 46:690–696.

Peeters, J.E., Charlier, G.J., & Raeymaekers, R. (1985) Scanning and transmission electron microscopy of attaching effacing *Escherichia coli* in weanling rabbits. *Veterinary Pathology* 22:54–59.

Peeters, J.E., Geeroms, R., & Glorieux, B. (1984) Experimental *Escherichia coli* enteropathy in weanling rabbits: clinical manifestations and pathological findings. *Journal of Comparative Pathology* 94:521–528.

Peeters, J.E., Geeroms, R., & Orskov, F. (1988) Biotype, serotype, and pathogenicity of attaching and effacing enteropathogenic *Escherichia coli* strains isolated from diarrheic commercial rabbits. *Infection and Immunity* 56:1442–1448.

Peeters, J.E., Pohl, P., Okerman, L., & Devriese, L.A. (1984) Pathogenic properties of *Escherichia coli* strains isolated from diarrheic commercial rabbits. *Journal of Clinical Microbiology* 20:34–39.

Prohaszka, L. & Baron, F. (1981) Studies on *E. coli*-enteropathy in weanling rabbits. *Zentralblatt fur Veterinarmedizin B* 28:102–110.

Schauer, D.B., McCathey, S.N., Daft, B.M., Jha, S.S., Tatterson, L.E., Taylor, N.S., & Fox, J.G. (1998) Proliferative enterocolitis associated with dual infection with enteropathogenic *Escherichia coli* and *Lawsonia intracellularis* in rabbits. *Journal of Clinical Microbiology* 36:1700–1703.

Swennes, A.G., Buckley, E.M., Parry, N.M.A., Madden, C.M., Garcia, A., Morgan, P.B., Astrofsky, K.M., & Fox, J.G. (2012) Enzootic enteropathogenic *Escherichia coli* infection in laboratory rabbits. *Journal of Clinical Microbiology* 50:2353–2358.

Takeuchi, A., Inman, L.R., O'Hanley, P.D., Cantey, J.R., & Lushbaugh, W.B. (1978) Scanning and transmission electron microscopic study of *Escherichia coli* O15 (RDEC-1) enteric infection in rabbits. *Infection and Immunity* 19:686–694.

Thouless, M.E., DiGiacomo, R.F., & Deeb, J.B. (1996) The effect of combined rotavirus and *Escherichia coli* infections in rabbits. *Laboratory Animal Science* 46:381–385.

Von Moll, I.K. & Cantey, J.R. (1997) Peyer's patch adherence of enteropathogenic *Escherichia coli* strains in rabbits. *Infection and Immunity* 65:3788–3793.

Enterohemorrhagic *Escherichia coli*

Garcia, A., Bosques, C.J., Wishnok, J.S., Feng, Y., Karalius, B.J., Butterton, J.R., Schauer, D.B., Rogers, A.B., & Fox, J.G. (2006) Renal injury is a consistent finding in Dutch Belted rabbits experimentally infected with enterohemorrhagic *Escherichia coli*. *Journal of Infectious Diseases* 193:1125–1134.

Garcia, A. & Fox, J.G. (2003) The rabbit as a new reservoir host of enterohemorrhagic *Escherichia coli*. *Emerging Infectious Diseases* 9:1592–1597.

Garcia, A., Marini, R.P., Vitsky, A., Knox, K.A., Taylor, N.S., Schauer, D.B., & Fox, J.G. (2002) A naturally-occurring rabbit model of enterohemorrhagic *Escherichia coli*-induced disease. *Journal of Infectious Diseases* 186:1682–1686.

Panda, A., Tatarov, I., Melton-Celsa, A.R., Kolappaswamy, K., Kriel, E.H., Petkov, D., Coksaygan, T., Livio, S., McLeod, C.G., Nataro, J.P., O'Brien, A.D., & DeTolla, L.J. (2010) *Escherichia coli* O157: H7 infection in Dutch Belted and New Zealand White rabbits. *Comparative Medicine* 60:31–37.

Francisella tularensis Infection: Tularemia, "Rabbit Fever"

Gyuranecz, M., Szeredi, L., Makrai, L., Fodor, L., Meszaros, A.R., Szepe, B., Fuleki, M., & Erdelyi, K. (2010) Tularemia of European Brown Hare (*Lepus europaeus*); a pathological, histopathological, and immunohistochemical study. *Veterinary Pathology* 47:958–963.

Fusobacterium necrophorum Infection

Seps, S.L., Battles, A.H., Nguyen, L., Wardrip, C.L., & Li, X. (1999) Oropharyngeal necrobacillosis with septic thrombophlebitis and pulmonary embolic abscesses: Lemierre's Syndrome in a New Zealand White rabbit. *Contemporary Topics in Laboratory Animal Science* 38:44–46.

Helicobacter spp. Infection

Van den Bulck, K., Baele, M., Hermans, K., Ducatelle, R., Haesebrouck, F., & Decostere, A. (2005) First report on the occurrence of "*Helicobacter heilmannii*" in the stomach of rabbits. *Veterinary Research Communications* 29:271–279.

Van den Bulck, K., Decostere, A., Baele, M., Marechal, M., Ducatelle, R., & Haesebrouck, F. (2006) Low frequency of *Helicobacter* species in the stomachs of experimental rabbits. *Laboratory Animals* 40:282–287.

Klebsiella spp. Infection

Coletti, M., Passamonti, F., Del Rossi, E., Franciosini, M.P., & Setta, B. (2001) *Klebsiella pneumoniae* infection in Italian rabbits. *Veterinary Record* 149:626–627.

Nemet, Z., Szenci, O., Horvath, A., Makrai, L., Kis, T., Toth, B., & Biksi, I. (2011) Outbreak of *Klebsiella oxytoca* enterocolitis on a rabbit farm in Hungary. *Veterinary Record* 168:143 (ePub).

Lawsonia intracellaris Infection

Cooper, D.M. & Gebhart, C.J. (1998) Comparative aspects of proliferative enteritis. *Journal of the American Veterinary Medical Association* 212:1446–1451.

Duhamel, G.E., Klein, E.C., Elder, R.O., & Gebhart, C.J. (1998) Subclinical proliferative enteropathy in sentinel rabbits associated with *Lawsonia intracellularis*. *Veterinary Pathology* 35:300–303.

Hotchkiss, C.E., Shames, B., Perkins, S.E., & Fox, J.G. (1996) Proliferative enteropathy of rabbits: the intracellular *Campylobacter-*

like organism is closely related to *Lawsonia intracellularis*. *Laboratory Animal Science* 46:623–627.

Lim, J.J., Kim, D.H., Lee, J.J., Kim, D.G., Kim, S.H., Min, W.G., Chang, H.H., Rhee, M.H., & Kim, S. (2012) Prevalence of *Lawsonia intracellularis, Salmonella* spp. and *Eimeria* spp. in healthy and diarrheic pet rabbits. *Journal of Veterinary Medical Science* 74:263–265.

Schauer, D.B., McCathey, S.N., Daft, B.M., Jha, S.S., Tatterson, L.E., Taylor, N.S., & Fox, J.G. (1998) Proliferative enterocolitis associated with dual infection with enteropathogenic *Escherichia coli* and *Lawsonia intracellularis* in rabbits. *Journal of Clinical Microbiology* 36:1700–1703.

Schoeb, T.R. & Fox, J.G. (1990) Enterocolitis associated with intraepithelial *Campylobacter*-like bacteria in rabbits (*Oryctolagus cuniculus*). *Veterinary Pathology* 27:73–80.

Umemura, T., Tsuchitani, M., Totsuka, M., Narama, I., & Yamashiro, S. (1982) Histiocytic enteritis of rabbits. *Veterinary Pathology* 19:326–329.

Watarai, Yamoto, Y., Horiuchi, N., Kim, S., Omata, Y., Shirahata, T., & Furuoka, H. (2004) Enzyme-linked immunoabsorbent assay to detect *Lawsonia intracellularis* in rabbits with proliferative enteropathy. *Journal of Veterinary Medical Science* 66:735–737.

Watarai, M., Yamato, Y., Murakata, K., Kim, S., Omata, Y., & Furuoka, H. (2005) Detection of *Lawsonia intracellularis* using immunomagnetic beads and ATP bioluminescence. *Journal of Veterinary Medical Science* 67:449–451.

Watarai, M., Yoshiya, M., Sato, A., & Furuoka, H. (2008) Cultivation and characterization of *Lawsonia intracellularis* isolated from rabbit and pig. *Journal of Veterinary Medical Science* 70:731–733.

Listeria monocytogenes Infection: Listeriosis

Gray, M.L. & Killinger, A.H. (1966) *Listeria monocytogenes* and listeriosis. *Bacteriological Reviews* 30:309–382.

Murray, E.G.D., Webb, R.A., & Swann, M.B.R. (1926) A disease of rabbits characterized by a large mononuclear leucocytosis caused by a hitherto undescribed bacillus *Bacterium monocytogenes* (n. sp.). *Journal of Pathology and Bacteriology* 40:407–439.

Rodriguez-Calleja, J.M., Garcia-Lopez, I., Garcia-Lopez, M.L., Santos, J.A., & Otero, A. (2006) Rabbit meat as a source of bacterial foodborne pathogens. *Journal of Food Protection* 69:1106–1112.

Watson, G.L. & Evans, M.G. (1985) Listeriosis in a rabbit. *Veterinary Pathology* 22:191–193.

Moraxella bovis Infection

Soave, O.A., Dominguez, J., & Doak, R.L. (1977) *Moraxella bovis*-induced metritis and septicemia in a rabbit. *Journal of the American Veterinary Medical Association* 171:972–973.

Mycobacterium spp. Infection: Tuberculosis, Paratuberculosis

Angus, K.W. (1990) Intestinal lesions resembling paratuberculosis in a wild rabbit (*Oryctolagus cuniculus*). *Journal of Comparative Pathology* 103:101–105.

Beard, P.M., Rhind, S.M., Buxton, D., Daniels, M.J., Henderson, D., Pirie, A., Rudge, K., Greig, A., Hutchings, M.R., Stevenson, K., & Sharp, J.M. (2001) Natural paratuberculosis infection in rabbits in Scotland. *Journal of Comparative Pathology* 124:290–299.

Cobbett, L. (1913) Two cases of spontaneous tuberculosis in the rabbit caused by the avian tubercle bacillus. *Journal of Comparative Pathology* 26:33–45.

Gill, J.W. & Jackson, R. (1993) Tuberculosis in a rabbit: a case revisited. *New Zealand Veterinary Journal* 41:147.

Harkins, M.J. & Saleeby, E.R. (1928) Spontaneous tuberculosis of rabbits. *Journal of Infectious Diseases* 43:554–556.

Himes, E.M., Miller, S., Miller, L.D., & Jamagin, J.L. (1989) *Mycobacterium avium* isolated from a domestic rabbit with lesions in the central nervous system. *Journal of Veterinary Diagnostic Investigation* 1:76–78.

Ludwig, E., Reischl, U., Janik, D., & Hermanns, W. (2009) Granulomatous pneumonia caused by *Mycobacterium genavense* in a Dwarf rabbit (*Oryctolagus cuniculus*). *Veterinary Pathology* 46:1000–1002.

Maio, E., Carta, T., Balseiro, A., Sevilla, I.A., Romano, A., Ortiz, J.A., Vieira-Pinto, M., Carrido, J.M., de la Lastra, J.M.P., & Gortazar, C. (2011) Paratuberculosis in European wild rabbits from the Iberian peninsula. *Research in Veterinary Science* 91:212–219.

Mokresh, A.H. & Butler, D.G. (1990) Granulomatous enteritis following oral inoculation of newborn rabbits with *Mycobacterium paratuberculosis* of bovine origin. *Canadian Veterinary Journal* 54:313–319.

Nedeltchev, G.G., Raghunand, T.R., Jassal, M.S., Lun, S., Cheng, Q-J., & Bishai, W.R. (2009) Extrapulmonary dissemination of *Mycobacterium bovis* but not *Mycobacterium tuberculosis* in a bronchoscopic rabbit model of cavitary tuberculosis. *Infection and Immunity* 77:598–603.

Pasteurella multocida Infection

Corbeil, L.B., Strayer, D.S., Skaletsky, E., Wunderlich, A., & Sell, S. (1983) Immunity to pasteurellosis in compromised rabbits. *American Journal of Veterinary Research* 44:845–850.

Deeb, B.J., DiGiacomo, R.F., Bernard, B.L., & Silbernagel, S.M. (1990) *Pasteurella multocida* and *Bordetella bronchiseptica* infection in rabbits. *Journal of Clinical Microbiology* 28:70–75.

Dhillon, A.S. & Andrews, D.K. (1982) Abortions, stillbirths, and infant mortality in a commercial rabbitry. *Journal of Applied Rabbit Research* 5:97–98.

DiGiacomo, R.F., Deeb, B.J., Giddens, W.E., Jr, Bernard, B.L., & Chengappa, M.M. (1989) Atrophic rhinitis in New Zealand rabbits. *American Journal of Veterinary Research* 50:1460–1465.

DiGiacomo, R.F., Garlinghouse, E., & Van Hoosier, G.L., Jr (1983) Natural history of infection with *Pasteurella multocida* in rabbits. *Journal of the American Veterinary Medical Association* 183:1172–1175.

DiGiacomo, R.F., Jones, C.D., & Wathes, C.M. (1987) Transmission of *Pasteurella multocida* in rabbits. *Laboratory Animal Science* 37:621–623.

Dziva, F., Muhairwa, S.P., Bisgaard, M., & Christensen, H. (2008) Diagnostic and typing options for investigating diseases associated with *Pasteurella multocida*. *Veterinary Microbiology* 128:1–22.

Flatt, R.E., Deyoung, D.W., & Hogle, R.M. (1977) Suppurative otitis media in the rabbit: prevalence, pathology and microbiology. *Laboratory Animal Science* 27:343–346.

Glass, L.S. & Beasley, J.N. (1990) Infection with and antibody response to *Pasteurella multocida* and *Bordetella bronchiseptica* in immature rabbits. *Laboratory Animal Science* 39:406–410.

Glorioso, J.C., Jones, G.W., Rush, H.G., Pentler, L.J., Darif, C.A., & Coward, J.E. (1982) Adhesion of type A *Pasteurella multocida* to rabbit pharyngeal cells and its possible role in rabbit respiratory tract infections. *Infection and Immunity* 35:1103–1109.

Holmes, H.T., Patton, N.M., & Cheeke, P.R. (1983) The incidence of vaginal and nasal *Pasteurella multocida* in a commercial rabbitry. *Journal of Applied Rabbit Research* 6:95–96.

Holmes, H.T., Patton, N.M., & Cheeke, P.R. (1983) *Pasteurella* contaminated water valves: its incidence and implications. *Journal of Applied Rabbit Research* 6:123–124.

Jaglic, Z., Jeklova, E., Christensen, H., Leva, L., Register, K., Kummer, V., Kucerova, Z., Faldyna, M., Maskova, J., & Nedbalcova, K. (2011) Host response in rabbits to infection with *Pasteurella multocida* serogroup F strains originating from fowl cholera. *Canadian Journal of Veterinary Research* 75:200–208.

Jaglic, Z., Jeklova, E., Leva, L., Kummer, V., Kucerova, Z., Faldyna, M., Maskova, J., Nedbalcova, K., & Alexa, P. (2008) Experimental study of pathogenicity of *Pasteurella multocida* serogroup F in rabbits. *Veterinary Microbiology* 126:168–177.

Manning, P.J., Naasz, M.A., DeLong, D., & Leary, S.L. (1986) Pasteurellosis in laboratory rabbits: characterization of lipopolysaccharides of *Pasteurella multocida* by polyacrylamide gel electrophoresis, immunoblot techniques, and enzyme-linked immunosorbent assay. *Infection and Immunity* 53:460–463.

Percy, D.H., Karrow, N., & Bhasin, J.L. (1988) Incidence of *Pasteurella* and *Bordetella* infections in fryer rabbits: an abattoir survey. *Journal of Applied Rabbit Research* 11:245–246.

Percy, D.H., Prescott, J.F., & Bhasin, J.L. (1984) Characterization of *Pasteurella multocida* isolated from rabbits in Canada. *Canadian Journal of Comparative Medicine* 48:36–41.

Watson, W.T., Goldsboro, J.A., Williams, F.P., & Sueur, R. (1975) Experimental respiratory infections with *Pasteurella multocida* and *Bordetella bronchiseptica* in rabbits. *Laboratory Animal Science* 25:459–464.

Webster, L.T. (1926) Epidemiological studies on respiratory infections of the rabbit. VII. Pneumonias associated with bacterium lepisepticum. *Journal of Experimental Medicine* 43:555–572.

Zaoutis, T.E., Reinhard, G.R., Cioffe, C.J., Moore, P.B., & Stark, D.M. (1991) Screening rabbit colonies for antibodies to *Pasteurella multocida* by an ELISA. *Laboratory Animal Science* 41:419–422.

***Pseudomonas aeruginosa* Infection**

Garabaldi, B.A., Fox, J.G., & Musto, D.R. (1990) Atypical moist dermatitis in rabbits. *Laboratory Animal Science* 40:652–653.

McDonald, R.A. & Pinheiro, A.F. (1967) Water chlorination controls *Pseudomonas aeruginosa* in a rabbitry. *Journal of the American Veterinary Medical Association* 151:863–864.

***Salmonella* spp. Infection: Salmonellosis**

Harwood, D.G. (1989) *Salmonella typhimurium* infection in a commercial rabbitry. *Veterinary Record* 125:554–555.

Newcomer, C.E., Ackerman, J.I., Murphy, J.C., & Fox, J.G. (1984) The pathogenicity of *Salmonella mbandaka* in specific pathogen free rabbits. *Laboratory Animal Science* 34:588–591.

***Staphylococcus aureus* Infection**

Devriese, L.A., Hendrickx, W., Godard, C., Okerman, L., & Haesebrouck, F. (1996) A new pathogenic *Staphylococcus aureus* type in commercial rabbits. *Zentralblatt für Veterinarmedizin B* 43:313–315.

Hagen, K.W. (1963) Disseminated staphylococcal infection in young domestic rabbits. *Journal of the American Veterinary Medical Association* 142:1421–1422.

Hermans, K., Devriese, L.A., & Haesbrouck, F. (2003) Rabbit staphylococcosis: difficult solutions for serious problems. *Veterinary Microbiology* 91:57–64.

Okerman, L., Devriese, L.A., Maertens, L., Okerman, F., & Godard, C. (1984) Cutaneous staphylococcosis in rabbits. *Veterinary Record* 114:313–315.

Osebald, J.W. & Gray, D.M. (1960) Disseminated staphylococcal infection in wild jack rabbits. *Journal of Infectious Diseases* 106:91–94.

Snyder, S.B., Fox, J.G., Campbell, L.H., & Soave, O.A. (1976) Disseminated staphylococcal disease in the laboratory rabbit (*Oryctolagus cuniculus*). *Laboratory Animal Science* 26:86–88.

Vancraeynest, D., Haesebrouck, F., & Hermans, K. (2007) Multiplex PCR assay for the detection of high virulence rabbit *Staphylococcus aureus* strains. *Veterinary Microbiology* 121:368–372.

***Streptococcus* spp. Infection**

Ren, S.Y., Geng, Y., Wang, K.Y., Zhou, Z.Y., Liu, X.X., He, M., Peng, X., Wu, C.Y., & Lai, W.M. (2014) *Streptococcus agalactiae* infection in domestic rabbits, *Oryctolagus cuniculus*. *Transboundary and Emerging Diseases* 61 e92–e95.

***Treponema paraluis-cuniculi* Infection: Rabbit Syphilis**

Cunliffe-Beamer, T.L. & Fox, R.R. (1981) Venereal spirochaetosis of rabbits: description and diagnosis. *Laboratory Animal Science* 31:366B71.

Cunliffe-Beamer, T.L. & Fox, R.R. (1981) Venereal spirochaetosis of rabbits: epizootiology. *Laboratory Animal Science* 31:372–378.

DiGiacomo, R.F., Lukehart, S.A., Talburt, C.D., Baker-Zander, S.A., Condon, J., & Brown, C. (1984) Clinical course and treatment of venereal spirochetosis in New Zealand White rabbits. *British Journal of Venereal Diseases* 60:214–218.

DiGiacomo, R.F., Talburt, C.D., Lukehart, S.A., Baker-Zander, S.A., & Condon, J. (1983) *Treponema paraluis-cuniculi* infection in a commercial rabbitry: epidemiology and serodiagnosis. *Laboratory Animal Science* 33:562–566.

Saito, K. & Hasegawa, A. (2004) Clinical features of skin lesions in rabbit syphilis: a retrospective study of 63 cases (1999–2003). *Journal of Veterinary Medical Science* 66:1247–1249.

Saito, K., Tagawa, M., & Hasegawa, A. (2003) RPR test for serological survey of rabbit syphilis in companion rabbits. *Journal of Veterinary Medical Science* 63:797–799.

FUNGAL INFECTIONS

Aspergillus spp. Infection: Aspergillosis

Pulmonary aspergillosis, caused by *A. fumigatus*, *A. niger*, and *A. flavus*, is primarily of historical interest, but occurs sporadically among young rabbits. Infection is often subclinical, with pulmonary granulomas encountered in rabbits at necropsy. Granulomas consist of circumscribed inflammatory lesions with a central area of coagulation necrosis with mononuclear inflammatory cell response. Typical septate hyphae are evident, particularly with PAS or methenamine silver stains (Fig. 6.56). Pulmonary aspergillosis affects young rabbits, with elimination of the fungus as rabbits mature, leaving pulmonary scars. Older rabbits are experimentally resistant to infection. Disseminated cutaneous infection with *Aspergillus* spp. in young rabbits with pulmonary involvement has been described. Septate branching hyphae were abundant within cystic hair follicles.

Dermatophytosis: Ringworm

Clinical cases of dermatophytosis are uncommon in domestic rabbits. Disease is usually sporadic, but can

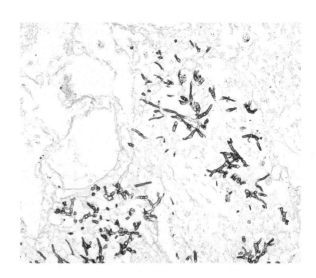

FIG. 6.56. *Lung from a rabbit kit with pulmonary aspergillosis, illustrating fungal hyphae (methenamine silver stain).*

also be epizootic within a rabbitry or colony. When present, lesions are usually located around the head and ears, sometimes with secondary spread to the paws. Affected areas are typically raised, circumscribed, and erythematous, with crusted surface and hair loss. *Trichophyton mentagrophytes* is most frequently involved, but *Microsporum canis* infections have also been recognized in rabbits. Microscopic examination of skin scrapings from the periphery of lesions cleared in 10% KOH should reveal the typical arthrospores. Examination of tissue sections for the characteristic fungi and culture on the appropriate media are both useful diagnostic procedures in confirming the diagnosis. On histopathology, characteristic changes include hyperkeratosis, epidermal hyperplasia, and folliculitis, with mononuclear and polymorphonuclear cell infiltration. Stains such as the methenamine silver and PAS staining procedures will demonstrate the typical arthrospores infesting infected hair shafts. Differential diagnoses include seasonal "molt," hair loss in does during nest building, "barbering" in group-housed juvenile rabbits, and acariasis.

Dermatophytes are readily transmitted to susceptible human contacts; thus careful screening, culling, and slaughter are recommended. If animals are to be treated, oral griseofulvin has been used with some success, but it is potentially teratogenic in pregnant does. Rabbits may harbor pathogenic dermatophytes, particularly *M. canis*, as an inapparent infection. Normal rabbits have also been found to be culture-positive for *T. verrucosum, M. nanum, M. gypseum, M. persicolor,* and *M. distortum.*

Encephalitozoon cuniculi Infection: Encephalitozoonosis; Microsporidiosis

"Infectious motor paralysis" attributed to a "protozoan parasite" was first reported in laboratory rabbits by Wright and Craighead in 1922. *Encephalitozoon cuniculi* is an obligate intracellular microsporidian that infects a variety of mammalian hosts, and very commonly infects the domestic rabbit. Because of its wide host range, humans are susceptible to zoonotic infection, and severe disease has been observed in immunosuppressed individuals. Taxonomists have historically disagreed on the classification for the organism, but genomic sequencing has now confirmed that *E. cuniculi* is a eukaryotic fungus within the phylum microsporidia. Gene sequencing among strains originating from different host species indicates identical gene content, but marked intraspecies genetic diversity. The prevalence of seropositive animals in some conventional rabbit populations is high, as well as among pet and wild rabbits. The organism is characterized by the presence of a coiled polar filament in the mature spore stage. Following the extrusion of the sporoplasm from the spore coat, the sporoplasm may then invade a susceptible host cell. Penetration may be due to the mechanical forces exerted by the extruded polar filament or due to an active migratory process by the sporoplasm. Following entry into the cell, multiplication

occurs in association with a cytoplasmic vacuole. Sporoblasts develop into mature spores, and finally the cell ruptures, releasing organisms that can then repeat the cycle.

Epizootiology and Pathogenesis

Transmission occurs through organisms excreted in the urine, as well as transplacentally. Rabbits are readily infected experimentally by the oral or respiratory route, and iatrogenic transmission through contaminated needles may also occur. Following ingestion/oral inoculation, spores appear to pass via infected mononuclear cells into the systemic circulation. Initially, target organs are those of high blood flow, such as lung, liver, and kidney. In rabbits inoculated orally with *E. cuniculi* and examined at 31 days postinoculation, moderate to marked lesions were demonstrated primarily in the lung, liver, and kidney, and occasionally in the myocardium. No lesions were present in the central nervous system at 1 month. At 3 months, moderate to severe lesions were evident histologically in the kidney, and changes were minimal in the lung, liver, and heart, but lesions were evident in the brain at this stage. Serum antibody titers may be detectable by 3–4 weeks and reach high titers by 6–9 weeks. Spores have been seen in the urine at 1 month and may be excreted in large numbers up to 2 months. Only small numbers are excreted thereafter. Shedding of spores is essentially terminated by 3 months. Spores survive for less than 1 week at 4°C but may remain viable for at least 6 weeks at 22°C.

Pathology

Infection is frequently subclinical, but rabbits may present with a variety of neurologic signs, including head tilt, ataxia, vestibular signs (circling, nystagmus, rolling), and occasionally behavioral changes. Uveitis and cataracts may be present in young rabbits. Infected animals are usually in good flesh. Lesions are frequently confined to the kidney and appear as focal, irregular, depressed areas 1–100 mm in diameter. In severely affected

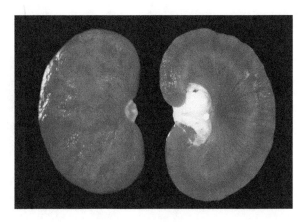

FIG. 6.57. *Kidneys from a rabbit with chronic encephalitozoonosis. There are multiple, irregular pitted, and depressed regions of the renal cortex.*

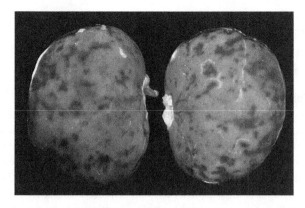

FIG. 6.58. *Kidneys from a rabbit with recent* Encephalitozoon *infection. There are multiple irregular dark red and depressed foci of the renal cortex.*

kidneys, lesions often coalesce with adjacent foci (Figs. 6.57 and 6.58). On cut surface, indistinct, linear, pale gray-white areas may extend into the underlying cortex. On histopathology, granulomatous lesions may be evident in the interstitium of the lung, kidney, and liver. In the lung, focal to diffuse interstitial pneumonitis, with mononuclear cell infiltration, may occur. Hepatic lesions are characterized by a focal granulomatous inflammatory response (Fig. 6.59), with periportal lymphocytic infiltration. Focal lymphocytic infiltrates may also occur in the myocardium. In the kidney, early lesions consist of focal to segmental interstitial nephritis, with degeneration and sloughing of tubular epithelial cells (Fig. 6.60). Lesions may be present at all levels of the renal tubule, with minimal involvement of the glomeruli. Using tissue Gram stains, spores are evident as ovoid, Gram-positive organisms approximately $1.5 \times 2.5–5\,\mu m$ in size. Staining procedures using carbol fuchsin will stain the organisms a distinct purple color. During early infection, spores may be present within epithelial cells, macrophages, inflammatory foci, or free within collecting tubules. In renal lesions of longer duration, interstitial fibrosis, collapse of the

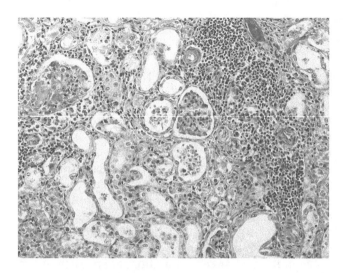

FIG. 6.60. *Kidney from a rabbit with encephalitozoonosis. There is infiltration of the interstitium with mononuclear leukocytes, degeneration of tubular epithelium, and cellular debris within tubular lumina.*

parenchyma, and mononuclear cell infiltration are typical changes, but the organism may no longer be detectable. When present, Gram-positive spores may be apparent in tubular epithelium or within tubular lumina (Fig. 6.61). In the central nervous system, lesions normally do not occur until at least 30 days postexposure. Changes include multifocal nonsuppurative meningitis and granulomatous encephalomyelitis, with astrogliosis and perivascular lymphocytic infiltration. Pseudocysts filled with organisms may be apparent (Fig. 6.62). Using appropriate stains, pseudocysts containing organisms may be evident as collections of spores within parasitized astroglia or as scattered organisms within granulomatous inflammatory foci. These lesions may also be present in the central nervous system in the absence of identifiable organisms. Severe malacia associated with intense inflammation may rarely be observed,

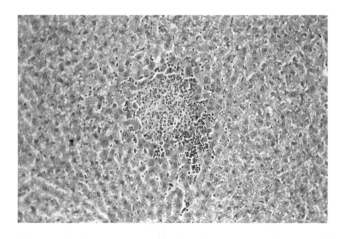

FIG. 6.59. *Focal nonsuppurative hepatitis associated with disseminated* Encephalitozoon *infection.*

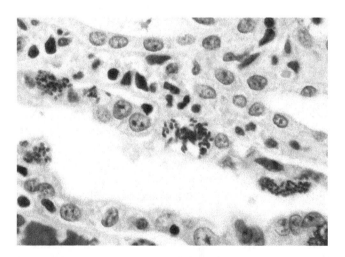

FIG. 6.61. Encephalitozoon *spores within renal tubular epithelium and tubular lumen of a rabbit with chronic encephalitozoonosis (Brown and Brenn stain).*

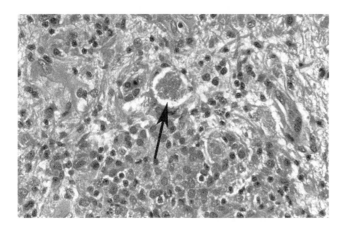

FIG. 6.62. *Focal granulomatous encephalitis associated with* chronic Encephalitozoon cuniculi *infection. Note the pseudocyst containing organisms (arrow).*

particularly in severely stressed or immunosuppressed rabbits. Lesions most frequently arise in the cerebrum, but may also occur in the brain stem, spinal cord, and cerebellum.

Phacoclastic uveitis (Fig. 6.63) and cataract formation (Fig. 6.64) occur in rabbits, and it is believed to follow transplacental infection. This syndrome is common among dwarf rabbits, but other breeds may be affected. On histological examination of the eye, keratitis, rupture of the lens capsule, and inflammatory cell infiltrates comprised of heterophils, foamy macrophages, and multinucleate giant cells are typical changes. The iris and ciliary body are infiltrated with lymphocytes and plasma cells. Using immunohistochemistry or tissue Gram stains, organisms may be identified, interspersed either around fragmented lens fibers or within macrophages.

Diagnosis
Identification of characteristic lesions and the demonstration of the organisms in tissue sections are the standard diagnostic procedures used to confirm the diagnosis. The organisms can be readily differentiated from protozoal infections, such as toxoplasmosis, by the

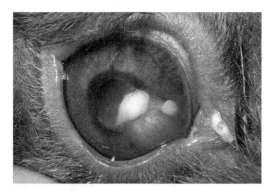

FIG. 6.63. *Phacoclastic uveitis in a rabbit infected with* Encephalitozoon cuniculi. *(Courtesy A. Strom, Veterinary Ophthalmology Service, UC Davis School of Veterinary Medicine.)*

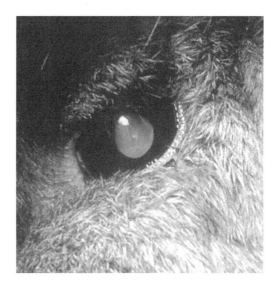

FIG. 6.64. *Dwarf rabbit with a cataract associated with* Encephalitozoon cuniculi *infection. Some breeds of dwarf rabbits appear to be particularly susceptible to congenital* E. cuniculi *infection.*

tissue tropisms and the staining properties of the organisms. Toxoplasma organisms are Gram-negative and do not stain with carbol fuchsin stains. An intradermal skin test has been used to detect infected rabbits, but serology has been the most widely used. Differential diagnoses for rabbits with neurologic signs include otitis interna, toxoplasmosis, and *Baylisascaris* migration.

Malassezia spp. Infection: Malasseziasis
Malassezia spp. (formerly *Pityrosporum* spp.) is rarely associated with disease in rabbits. Opportunistic overgrowth of *Malassezia* spp. yeast forms has been reported in an outbreak of sarcoptic mange involving 4% of rabbits in a rabbitry. *Malessezia cuniculi* has been validated as a new species and appears to be present as a component of the lipophilic microbiota of rabbit skin. The zoonotic significance of rabbit *Malassezia* is not known.

Pneumocystis oryctolagi sp. nov. Infection
Pneumocystis spp. are obligate extracellular yeast-like organisms that are now classified as members of the fungal kingdom. There is high genetic divergence among *Pneumocystis* species resulting from coevolution within their various mammalian hosts. Each species is host-specific, including *P. jirovecii* in humans, *P. carinii* and *P. wakefieldae* in rats, *P. murina* in mice, and *P. oryctolagi* in rabbits. The list of genetically distinct *Pneumocystis* species is likely to grow with genetic analysis of *Pneumocystis* from other host species.

Epizootiology and Pathogenesis
Pneumocystis oryctolagi organisms are typically restricted to the alveoli of the lung, and rabbits appear to become infected as neonates, presumably by inhalation or maternal grooming. The life cycle of *Pneumocystis* includes a trophic form, which replicates asexually by

binary fission, and sexual replication through formation of an ascus (cyst) containing 8 ascospores, plus several intermediate forms. Aerosol transmission is mediated by ascospores. Unlike other yeasts, *Pneumocystis* does not undergo budding. Trophic forms attach to type I pneumocytes. *Pneumocystis* spp. generally exist within their immunocompetent hosts as commensal organisms with minimal consequence. Infection becomes clinically significant under conditions in which the host is immunecompromised.

Pathology

Based on studies in Europe, subclinical pulmonary disease is very common in rabbits during the postweaning period. Rabbits have extensive diffuse pulmonary lesions that arise abruptly at weaning, evolve over the next 7–10 days, and then slowly resolve, with complete resolution within 3–4 weeks, corresponding to decline in pathogen levels. There is some evidence that intrauterine infections occur, and as early as the 10th day of pregnancy. Lesions described include pulmonary edema, congestion of alveolar vessels, thickening and hypercellularity of alveolar septa with infiltration of mononuclear and polymorphonuclear leukocytes, and exudation into alveolar lumina. During the early stages of infection, organisms can be demonstrated lining alveolar spaces in tissue sections using silver stains. Infection can also be confirmed by PCR and serology.

Deep Mycoses

Aside from pulmonary aspergillosis, deep mycoses are quite rare in domestic rabbits. A single case of adiaspiromycosis in a rabbit with pulmonary granulomata caused by *Emmonsia* spp. has been reported. Histoplasmosis has also been reported in 2 domestic rabbits. Affected animals had nodular cutaneous lesions. One case had disseminated disease, with multiple periocular, nasal, perioral, and prepucial alopecic nodules upon clinical presentation. Necropsy revealed additional involvement of other cutaneous sites, lymph node, and small intestine. Lesions featured dense infiltration of macrophages, with fewer numbers of heterophils and multinucleated giant cells. Both intracellular and extracellular yeast forms were apparent.

BIBLIOGRAPHY FOR FUNGAL INFECTIONS

Aspergillus Infection
Matsui, T., Taguchi-Ochi, S., Takano, M., Kuroda, S., Taniyama, H., & Ono, T. (1985) Pulmonary aspergillosis in apparently healthy young rabbits. *Veterinary Pathology* 22:200–205.
Patton, N.M. (1973) Cutaneous and pulmonary aspergillosis in rabbits. *Laboratory Animal Science* 25:347–350.

Dermatophytosis
Banks, K.L. and Clarkson, T.B. (1967) Naturally occurring dermatomycosis in the rabbit. *Journal of the American Veterinary Medical Association* 151:926–929.

Hagen, K.W. (1969) Ringworm in domestic rabbits: oral treatment with griseofulvin. *Laboratory Animal Care* 19:635–638.
Kraemer, A., Mueller, R.S., Werckenthin, C., Straubinger, R.K., & Hein, J. (2012) Dermatophytes in pet Guinea pigs and rabbits. *Veterinary Microbiology* 157:208–213.
Vogtsberger, L.M., Harroff, H.H., Pierce, G.E., & Wilkinson, G.E. (1986) Spontaneous dermatophytosis due to *Microsporum canis* in rabbits. *Laboratory Animal Science* 36:294–297.

Encephalitozoon cuniculi Infection
Baneux, P.J. & Pognan, F. (2003) In utero transmission of *Encephalitozoon cuniculi* strain type 1 in rabbits. *Laboratory Animals* 37:132–138.
Bywater, J.E.C. & Kellett, B.S. (1978) The eradication of *Encephalitozoon cuniculi* from a specific pathogen-free rabbit colony. *Laboratory Animal Science* 28:402–404.
Cox, J.C. & Gallichio, H.A. (1978) Serological and histological studies on adult rabbits with recent, naturally acquired encephalitozoonosis. *Research in Veterinary Science* 24:260–261.
Cox, J.C., Hamilton, R.C., & Attwood, H.D. (1979) An investigation of the route and progression of *Encephalitozoon cuniculi* infection in adult rabbits. *Journal of Protozoology* 26:260–265.
Csokai, J., Gruber, A., Kunzel, F., Tichy, A., & Joachim, A. (2009) Encephalitozoonosis in pet rabbits (*Oryctolagus cuniculus*): pathohistological findings in animals with latent infection versus clinical manifestation. *Parasitology Research* 104:629–635.
Flatt, R.E. & Jackson, S.J. (1970) Renal nosematosis in young rabbits. *Veterinary Pathology* 7:492–497.
Harcourt-Brown, F.M. & Holloway, H.K. (2003) Encephalitozoon infection in pet rabbits. *Veterinary Record* 152:427–431.
Kunzel, F. & Joachim, A. (2010) Encephalitozoonosis in rabbits. *Parasitology Research* 106:299–309.
Lyngset, A. (1980) A survey of serum antibodies to *Encephalitozoon cuniculi* in breeding rabbits and their young. *Laboratory Animal Science* 30:558–561.
Nast, R., Middleton, D.M., & Wheler, C.L. (1996) Generalized encephalitozoonosis in a Jersey wooley rabbit. *Canadian Veterinary Journal* 37:303–305.
Pakes, S.P., Shadduck, J.A., & Olsen, R.G. (1972) A diagnostic skin test for encephalitozoonosis (nosematosis) in rabbits. *Laboratory Animal Science* 22:870–877.
Pombert, J.F., Xu, J., Smith, D.R., Heiman, D., Young, S., Cuomo, C.A., & Weiss, L.M. (2013) Complete genome sequences from three genetically distinct strains reveal high intraspecies genetic diversity in the microsporidian *Encephalitozoon cuniculi*. *Eukaryotic Cell* 12:503–511.
Shadduck, J.A. & Pakes, S.P. (1971) Encephalitozoonosis (nosematosis) and toxoplasmosis. *American Journal of Pathology* 64:657–673.
Wright, J.H. & Craighead, E.M. (1922) Infectious motor paralysis in young rabbits. *Journal of Experimental Medicine* 36:135–140.

Ocular *Encephalitozoon* Infection
Ashton, N., Cook, C., & Clegg, F. (1976) Encephalitozoonosis (nosematosis) causing bilateral cataract in a rabbit. *British Journal of Ophthalmology* 60:618–631.
Giordano, C., Weigt, A,. Vercelli, A., Rondena, M., Grilli, G., & Giudice, C. (2005) Immunohistochemical identification of *Encephalitozoon cuniculi* in phacoclastic uveitis in four rabbits. *Veterinary Ophthalmology* 8:271–275.
Stiles, J., Didier, E., Ritchie, B., Greenacre, C., Willis, M., & Martin, C. (1997) *Encephalitozoon cuniculi* in the lens of a rabbit with phacoclastic uveitis: confirmation and treatment. *Veterinary Comparative Ophthalmology* 7:233–238.
Wolfer, J. (1992) Spontaneous lens capsule rupture in the rabbit. *Veterinary Pathology* 29:449.
Wolfer, J., Grahn, B., Wilcock, B., & Percy, D. (1993) Phacoclastic uveitis in the rabbit. *Progress in Comparative and Veterinary Ophthalmology* 3:92–97.

Malessezia spp. Infection

Cabanes, F.J., Vega, S., & Castella, G. (2011) *Malassezia cuniculi* sp. nov., a novel yeast species isolated from rabbit skin. *Medical Microbiology* 49:40–48.

Radi, Z.A. (2004) Outbreak of sarcoptic mange and malasseziasis in rabbits (*Oryctolagus cuniculus*). *Comparative Medicine* 54:434–437.

Pneumocystis oryctolagi Infection

Cere, N., Drouet-Viard, F., Dei-Cas, E., Chanteloup, N., & Coudert, P. (1997) In utero transmission of *Pneumocystis* sp. f. *oryctolagi*. *Parasite* 4:325–330.

Cere, N., Polack, B., Chanteloup, N.K., & Coudert, P. (1997) Natural transmission of *Pneumocystis carinii* in nonimmunosuppressed animals: early contagiousness of experimentally infected rabbits (*Oryctolagus cuniculus*). *Journal of Clinical Microbiology* 35:2670–2672.

Cushion, M.T. (2010) Are members of the fungal genus *Pneumocystis* (a) commensals; (b) opportunists; (c) pathogens; or (d) all of the above? *PLoS Pathogens* 6:e1001009.

Dei-Cas, E., Chabe, M., Moukhlis, R., Durand-Joly, I. Aliouat, E., Stringer, J.R., Cushion, M., Noel, C., de Hoog, G.S., Guillot, J., & Viscoglosi, E. (2006) *Pneumocystis oryctolagi* sp. nov., an uncultured fungus causing pneumonia in rabbits at weaning: review of current knowledge, and description of a new taxon on genotypic, phylogenetic and phenotypic bases. *FEMS Microbiology Reviews* 30:853–871.

Ortona, E., Visconti, E., Barca, S., Margutti, P., Mencarini, P., Zolfo, M., Tamburrini, E., & Siracusano, A. (1997) Cellular and humoral response in *Pneumocystis carinii* spontaneously infected rabbits. *Journal of Eukaryotic Microbiology* 44:49S.

Soulez, B., Dei-Cas, E., Charat, P., Mougeot, G,. Caillaux, M., & Camus, D. (1989) The young rabbit: a nonimmunosuppressed model for *Pneumocystis carinii* pneumonia. *Journal of Infectious Diseases* 160:355–356.

Tamburrini, E., Ortona, E., Visconti, E., Mencarini, P., Margutti, P., Zolfo, M., Barca, S., Peters, S.E., Wakefield, A.E., & Siracusano, A. (1999) *Pneumocystis carinii* infection in young non-immunosuppressed rabbits: kinetics of infection and of the primary specific immune response. *Medical Microbiology and Immunology* 188:1–7.

Deep Mycoses

Brandao, J., Woods, S., Fowlkes, N., Leissinger, M., Blair, R., Pucheu-Haston, C., Johnson, J., Phillipps, C.E., & Tully, T. (2014) Disseminated histoplasmosis (*Histoplasma capsulatum*) in a pet rabbit: case report and review of the literature. *Journal of Veterinary Diagnostic Investigation* 26:158–162.

Dvorak, J., Otcenaske, M., & Rasin, K. (1966) Adiaspiromycosis in mice and a laboratory rabbit. *Journal of the American Veterinary Medical Association* 149:932.

Frame, S.R., Mehdi, N.A., & Turek, J.J. (1989) Naturally occurring mucocutaneous histoplasmosis in a rabbit. *Journal of Comparative Pathology* 101:351–354.

PARASITIC DISEASES

Protozoal Infections
Cryptosporidium cuniculus *Infection: Cryptosporidiosis*

The very large *Cryptosporidium* group, although morphologically similar among members, has been a taxonomic challenge based on host range, biologic behavior, and morphology. Genetic sequencing has added more complexity to this issue. There is evidence of cophylogeny within specific hosts, but also considerable cross-species infectivity. Many *Cryptosporidium* spp., including *C. cuniculus*, have been traditionally named after the host species in which they were originally observed. Recent studies have shown that *C. cuniculus* has unique genetic sequences, and is now considered a validated species. It is most closely related to, but distinct from, *C. hominis*. Infections of rabbits are usually subclinical, and the organism is typically an incidental finding. When examined microscopically, the villi of the terminal small intestine may be shortened and blunted. Round to ovoid bodies are present within the brush border of enterocytes at the tips of villi. Changes on enterocytes are minimal and consist of elongation or shortening of microvilli adjacent to attachment sites. Recently, several outbreaks of cryptosporidiosis in humans have been associated with *C. cuniculi*, underscoring the zoonotic significance of this organism.

Eimeria *spp. Infections*

Intestinal coccidiosis

Enteric coccidia are important causes of clinical (or subclinical) disease in commercial rabbitries, resulting in weight loss and mortality. There are 10 recognized species of intestinal *Eimeria* in the rabbit. Based upon experimental inoculation of pathogen-free laboratory rabbits, *Eimeria* spp. can be divided into 5 overlapping groups according to pathogenicity: nonpathogenic (*E. coecicola*), slightly pathogenic (*E. perforans*, *E. exigua*, and *E. vejdovskyi*), mildly pathogenic or pathogenic (*E. media*, *E. magna*, *E. piriformis*, and *E. irresidua*), and highly pathogenic (*E. intestinalis* and *E. flavescens*). Each of these species targets specific segments of the intestinal

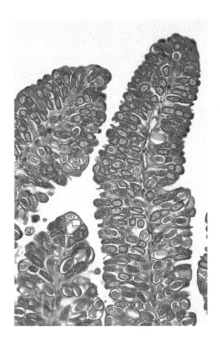

FIG. 6.65. *Small intestine from a juvenile rabbit with acute coccidiosis. Enterocytes contain large numbers of micro- and macrogametocytes and oocysts.*

tract (see Pakandl, 2009). Rabbits are usually coinfected with multiple *Eimeria* species. For example, all 10 species of intestinal *Eimeria* were found in young rabbits maintained at family farm rabbitries in Europe. As rabbits aged, *E. flavescens* and *E. piriformis* were predominant, and other species were rare. Disease severity depends upon infective dose, parasite species, immune status, and age of the rabbits. Enteritis is often accompanied by overgrowth of *E. coli* and presence of rotavirus, emphasizing the multifactorial nature of rabbit enteritis.

Epizootiology and Pathogenesis
Following passage in the feces, oocysts require 1 or more days to sporulate at room temperature before they become infective. Upon ingestion, sporulated oocysts (sporocysts) release sporozoites, which invade enterocytes and multiply by schizogony. In rabbits inoculated with sporocysts directly into the duodenum, excystation and the invasion of enterocytes occur as early as 10 minutes postinoculation. Sporozoites appear in the mucosa of the ileum within 6 hours, suggesting systemic rather than intraluminal migration. Depending on the species of *Eimeria*, 1 or more asexual cycles occur, followed by gametogony and oocyst passage in the feces. The prepatent period is from 5 to 12 days, depending on the species. There may be a phenomenal number of progeny from a single ingested oocyst. One oocyst of *E. magna* may produce over 25,000,000 oocysts in a susceptible host.

Rabbits most frequently develop clinical disease during the postweaning period. Rabbits younger than 20 days of age are highly resistant to infection, and can only be infected with very high doses of oocysts. This innate resistance is not fully understood, but has been attributed to factors in the milk, with age-related susceptibility evolving with changes in the intestinal environment attributed to consumption of plant feed. The most damaging stage in the life cycle is the sexual cycle, where there may be extensive destruction of enterocytes and cells in the lamina propria in affected sections of the gut. Because oocysts require sporulation at room temperature before they are infective, reingestion of the "night feces" (cecotrophy) does not play a role in the dissemination of the disease. Exposure to relatively small numbers of oocysts should result in a subclinical infection, with appropriate immune response. However, immunity to 1 species of *Eimeria* is unlikely to provide good protection against other species. In many commercial operations, the feed is routinely medicated with anticoccidials to control the disease. However, this should not be considered an acceptable substitute for rigid sanitation practices. In well-managed operations where anticoccidials are not used, control is dependent on rigorous sanitation practices.

Pathology
At necropsy, the perineal region and belly are frequently smeared with watery dark green to brown feces. The animal may be thin and dehydrated. Fecal losses of potassium result in hypokalemia. The cecum and colon contain dark green to brown watery, foul-smelling material. The mucosa of affected areas of the gut is congested and edematous, occasionally with hemorrhagic areas. Depending upon region of intestine involved, during acute coccidiosis, there is destruction of enterocytes, villus attenuation in affected areas of small intestine, denudation of cecal mucosa, and marked leukocytic infiltration of the lamina propria. With *E. intestinalis*, lesions are most severe at day 7–10 postinoculation with repair of the mucosa by day 12. Gametocytes and oocysts are usually evident in the intestinal mucosa in affected areas (Fig. 6.65). The higher pathogenic nature of *E. intestinalis* and *E. flavescens* has been attributed to infection of crypt epithelium by these species, resulting in failure of enterocyte regeneration and bacterial invasion.

Diagnosis
Fecal flotations, mucosal scrapings, and microscopic examination for oocysts are standard diagnostic procedures. An approximate oocyst count and oocyst speciation are recommended, particularly in view of the recognized variation in pathogenicity among species of *Eimeria*. A PCR assay has been developed for definitive identification of each of the 11 *Eimeria* species that infect domestic rabbits, including *E. stiedae* (below). In acute cases of coccidiosis, oocysts may not yet be present in the feces but will be evident in sections of the appropriate areas of small and large intestine. There is frequently a significant rise in the bacterial count, especially coliforms. Quantitative aerobic cultures are useful indices of disease, since aerobic coliform growth is minimal in the normal rabbit intestine. Differential diagnoses include *E. coli* and Salmonella enteritis, Lawsonia enteritis, Tyzzer's disease, clostridial enteropathies, viral enteritides, and mucoid enteropathy. Multiple factors often cocontribute to rabbit enteritis.

Hepatic Coccidiosis
Eimeria stiedae infections occur in both domestic and wild rabbits and represent an important cause of poor weight gains, disease, and mortality in commercial rabbitries.

Epizootiology and Pathogenesis
Following the ingestion of sporulated oocysts (sporocysts), sporozoites invade the duodenal mucosa and migrate to the lamina propria prior to systemic migration. Sporozoites have been demonstrated in the regional mesenteric lymph nodes within 12 hours postexposure and in the liver by 48 hours. Organisms have been reported to migrate to the liver in mononuclear cells via lymphatics. However, viable sporozoites have also been demonstrated in the peripheral blood and bone marrow in *E. stiedae*-inoculated rabbits, and the hematogenous route has been proposed as a means of

migration to the liver. In the liver, sporozoites invade the epithelial cells of the bile ducts and schizogony begins. Following the gametogeny, oocysts are formed, released into the bile ducts, and passed to the intestine. The prepatent period is approximately 15–18 days. Oocysts may be shed in the feces for up to 7 or more weeks. Oocysts are normally resistant to environmental change; thus, contaminated premises and fomites may be a source of infective sporulated oocysts for several months. *Eimeria stiedae* infections may be manifest either as clinical or subclinical disease and typically accompany intestinal *Eimeria* infections.

Weanling rabbits are most often affected. In the past, a significant number of livers collected from fryer rabbits in abattoirs have been condemned because of hepatic coccidiosis. A dose-related effect has been observed in experimentally infected animals. In young rabbits inoculated orally with varying numbers of sporocysts (100–100,000 per animal), mortality rates in animals that received either 10,000 or 100,000 sporocysts were 40 or 80%, respectively. No fatalities occurred at lower dosages. Significant variations in liver enzymes and blood chemistry have been observed during the course of the disease. Four stages have been proposed: (i) the initial stage of metabolic dysfunction that coincides with liver damage during schizogony; (ii) the cholestatic stage, with elevated transaminases and serum bilirubin; (iii) the stage of metabolic dysfunction, characterized by hypoglycemia and hypoproteinemia; and (iv) the period of immunodepression in heavily infected animals resulting in an inability to curtail the production of oocysts in the biliary system.

Pathology

Affected animals are frequently thin, potbellied, and lack body fat reserves. There may be dark brown to green soiling in the perineal region. Ascites is a variable finding. Depending on the degree of liver involvement, there may be hepatomegaly, and in severe cases, icterus. In the liver, there are variable numbers of raised, linear bosselated, yellow to pearl gray circumscribed lesions 0.5–2 cm in diameter scattered throughout the hepatic parenchyma. The gall bladder is thickened and contains viscid green bile and debris (Fig. 6.66). On cut surface, lesions contain fluid green to inspissated, dark green to tan material (Fig. 6.67). Microscopically, there may be marked dilation of bile ducts, extensive periportal fibrosis, and mixed inflammatory cell infiltration in the periportal regions. In affected bile ducts, there is hyperplasia of epithelium, with papillary projections lined by reactive epithelial cells overlying collagenous tissue stroma. Infiltrating periductal inflammatory cells include lymphocytes, macrophages, and a sprinkling of polymorphonuclear leukocytes. Large numbers of gametocytes and oocysts may be present in parasitized ducts (Fig. 6.68). In lesions of some duration, organisms may be sparse to absent in bile ducts, with prominent periportal fibrosis.

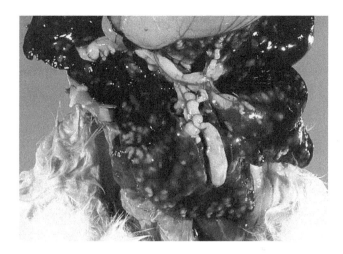

FIG. 6.66. *Liver from a juvenile rabbit with florid hepatic coccidiosis. In addition to the raised linear hepatic lesions, representing involved bile ducts, the gall bladder and common bile duct are dilated and contain flocculent material.*

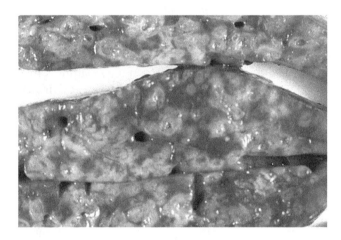

FIG. 6.67. *Cut surface of the liver from a rabbit with hepatic coccidiosis. Bile ducts are dilated with mural thickening and lumina are filled with inspissated material.*

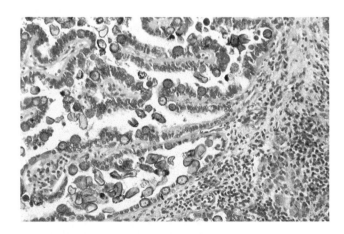

FIG. 6.68. *Hepatic bile duct of a rabbit with chronic hepatic coccidiosis, featuring proliferative cholangitis, periportal fibrosis, and inflammation. Bile ductular epithelium contains large numbers of microgametocytes, macrogametocytes, and oocysts.*

Diagnosis

The diagnosis can be confirmed at necropsy by wet mount preparations. Oocysts are usually readily observed in aspirates from the gall bladder or in impression smears of sectioned lesions. The characteristic proliferative biliary changes and organisms seen histologically are pathognomonic of the disease.

Giardia duodenalis *Infection*

Infection of rabbits with *G. duodenalis* is often subclinical, but several cases of enteritis have been associated with this organism in rabbits. The taxonomy of *Giardia* spp. is still in flux, but *G. duodenalis* is considered a valid species (syn. *G. lamblia* or *G. intestinalis*) that infects a wide range of mammals. Although isolates from various infected host species are morphologically indistinguishable, host-adapted *G. duodenalis* genotypes are recognized. A number of genetic "assemblages" have been recognized, and one major group, assemblage B, contains most human isolates and a rabbit isolate, underscoring the zoonotic potential of rabbit *G. duodenalis*.

Hepatozoon cuniculi *Infection*

Hepatozoon cuniculi is of minor significance, but has been reported in domestic rabbits. The nomenclature is historically based on the host (rabbit), and was originally named *Leucocytogregarina cuniculi*. The relationship to other Hepatozoon species is unknown. Gametocytes were observed in peripheral blood leukocytes and schizonts in the spleen of domestic rabbits. *Hepatozoon* spp. utilize an intermediate arthropod host, which has not been defined for rabbits, but fleas are suspected.

Sarcocystis cuniculi *Infection*

There are over 130 named species of *Sarcocystis*, nomenclature of which has been historically based upon association with various hosts. Thus, taxonomy is in complete flux, and it remains to be determined if *S. cuniculi* is a valid separate species. Typical *Sarcocystis* cysts have been observed as incidental findings in skeletal and cardiac muscle of domestic rabbits, and are very common in different species of wild rabbits (including *Oryctolagus*) and hares. Domestic rabbits may have a high prevalence of seroconversion to this organism, with no clinical disease. Rabbit *Sarcocystis* is infective to cats and back to rabbits, indicating that the definitive host is the cat.

Toxoplasma gondii *Infection: Toxoplasmosis*

Toxoplasma gondii infection has been documented in rabbits in many parts of the world. Serologic surveys indicate that infection is common, but clinical disease is rare. Toxoplasmosis is associated with contamination of feed and water by cat feces. In 1 reported outbreak of the disease, anorexia, pyrexia, and neurological disorders were the presenting signs. At necropsy, multiple foci of necrosis were found with a granulomatous inflammatory response in the lung, liver, and spleen. Tachyzoites and tissue cysts with PAS-positive bradyzoites were observed within thin PAS-negative cyst walls. No lesions were found in other organs, including brain. Another report found 25.4–51.2 μm cysts within the brain, but not other organs of a clinically ill rabbit. Wild and domestic meat rabbits are considered to pose a major source of infection for humans. In contrast to *Encephalitozoon cuniculi*, *T. gondii* tachyzoites and bradyzoites within cysts are Gram-negative.

Trypanosoma nabiasi *Infection: Trypanosomiasis*

Trypanosomiasis is indigenous to the wild European rabbit, and similar organisms are found in North American *Sylvilagus* rabbits. Infection with *T. nabiasi* has been found in Australian wild *Orytolagus* rabbits. Although it may have been carried with the original 24 rabbits that were introduced to Australia in 1859, it is more likely to have been carried with the rabbit flea, which was purposely introduced into the wild in 1968 for myxomatosis control. This trypanosome has been reported in European domestic rabbits, as well as outside of Europe. The vector is the rabbit flea, *Spilopsyllus cuniculi*, and transmission is via flea feces and ingestion of fleas during grooming. Upon infection, parasitemia increases rapidly, peaks around 20 days, then declines, and duration of infection is 4–8 months, followed by recovery. The organism is rabbit species specific and essentially nonpathogenic.

Nonpathogenic (Commensal) Intestinal Protozoa

The rabbit intestine contains *Chilomastix cuniculi*, *Monocercomonas cuniculi*, *Retortamonas cuniculi*, and *Entamoeba cuniculi*, among others, which are all nonpathogenic.

Helminth Infestations

Baylisascaris *spp. Larval Migrans*

The natural host of *Baylisascaris procyonis* is the raccoon. However, when an unnatural host such as a rabbit (or human) accidentally ingests infective eggs, a devastating cerebrospinal disorder may result. Hay or bedding contaminated with raccoon feces containing *B. procyonis* eggs is the usual source of the parasite. Following passage in raccoon feces, embryonation requires approximately 30 days before the eggs are infective. Eggs will remain infective for at least a year under appropriate environmental conditions. Following the accidental ingestion of embryonated eggs, the larvae are released in the intestine and undergo aggressive somatic and pulmonary migration. Larvae have a tropism for the brain stem. Typical neurological signs include torticollis, ataxia, circling, opisthotonus, and recumbency. If not euthanized, animals usually die as a result of the unremitting nervous signs. In addition, *B. columnaris*, the ascarid of skunks, may also cause similar disease, but is less common.

Pathology

Multiple, circumscribed, raised white nodules up to 1.5 mm in diameter may be found in the subepicardial and subendocardial regions of the heart and the serosal surface of the liver. Microscopic examination of the visceral lesions reveals focal granulomas, with mononuclear cells and heterophils infiltrating the area. Remnants of the parasite are often present within these lesions. In the central nervous system, lesions are most often present in the gray and white matter in the brain stem and cerebellar regions, but the cerebrum, including the hippocampus, may be involved. Sites of parasitic migration are characterized by extensive malacia and astrogliosis. Large numbers of Gitter cells and gemistocytic astrocytes may be present in lesions interpreted to be of several days' duration. Infiltrating inflammatory cells include lymphocytes, macrophages, eosinophils, and heterophils. Within the neuropil adjacent to the lesions, nematode larvae can be identified with characteristic excretory columns and lateral alae (Fig. 6.69). Because of active migratory behavior, larvae may not be found in association with inflammation, but can be found in other regions that have yet to develop an inflammatory response. Thus, if larval migrans is suspected, multiple tissue sections may need to be examined. The primary differential diagnosis is *Encephalitozoon cuniculi* infection, but that organism tends not to target the brain stem, and can be identified with tissue Gram stains.

Capillaria hepatica *Infestation*

Capillaria hepatica infects many species, including wild lagomorphs. It was observed in the livers of laboratory rabbits purchased from a commercial supplier in the United Kingdom. Gross findings included irregular white or yellow patches, streaks or small nodules visible on the surface, and cut sections of liver. Lesions included portal inflammation, dilated bile ducts, and fibrosis. The hepatic parenchyma contained multiple granulomas infiltrated with macrophages, eosinophils, and lymphocytes in association with multiple double-operculated ova. In 1 report, ova were also present in the bile ducts and gall bladder of infected rabbits. Wild rodents are the most common definitive hosts for *C. hepatica*.

Dirofilaria spp. *Infestation*

Dirofilariasis is common in wild lagomorphs, with *D. uniformis* adults localized within the connective tissue of the subcutis of the trunk and *D. scapiceps* localized around tendons of the hock and stifle. Both feature microfilaria in the blood, and are transmitted by mosquitoes. Infection of outdoor domestic rabbits in Canada is reported to be common. Rabbits can also be aberrant hosts for *D. immitis*, which develop in pulmonary arteries, but die and are associated with organized thrombi.

Passalurus ambiguus *Infestation: Pinworms*

Passalurus ambiguus is a very common parasite of domestic rabbits. Adult worms are located in the cecum and other areas of the large intestine (Fig. 6.70). The identification of the eggs on fecal flotation and/or the adult worms in feces or in the large intestine will confirm the diagnosis. Infections with moderate numbers of *Passalurus* are considered to be relatively harmless, although clinicians frequently elect to treat affected animals. However, impaired weight gains, poor breeding performance, and occasionally deaths have been attributed to heavy burdens of pinworms. *Dermatoxys veligera* is a common oxyurid in North American wild rabbits and may rarely infect domestic rabbits.

Toxocara canis *Infestation*

Rabbits, particularly wild rabbits, are widely recognized as paratenic hosts for the canine ascarid, *T. canis*, and are purported to pose a risk to humans when rabbit meat is consumed. However, no descriptions of natural cases in domestic rabbits could be found.

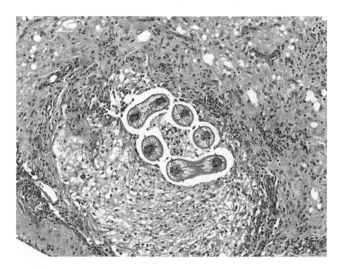

FIG. 6.69. *Cerebral* Baylisascaris *infestation in a New Zealand White rabbit. Note the focus of malacia and inflammation containing multiple cross sections of ascarid larvae with characteristic lateral alae.*

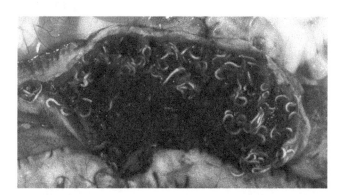

FIG. 6.70. *Opened cecum from a domestic rabbit with* Passalurus ambiguus *(pinworm) infestation.*

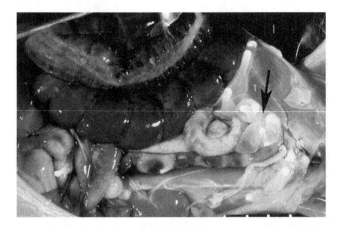

FIG. 6.71.   *Multiple* Taenia pisiformis *cysticerci (arrow) within the peritoneal cavity of a rabbit.*

Tapeworm Infestations

Several species of tapeworms infect wild lagomorphs, but adult tapeworms are rare in the domestic rabbit. The most common adult tapeworm of domestic rabbits is *Cittotaenia variabilis*, which attaches to the mucosa of the small intestine. Its intermediate hosts are believed to be orbatid mites. Infection occurs through ingestion of infested grass or hay. Wild lagomorphs are an important intermediate host for *Taenia pisiformis*, a parasite whose definitive hosts are wild canids. On occasion, cysticerosis may occur in domestic rabbits. The intermediate host stage is known as *Cysticercus pisiformis*. Upon ingestion of eggs, larvae hatch in the small intestine and migrate to the liver and blood stream. Cysticerci develop in the liver for a few weeks, and then find their way to the peritoneal cavity, where they attach to serosal surfaces (Fig. 6.71). Raised, light tan, focal to linear, solitary or multiple lesions up to 3 mm in diameter are present on the surface of the liver, and single or multiple cysticerci occupy the peritoneal and occasionally pleural surfaces. Liver lesions may have granulomatous inflammation with parasite fragments surrounded by fibrosis. *Taenia serialis*, another tapeworm of canids, also utilizes wild lagomorphs as its intermediate hosts, and is common in Australia. The intermediate stage of this tapeworm is a coenurus (*Coenurus serialis*), which contains multiple larval forms with scolesces. Infestation of pet rabbits has been reported, with coenurus cysts localized in various anatomical locations. One case in Australia featured exophthalmos due to a retrobulbar cyst and multiple coenurus cysts protruding from the conjunctiva. Notably, a similar case with conjunctival coenurus cysts was noted by the authors in California.

Other Gastrointestinal Helminth Infestations

Wild lagomorphs are host to several gastrointestinal nematodes, and although domestic rabbits are potentially susceptible, infections are rare. The gastric worms, *Graphidium strigosum* and *Obeliscoides cuniculi*, have been rarely found in domestic rabbits. Both are associated

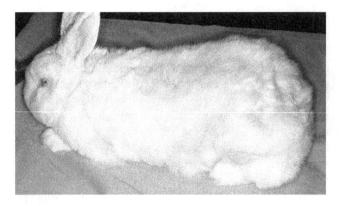

FIG. 6.72.   *New Zealand White rabbit with* Cheyletiella parasitovorax *infestation. Pruritus has resulted in patchy hair loss and cutaneous erythema.*

with gastritis. *Nematodirus leporis* and *Trichostrongylus calcaratus* have been rarely found as small intestinal nematodes in domestic rabbits, and are associated with enteritis in heavy infections. *Trichuris leporis* and *T. sylvilagus* are whipworms that may rarely be found in the cecum and large intestine of domestic rabbits. A number of other species infest wild lagomorphs, but have not been reported in domestic rabbits.

Ectoparasite Infestations

Cheyletiella parasitovorax *Infestation*

Cheyletiellid fur mites, in the authors' experience, are relatively common in laboratory rabbits. They may be present without producing obvious detectable disease. The relatively large and motile mites can be seen with the naked eye, resulting in the term "walking dandruff" for this infestation. When lesions are present, they are usually located on the dorsal trunk, scapular areas, and occasionally the ventral abdomen. They consist of areas of scaliness and hyperemia, with crusting and variable degrees of hair loss (Figs. 6.72 and 6.73). Pruritus is not intense, but careful observation reveals that rabbits are

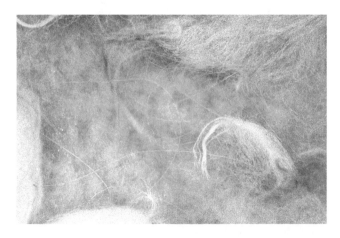

FIG. 6.73.   *Inguinal region of the rabbit represented in the previous figure, depicting alopecia and cutaneous erythema.*

pruritic and agitated. There may be a relatively high prevalence of these mites in some commercial rabbitries. Rabbits are susceptible to several species of *Cheyletiella* mites, but *C. parasitovorax* is the most common in North America. These mites can be acquired from and transmitted to other species of animals, and are readily transmissible to humans, where they induce pruritic dermatitis.

Demodex cuniculi *Infestation: Demodectic Mange*

In keeping with *Demodex* biology in other species, infestations in the rabbit are probably common and subclinical, although this has not been documented. Sporadic cases of demodictic mange have been noted in domestic rabbits, which had areas of alopecia with mild seborrhea sicca. Microscopic findings included acanthosis and orthokeratotic hyperkeratosis with typical follicular plugging with keratin debris and mites.

Leporacarus gibbus *Infestation*

Leporacarus gibbus, a fur mite, is probably more common than generally realized. Both pet and laboratory rabbits have been found to be infested. Infestation of rabbits is usually subclinical, and there is usually no evidence of movement of mites on the hair. Several reports have described alopecia and moist dermatitis of the dorsal neck and medial aspects of the hind feet, and 1 report described more generalized alopecia and dermatitis involving the neck, dorsum, flanks, and hind legs. The preferred site of attachment is on the underside of the tail. Mites tend to localize on the distal third of the hair shaft. Microscopic examination of hair samples is used for the identification of the parasites, but finding them is often challenging. Transmission to humans has been shown to result in pruritic dermatitis.

Psoroptes cuniculi *Infestation: Psoroptic Mange; Ear Canker*

The mites are obligate, nonburrowing parasites that chew and pierce the epidermal layers of the external ear, evoking a marked inflammatory response. The mite normally spends its entire life span in the external ear of the rabbit. The life cycle (egg to egg) is usually completed in around 3 weeks. Up to 10,000 mites may be present in a severely infested ear. In heavily parasitized ears, foul-smelling branlike crusts fill the external ear canal and extend up the ear (Fig. 6.74). The ear is often thickened and edematous. The mites can be easily demonstrated in wet mount preparations from the ear. Rarely, cutaneous lesions have been observed in the perineal region. Notably, *P. cuniculi* is not a parasite of wild rabbits, but rather was acquired during domestication of the rabbit. Its origin is generally believed to be the sheep mite, *P. ovis*, but recent molecular analyses suggest that *P. cuniculi*, *P. ovis*, and a number of other *Psoroptes* spp. are all synonyms of *P. equi*.

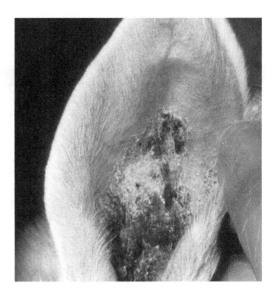

FIG. 6.74. *Auricular acariasis due to* Psoroptes cuniculi *infestation. The external ear canal contains accumulations of branlike serous crusts containing mites.*

Psorobia lagomorpha *Infestation*

There is a single report describing a new species of *Psorobia* (formerly *Psorergates*) in a 6-month-old Dutch rabbit. The affected rabbit had hyperkeratosis, scaling, and alopecia. Diagnosis was achieved by skin scrapings. The validity of this being a new species remains to be determined. Related *Psorobia* spp. are the "itch mites" of sheep and cattle.

Sarcoptes scabei *Infestion: Scabies*

Sarcoptes scabiei is a burrowing mite that inhabits the superficial layers of the skin of multiple host species, including humans. Female mites tunnel into the cornified layers and lay eggs that hatch and develop into larvae and later into nymphs. It is the feeding activity of these stages that evokes a hypersensitivity reaction, with subsequent hyperkeratosis, seborrhea, and hair loss. Alopecia with hyperkeratosis involving the face, nose, lips, ear margins, feet, abdomen, and external genitalia are typical presenting signs (Fig. 6.75 and 6.76). Pruritus is common, and self-mutilation may also occur. There is 1 report of an outbreak of sarcoptic mange in adult Holland lops rabbits with a concurrent yeast infection in the parasitized areas of the skin. The round to oval and budding forms of yeast were identified as members of the *Malassezia* spp. Diagnosis of sarcoptic mange is achieved by deep scrapings of affected skin, or by histopathology, in which mites can be visualized burrowing within the hyperkeratinized epidermis (Fig. 6.77). *Notoedres cati* has been found to cause cutaneous disease with a similar appearance and distribution as *Sarcoptes* in rabbits.

Trombiculid Mite Infestation: Chiggers

Several species of *Trombicula* can infest rabbits. Adult mites are free-living, and larvae are parasitic. Larvae

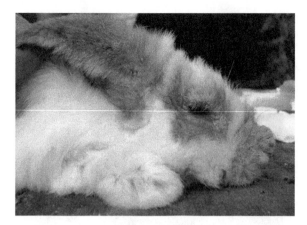

FIG. 6.75. *Young rabbit infested with* Sarcoptes scabei. *Note the perinasal, periocular, and auricular crusty lesions that are typical of scabies in the rabbit. (Source: Farmaki et al., 2009. Reproduced with permission from BMJ Publishing Group Ltd.)*

attach to the skin and form a tubular feeding structure around their mouth parts known as a stylosome. Their presence elicits intense pruritus. They tend to locate on the feet, ears, medial canthus, and perineaum of infested rabbits. *Dermanyssus gallinae* (red poultry mite) is also known to infest rabbits in contact with birds.

Haemodipsus ventriculosis *Infestation: Pediculosis*

Haemodipsus ventriculosis is the rabbit louse, which infests wild *O. cuniculus*, and occurs occasionally in domestic rabbits. Heavy infestations may result in anemia, weight loss, alopecia, pruritus, and pustular dermatitis.

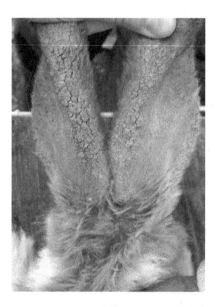

FIG. 6.76. *Ears of the rabbit with scabies in the previous figure, depicting severe hyperkeratosis. Source: Farmaki et al., 2009. Reproduced with permission from BMJ Publishing Group Ltd.*

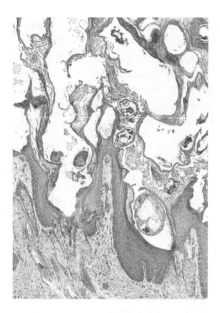

FIG. 6.77. *Marked hyperkeratosis with numerous* Sarcoptes *mites embedded in the keratinized debris. Note the spongiform appearance of the keratinized epithelium due to tunneling by mites. (Source: M.K. Keel, University of California, Davis, CA. Reproduced with permission from M.K. Keel.)*

Myiasis

Myiasis can be encountered in outdoor rabbitries, including *Cuterebra* spp. and "fly strike" of wounds, ear canker, hutch burn, and other exudative lesions.

Fleas

The major flea of the European rabbit is *Spilopsyllus cuniculi*, which was purposely introduced to Australia to facilitate transmission of myxomatosis. It can occasionally be found on cats. The most common fleas of North American domestic rabbits are *Cediopsylla simplex* (common eastern rabbit flea) and *Odontopsyllus multispinosus* (giant rabbit flea). Dog and cat *Ctenocephalides* fleas are also known to infest rabbits.

BIBLIOGRAPHY FOR PARASITIC DISEASES

General References for Parasitic Diseases

Pritt, S., Cohen, K., & Sedlack, H. (2012) Parasitic diseases. In: *The Laboratory Rabbit, Guinea Pig, Hamster and Other Rodents* (eds. M.A. Suckow, K.A. Stevensn, & R.P. Wilson), pp. 415–501. Elsevier, London.

Schoeb, T.R., Cartner, S.C., Baker, R.A., & Gerrity, L.G. (2007) Parasites of rabbits. In: *Flynn's Parasites of Laboratory Animals* (ed. D.G. Baker), pp. 451–500. Blackwell Publishing, Ames.

Van Praag, E. (2014) MediRabbit.com.

Protozoal Infections

Cryptosporidium cuniculus Infection

Hadfield, S.J. & Chalmers, R.M. (2012) Detection and characterization of *Cryptosporidium cuniculus* by real-time PCR. *Parasitology Research* 111:1385–1390.

Inman, L.R. & Takeuchi, A. (1979) Spontaneous cryptosporidiosis in an adult female rabbit. *Veterinary Pathology* 16:89–95.

Rehg, J.E., Lawton, G.W., & Pakes, S.P. (1979) *Cryptosporidium cuniculus* in the rabbit (*Oryctolagus cuniculus*). *Laboratory Animal Science* 29:656–660.

Robinson, G., Wright, S., Elwin, K., Hadfield, S.J., Katzer, F., Bartley, P.M., Hunter, P.R., Nath, M., Innes, E.A., & Chalmers, R.M. (2010) Redescription of *Cryptosporidium cuniculus* Inman and Takeuchi, 1979 (Apicomplexa: Cryptosporidiidae): morphology, biology and phylogeny. *International Journal of Parasitology* 40:1539–1548.

Eimeria spp. Infections: Intestinal and Hepatic Coccidiosis

Barriga, O.O. & Arnoni, J.V. (1979) *Eimeria stiedae*: weight, oocyst output, and hepatic function of rabbits with graded infections. *Experimental Parasitology* 48:407–414.

Barriga, O.O. & Arnoni, J.V. (1981) Pathophysiology of hepatic coccidiosis in rabbits. *Veterinary Parasitology* 8:201–210.

Drouet-Viard, F., Licois, D., Provot, D., & Coudert, P. (1994) The invasion of the rabbit intestinal tract by *Eimeria intestinalis* sporozoites. *Parasitology Research* 80:706–707.

Gregory, M.W. & Catchpole, J. (1986) Coccidiosis in rabbits: the pathology of *Eimeria flavescens* infection. *International Journal of Parasitology* 16:131–145.

Horton, R.J. (1967) The route of migration of *Eimeria stiedae* (Lindemann, 1865) sporozoites between the duodenum and bile ducts of the rabbit. *Parasitology* 57:9–17.

Oliviera, U.C., Fraga, J.S., Licois, D., Pakankl, M., & Gruber, A. (2011) Development of molecular assays for the identification of the 11 *Eimeria* species of the domestic rabbit (*Oryctolagus cuniculus*). *Veterinary Parasitology* 176:275–280.

Owen, D. (1970) Life cycle of *Eimeria stiedae*. *Nature* 227:304.

Pakandl, M. (2009) Coccida of rabbit: a review. *Folia Parasitologica* 56:153–166.

Peeters, J.E., Charlier, G., Antoine, O., & Mammerickx, M. (1984) Clinical and pathological changes after *Eimeria intestinalis* infection in rabbits. *Zentralblatt Veterinaermedizin (B)* 31:9–24.

Rutherford, R.L. (1943) The life cycle of four intestinal coccidia of the domestic rabbit. *Journal of Parasitology* 29:10–32.

Varga, I. (1982) Large-scale management systems and parasite populations: Coccidia in rabbits. *Veterinary Parasitology* 11:69–84.

Giardia duodenalis Infection

Sulaiman, I.M., Fayer, R., Bern, C., Gilman, R.H., Trout, J.M., Schantz, P.M., Das, P., Lai, A.A., & Xiao, L. (2003) Triosephosphate isomerase gene characterization and potential zoonotic transmission of *Giardia duodenalis*. *Emerging Infectious Diseases* 9:1434–1442.

Hepatozoon cuniculi Infection

Sangiorgi, A. (1914) *Leucocytogregarina cuniculi* n. sp. *Pathologica* 6:49.

Sarcocystis cuniculi Infection

Cerna, Z., Louckova, M., Nedvedova, H., & Vavra, J. (1981) Spontaneous and experimental infection of domestic rabbits by *Sarcocystis cuniculi* Brumpt 1913. *Folia Parasitologica* 28:313–318.

Trypanosoma nabiasi Infection

Hamilton, P.B., Stevens, J.R., Holz, P., Boag, B., Cooke, B., & Gibson, W.C. (2005) The inadvertent introduction into Australia of *Trypanosoma nabiasi*, the trypanosome of the European rabbit (*Oryctolagus cuniculus*), and its potential for biocontrol. *Molecular Ecology* 14:3167–3175.

Toxoplasma gondii Infection

Dubey, J.P. Brown, C.A., Carpenter, J.L., & Moore, J., III (1992) Fatal toxoplasmosis in domestic rabbits in the USA. *Veterinary Parasitology* 44:305–309.

Leland, M.M., Hubbard, G.B., & Dubey, J.P. (1992) Clinical toxoplasmosis in domestic rabbits. *Laboratory Animal Science* 42:318–319.

Sroka, J., Zwolinski, J,. Dutkiewicz, J,. Tos-Luty, S., & Latuszynska, J. (2003) Toxoplasmosis in rabbits confirmed by strain isolation: a potential risk of infection among agricultural workers. *Annals of Agricultural and Environmental Medicine* 10:125–128.

Helminth Infestations

Bartlett, C.M. (1984) Pathology and epizootiology of *Dirofilaria scapiceps* (Leidy, 1886) (Nematoda: Filarioidea) in *Sylvilagus floridanus* (J.A. Allen) and *Lepus americanus* Erxleben. *Journal of Wildlife Diseases* 20:197–206.

Dade, A.W., Williams, J.F., Whitenack, D.L., & Williams, C.S. (1975) An epizootic of cerebral nematodiasis in rabbits due to *Ascaris columnaris*. *Laboratory Animal Science* 25:65–69.

Duwel, D. & Brech, K. (1981) Control of oxyuriasis in rabbits by fenbendazole. *Laboratory Animals* 15:101–105.

Flatt, R.E. & Campbell, W.W. (1974) Cysticercosis in rabbits: incidence and lesions of the naturally occurring disease in young domestic rabbits. *Laboratory Animal Science* 24:914–918.

Kazacos, K.R., Reed, W.M., Kazacos, E.A., & Thacker, H.L. (1983) Fatal cerebrospinal disease caused by *Baylisascaris procyonis* in domestic rabbits. *Journal of the American Veterinary Medical Association* 183:967–971.

Mowat, V., Turton, J., Stewart, J. Lui, C.K., & Pilling, A.M. (2009) Histopathological features of *Capillaria hepatica* infection in laboratory rabbits. *Toxicologic Pathology* 37:661–666.

Narama, I., Tsuchitani, M., Umemura, T., & Kamiya, H. (1982) Pulmonary nodule caused by *Dirofilaria immitis* in a laboratory rabbit (*Oryctolagus cuniculus domesticus*). *Journal of Parasitology* 68:351–352.

Reed, S.D., Shaw, S., & Evans, D.E. (2009) Spinal lymphoma and pulmonary filariasis in a pet rabbit (*Oryctolagus cuniculus domesticus*). *Journal of Veterinary Diagnostic Investigation* 21:253–256.

Ectoparasitic Infestations

Flatt, R.E. & Weimers, J. (1976) A survey of fur mites in domestic rabbits. *Laboratory Animal Science* 26:758–761.

Demodex cuniculi Infestation

Harvey, R.G. (1990) *Demodex cuniculi* in dwarf rabbits (*Oryctolagus cuniculus*). *Journal of Small Animal Practice* 31:204–207.

Leporacarus gibbus Infestation

Burns, D.A. (1987) Papular urticaria produced by the mite *Listrophorus gibbus*. *Clinical and Experimental Dermatology* 12:200–201.

D'Ovidio, D. & Santoro, D. (2014) *Leporacarus gibbus* infestation in client-owned rabbits and their owners. *Veterinary Dermatology* 25:46e17.

Niekrasz, M.A., Curl, J.L., & Curl, J.S. (1998) Rabbit fur mite (*Listrophorus gibbus*) infestation of New Zealand White rabbits. *Contemporary Topics in Laboratory Animal Science* 37:73–75.

Patel, A. & Robinson, K.J.E. (1993) Dermatosis associated with *Listrophorus gibbus* in the rabbit. *Journal of Small Animal Practice* 34:409–411.

Printer, L. (1999) *Leporacarus gibbus* and *Spilopsyllus cuniculi* infestation in a pet rabbit. *Journal of Small Animal Practice* 40:220–221.

Psoroptes cuniculi Infestation

Bulliot, C., Mentre, V., Marignac, G., Polack, B., & Chermette, R. (2013) A case of atypical psoroptic mange in a domestic rabbit. *Journal of Exotic Pet Medicine* 22:400–404.

Curtis, S.K. (1991) Diagnostic exercise: moist dermatitis on the hind quarters of a rabbit. *Laboratory Animal Science* z41:623–624.

Zahler, M., Hendrikx, W.M., Essig, A., Rinder, H., & Gothe, R. (2000) Species of the genus *Psoroptes* (Acari: Psoroptidae): a taxonomic consideration. *Experimental and Applied Acarology* 24:213–225.

Sarcoptes scabei Infestation

Farmaki, R., Koutinas, A.F., Papazahariadou, M.G., Kasabalis, D., & Day, M.J. (2009) Effectiveness of a selamectin spot-on formulation in rabbits with sarcoptic mange. *Veterinary Record* 164:431–432.

Lin, S.L., Pinson, D.M., & Lindsey, J.R. (1984) Diagnostic exercise: mange due to *Sarcoptes scabei*. *Laboratory Animal Science* 34:353–355.

Radi, Z.A. (2004) Outbreak of sarcoptic mange and malasseziasis in rabbits (*Oryctolagus cuniculus*). *Comparative Medicine* 54:434–437.

NONINFECTIOUS GASTROINTESTINAL DISORDERS

The foregoing sections feature many viral and bacterial infectious diseases of the gastrointestinal tract of rabbits, which often occur in combination and affect the overall enteric physiology of the rabbit in a syndrome known as dysbiosis. It is a challenge for the pathologist to discern primary from secondary etiologies in rabbit enteric disease. A simple measure of dysbiosis is Gram stain and semiquantitative aerobic culture of the upper small intestine and cecum for *E. coli*, which is rarely present in the normal rabbit gut.

Mucoid Enteropathy

Mucoid enteropathy is recognized as a major disease in domestic rabbits, but it is inappropriate to consider it a primary disease. Gastric bloat, mucous discharge, and cecal impaction, which are the cardinal features of mucoid enteropathy, are nonspecific responses of the rabbit intestine to a number of deleterious factors. Clinical signs associated with the syndrome include bruxism, anorexia, lethargy, crouched stance, diarrhea, succussion splash, cecal impaction, and accumulation of large quantities of clear gelatinous mucus in the colon. Cecal impaction and mucous production occur most often in rabbits that live for 7–14 days after the onset of the syndrome. The morbidity is variable but may be high, particularly in rabbits affected during the postweaning period. There is usually a high mortality rate in affected animals regardless of the treatment. Rabbits 7–10 weeks of age are most often affected, but ages ranging from 5 weeks to adults may be involved in outbreaks of mucoid enteropathy.

Many theories have been proposed to explain the etiopathogenesis of mucoid enteropathy. Dietary factors have frequently been implicated. This condition was relatively uncommon prior to the feeding of high-energy commercial rations, and rabbits fed a high-carbohydrate/low-fiber diet have been shown to have a higher incidence of the syndrome than those fed diets high in fiber. Studies of the cecal microbial flora have revealed striking changes in rabbits with mucoid enteropathy. In normal animals, large numbers of ciliated protozoa and large, metachromatically staining bacilli are present in the cecal contents. Rabbits with mucoid enteropathy have a dramatic cecal dysbiosis. Large metachromatic bacilli and ciliated protozoa may be present in small numbers or completely absent, and there is a marked rise in coliform bacteria in the cecal contents. Microbial instability may occur more often in young animals, where homeostatic mechanisms are poorly developed, thus increasing susceptibility to dietary changes associated with weaning.

Pathology

The stomach is often distended with fluid and gas. The jejunum is frequently distended with translucent, watery fluid, and the cecum is often impacted with dried contents and gas. The colon is usually distended with characteristic clear, gelatinous mucus (Fig. 6.78). Microscopically, there is massive discharge of mucin from goblet cells in the mucosa of affected small and large intestine, with minimal or no inflammatory response. Goblet cells may be in different stages of mucin release. In the colon, crypts and the lumen of the gut are distended with mucus and mucous plugs (Fig. 6.79). Lesions are usually minimal to absent in the cecum. Mucoid enteropathy often accompanies or precedes viral and/or bacterial enteritides, or management problems that may lead to disruption of the intestinal microflora or function.

Gastric Dilation (Bloat) and Gastrointestinal Stasis

Acute gastric bloat, often accompanied by tympany of the intestine, is a life-threatening syndrome in rabbits. A number of factors are associated with bloat, including high-carbohydrate diet, dysautonomia, epizootic rabbit enteropathy (Fig. 6.33), mucoid enteropathy, and others. In 1 study, a significant majority of rabbits presenting with gastric bloat had accompanying intestinal obstruction due to bezoars, neoplasia, postsurgical adhesions, foreign bodies, tapeworm cysts, and others. Gastrointestinal stasis, including gastric and intestinal bloat, is secondary to a large number of factors, often in

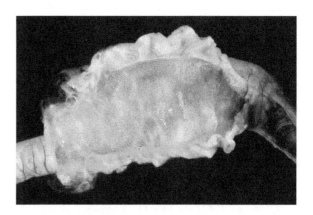

FIG. 6.78. *Sacculated colon from a juvenile rabbit with mucoid enteropathy. The opened bowel is filled with clear gelatinous material.*

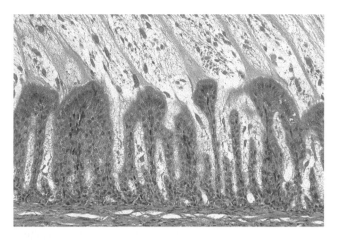

FIG. 6.79. *Colon from a rabbit with acute onset of mucoid enteropathy. Note the abundant mucous within the lumen and adherent to enterocytes, depletion of goblet cells, and lack of inflammation.*

combination, that cause anorexia, including dental disease, stress, infection, neoplasia, drug effects, restricted water and food intake, and so on. Once initiated, dysmotility leads to a downward spiral of abnormal colonic/cecal transit, maldigestion, and dysbiosis. Unrelieved tympany leads to hypovolemic shock.

Gastric Ulceration

Acute ulceration of the gastric fundus and pylorus is a common finding in rabbits. Studies have revealed that fundic ulcers are typically multifocal, small, shallow, and hemorrhagic (dark to black). Microscopic changes are minimal, indicating acute antemortem onset. In the majority of cases, fundic ulceration was associated with other significant disease. Pyloric ulcers generally occurred as single lesions, up to 1 cm in diameter, and were frequently the only lesion found. A significant number of pyloric ulcers perforate, with development of peritonitis. They tended to be associated with does in labor or the postparturient period, and tended not to occur in concert with fundic ulceration.

Trichobezoar: Hairball

Gastric trichobezoars are frequently present as an incidental finding at necropsy in rabbits that have died from other causes. Depending on the size, however, anorexia, wasting, and occasionally gastric rupture and death may occur in severely affected animals. Antemortem diagnosis is usually confirmed by palpation and sometimes by contrast radiography. Predisposing factors implicated include excessive grooming and hair chewing due to boredom, insufficient dietary roughage, poor gastric motility, and a sedentary lifestyle. "Outbreaks" of trichobezoars have been seen in laboratory rabbits raised in cold climates, and then introduced to warm indoor housing. They also tend to occur more frequently in sedentary rabbits, which may have decreased gastric motility. At necropsy, animals may be in fair to poor

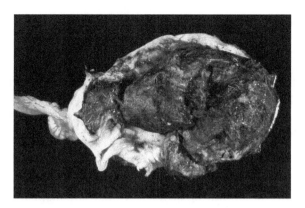

FIG. 6.80. *Trichobezoar filling the stomach of an adult New Zealand White rabbit. These masses can be intractably felt-like in consistency, resulting in gastric occlusion, anorexia, and death.*

condition. Large felt-like trichobezoars usually fill the stomach, extending into the pyloric region (Fig. 6.80). The intestinal tract usually contains scant ingesta. Hepatic lipidosis is a characteristic finding. Gastric rupture and peritonitis may occur. Trichobezoars have also been found in the large intestine of rabbits.

Gastric Pyloric Hypertrophy

Marked muscular hypertrophy of the pyloric sphincter (Fig. 6.81) resulting in interference with gastric emptying may be associated with weight loss. This syndrome has been noted in New Zealand White rabbits. It may be variably associated with trichobezoars, but the relationship of the 2 syndromes is not absolute.

Intestinal Obstruction and Rupture

Cecal impaction with abnormally firm masses of cecal content is a common cause of lower intestinal obstruction in rabbits. These masses often lodge at the fusus coli of the caudal end of the sacculated colon. Affected rabbits often have a chronic history of intestinal disorders with large, malformed feces. Diets with fine-particle indigestible fiber or diets with small fiber length predispose to this syndrome. Dry cecal content often occurs in association with

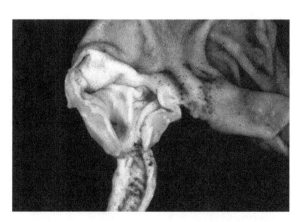

FIG. 6.81. *Muscular hypertrophy of the gastric pyloric sphincter of a New Zealand White rabbit, which can result in interference with gastric emptying and subsequent weight loss.*

mucoid enteropathy, dysautonomia, and other enteric diseases. Rabbits have also been found to develop obstruction of the jejunum or ileum with bezoars consisting of hair and fiber. Varying stages of obstruction with peritonitis and rupture were present. Affected rabbits tended to be overweight and an association with handling was noted. The problem was ameliorated by wrapping rabbits in towels as a restraint method.

Intestinal Plasmacytosis

A syndrome characterized by marked plasma cell infiltration in the intestinal tract of domestic rabbits has been described. The intestinal lesions have been identified in New Zealand White, Dutch Belted, and Watanabe rabbits used in research projects. Older animals are at risk, particularly rabbits used for antibody production or cholesterol studies. Affected animals are usually subclinical, and the changes are frequently detected only on histopathologic examination. The selective involvement of the intestinal tract and the nature of the cellular infiltrate are consistent with the response to antigenic stimuli at the local level. The etiology and pathogenesis are currently unknown.

Anorectal Polyps

Multiple polyps may arise in the anal region. Their etiology is unknown, and these polyps have been incorrectly termed anal papillomas.

Hepatic Lobe Torsion

A number of reports have documented torsion of liver lobes in domestic rabbits, including laboratory rabbits. Rabbits presented with anorexia, jaundice, abdominal pain, and bowel stasis. In other cases, torsion was encountered as an incidental finding.

Biliary Hyperplasia

A frequent incidental finding in laboratory rabbits as well as rodents is bile ductular hyperplasia with varying degrees of portal fibrosis.

BIBILIOGRAPHY FOR NONINFECTIOUS GASTROINTESTINAL DISORDERS

Mucoid Enteropathy
Haligur, M., Ozmen, O., & Demir, N. (2009) Pathological and ultrastructural studies on mucoid enteropathy in New Zealand White rabbits. *Journal of Exotic Pet Medicine* 18:224–228.

Lelkes, L. & Chang, C-L. (1987) Microbial dysbiosis in rabbit mucoid enteropathy. *Laboratory Animal Science* 37:757–764.

McLeod, C.G. & Katz, W. (1986) Toxic components in commercial rabbit feeds and their role in mucoid enteritis. *South African Journal of Science* 82:375–379.

Toofanian, F. & Targowski, S. (1983) Experimental production of rabbit mucoid enteritis. *American Journal of Veterinary Research* 44:705–708.

van Kruiningen, H.J. & Williams, C.B. (1972) Mucoid enteritis in rabbits: comparison to cholera and cystic fibrosis. *Veterinary Pathology* 9:53–77.

Gastric Dilation and Gastrointestinal Stasis
Harcourt-Brown, F.M. (2007) Gastric dilation and intestinal obstruction in 76 rabbits. *Veterinary Record* 161:409–414.

Gastric Ulceration
Collin, B.J. (1977) L'ulcere de stress par choc hypovolemique chez la lapine. *Zentralblatt fur Veterinarmedizin C* 6:94.

Hinton, M. (1980) Gastric ulceration in the rabbit. *Journal of Comparative Pathology* 90:475–481.

Ostler, D.C. (1961) The diseases of broiler rabbits. *Veterinary Record* 73:1237–1252.

Trichobezoar
Lee, K.P., et al. (1978) Acute peritonitis in the rabbit (*Oryctolagus cuniculi*) resulting from gastric trichobezoar. *Laboratory Animal Science* 28:202–204.

Wagner, J.E., et al. (1974) Spontaneous deaths in rabbits resulting from gastric trichobezoars. *Laboratory Animal Science* 24:826–830.

Gastric Pyloric Hypertrophy
Weisbroth, S.H. & Scher, S. (1975) Naturally occurring hypertrophic pyloric stenosis in the domestic rabbit. *Laboratory Animal Science* 25:355–360.

Intestinal Obstruction and Rupture
Jackson, G. (1991) Intestinal stasis and rupture in rabbits. *Veterinary Record* 129:287–289.

Intestinal Plasmacytosis
Li, X. (1996) Intestinal plasmacytosis in rabbits: a histologic and ultrastructural study. *Veterinary Pathology* 33:721–724.

Hepatic Lobe Torsion
Saunders, R., Redrobe, S., Barr, F., Moore, A.H., & Elliot, S.C. (2009) Liver lobe torsion in rabbits. *Journal of Small Animal Practice* 50:562.

Weisbroth, S.H. (1975) Torsion of the caudate lobe of the liver in *Oryctolagus cuniculus*. *Veterinary Pathology* 12:13–15.

Wenger, S., Barrett, E.L., Pearson, G.R., Sayers, I., Blakey, C., & Redrobe, S. (2009) Liver lobe torsion in three adult rabbits. *Journal of Small Animal Practice* 50:301–305.

Wilson, R. B., Holscher, M.A., & Sly, D.L. (1987) Liver lobe torsion in a rabbit. *Laboratory Animal Science* 37:506–507.

AGING AND MISCELLANEOUS DISORDERS

Hair Chewing: Barbering

Hair loss due to hair chewing (barbering) occurs commonly among young group-housed rabbits. Patchy alopecia may be present on the face and back, with no evidence of a concurrent dermatitis. Skin scrapings for microscopic examination and fungal culture are recommended in order to eliminate the possibility of dermatophytosis or ectoparasitism. Boredom and low-roughage diets have been implicated as contributing factors to this condition. Barbering should not be confused with periparturient does that normally pluck their own hair, usually from their dewlap, to prepare nests.

Wet Dewlap: Slobbers

Excess ptyalism occurs in heat-stressed rabbits and in rabbits with malocclusion. Secondary bacterial infections, including necrobacillosis (Schmorl's disease), may arise, particularly in does with large dewlaps.

Tooth Abscesses

Tooth root infections are common in rabbits, and a number of opportunistic bacteria can be isolated from them. Abscesses often develop capsules with fistulous tracks, and osteomyelitis with retrobulbar involvement make them refractory to treatment.

Hutch Burn

Urine scalding of the perineal region may be a problem in young rabbits housed in filthy conditions. The skin may be hyperemic and excoriated, with serous exudation. Lesions may be complicated by myiasis.

Pugilism

Fighting is common among group-housed male rabbits that have reached sexual maturity. Abrasions and hair loss are common in the combatants, including lacerations around the external genitalia. Rarely, aggressive males may mutilate both bucks and does. Injuries observed include skin abrasions and amputation of the tips of the ears.

Exfoliative Dermatosis and Sebaceous Adenitis

This condition has been reported to occur in several different breeds of pet rabbits. Typically, there is a non-pruritic scaling dermatosis with patchy to coalescing areas of alopecia and scaling (Fig. 6.82). Affected rabbits have proven to be refractory to a variety of treatments, including antimicrobial and anti-inflammatory drugs. Microscopic changes may include hyperkeratosis, follicular interface dermatitis, interface folliculitis, reduction in the numbers of sebaceous glands with destruction and lymphocytic infiltration, and perifollicular to diffuse dermal fibrosis. Differential diagnoses include malnutrition, dermatophytosis, ectoparasitism, and sebaceous adenitis. Exfoliative dermatosis is often found to

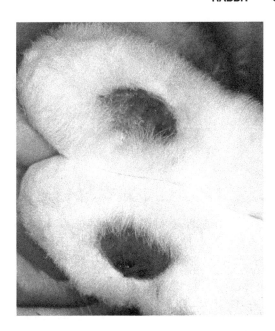

FIG. 6.83. *Bilateral pododermatitis (sore hock) in an adult rabbit.*

be associated with autoimmune hepatitis, thymoma, and cutaneous lymphoma in rabbits (see "Neoplasms"). Thus, it is important to pursue the possibility of the dermatosis having a paraneoplastic or neoplastic origin.

Pododermatitis: Sore Hocks

The plantar surface of rabbit feet is fully haired, but lesions consist of a circumscribed, ulcerated areas covered by granulation tissue and necrotic debris (Fig. 6.83). Purulent exudate may be adherent to the lesions. The problem is most commonly seen in heavy, mature adults. Poor sanitation, trauma from poor-quality, wire-bottom cages, and hereditary predisposition are factors that may influence the incidence of the disease. *Staphylococcus aureus* is the most frequent bacterium isolated from lesions.

Prolapse of the Deep Gland of the Third Eyelid

Swelling and protrusion of the third eyelid has been associated with prolapse of the deep bilobed gland of the third eyelid. Affected animals present with a unilateral or bilateral protrusion of the third eyelid from the medial canthus of the eye. Abnormal laxity of the connective tissue attaching the deep gland of the third eyelid to the bony orbital structures may be the underlying cause.

Vertebral Fracture and Degenerative Spinal Disease

Posterior paralysis due to vertebral fracture or dislocation occurs all too often in domestic rabbits. The axial and appendicular skeletons of domestic rabbits are relatively fragile in proportion to their muscle mass. An unsupported, sudden movement of the hind limbs

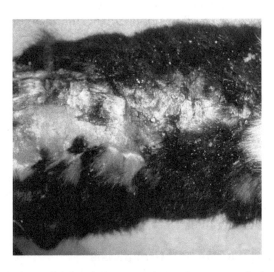

FIG. 6.82. *Rabbit with chronic exfoliative dermatosis and sebaceous adenitis. Note the marked scaling lesions and alopecia over the dorsal aspect of the body (Source: M. Taylor and K.E. Linder.)*

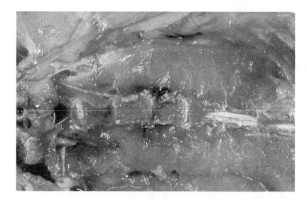

FIG. 6.84.   *Vertebral fracture in an adult rabbit due to improper restraint. Fractures typically occur in the lumbosacral region.*

may exert sufficient leverage on the lumbosacral junction to cause a vertebral fracture. Depending on the duration of the problem prior to euthanasia and necropsy, the hindquarters may be soiled with urine and fecal material consistent with incontinence. The site of the fracture (or luxation) is usually the lumbosacral region (L7) (Fig. 6.84). There may be extensive hemorrhage in the underlying psoas muscles. Changes vary from luxation to multiple fractures of the affected vertebra, with extensive damage to the lumbosacral spinal cord. Degenerative changes of the nucleus pulposis, usually involving the distal thoracic spinal segments, have been noted in rabbits as early as 3 months of age, with spondylosis among rabbits greater than 2 years of age.

Iatrogenic Nerve Damage

Following intramuscular injection of ketamine, xylazine, and acepromazine in the hind leg, rabbits were found to develop self-mutilation of digits. This syndrome was associated with inflammatory change and degeneration of the sciatic nerve in the region of the injections. Intrathecal injection of preservative-free ketamine has been shown to cause severe damage to the spinal cord and nerve roots, but ketamine with preservative did not. Long-term restraint of rabbits with hind leg extension was found to result in degeneration of sciatic nerves and skeletal muscle necrosis. Affected rabbits had transient hind leg paresis.

Tracheal Injury Following Intubation

Erosive to ulcerative tracheitis has been reported to occur in rabbits following tracheal intubation and inhalation anesthesia. The subjects were New Zealand White rabbits that were kept under general anesthesia for a period of 4–5 hours. Tracheal lesions have been identified in rabbits acquired from several different research facilities that had been subjected to this procedure. Clinically, stridor and mild cyanosis are the usual presenting signs in affected animals. At necropsy, changes may be confined to congestion of the tracheal mucosa. In more advanced cases, necrotic debris and blood are present

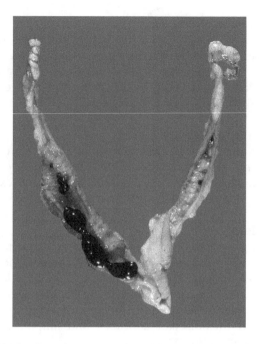

FIG. 6.85.   *Reproductive tract of a Californian breed doe with a history of intermittent vulvar bleeding due to rupture of endometrial venous aneurysms. Blood clots are present within the uterine lumina.*

on the tracheal mucosa. On histopathology, mucosal lesions are usually most extensive in the sections immediately distal to the larynx. Changes vary from multifocal mucosal ulceration to circumferential transmural ulceration of the tracheal mucosa.

Endometrial Venous Aneurysms

Multiple endometrial venous aneurysms have been associated with persistent urogenital bleeding. At necropsy, clotted blood is present in the uterine lumen (Fig. 6.85), and there are multiple blood-filled endometrial varices that consist of dilated, thin-walled veins (Fig. 6.86). These varices may rupture and bleed periodically into the uterine lumen, with subsequent hematuria. They have been observed in nonpregnant multiparous does. There is no evidence that predisposing factors, such as trauma or bleeding disorders, play a role in the disease.

Miscellaneous Genital Disorders

Cryptorchism may be occasionally encountered in bucks. In hot climates, bucks are prone to "seasonal infertility," and seasonal involution occurs in the testes of some bucks during the nonbreeding season (see "Anatomic Features"). Cystic endometrial hyperplasia is a relatively common disorder of aged does, and mucometra can be a sporadic finding. Because the uterine horns are completely separate with 2 cervices, mucometra may be unilateral or bilateral (Fig. 6.87).

Urinary Sludge and Urolithiasis

As noted previously, intestinal absorption of calcium in rabbits occurs in direct proportion to dietary intake, as intestinal uptake is not influenced by vitamin D. Renal

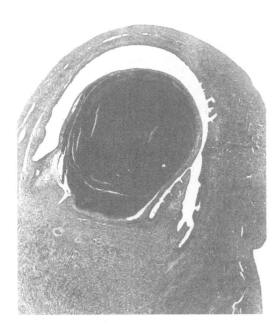

FIG. 6.86. *Section of uterus from the previous figure. Note the marked dilation of the endometrial vessel and thrombosis.*

calcium resorption and excretion are also in proportion to dietary intake, and regulated by parathyroid hormone, calcitonin, and vitamin D. When the resorptive capacity of the kidney is exceeded, calcium precipitates in the alkaline urine as calcium carbonate monohydrate, anhydrous calcium carbonate, and ammonium magnesium phosphate, resulting in the cloudy nature of rabbit urine in postweanling rabbits. When metabolic demand for calcium rises, the urine becomes less cloudy. When rabbits are fed high-calcium diets, such as diets rich in alfalfa, become dehydrated, or are suffering from other systemic disease, the likelihood of excess urinary mineral excretion takes on the characteristics of mud-like

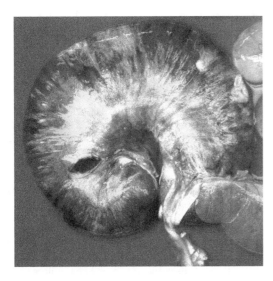

FIG. 6.87. *Uterine horn of a doe with mucometra. The uterine wall has been incised, and the uterus is surrounded by serosanguinous fluid from the lumen. Because the uterine horns and cervices in the rabbit are anatomically separate, mucometra may be unilateral or bilateral.*

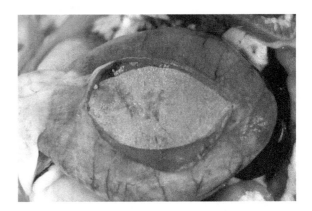

FIG. 6.88. *Urinary bladder of a rabbit that died of urinary obstruction due to massive accumulation of intractable urinary sludge, which has the consistency of modeling clay. This material can accumulate rapidly.*

"sludge." This can happen very rapidly, resulting in acute urinary obstruction. The urinary bladder fills with intractable material that has the consistency of modeling clay (Fig. 6.88). Rabbits may also develop true uroliths in the renal pelves, ureters, urinary bladder (Fig 6.89), or urethra, resulting in hydronephrosis, hematuria, and obstructive uropathy. Overweight and sedentary rabbits are at higher risk.

Miscellaneous Kidney Disorders
Chronic renal disease, analogous to similar syndromes in aged rodents, is common in aged rabbits. Hydronephrosis may occur in association with urolithiasis. Fibrosis, with or without nephrocalcinosis, is common in rabbits over 10 months of age. Abscesses, pyelonephritis, and neoplasia (lymphosarcoma) may all involve the kidneys.

Amyloidosis
Amyloidosis occurs sporadically among rabbits, and is most likely to be observed in older rabbits that have been

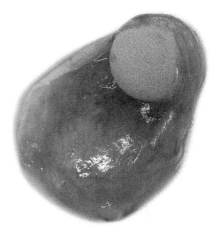

FIG. 6.89. *Urolithiasis of the urinary bladder in a rabbit. (Source: D. Imai, University of California, Davis, CA. Reproduced with permission from D. Imai.)*

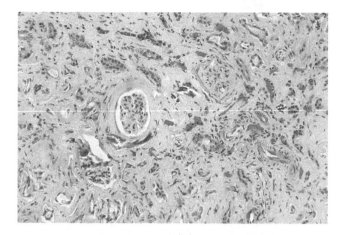

FIG. 6.90.   *Renal interstitial amyloidosis in a chronically immunized adult New Zealand White rabbit.*

hyperimmunized or in rabbits with chronic infections, including pododermatitis and pyometra. Amyloidosis can also be readily induced experimentally. The kidney is the most commonly affected organ, in which amyloid deposits can be found in glomeruli, cortical interstitial tissue, or medulla (Fig 6.90). Mild early cases involve interstitial deposition in the medulla. Glomerular and cortical deposition tend to occur when medullary involvement is more severe. Medullary deposition may be associated with papillary necrosis or nephrolithiasis. Stomach, intestine, spleen, myocardium, adrenals, liver, lungs, and other organs may also be involved. Deposits in most organs are frequently perivascular, except spleen, in which deposits may be perifollicular or around the periphery of germinal follicles.

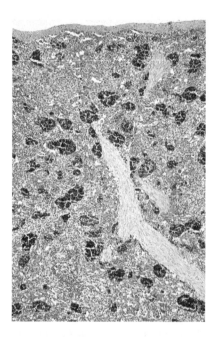

FIG. 6.91.   *Spleen of an adult rabbit with hemosiderin accumulation. This is a frequent incidental finding in aged rabbits.*

Splenic Hemosiderosis

Aged rabbits tend to accumulate hemosiderin pigment in their spleens (Fig 6.91), which is probably due to excess iron in their diet.

BIBLIOGRAPHY FOR AGING AND MISCELLANEOUS DISORDERS

Tooth Abscesses

Tyrrell, K.L., Citron, D.M., Jenkins, J.R., Goldstein, E.J.C., & the Veterinary Study Group (2002) Periodontal bacteria in rabbit mandibular and maxillary abscesses. *Journal of Clinical Microbiology* 40:1044–1047.

Exfoliative Dermatosis and Sebaceous Adenitis

Florizoone, K. (2005) Thymoma-associated exfoliative dermatitis in a rabbit. *Veterinary Dermatology* 16:281–284.

Florizoone, K., van der Luer, R., & van den Ingh, T. (2007) Symmetrical alopecia, scaling and hepatitis in a rabbit. *Journal of Veterinary Dermatology* 18:161–164.

Prelaud, A.R., Jassies-van der Lee, A., Mueller, R.S., van Zeeland, Y.R.A., Bettenay, S., Majzoub, M., Zenker, I., & Hein, J. (2012) Presumptive paraneoplastic exfoliative dermatitis in four domestic rabbits. *Veterinary Record* 172:155.

White, S.D., Campbell, T., Logan, A., Meredith, A., Schultheiss, P., Van Winkle, T., Moore, P.F., Naydan, D.K., & Mallon, F. (2000) Lymphoma with cutaneous involvement in three domestic rabbits (*Oryctolagus cuniculus*). *Veterinary Dermatology* 11:61–67.

White, S.D., Linder, K.D., Schultheiss, P., Scott, K.V., Garnett, P., Taylor, M., Best, S.J., Walder, E.J., Rosenkrantz, W., & Yaeger, J.A. (2000) Sebaceous adenitis in four domestic rabbits (*Oryctolagus cuniculus*). *Veterinary Dermatology* 11:53–60.

Prolapse of the Deep Gland of the Third Eyelid

Janssens, G., Simoens, P., Muylle, S., & Lauwers, H. (1999) Bilateral prolapse of the deep gland of the third eyelid in the rabbit: diagnosis and treatment. *Laboratory Animal Science* 49:105–109.

Vertebral Fracture and Degenerative Spinal Disease

Green, P.W., Fox, R.R., & Sokoloff, L. (1984) Spontaneous degenerative spinal disease in the laboratory rabbit. *Journal of Orthopedic Research* 2:161–168.

Jones, T., Lu, Y.S., Rehg, J., & Eckels, R. (1982) Diagnostic exercise: fracture of the lumbar vertebrae. *Laboratory Animal Science* 32:489–490.

Tracheal Injury Following Intratracheal Intubation

Nordin, U. & Lindholm, C.E. (1977) The vessels of the rabbit trachea and ischemia caused by cuff pressure. *Archives of Otorhinolaryngology* 215:11–24.

Nordin, U., Lindhom, C.E., & Wolgast, M. (1977) Blood flow in the rabbit tracheal mucosa under normal conditions and under the influence of tracheal intubation. *Acta Anesthesiologica Scandinavica* 21:81–94.

Phaneuf, L.R., Barker, S., Groleau, M.A., & Turner, P.V. (2006) Tracheal injury after intratracheal intubation and anesthesia in rabbit. *Journal of the American Association of Laboratory Animal Science* 45:67–72.

Iatrogenic Nerve Damage

Mendlowski, B. (1975) Neuromuscular lesions in restrained rabbits. *Veterinary Pathology* 12:378–386.

Vachon, P. (1999) Self-mutilation in rabbits following intramuscular ketamine-xylazine-acepromazine injections. *Canadian Veterinary Journal* 40:581–582.

Vranken, J.H., Troost, D., de Haan, P., Pennings, F.A., van der Vegt, M.H., Dijkgraaf, M.G., & Hollman, M.W. (2006) Severe toxic damage to the rabbit spinal cord after intrathecal administration of preservative-free S(+)-ketamine. *Anesthesiology* 105:813–818.

Endometrial Venous Aneurysms
Bray, M.V., Weir, E.C., Brownstein, D.G., & Delano, M.L. (1992) Endometrial venous aneurysms in three New Zealand White rabbits. *Laboratory Animal Science* 42:360–362.

Urinary Sludge and Urolithiasis
Eckermann-Ross, C. (2008) Hormonal regulation of calcium metabolism in the rabbit. *Veterinary Clinics of North America Exotic Animal Practice* 11:139–152.

Amyloidosis
Hinton, M. & Lucke, V.M. (1982) Histological findings in amyloidosis or rabbits. *Journal of Comparative Pathology* 92:285–294.
Hinton, M. & Lucke, V.M. (1982) Ultrastructure of the kidney in amyloidosis of rabbits. *Journal of Comparative Pathology* 92:295–300.
Hofmann, J.R. Jr. & Hixson, C.J. (1986) Amyloid A protein deposits in a rabbit with pyometra. *Journal of the American Veterinary Medical Association* 189:1155–1156.

Miscellaneous Kidney Disorders
Hinton, M. (1981) Kidney disease in the rabbit: a histological survey. *Laboratory Animals* 15:263–265.

NUTRITIONAL, METABOLIC AND TOXIC DISORDERS

Cystic Mastitis

Sterile fluctuant cysts with swollen teats may involve any mammary gland in rabbits of both sexes and all ages. These changes wax and wane with the hormone status, and disappear during estrus, pregnancy, pseudopregnancy, or lactation and reappear in the resting postlactation period. In virgin females, they disappear with first estrus. They are purported to progress to neoplasia. Ovariohysterectomy has been noted to ameliorate the disease. Microscopically, ducts are dilated and lined by flattened or hyperplastic epithelium and in some, epithelium is lost with associated inflammation. In 1 report, these changes were noted in aged nulliparous New Zealand White rabbits in association with prolactin-secreting pituitary adenomas.

Pregnancy Toxemia

Pregnancy toxemia is a poorly characterized condition that occurs in does, usually during the last week of pregnancy or the immediate postpartum period. Obesity and fasting are important predisposing factors. The disease is characterized by low morbidity and high mortality. Multiparous does are especially at risk, and metabolic toxemia may also occur on occasion in obese, "stressed," nonpregnant rabbits. Obesity, hereditary predisposition, impaired blood flow to the uterus, and pituitary dysfunction are factors implicated in this disease. There is 1 report of pregnancy toxemia and concurrent pancreatitis in a New Zealand White doe. Clinical manifestations of the disease are variable and may include incoordination, abortions, and coma. Most does fail to respond to treatment. In the typical case of pregnancy toxemia, mobilization of fat deposits for energy results in metabolic acidosis and ketosis, depression, and death. At necropsy, animals are usually obese, with marked fatty infiltration of the liver and adrenal glands.

Hypocalcemic Tetany in Lactating Does

There is a marked drain on serum calcium levels in does during the first month of lactation that can result in hypocalcemia and tetany. In 1 report in which rabbits were fed a commercial diet and hay, 6 of 31 Fauve de Bourgogne does were found lying on their side, and had signs that included ear flapping, jerking of posterior limbs, and muscle tremors. Plasma calcium levels were measured in affected rabbits, and found to be 5.8 ± 0.4 mg/dl, whereas plasma calcium in nonlactating control does was 13.8 ± 0.2 mg/dl.

Hypercalcemic Arteriosclerosis

As noted previously, rabbits absorb calcium in proportion to levels in their diet, and depend upon renal excretion for regulation of serum calcium levels. They are, therefore, vulnerable to hypercalcemia when confronted with severe renal disease (chronic renal disease, lymphosarcoma, etc.), which can be exacerbated by secondary hyperparathyroidism and excess dietary vitamin D. Hypercalcemia results in metastatic mineralization of blood vessels (Fig. 6.92) and other tissues, including pulmonary interstitium, and kidneys (nephrocalcinosis). Arterial lesions include mineral deposition in the tunica media, with macrophage infiltration and smooth muscle degeneration. The early mineral composition of aortic lesions was found to contain calcium phosphate, dicalcium phosphate dehydrate, and octacalcium phosphate, with later development of

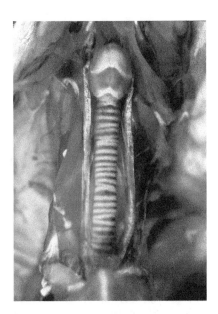

FIG. 6.92. *Metastatic mineralization of the carotid arteries in a rabbit with hypercalcemia secondary to chronic renal disease.*

hydroxyapatite crystals. In an atherogenesis study, rabbits were shown to develop dystrophic mineralization of atheromatous lesions, without disturbing calcium and phosphorous homeostasis, or mineralization of other tissues.

Nutritional Secondary Hyperparathyroidism

Chronic nutritional hypocalcemia with secondary hyperparathyroidism and decreased bone mass has been reported in rabbits fed a diet deficient in calcium. It was rapidly reversible with appropriate calcium supplementation. Dental disorders, similar to vitamin D deficiency, may also occur.

Atherosclerosis/Hypercholesterolemia

Rabbits are highly susceptible to hypercholesterolemia when fed high-cholesterol diets. Rabbits are unable to increase excretion of sterols, resulting in an enhanced hepatic export of cholesteryl ester-rich lipoproteins into the bloodstream. Hypercholesterolemia, in association with LDL and beta-VDL, is induced within a few days of feeding a high-cholesterol diet. Arterial plaques, ranging from fatty streaks to atheromas, arise in the aorta and coronary arteries. The aortic arch and thoracic aorta are predisposed at lower doses, whereas the entire aorta may be involved with higher dietary doses. Microscopic evidence of myocardial infarction is common. New Zealand White rabbits are the most frequently used breed of rabbit, but long-term experiments are hampered because of cholesterol-induced hepatopathy, which includes severe hepatic lipidosis (Fig. 6.93) and hepatocellular necrosis, with bile stasis and icterus. A number of inbred and transgenic rabbits have been developed for atherosclerosis research. Watanabe heritable hyperlipidemic (WHHL) rabbits have been particularly well studied.

Homozygous WHHL rabbits have a genetic deficiency of LDL receptors, and develop atherosclerotic arterial plaques and xanthomatous lesions in the digital joints, pia, and eye. WHHL rabbits develop atherosclerosis without feeding high-cholesterol diets.

Xanthomatosis/Hypercholesterolemia

Because of the prevalence of research on atherosclerosis using rabbits, including outbred New Zealand White rabbits, hypercholesterolemic rabbits may develop a number of nonvascular lesions of note. Dermal xanthomas have been shown to arise in the upper dermis, which was infiltrated with lipid-laden macrophages, as well as vascular pericytes throughout the dermis. Infiltration of lipid-laden macrophages or lipidosis arises in many tissues, including muscle, heart, lung, choroid plexus, kidney, gastrointestinal tract, and endocrine organs. Lipid keratopathy has been frequently reported in rabbits, including rabbits fed a commercial diet. Typically, the corneoscleral junction may be irregularly infiltrated with yellowish-white granular opacities, representing lipid-laden xanthoma cells. Xanthoma cells may also commonly infiltrate other regions of the eye. They can be seen grossly involving the iris (Fig. 6.94), and microscopically involving ciliary body, choroids, and sclera (Fig. 6.95). In 1 report of a rabbit fed a high-cholesterol diet, lipid-laden macrophages were not only observed in the eye, but also the dermis, lung, lymphoid tissue, and choroid plexus of the brain.

Vitamin A Toxicity or Deficiency

The clinical manifestations of vitamin A toxicity or deficiency are similar in domestic rabbits to those of other species, and are characterized by poor conception rates, congenital anomalies, fetal resorptions, abortion, and weak, thin kits. Congenital defects associated with hypervitaminosis A include microencephaly, hydrocephalus, and cleft palate. Rabbits are unique in that they can convert 100% of dietary beta-carotene into retinol. A case of hyperostotic polyarthropathy, presumptively diagnosed as hypervitaminosis A, has been reported in a pet rabbit that was chronically fed a diet of carrots.

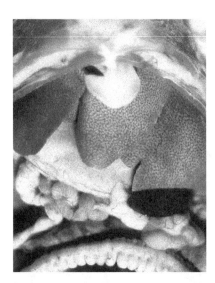

FIG. 6.93.   *Hepatic lipidosis in a New Zealand White rabbit fed a high-cholesterol diet. Rabbits are unable to increase excretion of sterols in the bile in response to high cholesterol in the diet, resulting in hypercholesterolemia, hepatic lipidosis, and icterus.*

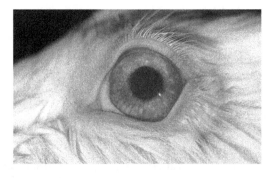

FIG. 6.94.   *Iridial xanthomatosis in a New Zealand White rabbit fed a high-cholesterol diet.*

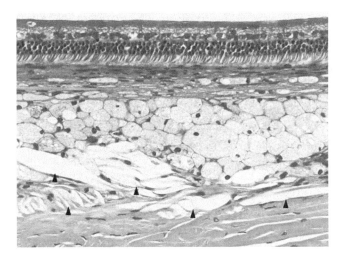

FIG. 6.95. *Xanthoma cells and cholesterol clefts (arrow heads) in periocular tissue of a rabbit with hypercholesterolemia. (Source: Kouchi et al. 2006. Reproduced with permission from Wiley.)*

Vitamin D Toxicity or Deficiency

The requirement for vitamin D is lower in rabbits compared to other mammals, and they are therefore prone to vitamin D intoxication. The problem usually arises when rabbits are fed an improperly formulated diet. Affected rabbits are anorectic with weight loss. They manifest muscle weakness and paresis. Histologic changes include medial degeneration and mineralization of major arteries. Mineralization of the glomerular tufts, basement membranes, and tubules of the kidney may also occur. In the long bones, there is deposition of basophilic material on the periosteal and endosteal surfaces, medullary trabeculae, and Haversian systems. In contrast, vitamin D deficiency presents as anemia, immunodeficiency, and osteomalacia. Dental disorders may also arise, with overgrowth and ridging of the incisor teeth and distorted growth of the premolar and molar teeth.

Vitamin E Deficiency

There are several reports of nutritional muscular dystrophy due to vitamin E deficiency. In addition to stiffness and muscle weakness, neonatal mortality and infertility are manifestations of vitamin E deficiency in domestic rabbits. At necropsy, pale mineralized streaks may be present in musculature, such as the diaphragm, paravertebral regions, and hind limbs. Typical changes seen microscopically are hyaline degeneration of affected myofibers and clumping and mineralization of the sarcoplasm. Macrophages may be present in reactive areas. Collapse of sarcolemmal sheaths and interstitial fibrosis frequently occur in lesions of some duration.

Copper Toxicosis

Copper sulfate is often added to rabbit feed as a supplement. Copper is generally well tolerated, but rabbits are considered to be sensitive to copper. A number of cases of copper toxicosis have been reported in domestic

rabbits. Acute toxicity was associated with hemolytic anemia with intravascular hemolysis, erythrophagocytosis in the spleen, hepatic centrilobular to midzonal necrosis, and hematuria with tubular casts. Periportal fibrosis and biliary hyperplasia have also been noted. Hepatocytes and Kupffer cells contained blue-green cytoplasmic granules that stained positive with rhodanine stain. In 1 outbreak, shipping stress and dietary change appeared to precipitate disease.

Fluoride Toxicosis: Osteofluorosis

Moderate to severe osseous proliferations of the extremities (Fig. 6.96) and mandibles were observed among growing rabbits in 2 European rabbitries. Bones had periosteal and endosteal hyperostosis. In addition, affected rabbits had marked proliferation of gastric and duodenal mucosa, but it is unclear if the gastrointestinal lesions were related. Bone ash analysis revealed high levels of fluoride reaching over 20 times the normal level. The source of the fluoride was pelleted feed produced by 2 different feed mills. Other outbreaks of osteofluorosis have been reported in rabbits from Mexico.

Lead Toxicosis

With the propensity of rabbits to chew foreign items including painted objects, it is not surprising that lead toxicosis is common among "free-ranging" pet rabbits, but can also occur in commercial and laboratory rabbits in cage environments with lead components (solder).

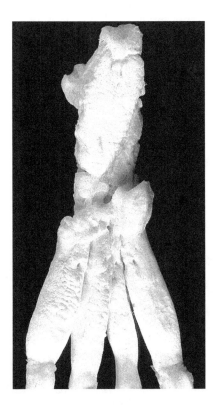

FIG. 6.96. *Hyperostosis of the tarsus and metatarsus of a rabbit with chronic fluoride toxicosis. (Source: Bock et al. 2007. Reproduced with permission from SAGE Publications.)*

Clinical signs include anorexia, tremors, seizures, torticollis, blindness, and ataxia. In fatal cases of lead toxicosis, myocardial degeneration, multifocal hepatic necrosis, renal tubular degeneration, and hemoglobin casts in renal tubules are microscopic findings. Features of anemia include reticulocytosis, nucleated erythrocytes, hypochromasia, basophilic stippling, poikilocytosis, and anisocytosis. Chronically affected rabbits may be immunosuppressed. Diagnosis is confirmed with blood lead concentrations. Toxicosis is considered positive with blood levels greater than 30 μg/dl, but lower levels may be considered abnormal in chronic toxicosis. Chronic toxicosis is also reported to be associated with gastrointestinal stasis or diarrhea. In cases diagnosed antemortem, removal of all lead from the gastrointestinal tract is recommended prior to the administration of chelating agents, since chelation will enhance the absorption of any lead present in the gastrointestinal tract.

Aflatoxicosis

Aflatoxicosis was reported in an incident involving a large number of Angora rabbitries in India. Affected rabbits were anorectic, lost weight, and became jaundiced within 3–4 days of disease onset. Mortality was highest in juvenile rabbits. Livers were congested, icteric, and gall bladders were distended with inspissated bile. Microscopic findings featured hepatocellular degeneration, periportal fibrosis, and regenerative foci. The toxin was identified as aflatoxin B1 contamination of feed. Coagulation defects develop during B1 aflatoxicosis in the rabbit, with diminished synthesis of coagulation factors, or in the case of severe hepatic necrosis, intravascular coagulation, and consumption of coagulation factors take place. Among various species, rabbits are among the most highly sensitive to aflatoxin B1.

Poisonous Plant Toxicity

Through their innate curiosity or contamination of pelleted feed or hay, rabbits are subject to inadvertent toxicity upon ingestion of any one of a very large list of common toxic plants that reside out of doors or as houseplants. The list is far too extensive to cover, and the reader is referred to various rabbit fancier Web sites for access to further information.

Drug Toxicoses

In-depth coverage of suitable drugs for use in rabbits and side effects that may be encountered can be found in *Textbook of Rabbit Medicine* by Molly Varga and in a review entitled *Clinical Toxicoses of Domestic Rabbits* by Matthew Johnston. A few adverse effects of commonly used drugs are listed below.

Cardiomyopathy Associated with Ketamine/Xylazine Administration

Multifocal myocardial degeneration with interstitial fibrosis has been observed in Dutch Belted rabbits following the administration of a ketamine/xylazine combination. A similar effect was found in New Zealand White rabbits given ketamine with the alpha$_2$ agonist detomidine or detomidine alone. This change is attributed to ischemia secondary to vasoconstriction with reduction in coronary blood flow, with subsequent myocardial degeneration and fibrosis. Collateral circulation in the myocardium is limited in this species. In lesions of recent onset, there is degeneration of myofibers with mononuclear and polymorphonuclear leukocytic infiltration. In lesions of some duration, there is loss of myofibers and marked interstitial fibrosis. Borderline vitamin E deficiency could also contribute to the development of the myocardial lesions.

Fluoroquinolone Arthropathy

Baytril (enrofloxacin) is a safe and efficacious fluoroquinilone antibiotic for use in rabbits, but arthropathy is a notable side effect that has been documented in juvenile New Zealand White rabbits. The arthropathy features development of vesicular lesions in the articular cartilage of large weight-bearing joints.

Ionophore Toxicity

Ionophore drugs are commonly used as coccidiostats in rabbit feed. Outbreaks of narasin poisoning with high mortality have occurred when rabbits were fed a pelleted ration to which poultry ration premix was added. Rabbits became anorectic, weak, and had impaired walking, diarrhea, respiratory distress, and opisthotonus. Microscopic findings included myofiber necrosis and regeneration in skeletal muscles, with milder changes in myocardium. Some of the drugs used for poultry may not work as well in rabbits.

Telazol Nephrotoxicity

The anesthetic Telazol is used as an intramuscular anesthetic in a variety of species. Low (32 mg/kg; recommended dose) to high doses (64 mg/kg) in rabbits resulted in elevated blood urea nitrogen at 4 days after administration. Necropsy revealed marked multifocal nephrosis and nephrocalcinosis in both dose groups, but most severe in the high-dose group.

Antibiotic "Toxicity"

A number of antibiotics, including clindamycin, erythromycin, and oral beta-lactam antibiotics are associated with induction of enteric dysbiosis and Clostridial enterotoxemia (see "Clostridial Diseases").

BIBLIOGRAPHY FOR NUTRITIONAL, METABOLIC, AND TOXIC DISORDERS

General Reference for Nutritional, Toxic, and Metabolic Diseases
Varga, M. (2013) *Textbook of Rabbit Medicine*, 2nd edn. Elsevier.

Cystic Mastitis
Atherton, J., Griffiths, L., & Williams, A. (1999) Cystic mastitis in the female rabbit. *Veterinary Record* 145:648.

Fifer, C.L. (1934) The breast. I. Lesions in rabbits resembling chronic cystic mastitis. *Archives of Surgery* 29:555–559.

Hughes, J.E., Chapman, W.L., & Prasse, K.W. (1981) Cystic mammary disease in rabbits. *Journal of the American Veterinary Medical Association* 178:138–139.

Lipman, N.S., Zhao, Z.B., Andrutis, K.A., Hurley, R.J., Fox, J.G., & White, H.J. (1994) Prolactin-secreting pituitary adenomas with mammary dysplasia in New Zealand White rabbits. *Laboratory Animal Science* 44:114–120.

Pregnancy Toxemia
Greene, H.S.N. (1937) Toxemia of pregnancy in the rabbit: clinical manifestations and pathology. *Journal of Experimental Medicine* 65:809–832.

Hypocalcemic Tetany in Lactating Does
Barlet, J.-P. (1980) Plasma calcium, inorganic phosphorus and magnesium levels in pregnant and lactating does. *Reproduction Nutrition Development* 20:647–651.

Hypercalcemic Arteriosclerosis
Ngatia, T.A., Mugera, G.M., Njiro, S.M., Kuria, J.K.N., & Carles, A.B. (1989) Arteriosclerosis and related lesions in rabbits. *Journal of Comparative Pathology* 101:279–286.

Rokita, E., Cichocki, T., Divoux, S., Gonsior, B., Hofert, M., Jarczyk, L., & Strzalkowski, A. (1992) Calcification of the aortic wall in hypercalcemic rabbits. *Experimental and Toxicologic Pathology* 44:310–316.

Rokita, E., Cichocki, T., Heck, D., Jarczyk, L., & Strzalkowski, A. (1991) Calcification of aortic wall in cholesterol-fed rabbits. *Atherosclerosis* 87:183–193.

Shell, L.G. & Saunders, G. (1989) Arteriosclerosis in a rabbit. *Journal of the American Veterinary Medical Association* 194:679–680.

Nutritional Secondary Hyperparathyroidism
Bas, S., Bas, A., Lopez, I., Estepa, J.C., Rodriguez, M., & Aguilera-Tejero, E. (2005) Nutritional secondary hyperparathyroidism in rabbits. *Domestic Animal Endocrinology* 28:380–390.

Harcourt-Brown, F.M. (1996) Calcium deficiency, diet and dental disease in pet rabbits. *Veterinary Record* 139:567–571.

Mehorotra, M,. Gupta, S.K., Kumar, K., Awasthi, P.K. Dubey, M., Pandey, C.M., & Godbole, M.M. (2006) Calcium deficiency-induced secondary hyperparathyroidism and osteopenia are rapidly reversible with calcium supplementation in growing rabbit pups. *British Journal of Nutrition* 95:582–590.

Atherosclerosis/Hypercholesterolemia
Aliev, G. & Burnstock, G. (1998) Watanabe rabbits with heritable hypercholesterolemia: a model of atherosclerosis. *Histology and Histopathology* 13:797–817.

Bocan, T.M., Mueller, S.B., Mazur, M.J., Uhlendorf, P.D., Brown, E.Q., & Kieft, K.A. (1993) The relationship between the degree of dietary-induced hypercholesterolemia in the rabbit and atherosclerotic lesion formation. *Atherosclerosis* 102:9–22.

Kolodgie, F.D., Katocs, A.S., Jr, Largis, E.E., Wrenn, S.M., Cornhill, L.F., Herderick, E.E., Lee, S.J., & Virmami, R. (1996) Hypercholesterolemia in the rabbit induced by feeding graded amounts of low-level cholesterol. *Arteriosclerosis, Thrombosis, and Vascular Biology* 16:1454–1464.

Xanthomatosis/Hypercholesterolemia
Fallon, M.T., Reinhard, M.K., DaRif, C.A., & Schoeb, T.R. (1988) Diagnostic exercise: eye lesions in a rabbit. *Laboratory Animal Science* 38:612–613.

Garibaldi, B.A. & Pequet Goad, M.E. (1988) Lipid keratopathy in the Watanabe (WHHL) rabbit. *Veterinary Pathology* 25:173–174.

Kouchi, M., Ueda, Y., Horie, H., & Tanaka, K. (2006) Ocular lesions in Watanabe heritable hyperlipidemic rabbits. *Veterinary Ophthalmology* 9:145–148.

Prior, J.T., Kurtz, D.M., & Ziegler, D.D. (1961) The hypercholesterolemic rabbit: an aid to understanding arteriosclerosis in man? *Archives of Pathology* 71:672–684.

Roth, S.I., Stock, L., Siel, J.M., Mendelsohn, A., Reddy, C., Preskill, D.G., & Ghosh, S. (1988) Pathogenesis of experimental lipid keratopathy: an ultrastructural study of an animal model system. *Investigative Ophthalmology and Visual Science* 29:1544–1551.

Sebesteny, A., Sheraidah, G.A.K., Trevan, D.J., Alexander, R.A., & Ahmed, A.I. (1985) Lipid keratopathy and atheromatosis in an SPF laboratory rabbit colony attributable to diet. *Laboratory Animals* 19:180–188.

Vitamin Toxicity/Deficiency
DiGiacomo, R.F., Deeb, B.J., & Anderson, R.J. (1992) Hypervitaminosis A and reproductive disorders in rabbits. *Laboratory Animal Science* 42:250–254.

Frater, J. (2001) Hyperostotic polyarthropathy in a rabbit: suspected case of chronic hypervitaminosis A from a diet of carrots. *Australian Veterinary Journal* 79:608–611.

Ringler, D.H. & Abrams, G.D. (1970) Nutritional muscular dystrophy and neonatal mortality in a rabbit breeding colony. *Journal of the American Veterinary Medical Association* 157:1928–1934.

Ringler, D.H. & Abrams, G.D. (1971) Laboratory diagnosis of vitamin E deficiency in rabbits fed a faulty commercial ration. *Laboratory Animal Science* 21:383–388.

St Claire, M.B., Kennett, M.J., & Besch-Williford, C.L. (2004) Vitamin A toxicity and vitamin E deficiency in a rabbit colony. *Contemporary Topics in Laboratory Animal Science* 43:26–30.

Stevenson, R.G., Palmer, N.C., & Finley, G.G. (1976) Hypervitaminosis D in rabbits. *Canadian Veterinary Journal* 17:54–57.

Yamimi, B. & Stein, S. (1989) Abortion, stillbirth, neonatal death, and nutritional myodegeneration in a rabbit breeding colony. *Journal of the American Veterinary Medical Association* 194:561–562.

Zimmerman, T.E., Giddens, W.E., Jr, DiGiacomo, R.F., & Ladiges, W.C. (1990) Soft tissue mineralization in rabbits fed a diet containing excess vitamin D. *Laboratory Animal Science* 40:212–214.

Copper, Fluoride, and Lead Toxicity
Bock, P., Peters, M., Bago, Z., Wolf, P., Thiele, A., & Baumgartner, W. (2007) Spontaneously occurring alimentary osteofluorosis associated with proliferative gastroduodenopathy in rabbits. *Veterinary Pathology* 44:703–706.

Cooper, G.L., Bickford, A.A., Charlton, B.R., Galey, F.D., Willoughby, D.H., & Grobner, M.A. (1996) Copper poisoning in rabbits associated with acute intravascular hemolysis. *Journal of Veterinary Diagnostic Investigation* 8:394–396.

DeCubellis, J. & Graham, J. (2013) Gastrointestinal disease in guinea pigs and rabbits. *Veterinary Clinics of North America Exotic Animal Practice* 16:421–435.

Gerken, D.F. & Swartout, M.S. (1986) Blood lead concentrations in rabbits. *American Journal of Veterinary Research* 47:2674–2675.

Hood, S., Kelly, J., McBurney, S., & Burton, S. (1997) Lead toxicosis in 2 dwarf rabbits. *Canadian Veterinary Journal* 38:721–722.

Johnston, M.S. (2008) Clinical toxicoses of domestic rabbits. *Veterinary Clinics of North America Exotic Animal Practice* 11:315–326.

Koller, L.D. (1973) Immunosuppression produced by lead, cadmium and mercury. *American Journal of Veterinary Research* 34:1457–1458.

Ramirez, C.J., Kim, D.Y., Hanks, B.C., & Evans, T.J. (2013) Copper toxicosis in New Zealand White rabbits (*Oryctolagus cuniculus*). *Veterinary Pathology* 50:1135–1138.

Swartout, M.S. & Gerken, D.F. (1987) Lead-induced toxicosis in two domestic rabbits. *Journal of the American Veterinary Medical Association* 191:717–719.

Vinlove, M.P., Britt, J., & Cornelium, J. (1992) Copper toxicity in a rabbit. *Laboratory Animal Science* 42:614–615.

Aflatoxicosis

Baker, D.C. & Green, R.A. (1987) Coagulation defects of aflatoxin intoxicated rabbits. *Veterinary Pathology* 24:62–70.

Krishna, L., Dawra, R.K., Vaid, J., & Gupta, V.K. (1991) An outbreak of aflatoxicosis in Angora rabbits. *Veterinary and Human Toxicology* 33:159–161.

Makkar, H.P.S. & Singh, B. (1991) Aflatoxicosis in rabbits. *Journal of Applied Rabbit Research* 14:218–221.

Drug Toxicoses

Brammer, D.W., Doerning, B.J., Chrisp, C.E., & Rush, H.G. (1991) Anesthetic and nephrotoxic effects of Telazol in New Zealand White rabbits. *Laboratory Animal Science* 41:432–435.

Hurley, R.J., Marini, R.P., Avison, D.L., Murphy, J.C., Olin, J.M., & Lipton, N.S. (1994) Evaluation of detomidine anesthetic combinations in the rabbit. *Laboratory Animal Science* 44:472–478.

Marini, R.P., Li, X., Harpster, N.K., & Dangler, C. (1999) Cardiovascular pathology possibly associated with ketamine/xylazine anesthesia in Dutch Belted rabbits. *Laboratory Animal Science* 49:153–160.

Salles, M.S., Lombardo de Barros, C.S., & Barros, S.S. (1994) Ionophore antibiotic (narasin) poisoning in rabbits. *Veterinary and Human Toxicology* 36:437–444.

Sharpnack, D.D., Mastin, J.P., Childress, C.P., & Henningsen, G.M. (1994) Quninolone arthropathy in juvenile New Zealand White rabbits. *Laboratory Animal Science* 44:436–442.

GENETIC DISORDERS

Considering the large number of relatively inbred breeds of rabbits, it is not surprising that rabbits may be afflicted with a number of hereditary disorders. A few disorders that are likely to be encountered, particularly in laboratory rabbits, are summarized in the following sections.

Congenital Glaucoma: Buphthalmia

This condition occurs most frequently in New Zealand White rabbits. Buphthalmia is characterized clinically by enlargement of 1 or both eyes, with subsequent corneal opacity. Abnormalities may occur within the first few weeks of life, but usually they are first evident by 3–5 months of age. The primary defect has been identified as an absence or underdevelopment of the outflow channels, with incomplete cleavage of the iridocorneal angles. With impaired drainage of aqueous humor from the anterior chamber, the increased intraocular pressure results in megaloglobus, increased corneal diameter, and protrusion of the corneal contours (Fig. 6.97). The sclera is relatively immature at this stage and thus expands to accommodate the increased volume of aqueous humor within the globe. The defect is inherited as an autosomal recessive allele, with incomplete penetrance. Therefore, some animals that are homozygous for the *bu/bu* gene may show no evidence of the disease. Buphthalmia does not appear to cause discernable discomfort in affected animals.

Anterior Corneal Dystrophy

Although rarely noticed or reported, anterior corneal dystrophy has been described in a closed colony of Dutch Belted rabbits, but is also seen by others in this

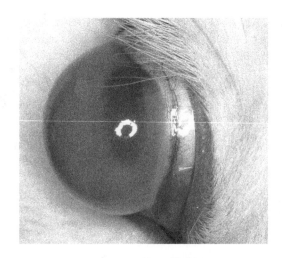

FIG. 6.97. *Buphthalmia in a New Zealand White rabbit. There is marked distention of the cornea of the affected eye.*

breed. Affected rabbits had unilateral or bilateral focal linear or plaque-like epithelial and subepithelial opacities of the central and paracentral corneas. Basement membranes were thickened and irregular, and adjacent stroma revealed disorganized collagen lamellae. Epithelium was often thin and disorganized in affected areas. Corneal dystrophy has also been reported in New Zealand White rabbits, but may differ in that epithelium and basement membranes were normal. These syndromes, particularly the former, are likely to have a genetic basis. They are of import for this text because both breeds are commonly used as laboratory animals, and such lesions have consequences for toxicology research. Lipid keratopathy is also common in hyperlipidemic rabbits, which has a genetic basis in the Watanabe rabbit with heritable hypercholesterolemia (see Atherosclerosis/Hypercholesterolemia and "Xanthomatosis/Hypercholesterolemia").

Ocular Cataracts

Spontaneous cataracts are a common finding in rabbits of various breeds. Fetal and congenital cataracts have been reported, and cataracts are known to occur in association with *Encephalitozoon cuniculi* infection of the lens and anterior segment of the eye. A recent study examined the eyes of NZW and NZW × New Zealand Red F1 hybrid rabbits and found that the incidence of cataracts was consistent with an autosomal recessive genetic disorder in NZW rabbits, with a significantly lower incidence in hybrids. Males and females were equally affected, and there was no indication that incidence increased with age. The primary differential diagnosis is cataracts associated with *E. cuniculi*.

Malocclusion

Maxillary brachygnathia (erroneously termed mandibular prognathism) is the most common genetic disorder in domestic rabbits. The defect is inherited as an autosomal recessive trait. Normally, occlusion brings the lower

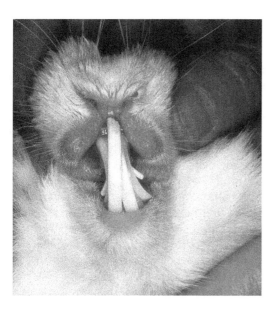

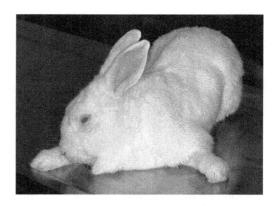

FIG. 6.99.   Splay leg in a preweanling rabbit. Affected rabbits are otherwise normal and the condition can be improved by housing the rabbit on more tractable surfaces. (Source: S. Vandewoulde, Colorado State University, Fort Collins, CO. Reproduced with permission from S. Vandewoude.)

FIG. 6.98.   Overgrowth of incisor and peg teeth in a New Zealand White rabbit due to genetically inherited brachygnathism of the maxillary bones.

incisor teeth into apposition against the upper secondary incisors (peg teeth) located behind the large upper incisors. In rabbits with maxillary brachygnathia, the maxilla is abnormally short relative to the mandible. The overshot lower jaw results in misalignment, failure of the incisors to wear normally, and impaired mastication. In domestic rabbits, growth of the combined lengths both the upper and lower incisors has been shown to be over 20 cm/year. Thus, malocclusion will cause overgrowth of the incisors in a relatively short period of time (Fig. 6.98). Although not as evident as malocclusion of the incisors, malocclusion of premolar and molar teeth with overgrowth also occurs in rabbits. Dietary deficiencies may also be a contributing factor. Overgrowth with ridging of the incisors and distortion of the cheek teeth has been observed in rabbits fed a diet deficient in calcium and vitamin D.

Splay Leg

Preweanling rabbits may develop a condition in which the front legs, hind legs, or all 4 legs splay to the side (Fig. 6.99). It is generally believed that the condition has a recessive genetic basis, but it involves various breeds of rabbits. It is exacerbated when kits are raised on substrates that do not provide adequate traction, and can be ameliorated if traction is provided. Morphologic changes in the hind legs include coxofemoral subluxation, shallow acetabula, lateral patellar luxation, valgus deformity, and bowing of the tibia.

Megacolon-Syndrome of Spotted Rabbits

The megacolon-syndrome is associated with an incomplete dominant mutant allele of the English spotting locus (En) that determines spotted coat phenotype in breeds such as the English Spot and the Checkered Giant when the allele is homozygous. The syndrome can affect any rabbit with the spotted phenotype carrying this mutation. Albino rabbits with this gene mutation do not manifest the coat color phenotype, but can suffer from the disease. Homozygous rabbits are "subvital" due to a megacolon-syndrome, which is not congenital, but rather progresses with age of the rabbit. The pathophysiology has not been extensively investigated, but affected rabbits appear to have a sodium absorption defect in the cecum and 1 study noted a relative hypogangliosis in the distal parts of the gut. Rabbit fanciers refer to this as "cow pie syndrome" since fecal pellets are much larger and poorly formed and cecotrophs are atypically large and torpedo-shaped.

Polycystic Kidney Disease

Polycystic kidney disease was reported in adult New Zealand White rabbits from multiple commercial sources. Cysts were found within the cortex, less than 2 mm in diameter, and often not noted grossly. Microscopically, dilation of Bowman's space and/or proximal tubules, irregular thickening and splitting of basement membranes, and expansion of cortical and medullary interstitium were observed. This syndrome was suspected to have a genetic basis. An autosomal recessive inheritance of cortical renal cysts was noted in partially inbred IIIvo rabbits, which had featured single to several hundred small cortical cysts, which arose in rabbits after 1 month of age.

BIBLIOGRAPHY FOR GENETIC DISORDERS

Congenital Glaucoma: Buphthalmia

Burrows, A.M., Smith, T.D., Atkinson, C.S., Mooney, M.P., Hiles, D.A., & Losken, H.W. (1995) Development of ocular hypertension in congenitally buphthalmic rabbits. *Laboratory Animal Science* 45:443–444.

Hanna, B.L., Sawin, P.B., & Sheppard, L.B. (1962) Recessive buphthalmos in the rabbit. *Genetics* 47:519–529.

Tesluk, G.C., Peiffer, R.L., & Brown, D. (1982) A clinical and pathological study of inherited glaucoma in New Zealand White rabbits. *Laboratory Animals* 16:234–239.

Anterior Corneal Dystrophy

Moore, C.P., Dubielzig, R., & Glaza, S.M. (1987) Anterior corneal dystrophy of American Dutch Belted rabbits: biomicroscopic and histopathologic findings. *Veterinary Pathology* 24:28–33.

Port, C.D. & Dodd, D.C. (1983) Two cases of corneal epithelial dystrophy in rabbits. *Laboratory Animal Science* 33:587–588.

Ocular Cataracts

Gelatt, K.N. (1975) Congenital cataracts in a litter of rabbits. *Journal of the American Veterinary Medical Association* 167:598–599.

Munger, R.J., Langevin, N., & Podval, J. (2002) Spontaneous cataracts in laboratory rabbits. *Veterinary Ophthalmology* 5:177–181.

Weisse, I., Niggeschultz, A., & Stotzer, H. (1974) Spontane, congenitale Katarakte bei Ratte, Maus und Kaninchen. *Archives of Toxicology* 32:199–207.

Malocclusion

Fox, R.R. & Crary, D.D. (1971) Mandibular prognathism in the rabbit: genetic studies. *Journal of Heredity* 62:23–27.

Verstraete, F.J.M. (2003) Advances in diagnosis and treatment of small exotic mammal dental disease. *Seminars in Avian and Exotic Pet Medicine* 12:37–48.

Zeman, W.V. & Fielder, F.G. (1969) Dental malocclusion and overgrowth in rabbits. *Journal of the American Veterinary Medical Association* 155:1115–1119.

Splay Leg

Arendar, G.M. & Milch, R.A. (1966) Splay-leg—a recessively inherited form of femoral neck anteversion, femoral shaft torsion and subluxation of the hip in the laboratory lop rabbit: its possible relationship to factors involved in so-called "congenital dislocation" of the hip. *Clinical Orthopaedics and Related Research* 44:221–229.

Innes, J.R.M. & O'Steen, W.K. (1957) Splayleg in rabbits: an inherited disease analogous to joint dysplasia in children and dogs. *Laboratory Investigation* 6:171–186.

Joosten, H.F.P., Wirtz, P., Verbeek, H.O.F., & Hoekstra, A. (1981) Splayleg: a spontaneous limb defect in rabbits—genetics, gross anatomy, and microscopy. *Teratology* 24:87–104.

Owiny, J.R., Vandewoude, S., Painter, J.T., Norrdin, R.W., & Veermachaneni, D.N.R. (2001) Hip dysplasia in rabbits: association with nest box flooring. *Comparative Medicine* 51:85–88.

Megacolon-Syndrome of Spotted Rabbits

Bodeker, D., Turck, O., Loven, E., Wieberneit, D., & Wegner, W. (1995) Pathophysiological and functional aspects of the megacolon-syndrome of homozygous spotted rabbits. *Zentralblatt Veterinarmedizin A* 42:549–559.

Gerlitz, S., Wessel, G., Wieberneit, D., & Wegner, W. (1993) The problems of breeding spotted rabbits. 3. Variability of the pigmentation grade, ganglionic intestinal wall supply, relationship to pathogenesis-animal breeding and animal welfare aspects. *Deutsche tierarztliche Wochenscrift* 100:237–239.

Wiebernett, D. & Wegner, W. (1995) Albino rabbits can suffer from megacolon-syndrome when they are homozygous for the "English Spot" gene (En/En). *World Rabbit Science* 3:19–26.

Polycystic Kidney Disease

Fox, R.R., Krinsky, W.L., & Crary, D.D. (1971) Hereditary cortical renal cysts in the rabbit. *Journal of Heredity* 62:105–109.

Mauer, K.J., Marini, R.P., Fox, J.G., & Rogers, A.B. (2004) Polycystic kidney syndrome in New Zealand White rabbits resembling human polycystic kidney disease. *Kidney International* 65:482–489.

NEOPLASMS

Rabbits develop numerous types of neoplasia, details of which can be found in the General References. Common tumors that are likely to be encountered are summarized in the following sections.

Uterine Adenocarcinoma

Uterine adenocarcinoma is the most commonly encountered spontaneous neoplasm occurring in *O. cuniculus*. The relatively low incidence of this tumor seen in most commercial rabbitries and research facilities is due to the fact that these animals are usually relatively young. In 1 study, the incidence of uterine adenocarcinoma in does 2–3 years of age was around 4%, and in does 5–6 years of age, around 80%. Thus, there is a striking increase in the incidence of uterine tumors with increasing age. A variety of breeds are affected. Cystic endometrial hyperplasia is often found in the rabbit uterus, and believed to be antecedent to neoplastic progression.

On gross examination, the tumors appear as nodular, frequently multicentric masses that often involve both uterine horns (Fig. 6.100). On the cut surface, masses are firm, frequently with a cauliflower-like surface and central necrosis. Serosal implantation and metastases to the lung (Fig. 6.101) and liver often occur. Typical microscopic changes of the tumor are those of an adenocarcinoma, with invasion of the underlying layers forming acinar and tubular structures (Fig. 6.102). In rapidly growing tumors, necrotic areas are frequently observed. Metastases and tumor implants are similar to the primary neoplasm, often with a prominent stromal component.

Lymphosarcoma: Lymphoma

Neoplasms of lymphocytic origin are the most common malignancy encountered in juvenile and young adult rabbits. Anemia, low hematocrit, and terminally elevated BUN (due to kidney involvement) are typical changes seen clinically. Leukemia occasionally occurs, particularly during the terminal stages of the disease. In 1 rabbit strain, an autosomal recessive gene has been implicated as a factor in susceptibility to the disease. Others have speculated on the relationship of rabbit endogenous retrovirus (cause and effect never proven).

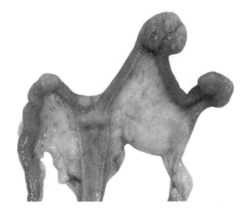

FIG. 6.100. *Uterine adenocarcinomas in an aged doe. These tumors are often multicentric, involving both uterine horns. (Source: D. Imai, University of California, Davis, CA. Reproduced with permission from D. Imai.)*

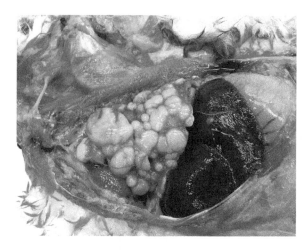

FIG. 6.101. *Metastatic uterine adenocarcinoma in the lung of an aged doe. Uterine adenocarcinomas frequently metastasize to the lungs. (Source: B.G. Caserto, Cornell University, Itaca, NY. Reproduced with permission from B.G. Caserto.)*

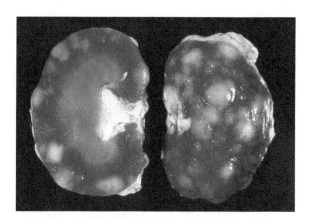

FIG. 6.103. *Kidneys from a young rabbit with lymphosarcoma. Multiple pale nodular masses are visible in the cortex, a frequent finding in lapine lymphosarcoma.*

Lymphosarcoma in the rabbit has unique patterns of organ involvement. Gross findings usually include pale kidneys with irregular cortical surfaces, enlarged GALT and mesenteric lymph nodes, hepatosplenomegaly, and patches of pale bone marrow. Nodular masses in the subcutis, lung, and eye involvement may occur. The most pathognomonic feature is renal involvement. On cut surface, changes are typically confined to the renal cortices (Fig. 6.103). Involvement of the GALT (pharyngeal tonsils, stomach mucosa, Peyer's patches, appendix, mesenteric lymph node, etc.) is frequent (Fig. 6.104). The wall of the stomach may be markedly thickened, with irregular surface plaques and mucosal ulceration. Examination of bone marrow will often reveal involvement (Fig. 6.105). The liver and spleen are often enlarged, pale, and swollen. Enlarged peripheral lymph nodes and pulmonary nodules may also be encountered. On histopathology, there are diffuse infiltrates of

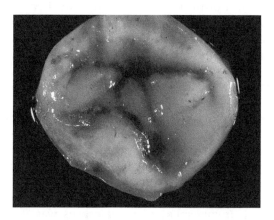

FIG. 6.104. *Diffuse mural thickening of the cecal appendix in a rabbit with lymphosarcoma. Lymphosarcoma most frequently arises in gut-associated lymphoid tissue in rabbits. (Source: D. Imai, University of California, Davis, CA. Reproduced with permission from D. Imai.)*

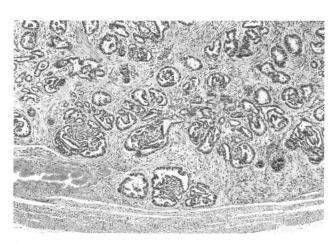

FIG. 6.102. *Uterine adenocarcinoma from an aged New Zealand White doe. Note the invasive glandular structures lined by neoplastic epithelium.*

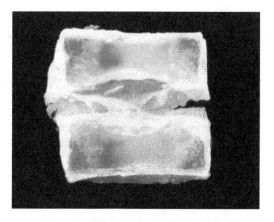

FIG. 6.105. *Vertebral bone from a rabbit with lymphosarcoma. Note the pale bone marrow due to neoplastic involvement. The bone marrow is a frequent site of involvement in lapine lymphosarcoma, but is seldom examined.*

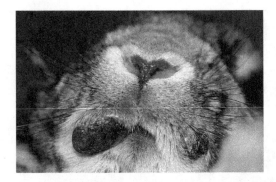

FIG. 6.106. *Cutaneous nodules involving the muzzle of a rabbit with cutaneous lymphoma. These multicentric tumors are populated by pleomorphic cells infiltrating the dermis without epitheliotropism, and arise on various sites of the body. (Source: Ritter et al. 2012. reproduced with permission from SAGE Publications.)*

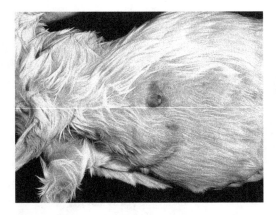

FIG. 6.107. *Mammary adenocarcinoma in an aged New Zealand White doe.*

lymphoblastic cells in the affected regions of stomach or intestine and in the interstitial regions of the renal cortex, with distortion of the normal architecture and relative sparing of the glomeruli. In the liver, there are periportal to diffuse sinusoidal infiltrates of neoplastic cells. Diffuse infiltration may occur in the spleen, lymph nodes, bone marrow, uveal tract, adrenal gland, and ovary. B-cell, T-cell, and mixed lymphoid cell populations have been documented.

Diffuse large B-cell and T-cell-rich B-cell lymphomas, presenting as one or more nodules (Fig. 6.106) on various locations of the body, have recently been reported in adult pet rabbits of various breeds in Europe, but not domestic rabbits from North America. The subcutis and dermis were infiltrated, but epitheliotropism was not observed. Involvement of other organs was variable. Neoplastic infiltrates were described as highly pleomorphic and often contained multinucleated giant cells. These differ from epitheliotropic T-cell lymphomas, which have been associated with exfoliative dermatosis in rabbits. In such cases, neoplastic cells infiltrated both the dermis and epidermis, with infiltration of distant organs.

Thymoma

Thymomas are uncommon, but well represented among neoplasms in domestic rabbits. They arise in rabbits between 1 and 4 years of age, and are often found as incidental findings at necropsy. Rabbits may present with dyspnea due to an anterior mediastinal mass. Rarely, thymomas may become metastatic. More commonly, paraneoplastic syndromes may arise. Concurrent hypercalcemia, exfoliative dermatosis, and periodic exophthalmos have all been reported as paraneoplastic syndromes associated with thymomas in rabbits.

Mammary Adenomas and Carcinomas

Glandular tumors of the mammary gland (Fig 6.107) are relatively frequent in multiple breeds of rabbits, including laboratory rabbits, arising around 3–4 years of age.

The majority of mammary tumors are carcinomas, including tubular, papillary, tubulopapillary, solid, adenosquamous, comedo, complex, ductal, cribriform, anaplastic, and spindle cell carcinomas. Cystic mastitis is conjectured as a prelude to neoplastic transformation from benign adenomas to adenocarcinomas. Metastasis to regional lymph nodes and lungs, as well as other organs, has been reported.

Bile Duct Adenomas and Adenocarcinomas

Bile duct tumors are the fourth most common reported tumor in rabbits. They are usually found incidentally at necropsy in older rabbits and appear as solitary or multiple cystic lesions filled with thick yellow to tan fluid.

Pseudo-odontoma: Odontoma

Odontomas are tumors of odontogenic origin that feature both epithelial and mesenchymal cells of tooth origin that are well differentiated (Fig. 6.108). When the cells within these masses are disorganized to the extent that they do not resemble a tooth, they are termed complex odontomas. Such tumors arise rarely from the elodont tooth roots of rabbits and rodents (and are particularly common in prairie dogs). They are not

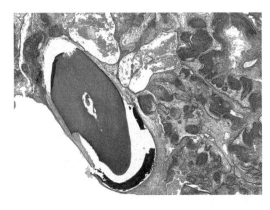

FIG. 6.108. *Pseudo-odontoma arising from the elodont incisor tooth root of an aged rabbit. These lesions contain various tooth germ elements, and are often diagnosed as odontomas, but are probably hamartomas.*

true neoplasms, but are rather believed to be hamartomas. Thus, the term pseudo-odontoma is the most appropriate descriptor of this syndrome.

Other Neoplasms

Like any species, rabbits develop sporadic cases of neoplasia involving virtually any tissue. Although not as common in commercial and laboratory rabbits because of their relatively younger age, a variety of neoplasms are found in aging pet rabbits. See Heatley and Smith, and Tinkey et al. for more comprehensive reviews on rabbit neoplasia, and von Bomhard et al. for cutaneous neoplasia in rabbits.

BIBLIOGRAPHY FOR NEOPLASMS

General References for Neoplasms
Heatley, J.J. & Smith, A.N. (2004) Spontaneous neoplasms of lagomorphs. *Veterinary Clinics of North America Exotic Animal Practice* 7:561–577.
Tinkey, P.T., Uthamanthil, R.K., & Weisbroth, S.H. (2012) Rabbit neoplasia. In: *The Laboratory Rabbit, Guinea Pig, Hamster and Other Rodents* (eds. M.A. Suckow, K.A. Stevensn, & R.P. Wilson), pp. 447–501. Elsevier.
Von Bomhard, W., Goldschmidt, M.H., Shofer, F.S., Perl, L., Rosenthal, K.L., & Mauldin, E.A. (2007) Cutaneous neoplasms in pet rabbits: a retrospective study. *Veterinary Pathology* 44:579–588.

Uterine Adenocarcinoma
Asakawa, M.G., Goldschmidt, M.H., Une, Y., & Nomura, Y. (2008) The immunohistochemical evaluation of estrogen receptor-alpha and progesterone receptors of normal, hyperplastic, and neoplastic endometrium in 88 pet rabbits. *Veterinary Pathology* 45:217–225.
Green, H.S.N. (1958) Adenocarcinoma of the uterine fundus in the rabbit. *Annals of the New York Academy of Science* 75:535–542.

Lymphosarcoma
Fox, R.R., Meier, H., Crary, D.D., Meyers, D.D., Norberg, R.F., & Laird, C.W. (1970) Lymphosarcoma in the rabbit: genetics and pathology. *Journal of the National Cancer Institute* 45:719–730.

Gomez, L., Gazquez, A., Roncero, V., Sanchez, C., & Duran, M.E. (2002) Lymphoma in a rabbit: histopathological and immunohistochemical findings. *Journal of Small Animal Practice* 43:224–226.
Ishikawa, M., Maeda, H., Kondo, H., Shibuya, H., Onuma, M., & Sato, T.A. (2007) A case of lymphoma developing in the rabbit cecum. *Journal of Veterinary Medical Science* 69:1183–1185.
Kolappaswamy, K., Kriel, E.H., McLeod, C.G., & DeTolla, L.J. (2006) Intermittent inappetence and fur loss in a New Zealand White rabbit. *Laboratory Animals (NY)* 35:19–20.
Reed, S.D., Shaw, S., & Evans, D.E. (2009) Spinal lymphoma and pulmonary filariasis in a pet rabbit (*Oryctolagus cuniculus domesticus*). *Journal of Veterinary Diagnostic Investigation* 21:253–256.
Ritter, J.M., von Bomhard, W., Wise, A.G., Maes, R.K., & Kiupel, M. (2012) Cutaneous lymphomas in European pet rabbits. *Veterinary Pathology* 49:846–851.
Toth, L.A., Olson, G.A., Wilson, E., Rehg, J.E., & Claassen, E. (1990) Lymphocytic leukemia and lymphosarcoma in a rabbit. *Journal of the American Veterinary Medical Association* 197:627–629.
Volopich, S., Gruber, A., Hassan, J., Hittmair, K.M., Schwendenwein, I., & Nell, B. (2005) Malignant B-cell lymphoma of the Harder's gland in a rabbit. *Veterinary Ophthalmology* 8:259–263.
White, S.D., Campbell, T., Logan, A., Meredith, A., Schultheiss, P., Van Winkle, T., Moore, P.F., Naydan, D.K., & Mallon, F. (2000) Lymphoma with cutaneous involvement in three domestic rabbits (*Oryctolagus cuniculus*). *Veterinary Dermatology* 11:61–67.

Thymoma
Florizoone, K. (2005) Thymoma-associated exfoliative dermatitis in a rabbit. *Veterinary Dermatology* 16:281–284.
Vernau, K.M., Grahn, B.H., Clarke-Scott, H.A., & Sullivan, N. (1995) Thymoma in a geriatric rabbit with hypercalcemia and periodic exophthalmos. *Journal of the American Veterinary Medical Association* 206:820–822.
Wagner, F., Beinecke, A., Fehr, M., Brunkhorst, N., Mischke, R., & Gruber, A.D. (2005) Recurrent bilateral exophthalmos associated with metastatic thymic carcinoma in a pet rabbit. *Journal of Small Animal Practice* 46:369–370.

Mammary Adenoma and Adenocarcinoma
Baba, N. & Von Haam, E. (1972) Animal model: spontaneous adenocarcinoma in aged rabbits. *American Journal of Pathology* 68:653–656.
Baum, B. & Hewicker-Trautwein, M. (2015) Classification and epidemiology of mammary tumours in pet rabbits (*Oryctolagus cuniculus*). *Journal of Comparative Pathology* 152:291–298.

Index

Pathology of Laboratory Rodents and Rabbits, Fourth Edition. Stephen W. Barthold, Stephen M. Griffey, and Dean H. Percy.
© 2016 John Wiley & Sons, Inc. Published 2016 by John Wiley & Sons, Inc.